AF412338

Statistics for Biology and Health

Series Editors
M. Gail
K. Krickeberg
J. Samet
A. Tsiatis
W. Wong

For further volumes:
www.springer.com/series/2848

Gang Zheng · Yaning Yang · Xiaofeng Zhu · Robert C. Elston

Analysis of Genetic Association Studies

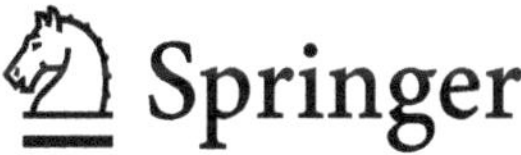 Springer

Gang Zheng
Bethesda, MD, USA

Yaning Yang
School of Management, Dept. Statistics &
    Finance
University of Science & Technology of
    China
Hefei, Anhui, People's Republic of China

Xiaofeng Zhu
School of Medicine, Dept. Epidemiology &
    Biostatistics
Case Western Reserve University
Cleveland, OH, USA

Robert C. Elston
School of Medicine, Dept. Epidemiology &
    Biostatistics
Case Western Reserve University
Cleveland, OH, USA

Statistics for Biology and Health Series Editors
M. Gail
National Cancer Institute
Bethesda, MD, USA

K. Krickeberg
Le Châtelet
Manglieu, France

J. Samet
Department of Preventive Medicine
Keck School of Medicine
University of Southern California
Los Angeles, CA, USA

A. Tsiatis
Department of Statistics
North Carolina State University
Raleigh, NC, USA

W. Wong
Department of Statistics
Stanford University
Stanford, CA, USA

ISSN 1431-8776   Statistics for Biology and Health
ISBN 978-1-4614-2244-0   e-ISBN 978-1-4614-2245-7
DOI 10.1007/978-1-4614-2245-7
Springer New York Dordrecht Heidelberg London

Library of Congress Control Number: 2011946278

Printed on acid-free paper

Springer is part of Springer Science+Business Media (www.springer.com)

To my mother: GZ

To my parents, Min and Qiutong: YY

To family: Fang, Luke, Jimmy and Helen: XZ

To all my numerous former students and family: RCE

Preface

We started writing this book two years ago targeting it not only as a graduate level text book in statistical genetics and genetic epidemiology, especially for genetic association studies, but also as a reference book for the analysis of genetic association studies. As a text book for graduate students in statistics, biostatistics, genetics and genetic epidemiology, in addition to covering various topics in this subject, we wanted to cover details of the various derivations as well as illustrate detailed step-by-step applications through both real examples and simulations. We hope this book can serve as a bridge from taking classes in statistical genetics and genetic epidemiology to conducting independent research in this area. As a reference, we wanted to cover a broad range of topics in genetic association studies, both population-based and family-based, but we focus mostly on population-based case-control association studies. The book should also be useful for other statisticians or readers who are not familiar with the subject.

The book covers many technical details, and the breadth of coverage gives the option to pick and choose what interests the reader most. The book contains thirteen chapters in six parts and we give here a brief introduction to each part. In the first part, we have two introductory chapters. The probability and statistical background required for this book is covered in the first chapter, while the second chapter covers the basic genetic and genetic epidemiology terminology necessary to understand the rest of the book. Readers who are familiar with the material in either of these two background chapters can skip one or both of them.

Part II of the book comprises four chapters. Chapters 3 and 4 cover single-marker analysis for case-control data in unmatched and matched designs, respectively. In Chap. 3, we introduce both genotype-based tests (including trend tests and Pearson's chi-squared test) and the allele-based test, and inference in terms of odds ratios. Their relation to each other and their relation to a logistic regression model are discussed. Exact tests for association and tests using the deviation from Hardy-Weinberg proportions to detect association are studied. How to simulate case-control data with or without covariates is also studied. In Chap. 4, we focus on matched designs under 1: m or variable matching. Results for the matched trend test and the matched Hardy-Weinberg disequilibrium test are derived. Chapter 5 covers Bayesian analysis of case-control genetic association studies. Bayesian analysis plays an important role in the analysis of genetic association studies, especially in reporting results from genome-wide association studies. We focus on calculating Bayes factors and their approximations, derivations of approximate Bayes factors with or without covariates, coding genotypes in Bayesian analysis, and the choice of priors. We assume the underlying genetic model is known in all these three chapters. In Chap. 6, however, we assume the genetic model is unknown and study robust procedures for association studies. The maximin efficiency robust test, maximum-type statistics (including MAX3), constrained likelihood ratio test, tests based on genetic model selection or exclusion, and minimum p-values are considered.

Part III, comprising Chaps. 7 and 8, covers multi-marker analysis. We study haplotype analysis in Chap. 7 and gene-gene interactions in Chap. 8. Part IV contains three additional chapters on related topics. Population stratification is an important topic in the analysis of case-control data and is covered in Chap. 9. The impact of population stratification and various approaches to correct for it are discussed. Chapter 10 discusses gene-environment interactions with different genetic models, illustrated with real examples. Power and sample size calculations are important when designing an association study. In Chap. 11 we consider the power and sample size calculations for single marker analysis using the trend test with perfect or imperfect linkage disequilibrium, and for Pearson's chi-squared test. We also cover power for gene-gene and gene-environment interactions using an existing publicly available Power Program. An introduction to genome-wide association studies, popular since 2005, is presented as Chap. 12 in Part V. This brief introduction discusses quality control, analysis strategy, genome-wide scans, ranking, and replication.

An introduction to family-based association studies is given in Chap. 13, the last part of the book. Although we still focus on association studies, we also briefly discuss linkage analysis, including the original and revised Haseman-Elston regression models and linkage studies using affected sibpairs. We focus on the transmission disequilibrium test (TDT) and family-based association tests (FBAT). Both binary and quantitative traits are studied.

One challenge in writing this book has been how to balance the overall coverage, technical details and applications. Although we have tried to cover most topics of association studies, some topics, especially those recently developed since we started writing this book, including the analysis of imputed SNPs, copy number variants and the detection of rare variants, are not covered. The analysis of family data is reduced to one chapter. Moreover, the book focuses more on technical details and presenting application results than on demonstrating them with programs or the use of software. Almost all illustrations presented in the book, including figures and tables, were obtained by running our own programs, which were written using a combination of SAS, R, S-Plus, Maple, S.A.G.E., and other existing programs or software. Therefore it is not easy to present all the programs used in this book, although some illustrations are given. Selected materials can be used for one-semester or a one-year course in statistical genetics together with other supplementary reading materials.

We would like to thank John Kimmel, the former senior editor of statistics at Springer, and Marc Strauss, the current editor, for their support and unending patience. We are grateful to Han Zhang for collecting some references and Huizhen

Qin for producing a figure; to Prakash Gorroochurn, Neal Jeffries, Jungnam Joo, Qizhai Li, and Yong Zang for reading and commenting on some of the chapters. Gang Zheng thanks Joseph Gastwrith and Nancy Geller for their strong support of this project, and Zhaohai Li for teaching him statistical genetic at George Washington University. Yaning Yang also acknowledges the continuous encouragement from Zhiliang Ying and Jurg Ott.

Maryland, Anhui and Cleveland   Gang Zheng
                                                                          Yaning Yang
                                                                          Xiaofeng Zhu
                                                                          Robert C. Elston

Acknowledgements

The work of Gang Zheng is in his private capacity. The views expressed do not necessarily represent the views of NIH, DHHS, or the United States.

Contents

Part V Introduction to Genome-Wide Association Studies

Part VI Introduction to Family-Based Association Studies

Acronyms

ABF	Approximate Bayes factor
ADD	Additive model
AIM	Ancestry informative marker
ARE	Asymptotic relative efficiency
BF	Bayes factor
BFDP	Bayesian false discovery probability
BIC	Bayesian information criterion
CATT	Cochran-Armitage trend test
CDF	Cumulative distribution function
CI	Confidence interval
CLRT	Constrained likelihood ratio test
CNV	Copy number variant
Corr	Correlation
Cov	Covariance
CR	Cryptic relatedness
DOM	Dominant model
ECM	Expectation/conditional maximization
FBAT	Family based association test
FDR	False discovery rate
GC	Genomic control
GEE	Generalized estimating equation
GHRR	Genotype-based haplotype relative risk
GLM	Generalized linear model
GME	Genetic model exclusion
GMS	Genetic model selection
GRR	Genotype relative risk
GWAS	A genome-wide association study or genome-wide association studies
HE	Haseman-Elston regression
HHRR	Haplotype relative risk
HWE	Hardy-Weinberg equilibrium
HWD	Hardy-Weinberg disequilibrium

HWDTT	Hardy-Weinberg disequilibrium trend test
IBD	Identity by descent
IID	Independent and identically distributed
ILP	Inductive logic programming
LD	Linkage disequilibrium
LRT	Likelihood ratio test
MAF	Minor allele frequency
MAP	Maximum a posteriori
MAX	Maximum of a test over all genetic models
MAX3	Maximum of a test over three genetic models
MCMC	Markov Chain Monte Carlo
MDR	Multifactor dimensionality reduction
MDS	Multidimensional scaling
MDT	Matching disequilibrium test
MERT	Maximin efficiency robust test
MGRR	Matched genotype relative risk
MLE	Maximum likelihood estimate
MLS	Maximum lod score
MTT	Matched trend test
MUL	Multiplicative model
OR	Odds ratio
PC	Principal component
PCA	Principal component analysis
PDF	Probability density function
PPA	Posterior probability of association
PS	Population stratification
QTDT	Quantitative transmission disequilibrium test
QTL	Quantitative trait locus
REC	Recessive model
RR	Relative risk
SA	Structural association
S.A.G.E.	Statistical Analysis for Genetic Epidemiology
SNP	Single nucleotide polymorphism
ST	Score test
TDT	Transmission disequilibrium test
Var	Variance
VIF	Variance inflation factor
WT	Wald test

Part I
Background

Chapter 1
Introduction to Probability Theory and Statistics

Abstract Basic probability theory and statistical models and procedures for the analysis of genetic studies are covered in Chap. 1. This chapter starts with an introduction to basic distribution theory and common distributions that are used in the book, including the uniform, multinomial, normal, t-, F-, Beta, Gamma, chi-squared and hypergeometric distributions. The basic distributions for order statistics are also given. Several types of stochastic convergence used in the book are summarized. Maximum likelihood estimation and its large sample properties are discussed. Various tests, including the efficient Score test, likelihood ratio test and Wald test, are studied with or without nuisance parameters. Multiple testing issues related to testing association with multiple genetic markers and related to hypothesis testing with an unknown genetic model are briefly reviewed. This chapter also covers the Delta method, the EM algorithm, basic concepts of sample size and power calculations, and asymptotic relative efficiency.

Applications of classical probability and statistical techniques to the analysis of genetic data date back to at least 1918 when R.A. Fisher studied the correlation between relatives under Mendelian inheritance. It should be recognized, however, that Gregor Mendel's *Experiments on Plant Hybridization* presented at the meetings of the Natural History Society of Brünn in 1865 was highly statistical in nature. Since then, probability theory and statistical methods have played important roles in the analysis of genetic data. Basic probability theory and statistical models and procedures for the analysis of case-control genetic association studies are covered in this chapter.

We start with an introduction to basic probability theory and common distributions that are used in this book, including the uniform, multinomial, normal, t-, F-, Beta, chi-squared and hypergeometric distributions. The basic distributions for order statistics are also discussed. We then review several stochastic convergences used in this book.

Maximum likelihood estimation and its large sample properties are discussed. Test statistics, including the efficient Score test, likelihood ratio test, and Wald test are studied with or without nuisance parameters. Multiple testing issues related to testing association with multiple genetic markers or related to hypothesis testing with an unknown genetic model are briefly reviewed. We also cover the Delta

G. Zheng et al., *Analysis of Genetic Association Studies*,
Statistics for Biology and Health,
DOI 10.1007/978-1-4614-2245-7_1, © Springer Science+Business Media, LLC 2012

method, the EM algorithm, an introduction to sample size and power calculations, and asymptotic relative efficiencies.

1.1 Basic Probability Theory

1.1.1 Introduction

Denote a random variable by X and its realization (observation) by x. Let Ω be the sample space for X. The cumulative distribution function (CDF) of X is defined as $F(x) = \Pr(X \leq x)$ for $x \in \Omega$. We use the notation: $X \sim F(x)$. We only consider two types of random variables. One is a continuous random variable whose CDF $F(x)$ has a continuous derivative at every $x \in \Omega$. The derivative of $F(x)$ is then called the probability density function (PDF) of X, denoted by $f(x)$. Hence, $F(x) = \int_{-\infty}^{x} f(y)dy$ and $F(x)$ is continuous at every $x \in \Omega$. The kth moment of X is given by $E(X^k) = \int x^k f(x)dx$. The second type is a discrete random variable, which only takes on a finite or countable number of values, e.g. $X = x_1, x_2, \dots$. Thus, $\Omega = \{x : x_1, x_2, \dots\}$. Its distribution function (or probability mass function) is denoted by $\Pr(X = x_i)$ for $i = 1, 2, \dots$. Hence, $F(x) = \sum_{x_i \leq x} \Pr(X = x_i)$, and the kth moment is given by $E(X^k) = \sum_{x_i} x_i^k \Pr(X = x_i)$. For both continuous and discrete random variables, the mean and variance of X are given by $E(X)$ and $\text{Var}(X) = E(X^2) - \{E(X)\}^2$, respectively. Note that $F(x)$ is non-decreasing and strictly increasing for a continuous random variable as defined above. In most of our applications, $\Omega = (-\infty, \infty)$, $(0, 1)$, or $(0, \infty)$ for continuous random variables. Unless the sample space Ω is $(0, 1)$ or $(0, \infty)$, we always use $\Omega = (-\infty, \infty)$ to display formulas.

The joint CDF of two continuous random variables X_1 and X_2 is given by $F(x_1, x_2) = \Pr(X_1 \leq x_1, X_2 \leq x_2)$ with the PDF denoted by $f(x_1, x_2)$, where

$$F(x_1, x_2) = \int_{-\infty}^{x_2} \left\{ \int_{-\infty}^{x_1} f(y_1, y_2)dy_1 \right\} dy_2.$$

For two discrete random variables, the joint distribution function is

$$F(x_1, x_2) = \sum_{y_1 \leq x_1, y_2 \leq x_2} \Pr(X_1 = y_1, X_2 = y_2).$$

In this book, we only consider joint distributions of random variables of the same type. Two random variables are independent if, for any x_1 and x_2, $F(x_1, x_2) = F(x_1)F(x_2)$. The covariance of the two random variables X_1 and X_2 is defined as

$$\text{Cov}(X_1, X_2) = E[\{X_1 - E(X_1)\}\{X_2 - E(X_2)\}],$$

which equals $\int \int \{x_1 - E(X_1)\}\{x_2 - E(X_2)\} f(x_1, x_2)dx_2dx_2$ for continuous random variables or $\sum_{x_1, x_2} \{x_1 - E(X_1)\}\{x_2 - E(X_2)\} \Pr(X_1 = x_1, X_2 = x_2)$ for discrete random variables. It can be shown that $\text{Cov}(X_1, X_2) = E(X_1 X_2) - E(X_1)E(X_2)$, where the integration in $E(X_1X_2)$ is with respect to the joint distribution. The correlation between X_1 and X_2 is defined as

$$\text{Corr}(X_1, X_2) = \frac{\text{Cov}(X_1, X_2)}{\sqrt{\text{Var}(X_1)\text{Var}(X_2)}}.$$

If X_1 and X_2 are independent, $\text{Cov}(X_1, X_2) = 0$ and $\text{Corr}(X_1, X_2) = 0$. The converse, however, is not always true.

For a continuous random variable $X \sim F(x)$, the pth quantile of $F(x)$, denoted by x_p, is given by $x_p = F^{-1}(p)$ for $p \in (0, 1)$. Here x_p is also called the $100p$th percentile of $F(x)$. For a discrete random variable, $x_p = \sup\{x : F(x) \le p\}$. That is, the largest value of x such that $F(x) \le p$.

1.1.2 Marginal and Conditional Distributions

Given the joint PDF or the joint distribution function of X_1 and X_2, the PDF and distribution function of X_2 can be obtained, respectively, from

$$f(x_2) = \int_{-\infty}^{\infty} f(x_1, x_2)dx_1,$$

$$\Pr(X_2 = x_2) = \sum_{x_1} \Pr(X_1 = x_1, X_2 = x_2),$$

which are also referred to as the marginal PDF and marginal distribution function of X_2 with respect to the joint PDF and joint distribution function. Let E_1 and E_2 be two events. Then the following conditional probability can be used to define the conditional distribution

$$\Pr(E_2|E_1) = \Pr(E_1, E_2)/\Pr(E_1), \quad \text{provided } \Pr(E_1) \ne 0.$$

If we substitute E_i with $\{X_i = x_i\}$, we obtain the conditional distribution function for $X_2 = x_2$ given $X_1 = x_1$. For the continuous random variables X_1 and X_2, we have $f(x_2|x_1) = f(x_1, x_2)/f(x_2)$. Thus, if X_1 and X_2 are independent, $\Pr(X_2 = x_2|X_1 = x_1) = \Pr(X_2 = x_2)$ or $f(x_2|x_1) = f(x_2)$.

Suppose the conditional distribution of X_2 given $X_1 = x_1$ is given by $f(x_2|x_1)$ or $\Pr(X_2 = x_2|X_1 = x_1)$. Then the conditional expectation of X_2 given $X_1 = x_1$ is given by

$$E(X_2|X_1 = x_1) = \int x_2 f(x_2|x_1)dx_2,$$

$$E(X_2|X_1 = x_1) = \sum_{x_2} x_2 \Pr(X_2 = x_2|X_1 = x_2).$$

Note that $E(X_2|X_1)$ itself is a random variable. Therefore, we can calculate its mean and variance. The following results are useful (Problem 1.5):

$$E(X_2) = E\{E(X_2|X_1)\}, \tag{1.1}$$

$$\mathrm{Var}(X_2) = \mathrm{Var}\{E(X_2|X_1)\} + E\{\mathrm{Var}(X_2|X_1)\}. \tag{1.2}$$

We have not indicated parameters in the CDF $F(x)$ and PDF $f(x)$. For many applications, a parameter or a vector of parameters θ appear in $F(x)$ and $f(x)$. In this case, we denote them by $F(x|\theta)$ and $f(x|\theta)$, respectively.

1.1.3 Basic Distributions

Some basic statistical distributions are now considered, including the uniform distribution, multinomial (including binomial), normal, multivariate normal, chi-squared, t-, F-, Beta, Gamma, and hypergeometric distributions. These distributions are used in subsequent chapters. A symbol is given to indicate a distribution, which is also often used to indicate a variate following the same distribution. For example, $N(0, 1)$ is used to present the standard normal distribution as well as a variate following the standard normal distribution. Otherwise the capital letter X is used to indicate a random variable and the lower case x is a realization of the random variable X.

The Uniform Distribution

A random variate X is said to follow the uniform distribution on $(0, 1)$, denoted by $X \sim U(0, 1)$, if it has the PDF

$$f(x) = 1 \quad \text{for } x \in (0, 1),$$

and 0 for $x \notin (0, 1)$. The CDF is $F(x) = x$ for $x \in (0, 1)$, 0 if $x \leq 0$, and 1 if $x \geq 1$. The mean and variance of X are $E(X) = 1/2$ and $\mathrm{Var}(X) = 1/12$. The random variate $X \sim U(0, 1)$ is also called the unit rectangular variate.

Let Y be any continuous random variable with a CDF $F(y)$. Then the random variable $X = F(Y) \sim U(0, 1)$ because, for any $x \in (0, 1)$,

$$\Pr(X \leq x) = \Pr(F(Y) \leq x) = \Pr(Y \leq F^{-1}(x)) = F(F^{-1}(x)) = x.$$

It follows that if $X \sim U(0, 1)$, $F^{-1}(X) \sim F(x)$.

The Multinomial Distribution

Assume that n independent experiments or trials are conducted. Each experiment has one of L outcomes. The probabilities of the L outcomes are the same among each of the n experiments and are denoted by $p_1, \ldots, p_L$ with $p_1 + \cdots + p_L = 1$. Among the n experiments, the count of each outcome is obtained. The counts of the L outcomes are denoted by $X_1, \ldots, X_L$, which represent a random sample $X = (X_1, \ldots, X_L)$ drawn from the multinomial distribution, denoted by $X \sim Mul(n; p_1, p_2, \ldots, p_L)$. The distribution function for $X = (X_1, \ldots, X_L)$ can be written as

$$\Pr(X = x) = \Pr(X_1 = x_1, \ldots, X_L = x_L) = \frac{n!}{x_1! \cdots x_L!} p_1^{x_1} \cdots p_L^{x_L}, \quad 0 \le x_i \le n,$$

where $p_L = 1 - (p_1 + \cdots + p_{L-1})$ and $x_1 + \cdots + x_L = n$.

The binomial distribution is a special case with $L = 2$, where the two outcomes are often termed "success" and "failure". The binomial distribution is denoted by $B(n; p)$, where $p_1 = p$ and $p_2 = 1 - p$. For the binomial random variable X (the number of successes in n trials) with the probability of success p, the distribution function can be written as

$$\Pr(X = x) = \frac{n!}{x!(n - x)!} p^x (1 - p)^{n-x}, \quad 0 \le x \le n.$$

Let X_i be the number of ith outcomes of a multinomial random variable. The mean and variance of X_i are given by $\mathrm{E}(X_i) = np_i$ and $\mathrm{Var}(X_i) = p_i(1 - p_i)/n$. The covariance of two outcomes X_i and X_j is given by $\mathrm{Cov}(X_i, X_j) = -p_i p_j/n$ for $i \ne j$. Thus,

$$\mathrm{Corr}(X_i, X_j) = -\sqrt{\frac{p_i p_j}{(1 - p_i)(1 - p_j)}}.$$

The Normal Distribution

The normal distribution is the most commonly used distribution in statistics. Let X be a random variable that follows a normal distribution. Then the PDF of X is given by

$$f(x) = \frac{1}{\sqrt{2\pi\sigma^2}} e^{-\frac{1}{2}\left(\frac{x - \mu}{\sigma}\right)^2}, \quad x \in (-\infty, \infty), \tag{1.3}$$

where μ is the mean (location) of X and σ is the standard deviation (scale) of X. The normal distribution is denoted by $X \sim N(\mu, \sigma^2)$, where σ^2 is the variance of X. A special case with $\mu = 0$ and $\sigma^2 = 1$ is called the standard normal distribution. The symbols $\phi(x)$ and $\Phi(x)$ are used for the PDF and CDF of $N(0, 1)$. The normal distribution plays an important role in large sample statistical inference (estimation and hypothesis testing). It is used to construct confidence intervals and calculate the power and sample size in the design of genetic studies. Normal densities with $(\mu, \sigma) = (0, 1)$ and $(2, 1.5)$ are plotted in Fig. 1.1.

Fig. 1.1 Normal density
plots: The *solid curve* is the
standard normal density
$N(0, 1)$ and the *dotted curve*
is $N(2, 1.5^2)$ with the
location parameter $\mu = 2$ and
the scale parameter $\sigma = 1.5$

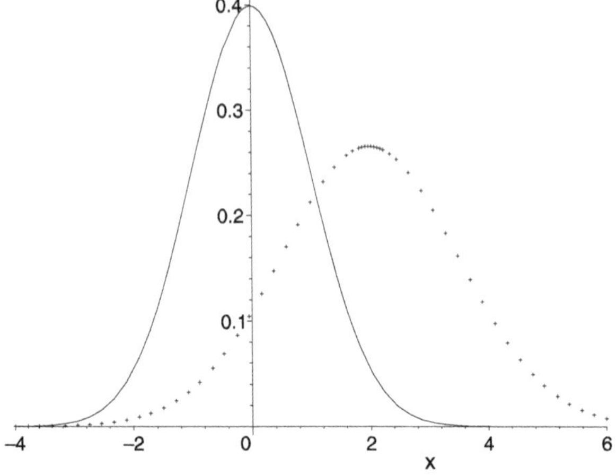

The Multivariate Normal Distribution

The multivariate normal distribution is a generalization of the normal distribution.
Let $\mathbf{X} = (X_1, \ldots, X_p)^T$ be a p-dimensional random vector, where T is a matrix
transpose. Denote $\mathbf{x} = (x_1, \ldots, x_p)^T$ and $\mu = (\mu_1, \ldots, \mu_p)^T$. Let $\Sigma = \mathrm{Var}(\mathbf{X})$ be
the $p \times p$ covariance matrix of $\mathbf{X}$, whose (i, j)th element is $E\{X_i - E(X_i))(X_j - E(X_j)\}$. The covariance matrix is positive definite. That is, for any real-valued vector $\mathbf{a} \neq \mathbf{0}$, $\mathbf{a}^T \Sigma \mathbf{a} > 0$. The random vector $\mathbf{X}$ is said to have the multivariate normal
distribution $N_p(\mu, \Sigma)$ if its PDF has the form

$$f(x_1, \ldots, x_p) = \frac{1}{(2\pi)^{p/2} |\Sigma|^{1/2}} \exp\{-(x - \mu)^T \Sigma^{-1}(x - \mu)/2\},$$

where $|\Sigma|$ is the determinant of Σ. The above PDF reduces to (1.3) when $p = 1$
and $\Sigma = \sigma^2$. When $p = 2$, $\mathbf{X}$ is said to follow a bivariate normal distribution. The
covariance matrix for the bivariate normal distribution can be written as

$$\Sigma = \begin{bmatrix} \sigma_1^2 & \rho_{12}\sigma_1\sigma_2 \\ \rho_{12}\sigma_1\sigma_2 & \sigma_2^2 \end{bmatrix},$$

where $\sigma_i^2 = \mathrm{Var}(X_i)$ and $\rho_{12} = \mathrm{Corr}(X_1, X_2)$.

Let $p = 2$. Given $X_2 = x_2$, the conditional distribution of X_1 is normal with
mean $\mu_1 + \rho_{12}\sigma_1(x_2 - \mu_2)/\sigma_2$ and variance $\sigma_1^2(1 - \rho_{12}^2)$, denoted by

$$X_1 | X_2 = x_2 \sim N\left(\mu_1 + \rho_{12}\frac{\sigma_1}{\sigma_2}(x_2 - \mu_2), \sigma_1^2(1 - \rho_{12}^2)\right). \tag{1.4}$$

Note that (1.4) can be used to generate bivariate normal random variates.

For a general $p \geq 2$, we can decompose $\mathbf{X} = (\mathbf{X_1}, \mathbf{X_2})^T$, where $\mathbf{X_i}$ is a p_i-dimensional random vector and $p_1 + p_2 = p$. Accordingly, $\mu = (\mu_1, \mu_2)^T$ and

$$\Sigma = \begin{bmatrix} \Sigma_{11} & \Sigma_{12} \\ \Sigma_{12} & \Sigma_{22} \end{bmatrix},$$

where $|\Sigma_{22}| > 0$. Then the conditional distribution of $\mathbf{X_1}$ given $\mathbf{X_2} = \mathbf{x_2}$ is the p_1-dimensional normal with mean and covariance matrix matrix given by

$$E(\mathbf{X_1}|\mathbf{X_2} = \mathbf{x_2}) = \mu_1 + \Sigma_{12}\Sigma_{22}^{-1}(\mathbf{x_2} - \mu_2)$$

and

$$\text{Var}(\mathbf{X_1}|\mathbf{X_2} = \mathbf{x_2}) = \Sigma_{11} - \Sigma_{12}\Sigma_{22}^{-1}\Sigma_{21}.$$

Chi-Squared Distribution

Let Y_l, $l = 1, \ldots, L$, be independent random variables from $N(0, 1)$. Then $X = \sum_{l=1}^{L} Y_l^2$ has a central chi-squared distribution with L degrees of freedom, denoted by $X \sim \chi_L^2$. Its PDF is given by

$$f(x) = \frac{x^{L/2-1}}{2^{L/2}\Gamma(L/2)}e^{-x/2},$$

where $\Gamma(L/2)$ is the gamma function with argument $L/2$, which is given by $\Gamma(x) = \int_0^\infty t^{x-1}e^{-x}dx$. The mean and variance of X are L and $2L$, respectively. The chi-squared distributions with 1, 2 and 4 degrees of freedom are frequently used in subsequent chapters in testing hypothesis.

On the other hand, if $Y_l \sim N(\mu_l, 1)$ for $l = 1, \ldots, L$. Then $X = \sum_{l=1}^{L} Y_l^2$ has a non-central chi-squared distribution with L degrees of freedom and the non-centrality parameter is $\delta = \sum \mu_l^2$. The non-central chi-squared distribution is often used to calculate the power of a statistic with a chi-squared distribution. Plots of central chi-squared densities with different degrees of freedom are given in Fig. 1.2. We always use chi-squared distribution to refer to a central chi-squared distribution unless "non-central" is specified.

The F-Distribution

The F-distribution with shape parameters s and t is the ratio of two variates following chi-squared distributions with s and t degrees of freedom, respectively. The shape parameters of the F-distribution are often referred to as the degrees of freedom, which are positive integers. The PDF of the F-distribution with s and t degrees of freedom can be written as

$$f(x|s, t) = \frac{\Gamma((s+t)/2)(s/t)^{s/2}x^{(s-2)/2}}{\Gamma(s/2)\Gamma(t/2)(1 + xs/t)^{(s+t)/2}}.$$

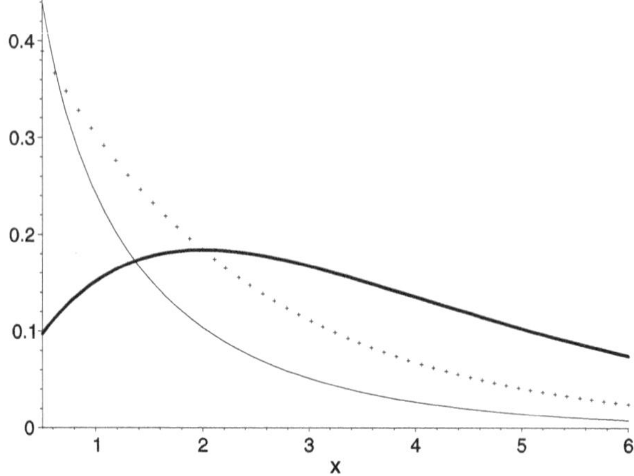

Fig. 1.2 Chi-squared density plots with degrees of freedom 1 (the *solid curve*), 2 (the *dotted curve*) and 4 (the *thick curve*)

Let X follow the F-distribution with s and t degrees of freedom, denoted by $F(s,t)$. The mean and variance of X are respectively $t/(t-2)$ when $t > 2$ and $2t^2(s+t-2)/\{s(t-2)^2(t-4)\}$ when $t > 4$. Let Y_s and Y_t follow chi-squared distributions with s and t degrees of freedom, respectively. Then $(Y_s/s)/(Y_t/t)$ follows $F(s,t)$. When both s and t go to infinity, $F(s,t)$ converges to $N(0,1)$ in distribution. When t goes to infinity, $F(s,t)$ converges to χ_s^2 in distribution. Convergence in distribution is used here, which will be defined with other stochastic convergences in Sect. 1.1.5.

The t-Distribution

The t-distribution, also called Student's t-distribution, has a shape parameter d, which is a positive integer and referred to as the degrees of freedom. Its PDF can be written as

$$f(x|d) = \frac{\Gamma((d+1)/2)}{\sqrt{\pi d}\,\Gamma(d/2)(1+x^2/d)^{(d+1)/2}},$$

where $d > 1$. When $d = 1$, the t-distribution corresponds to the Cauchy distribution. The t-distribution has mean 0 when $d > 1$ and variance $d/(d-2)$ when $d > 2$.

Let X follow a t-distribution with d degrees of freedom. Then X is related to the F-distribution by $X^2 \sim F(1,d)$, related to the chi-squared distribution by $X^2 \sim \chi_1^2/(\chi_d^2/d)$, and related to the normal distribution by $X \sim N(0,1)/\sqrt{\chi_d^2/d}$. When d goes to infinity, the t-distribution converges to the normal distribution. Figure 1.3 plots the normal density $N(0,1)$ and the t-densities with 1 and 5 degrees of freedom.

The Hypergeometric Distribution

Consider a finite population of size n, from which a random sample of size $m < n$ is drawn. Suppose the finite population consists of two types of sample outcomes

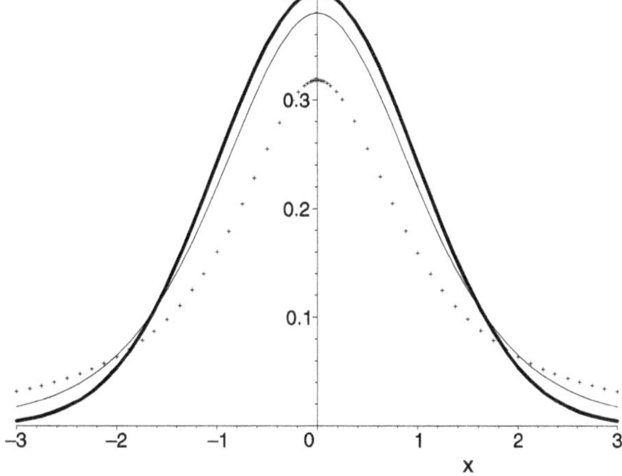

Fig. 1.3 Plots of the densities of normal $N(0, 1)$ (the *thick curve*) and t distributions with 1 (the *dotted curve*) and 5 (the *solid curve*) degrees of freedom

Table 1.1 The hypergeometric distribution with x successes

Sets of	Sampled	Not sampled	Total
Black balls	x	$s - x$	s
White balls	$m - x$	$n - m + x - s$	$n - s$
Total	m	$n - m$	n

(e.g., black balls and white balls). Suppose there are s black balls and $n - s$ white balls. One is interested in calculating the probability of drawing x black balls among m draws. The number of black balls among m draws follows the hypergeometric distribution. The probability of obtaining x black balls among m draws is given by

$$\Pr(x) = \frac{\binom{m}{x}\binom{n-m}{s-x}}{\binom{n}{s}} = \frac{m!(n-m)!s!(n-s)!}{x!(m-x)!(s-x)!(n-m-s+x)!n!},$$

where $\max(0, s + m - n) \le x \le \max(m, s)$. The mean and variance of a hypergeometric random variable X are sm/n and $sm(n-m)(n-s)/\{n^2(n-1)\}$, respectively.

The hypergeometric distribution can be displayed in a 2×2 table as in Table 1.1. The probability $\Pr(x)$ is the probability of obtaining a 2×2 table given the four margins: s, $n - s$, m, and $n - m$. This probability is used when Fisher's exact test for association of the 2×2 table is studied in Chap. 3.

Beta and Gamma Distributions

The Beta distribution has two shape parameters $u > 0$ and $v > 0$. A variate with the Beta distribution is denoted by $\text{Beta}(u, v)$. The PDF is given by

$$f(x|u, v) = x^{u-1}(1 - x)^{v-1}/B(u, v),$$

where $B(u, v)$ is the Beta function with arguments u and v, given by

$$B(u, v) = \int_0^1 y^{u-1}(1 - y)^{v-1} dy = \frac{\Gamma(u)\Gamma(v)}{\Gamma(u + v)}.$$

The mean and variance of Beta(u, v) are $u/(u + v)$ and $uv/\{(u + v)^2(u + v + 1)\}$. Beta$(1, 1)$ is the uniform distribution on $(0,1)$.

The Gamma distribution includes many common distributions as special cases (e.g., a chi-squared distribution). Its PDF is given by

$$f(x|u, v) = (x/u)^{v-1} \exp(-x/u)/\{u\Gamma(v)\}, \quad u > 0, \ v > 0.$$

A variate with the Gamma distribution is denoted as Gamma(u, v).

For integer v, the variate Gamma(u, v) can be generated from $\sum_{i=1}^v -u \log(U_i)$ where $U_i \sim U(0, 1)$ are independent unit rectangular variates. The identity

$$\text{Beta}(u, v) = \frac{\text{Gamma}(1, u)}{\text{Gamma}(1, u) + \text{Gamma}(1, v)}$$

is often used to generate variates with the Beta distribution.

1.1.4 Order Statistics

Let $X_1, \ldots, X_n$ be a random sample drawn from $F(x)$ with the PDF $f(x)$. Then $X_1, \ldots, X_n$ are referred to as independent and identically distributed (IID). Rank $X_1, \ldots, X_n$ in ascending order, denoted by $X_{(1:n)} \leq \cdots \leq X_{(n:n)}$. The ordered samples are order statistics. That is, $X_{(1:n)}, \ldots, X_{(n:n)}$ are order statistics of random samples $X_1, \ldots, X_n$.

The Distribution of a Single Order Statistic

Let i be any number between 1 and n. The PDF of $X_{(i:n)}$ can be obtained from the multinomial distribution. Once the random variable $X_{(i:n)}$ is observed as $X_{(i:n)} = x$, the sample space of X can be divided into three portions: the one containing $X_{(i:n)} = x$ chosen from $X_1, \ldots, X_n$ with probability $f(x)$, the second one containing $i - 1$ observations chosen from $X_1, \ldots, X_n$ whose values are smaller than x and each with probability $F(x)$, and the third one containing $n - i$ observations chosen from $X_1, \ldots, X_n$ whose values are greater than x and each with probability $1 - F(x)$. Hence, the PDF of $X_{(i:n)}$ can be written as

$$f_{i:n}(x) = \frac{n!}{(i - 1)!(n - i)!}\{F(x)\}^{i-1} f(x)\{1 - F(x)\}^{n-r}, \quad x \in (-\infty, \infty).$$

When $i = 1$ and $i = n$, $X_{(1:n)}$ and $X_{(n:n)}$ are the smallest and largest order statistics. Their CDFs can also be directly obtained as follows:

$$\Pr(X_{(1:n)} \le x) = 1 - \Pr(X_1 > x, \ldots, X_n > x) = 1 - \{1 - F(x)\}^n,$$

$$\Pr(X_{(n:n)} \le x) = \Pr(X_1 \le x, \ldots, X_n \le x) = \{F(x)\}^n.$$

The Distribution of Two Order Statistics

Let $X_{(i:n)}$ and $X_{(j:n)}$ be two order statistics, $1 \le i < j \le n$. The joint PDF of $X_{(i:n)}$ and $X_{(j:n)}$ can be obtained as follows. Assume the values of $X_{(i:n)}$ and $X_{(j:n)}$ are observed as x_i and x_j, respectively. Then the sample space is divided into five portions: in addition to the two portions containing $X_{(i:n)} = x_i$ with probability $f(x_i)$ and $X_{(j:n)}$ with probability $f(x_j)$, it also contains the portion with $i - 1$ samples smaller than x_i each with probability $F(x_i)$, $j - i - 1$ samples between x_i and x_j each with probability $F(x_j) - F(x_i)$, and $n - j$ samples greater than x_j each with probability $1 - F(x_j)$. Thus, the joint PDF for $(X_{(i:n)}, X_{(j:n)})$ can be written as

$$f_{ij:n}(x_i, x_j) = \frac{n!}{(i-1)!(j-i-1)!(n-j)!}$$
$$\times \{F(x_i)\}^{i-1}\{F(x_j) - F(x_i)\}^{j-i-1}\{1 - F(x_j)\}^{n-j} f(x_i) f(x_j),$$

where $-\infty < x_i < x_j < \infty$.

Remarks

The joint distribution for any collection of order statistics can be obtained similarly. The joint PDF of all order statistics is given by (Problem 1.1)

$$f_{1 \cdots n:n}(x_1, \ldots, x_n) = n! \prod_{i=1}^{n} f(x_i), \quad x_1 < \cdots < x_n.$$

Although $X_1, \ldots, X_n$ are independent, the order statistics are dependent. For example, $f_{ij:n}(x_i, x_j) \ne f_{i:n}(x_i) f_{j:n}(x_j)$. The conditional density of $X_{(j:n)}$ given $X_{(i:n)}$ can be written as $f_{j|i:n}(x_j|x_i) = f_{ij:n}(x_i, x_j)/f_{i:n}(x_i)$. Then it can be shown that (Problem 1.2) the order statistics have the following Markov Chain property,

$$f_{j|1 \cdots j-1:n}(x_j|x_1, \ldots, x_{j-1}) = f_{j|j-1:n}(x_j|x_{j-1}).$$

That is, conditional on $X_{(j-1:n)}$, $X_{(j:n)}$ and $(X_{(1:n)}, \ldots, X_{(j-2:n)})$ are independent.

Suppose $X \sim F(x)$ with continuous PDF $f(x)$, which is positive for any $x \in \Omega$. The pth quantile (or $100p$th percentile) is denoted by $x_p = F^{-1}(p)$. Let $X_{(r:n)}$ be the rth order statistic, $1 < r < n$. If $r/n \to p \in (0, 1)$ as $n \to \infty$, then

$$\sqrt{n}(X_{(r:n)} - x_p) \to N(0, \sigma_p^2) \tag{1.5}$$

in distribution, where $\sigma_p^2 = p(1 - p)/f^2(x_p)$.

1.1.5 Convergence

We use two basic types of stochastic convergence in this book: convergence in distribution, which is also called weak convergence or convergence in law, and convergence in probability. Another type of convergence that we do not use in this book is convergence almost surely (a.s.). We review these three types of convergence using univariate random variables. The results hold for multivariate random variables with some notational modifications.

Let $\{X_n; n \geq 1\}$ be a sequence of random variables and X be a random variable whose CDF is $F(x) = \Pr(X \leq x)$. Let Ω be the sample space of X. The sequence $\{X_n; n \geq 1\}$ is said to converge in distribution to X if

$$\lim_{n \to \infty} \Pr(X_n \leq x) = F(x)$$

for every $x \in \Omega$ at which $F(x)$ is continuous. The sequence $\{X_n; n \geq 1\}$ is said to converge in probability to X if, for any $\varepsilon > 0$,

$$\lim_{n \to \infty} \Pr(|X_n - X| > \varepsilon) = 0.$$

For comparison, $\{X_n; n \geq 1\}$ converge to X a.s. if

$$\Pr\left(\lim_{n \to \infty} |X_n - X| = 0\right) = 1.$$

The following properties are useful.

1) A sequence $\{X_n; n \geq 1\}$ converges to X in distribution if and only if

$$\lim_n \mathrm{E}\{f(X_n)\} = \mathrm{E}\{f(X)\}$$

   for all continuous and bounded functions f.
2) For a continuous function $g(x)$, $X_n \to X$ in distribution (in probability, a.s.) implies $g(X_n) \to g(X)$ in distribution (in probability, a.s.).
3) $X_n \to X$ a.s. implies $X_n \to X$ in probability, which implies $X_n \to X$ in distribution.
4) (Slutsky's Theorem) If $X_n \to X$ in distribution and $Y_n \to c$ in distribution, where c is a constant, then $X_n + Y_n \to X + c$ in distribution, $X_n Y_n \to cx$ in distribution, and $X_n / Y_n \to X/c$ in distribution.
5) If $X_n \to X$ in distribution and $|X_n - Y_n| \to 0$ in probability, then $Y_n \to X$ in distribution.

Note that property 1) shows that convergence in distribution does not imply convergence in moments.

1.2 Statistical Inference

1.2.1 Estimation and Confidence Intervals

Maximum Likelihood Estimate

When a random sample of size n, $x_1, \ldots, x_n$, is drawn from $F(x|\theta)$ with parameter θ, one of the goals of statistical inference is to estimate the parameter θ using the observations. In the binomial distribution $B(n; p)$, $\theta = p$, the probability of success, and in the normal distribution $N(\mu, \sigma^2)$, $\theta = (\mu, \sigma^2)^T$, its mean and variance.

We focus on the maximum likelihood estimate (MLE). To find the MLE, the likelihood function is first obtained, which is given by

$$L(\theta|x_1, \ldots, x_n) = \prod_{i=1}^{n} f(x_i|\theta),$$

where $f(x|\theta)$ is the PDF or the distribution function. We often use $L(\theta)$ for the likelihood function. An estimate of θ, denoted by $\widehat{\theta}$, is the MLE for θ if it maximizes the likelihood function. Denote the parameter space as Θ, e.g., $\Theta = (0, 1)$ for the binomial probability p. Then the MLE $\widehat{\theta}$ satisfies

$$L(\widehat{\theta}) = \max_{\theta \in \Theta} L(\theta). \tag{1.6}$$

We may also write

$$\widehat{\theta} = \arg\max_{\theta \in \Theta} L(\theta) = \arg\max_{\theta \in \Theta} l(\theta),$$

where $l(\theta) = \log L(\theta)$ is the log-likelihood function. If the base of the log function is not specified, the natural log is used throughout this book.

To find the MLE satisfying (1.6) may not be trivial. It is often solved from the following equation

$$\frac{d}{d\theta} l(\theta) = 0.$$

Note that when θ contains multiple parameters, the derivative $d/d\theta$ in the above equation becomes a partial derivative, which is evaluated for each element of θ.

Let $X \sim B(n; p)$ with an observation x. Then $l(p) = c(x, n) + x \log p + (n - x) \log(1 - p)$, where $c(x, n)$ does not contain the parameter p. Thus, we solve

$$\frac{dl(p)}{dp} = \frac{x}{p} - \frac{n - x}{1 - p} = 0,$$

from which we obtain the MLE for p as $\widehat{p} = x/n$. This estimate is unbiased, that is, $\mathrm{E}(\widehat{p}) = p$, with variance $\mathrm{Var}(\widehat{p}) = p(1 - p)/n$. Similarly, if $(x_1, \ldots, x_L) \sim Mul(n; p_1, \ldots, p_L)$ with $\sum_{l=1}^{L} x_l = n$, the MLE for p_l is $\widehat{p}_l = x_l/n$ with mean and variance $E(\widehat{p}_l) = p_l$ and $Var(\widehat{p}_l) = p_l(1 - p_l)/n$ for $l = 1, \ldots, L$. Here, $\widehat{p}_l$ is also an unbiased estimate for p_l. For any two MLEs $\widehat{p}_i$ and $\widehat{p}_j$, their covariance is $Cov(\widehat{p}_i, \widehat{p}_j) = -p_i p_j/n$ for $i \neq j$.

Let $X_1, \ldots, X_n \sim N(\mu, \sigma^2)$ with observations $x_1, \ldots, x_n$. Then the MLEs for μ and σ^2 are

$$\widehat{\mu} = \frac{1}{n} \sum_{i=1}^{n} x_i = \bar{x} \quad \text{and} \quad \widehat{\sigma}^2 = \frac{1}{n} \sum_{i=1}^{n} (x_i - \bar{x})^2.$$

This MLE of σ^2 is biased, but the estimate

$$s^2 = \frac{1}{n-1} \sum_{i=1}^{n} (x_i - \bar{x})^2$$

is unbiased for σ^2. It is known that $\bar{x}$ and s^2 are independent and that $\sqrt{n}\bar{x}/s$ follows a t-distribution with $n - 1$ degrees of freedom.

Properties of Maximum Likelihood Estimate

Let $x_1, \ldots, x_n$ be a random sample from $F(x|\theta)$ and $\widehat{\theta}$ be the MLE for θ. Under some regularity conditions, the MLE uniquely exists and satisfies the following large sample property:

$$\sqrt{n}(\widehat{\theta} - \theta) \rightarrow N\left(0, \frac{1}{I_1(\theta)}\right). \tag{1.7}$$

The above result can be interpreted as the distribution of $\sqrt{n}(\widehat{\theta} - \theta)$ converging to $N(0, I_1^{-1}(\theta))$, where $I_1(\theta)$ is the Fisher information about θ contained in a single observation, given by

$$I_1(\theta) = E\left(\frac{d}{d\theta} l(\theta)\right)^2 = -E\left(\frac{d^2}{d\theta^2} l(\theta)\right), \quad X \sim F(x|\theta).$$

The Fisher information about θ contained in a random sample of size n, denoted by $I_n(\theta)$, is n times that in a single observation. That is, $I_n(\theta) = nI_1(\theta)$. $I_n(\theta)$ is also called the expected Fisher information, while $i_n(\theta) = -d^2 l(\theta)/d\theta^2$ is the observed Fisher information. The subscript n in $I_n(\theta)$ and $i_n(\theta)$ may be omitted if this does not cause confusion. The MLE $\widehat{\theta}$ is a consistent estimate of θ, i.e., $\widehat{\theta} \rightarrow \theta$ in probability as $n \rightarrow \infty$. In addition, the MLE is also optimal in the sense that its asymptotic variance reaches the Cramer-Rao lower bound. Under some regularity conditions, the variance of a consistent estimate of θ has a lower bound $1/\{nI_1(\theta)\}$.

When θ contains multiple parameters, $I_n(\theta)$ and $i_n(\theta)$ can be written as

$$I_n(\theta) = \mathrm{E}\left\{\left(\frac{\partial}{\partial\theta}l(\theta)\right)\left(\frac{\partial}{\partial\theta}l(\theta)\right)^T\right\} = -\mathrm{E}\left(\frac{\partial^2 l(\theta)}{\partial\theta\,\partial\theta^T}\right),$$

$$i_n(\theta) = -\frac{\partial^2 l(\theta)}{\partial\theta\,\partial\theta^T}.$$

Under suitable regularity conditions, $I_n(\theta)$ and $i_n(\theta)$ are both positive definite for $\theta \in \Theta$.

Let $X \sim B(n; p)$. Then, $\partial^2 l(p)/\partial p^2 = -x/p^2 - (n-x)/(1-p)^2$. Thus,

$$-\mathrm{E}\left(\frac{\partial^2}{\partial p^2}l(\theta)\right) = np/p^2 + n(1-p)/(1-p)^2 = n/(p(1-p)) = I_n(p).$$

Hence,

$$\sqrt{n}(\widehat{p} - p) \to N(0, p(1-p)).$$

For comparison, $i_n(p) = x/p^2 + (n-x)/(1-p)^2$.

For the multinomial distribution,

$$\sqrt{n}\begin{bmatrix} \widehat{p}_1 - p_1 \\ \widehat{p}_2 - p_2 \\ \vdots \\ \widehat{p}_L - p_L \end{bmatrix} \to N_L\left(\begin{bmatrix} 0 \\ 0 \\ \vdots \\ 0 \end{bmatrix}, \begin{bmatrix} p_1(1-p_1) & -p_1 p_2 & \cdots & -p_1 p_L \\ -p_2 p_1 & p_2(1-p_2) & \cdots & -p_2 p_L \\ \vdots & \vdots & \cdots & \vdots \\ -p_L p_1 & -p_L p_2 & \cdots & p_L(1-p_L) \end{bmatrix}\right).$$

Confidence Intervals

The MLE $\widehat{\theta}$ for θ is referred to as a point estimate. To incorporate the uncertainty of the point estimate, a common approach is to report a confidence interval (CI). A $100(1-\alpha)\%$ CI for θ is an interval (a, b) such that

$$\Pr(\theta \in (a, b)) = 1 - \alpha$$

asymptotically holds for the true value of θ. The CI can be obtained from the exact distribution of a pivotal statistic or based on the large sample property of the estimate.

Suppose $X_1, \ldots, X_n$ are independent and identically distributed random variables with finite second moments. Denote $\mu = \mathrm{E}(X_1)$ and $\sigma^2 = \mathrm{Var}(X_1)$. Then $\bar{X} = \sum_{i=1}^{n} X_i/n$ is asymptotically normally distributed and

$$\sqrt{n}(\bar{X} - \mu) \to N(0, \sigma^2) \tag{1.8}$$

in distribution. The result (1.8) is due to the central limit theorem (CLT).

Suppose $x_1, \ldots, x_n$ is a random sample drawn from $N(\mu, \sigma^2)$. Then the estimates of μ and σ^2 are $\bar{x}$ and s^2. Then, $\sqrt{n}(\widehat{\mu} - \mu) \to N(0, \sigma^2)$ in distribution. Thus, $\sqrt{n}(\widehat{\mu} - \mu)/s \to t_{n-1}$ in distribution and

$$\Pr(\sqrt{n}|\bar{x} - \mu|/s < t_{1-\alpha/2}(n-1)) = 1 - \alpha,$$

where $t_{1-\alpha/2}(n-1)$ is the $100(1-\alpha/2)$th percentile of t_{n-1}. Hence, the $100(1-\alpha)\%$ CI for μ is given by

$$\bar{x} \pm t_{1-\alpha/2}(n-1)s/\sqrt{n}.$$

Note that when n is large, $t_{1-\alpha/2}(n-1)$ is approximately equal to $z_{1-\alpha/2}$, the $100(1-\alpha/2)$th percentile of $N(0,1)$.

Let $\widehat{\theta}$ be the MLE for a single parameter θ. From (1.7), $\sqrt{I_n(\theta)}(\widehat{\theta} - \theta)$ has an approximate $N(0,1)$. Then, asymptotically,

$$\Pr\left(\sqrt{I_n(\theta)}|\widehat{\theta} - \theta| < z_{1-\alpha/2}\right) = 1 - \alpha.$$

The above equation holds asymptotically if we replace θ in $I_n(\theta)$ by the MLE $\widehat{\theta}$, i.e.,

$$\Pr\left(\sqrt{I_n(\widehat{\theta})}|\widehat{\theta} - \theta| < z_{1-\alpha/2}\right) = 1 - \alpha.$$

from which the CI is

$$\widehat{\theta} \pm z_{1-\alpha/2}/\sqrt{I_n(\widehat{\theta})}.$$

Let $X \sim B(n; p)$. Then $\widehat{p} = x/n$ and $I_n(p) = n/(p(1 - p))$. Thus, $I_n(\widehat{p}) = n^3/(x(n - x))$. Note that $i_n(\widehat{p}) = n^3/(x(n - x))$ as well. The 95% CI for p is

$$x/n \pm 1.96\sqrt{x(n - x)/n^3}.$$

1.2.2 Testing Hypotheses

Introduction

Hypothesis testing considers a null hypothesis H_0 and an alternative hypothesis H_1. For example, to test for association between a genetic marker and a disease, the null hypothesis is "H_0: There is no association", and the alternative hypothesis is "H_1: There is association between the genetic marker and the disease". More specifically, the genetic association can be measured by the odds ratio (see Chap. 2 and Chap. 3). Denote the log odds ratio by θ. Then the null hypothesis of no association is $H_0 : \theta = 0$ and the alternative hypothesis of association is equivalent to $H_1 : \theta \neq 0$. This alternative hypothesis is two-sided because the direction under an association is not specified. That is, which of the two alleles is the risk allele is unknown. If the risk allele is known, a one-sided alternative can be used and is given by either $H_1 : \theta > 0$ or $H_1 : \theta < 0$.

In some cases, the parameter θ is a vector, which contains multiple parameters, for example, $\theta = (\theta_1, \theta_2)^T$. However, the null hypothesis may be written as $H_0 : \theta_1 = 0$ where θ_2 is not specified. In this case, θ_2 is often called a nuisance parameter because only the parameter θ_1 is of interest. A hypothesis is simple if all the values of unknown parameters are specified, while a hypothesis is composite if it does not specify all the values of the parameters. For example, if θ is an unknown scalar parameter, the alternative hypothesis $H_1 : \theta = 1.5$ is simple while $H_1 : \theta > 0$ is composite.

Here we review classical hypothesis testing (a frequentist approach). Bayesian hypothesis testing using Bayes factors will be discussed in Chap. 5.

Type I and Type II Errors

The Type I and Type II errors are often specified in classical hypothesis testing. The Type I error refers to rejecting the null hypothesis when it is true, while the Type II error refers to failure to reject the null hypothesis when the alternative is true. In other words,

$$\Pr(\text{Type I error}) = \Pr(\text{reject } H_0 | H_0),$$

$$\Pr(\text{Type II error}) = \Pr(\text{accept } H_0 | H_1).$$

Given simple hypotheses and a sample size, it is not possible to make both probabilities of Type I and Type II errors as small as possible. In practice, one may limit the probability of making a false positive error. Therefore, a significance level α is prespecified to control the Type I error, i.e., $\Pr(\text{Type I error}) \leq \alpha$. For testing a single null hypothesis, $\alpha = 0.05$ is often chosen, so that the rejection rate is no more than 5% when H_0 is true.

Once the null and alternative hypotheses are specified and α is chosen, a test statistic, denoted by T, is identified and calculated using the observed data. Then the asymptotic null distribution of the test statistic is derived to find the critical value C such that the probability that the test statistic is greater than C is less than or equal to α under H_0. Then T is compared with C. Usually, the null hypothesis is rejected if $T > C$ and the null hypothesis is accepted if $T < C$. When more than one test statistic is available, given the same significance level α, the test statistic with smaller probability of Type II error is more powerful. For a given sample size and α, the power of a test statistic is defined as 1 minus the probability of its Type II error. We use β and π to indicate the probability of Type II error and power. Thus, $\pi = 1 - \beta$.

P-Value

The p-value is commonly used in classical significance testing. It is the smallest significance level with which one can reject the null hypothesis. That is, if the significance level α is less than the p-value, one will accept the null hypothesis. Denote the p-value of a test statistic T by p. Assume, under H_0, $T \sim F(x)$. In addition, assume $T > 0$. Let $X \sim F(x)$, the same distribution for T and continuous. Then the p-value is given by

$$p = \Pr(X > T \mid H_0) = 1 - F(T).$$

For $t \in (0, 1)$,

$$\Pr(p < t) = \Pr(T > F^{-1}(1 - t)) = 1 - F(F^{-1}(1 - t)) = 1 - (1 - t) = t.$$

Thus, under H_0, the p-value follows the uniform distribution in $(0, 1)$, i.e., $p \sim U(0, 1)$.

If $T \sim N(0, 1)$ under H_0 and the two-sided alternative is used, then the p-value can be written as

$$p = 2\Pr(Z > |T|) = 2\{1 - \Phi(|T|)\},$$

where $Z \sim N(0, 1)$. If the alternative is one-sided, then the p-value is given by

$$p = \Pr(Z > T) = 1 - \Phi(T).$$

In applications, the p-value is often reported. For testing a single hypothesis, a p-value less than 0.0001 would be regarded as a very significant one. If the significance level α is specified, then the null hypothesis is rejected if $p < \alpha$. Note that the p-value only depends on the distribution of the test statistic, it does not depend on the sample size given the test statistic.

1.2.3 Likelihood-Based Test Statistics: Without a Nuisance Parameter

Let $X_1, \ldots, X_n$ be independent, identically distributed random variables with the CDF $F(x|\theta)$ and the PDF $f(x|\theta)$, where $\theta = (\theta_1, \ldots, \theta_d)^T$ is the vector of the unknown parameters. We test $H_0 : \theta = \theta_0 = (\theta_{10}, \ldots, \theta_{d0})^T$. The likelihood function is denoted by $L(\theta) = \prod_i f(X_i|\theta)$. The log-likelihood function is given by $l(\theta) = \sum_{i=1}^{n} \log f(X_i|\theta)$. Under H_0, the log-likelihood function is $l(\theta_0)$. Denote

$$l'(\theta) = \frac{\partial l(\theta)}{\partial \theta^T} = \left(\frac{\partial l(\theta)}{\partial \theta_1}, \ldots, \frac{\partial l(\theta)}{\partial \theta_d} \right)^T_{d \times 1},$$

$$l''(\theta) = \frac{\partial^2 l(\theta)}{\partial \theta \partial \theta^T} = \left[\frac{\partial^2 l(\theta)}{\partial \theta_i \partial \theta_j} \right]_{d \times d}.$$

The Score function is defined as $U(\theta) = l'(\theta)$ and the observed Fisher information matrix is given by $i_n(\theta) = -l''(\theta)$. Note that "Score" is used in the Score function and Score statistic throughout this book. This is to distinguish it from the scores used in the trend test in Chap. 3. Denote the MLE of θ by $\widehat{\theta}$, which satisfies $U(\widehat{\theta}) = l'(\widehat{\theta}) = 0$.

Score Test

To test $H_0 : \theta = \theta_0$, the Score statistic can be written as

$$\text{ST} = U(\theta_0)^T i_n^{-1}(\theta_0) U(\theta_0) = U(\theta_0)^T \{-l''(\theta_0)\}^{-1} U(\theta_0) \sim \chi_d^2 \quad \text{under } H_0.$$

Wald Test

The Wald test is also called the maximum likelihood test. It is based on the large sample property of the MLE $\widehat{\theta}$, $\widehat{\theta} - \theta \approx N_d(0, i_n^{-1}(\theta))$, where θ is the true value. The Wald statistic for $H_0 : \theta = \theta_0$ can be written as

$$\text{WT} = (\widehat{\theta} - \theta_0)^T i_n(\widehat{\theta})(\widehat{\theta} - \theta_0) = (\widehat{\theta} - \theta_0)^T \{-l''(\widehat{\theta})\}(\widehat{\theta} - \theta_0) \sim \chi_d^2 \quad \text{under } H_0.$$

Likelihood Ratio Test

To test $H_0 : \theta = \theta_0$, the likelihood ratio test (LRT) is based on the likelihood ratio and is given by

$$\text{LRT} = 2\log \frac{L(\widehat{\theta})}{L(\theta_0)} = 2l(\widehat{\theta}) - 2l(\theta_0) \sim \chi_d^2 \quad \text{under } H_0.$$

1.2.4 Likelihood-Based Test Statistics: With a Nuisance Parameter

In genetic association studies, nuisance parameters are often present. For example, in the analysis of gene-environment interaction, we may be interested in testing only the gene-environment interaction and treat the odds ratios of the main genetic and environmental effects as nuisance parameters. When applying a logistic regression model to test for association between a genetic susceptibility and a disease using case-control data, the intercept in the logistic regression model is a nuisance parameter.

In general, we assume the parameter θ is decomposed into $\theta = (\psi, \eta)^T$. We test $H_0 : \psi = \psi_0$ without specifying η, a nuisance parameter. Let the log-likelihood function be $l(\theta)$. Denote the MLE as $\widehat{\theta} = (\widehat{\psi}, \widehat{\eta})^T$, which maximizes $l(\theta) = l(\psi, \eta)$ without any restriction, and the restricted MLE as $\widetilde{\theta} = (\psi_0, \widetilde{\eta})^T$, which maximizes $l_0(\theta) = l(\psi_0, \eta)$ under H_0. Note that $\widehat{\psi} \neq \widetilde{\psi}$.

The Score function $U(\theta)$ can be written as

$$U(\theta) = \begin{bmatrix} U_\psi(\theta) \\ U_\eta(\theta) \end{bmatrix} = \begin{bmatrix} \frac{\partial l(\theta)}{\partial \psi} \\ \frac{\partial l(\theta)}{\partial \eta} \end{bmatrix}.$$

Decompose the observed Fisher information matrix $i_n(\theta)$ according to $(\psi, \eta)^T$ as

$$i_n(\theta) = -\frac{\partial^2 l(\theta)}{\partial\theta\,\partial\theta^T} = \begin{bmatrix} i_{\psi\psi}(\theta) & i_{\psi\eta}(\theta) \\ i_{\eta\psi}(\theta) & i_{\eta\eta}(\theta) \end{bmatrix}.$$

Denote the inverse of $i_n(\theta)$ as

$$i_n^{-1}(\theta) = \begin{bmatrix} i^{\psi\psi}(\theta) & i^{\psi\eta}(\theta) \\ i^{\eta\psi}(\theta) & i^{\eta\eta}(\theta) \end{bmatrix}.$$

Then the Score test for $H_0 : \psi = \psi_0$ is given by

$$\text{ST} = U_\psi^T(\tilde{\theta}) i^{\psi\psi}(\tilde{\theta}) U_\psi(\tilde{\theta}) \sim \chi_d^2 \quad \text{under } H_0, \tag{1.9}$$

where d is the dimension of ψ. The Wald test for $H_0 : \psi = \psi_0$ can be written as

$$\text{WT} = (\widehat{\psi} - \psi_0)^T \{i^{\psi\psi}(\widehat{\theta})\}^{-1} (\widehat{\psi} - \psi_0) \sim \chi_d^2 \quad \text{under } H_0. \tag{1.10}$$

The LRT is given by

$$\text{LRT} = 2l(\widehat{\theta}) - 2l_0(\tilde{\theta}) \sim \chi_d^2 \quad \text{under } H_0. \tag{1.11}$$

When the nuisance parameter η vanishes, the above three tests become the ones discussed in Sect. 1.2.3.

1.2.5 Multiple Testing

Suppose the conventional significance level $\alpha = 0.05$ is used to test a single null hypothesis. When multiple hypothesis testing is conducted, each at the α level, the probability of rejecting at least one null hypothesis is expected to be greater than α. It is common in genetic association studies to test association with several genetic markers. Suppose M markers are tested. Then the null hypothesis is that no marker is associated with the disease, and the alternative hypothesis is at least one of the markers is associated with the disease. Two commonly used methods, Bonferroni correction and control of the false positive rate, are discussed in this section to correct for such multiple testing issues.

A second multiple testing issue arises when the data generating model is unknown, even if only a single null hypothesis is tested. In this case, when the trend test is used, the test result depends on the choice of a model underlying the data. In practice, the true model is unknown. Therefore, several models may be assumed and the Score statistics for each of these models are applied. Then, only the best result (e.g., the smallest p-value) among these Score statistics may be reported. This multiple testing issue may not be recognized if the number of test statistics or analyses that have been tried is not reported. To resolve this type of multiple testing, the correlations among the test statistics have to be derived. Then asymptotic distribution theory or Monte-Carlo approaches can be used to correct for inflated Type I errors caused by the multiple testing procedure.

Bonferroni Correction

Bonferroni correction is one of the most common approaches to control the family-wise error rate. To apply a Bonferroni correction when testing M null hypotheses, each null hypothesis is tested at the level α/M. If one of the M tests is significant at the α/M level, the null hypothesis is rejected, and the overall Type I error would be controlled at the α level.

Let T_i be the ith test for the ith null hypothesis with level α/M. Denote its critical value by C_i. Thus, under H_0, $\Pr(T_i > C_i) = \alpha/M$. Hence, under H_0, the Type I error to incorrectly reject H_0 is

$$\Pr(\text{reject } H_0) = \Pr\left(\bigcup_{i=1}^{M}(T_i > C_i)\right) \leq \sum_{i=1}^{M}\Pr(T_i > C_i) = \sum_{i=1}^{M}\alpha/M = \alpha.$$

It is known that Bonferroni correction is conservative because it assigns equal level α/M to each null hypothesis. The loss of power using Bonferroni correction is substantial when the statistics for testing M hypotheses are highly correlated. On the other hand, when the test statistics are nearly independent, Bonferroni correction is a reasonable approach to use.

False Discovery Rate

In contrast to Bonferroni correction to control the family-wise error rate, which tests each of M hypotheses at the α/M level, an alternative approach is to control the false discovery rate (FDR). The FDR approach is to control the expected proportion of true null hypotheses among the rejected null hypotheses.

Suppose there are M_0 non-true null hypotheses among a total of M hypotheses. Assume $R > 0$ null hypotheses are rejected, among which V are true null hypotheses. Then the FDR is defined as $E(V/R)$. To control the FDR, we keep $E(V/R)$ below a given threshold α. One simple procedure to control the FDR is as follows. Assume the M test statistics are independent or positively correlated. Then, first calculate all the p-values for testing M hypotheses, denoted by $p_1, \ldots, p_M$. Next, order these p-values in ascending order to obtain order statistics: $p_{(1:M)} < \cdots < p_{(M:M)}$.

For a given threshold level α, find the largest k such that $p_{(k:M)} \leq k\alpha/M$. Finally, reject the k null hypotheses corresponding to $p_{(1:M)}, \ldots, p_{(k:M)}$.

Note that, in the above simple approach, in order to reject at least one null hypothesis, the smallest p-value has to be smaller than the Bonferroni-corrected significance level α/M. Therefore, any null hypothesis that is rejected under Bonferroni correction will be rejected using the FDR when the same threshold level is used. The FDR approach is often more powerful than the Bonferroni correction to reject the null hypothesis when the alternative hypothesis is true.

When the Data Generating Model Is Unknown

When testing a single hypothesis, the data generating model is unknown. A family of plausible models is available. For each model in the family, an asymptotically normally distributed test statistic is obtained. Multiple testing may be conducted if the null hypothesis is tested for each model and the corresponding p-value is obtained. In this case, the FDR approach cannot be applied, and Bonferroni correction is still too conservative because all tests under various genetic models are positively correlated.

When the asymptotic null correlations among the test statistics can be obtained, a common approach to control Type I error is to calculate the maximum statistic over all statistics under various genetic models, or equivalently to find the minimum p-value. Then the asymptotic null distributions for the maximum statistic or the minimum p-value can be found using an asymptotic multivariate normal distribution and the asymptotic null covariance matrix. For case-control genetic association studies, see Chap. 6. In Chap. 8 and Chap. 10, we also mention multiple testing issues due to model uncertainty in the analysis of gene-gene and gene-environment interactions.

1.3 The Delta Method

The Delta method is a useful tool to derive the asymptotic variance and large sample distribution for some estimates and test statistics. Let T be a test statistic or an estimator (e.g., the MLE) such that, asymptotically, $\sqrt{n}(T - \theta) \to N(0, \sigma^2)$. Then, for a continuously differentiable function g, $\sqrt{n}(g(T) - g(\theta))$ has the same asymptotic distribution as the random variate $\sqrt{n}g'(\theta)(T - \theta)$. That is,

$$\sqrt{n}(g(T) - g(\theta)) \to N(0, \{g'(\theta)\}^2\sigma^2).$$

$g(T)$ can be approximated from a Taylor expansion around θ. The above result also implies that the asymptotic variance of $g(T)$ is given by $\mathrm{Var}(g(T)) = \{g'(\theta)\}^2 \mathrm{Var}(T) = \{g'(\theta)\}^2\sigma^2$. When $g'(\theta) = 0$, the Taylor expansion to a higher order term is required, for example,

$$g(T) = g(\theta) + g'(\theta)(T - \theta) + \frac{1}{2}g''(\theta^*)(T - \theta)^2,$$

where θ^* is between θ and T. In this case, the asymptotic distribution is no longer normally distributed.

The above one-dimensional Taylor expansion can be modified to a high dimensional expansion. Let g be a real-valued function of the k dimensional statistic or estimator T. Let t_i and θ_i be the ith coordinates of T and θ, respectively, $i = 1, \ldots, k$. Then

$$g(T) - g(\theta) = \sum_{i=1}^{k} \frac{\partial g(\theta)}{\partial t_i}(t_i - \theta_i) + \frac{1}{2}\sum_{i,j} \frac{\partial^2 g(\theta^*)}{\partial t_i \partial t_j}(t_i - \theta_i)(t_j - \theta_j),$$

where θ_i^* is the ith coordinate of θ^* which is between t_i and θ_i for $i = 1, \ldots, k$.

1.4 The Newton-Raphson Method

The Newton-Raphson method is commonly used in numerical analysis to find the root of an equation $g(\theta) = 0$. When $g = \sum_{i=1}^{n} f'(X_i|\theta)/f(X_i|\theta)$ and $f(x|\theta)$ is the density function, the root is the MLE of θ. The Newton-Raphson method is a one-step approximation given the previous estimate of θ. Suppose at step i, given $\widehat{\theta}_{i-1}$,

$$g(\theta_i) = g(\widehat{\theta}_{i-1}) + g'(\widehat{\theta}_{i-1})(\theta_i - \widehat{\theta}_{i-1}) + \cdots.$$

From $g(\theta_i) = 0$, one obtains an approximate estimate of θ at step i as

$$\widehat{\theta}_i = \widehat{\theta}_{i-1} - \{g'(\widehat{\theta}_{i-1})\}^{-1}g(\widehat{\theta}_{i-1}),$$

which forms the iteration step, where $\widehat{\theta}_0$ can be an initial guess or some simple estimate.

If the iteration converges (it may not), then the solution may be at a maximum, at a minimum, or at a saddle point. This can cause problems when using the Newton-Raphson method to find MLEs.

1.5 The EM Algorithm

The EM algorithm was originally developed to maximize the likelihood function with incomplete observations. It contains two steps. One is an expectation step (the E-step) and the other is a maximization step (the M-step).

Let $X = (X_1, \ldots, X_n)$ be a random sample with the PDF $f(x|\theta)$. The log-likelihood function is denoted by $l(\theta|X) = \sum_{i=1}^{n} \log f(X_i|\theta)$. The MLE of θ, denoted by $\widehat{\theta}$, is given by $\widehat{\theta} = \arg\max_\theta l(\theta|X)$. Consider augmenting the data with Y with the joint density $f(x, y|\theta)$ and the complete log-likelihood function $l(\theta|X, Y)$. Let

$$Q(\theta|\theta_{(i)}, X) = \mathrm{E}_{\theta_{(i)}}\{l(\theta|X, Y)\},$$

where the expectation is with respect to the conditional density $f(y|\theta_{(i)}, x)$. The EM algorithm is an iterative procedure. Start with some initial estimate of θ. In the E-step, compute the expectation $Q(\theta|\widehat{\theta}_{(i)}, X) = E_{\widehat{\theta}_{(i)}}\{l(\theta|X, Y)\}$, the expectation being with respect to $f(y|\widehat{\theta}_{(i)}, x)$. Then in the M-step, maximize $Q(\theta|\widehat{\theta}_{(i)}, X)$ with respect to θ. Denote $\widehat{\theta}_{(i+1)} = \arg\max_\theta Q(\theta|\widehat{\theta}_{(i)}, X)$. The iteration continues until a fixed point of Q is obtained. This iteration process generates a sequence of estimates $\widehat{\theta}_{(i)}$ such that $l(\widehat{\theta}_{(i+1)}|X) \geq l(\widehat{\theta}_{(i)}|X)$.

Applying the EM algorithm to ABO allele frequencies assuming Hardy-Weinberg equilibrium proportions is a typical example (see Bibliographical Comments). Here we consider an example from a linkage study using affected sibpairs. For n sibpairs, the data (x_0, x_1, x_2) follow a multinomial distribution

$$(x_0, x_1, x_2) \sim Mul(n; p_0, p_1, p_2),$$

where $p_0 = (1 - \theta)/4$, $p_1 = r\theta + (1 - \theta)/2$, $p_2 = (1 - r)\theta + (1 - \theta)/4$, where $\theta \in [0, 1]$ is an unknown parameter and $r \in [0, 1/2]$ is known. The null hypothesis of no linkage corresponds to $H_0 : \theta = 0$ under which r is not defined. Under the alternative hypothesis, r corresponds to an underlying genetic model. The observed-data likelihood function is proportional to

$$L(\theta|x) = (1 - \theta)^{x_0}\{r\theta + (1 - \theta)/2\}^{x_1}\{(1 - r)\theta + (1 - \theta)/4\}^{x_2}.$$

The MLE of θ has no closed form. To apply the EM algorithm, we augment x to $(x_0, y_1, y_2, y_3, y_4)$ as follows

$$(x_0, y_1, y_2, y_3, y_4) \sim Mul\left(n; \frac{1 - \theta}{4}, r\theta, \frac{1 - \theta}{2}, (1 - r)\theta, \frac{1 - \theta}{4}\right),$$

where $y_1 + y_2 = x_1$ and $y_3 + y_4 = x_2$. The complete-data likelihood function is proportional to

$$L(\theta|x, y) = \theta^{y_1+y_3}(1 - \theta)^{x_0+y_2+y_4}.$$

Therefore, given $\widehat{\theta}_{(i)}$, in the E-step

$$Q(\theta|\widehat{\theta}_{(i)}, x)$$

$$= E_{\widehat{\theta}_{(i)}}(\log L(\theta|x, y))$$

$$= \left\{\frac{r\widehat{\theta}_{(i)}x_1}{r\widehat{\theta}_{(i)} + \frac{1}{2}(1 - \widehat{\theta}_{(i)})} + \frac{(1 - r)\widehat{\theta}_{(i)}x_2}{(1 - r)\widehat{\theta}_{(i)} + \frac{1}{4}(1 - \widehat{\theta}_{(i)})}\right\}\log\theta$$

$$+ \left\{x_0 + \frac{\frac{1}{2}(1 - \widehat{\theta}_{(i)})x_1}{r\widehat{\theta}_{(i)} + \frac{1}{2}(1 - \widehat{\theta}_{(i)})} + \frac{\frac{1}{4}(1 - \widehat{\theta}_{(i)})x_2}{(1 - r)\widehat{\theta}_{(i)} + \frac{1}{4}(1 - \widehat{\theta}_{(i)})}\right\}\log(1 - \theta).$$

$$(1.12)$$

Denote the above equation by

$$Q(\theta|\widehat{\theta}_{(i)}, x) = u(\widehat{\theta}_{(i)}, x)\log\theta + v(\widehat{\theta}_{(i)}, x)\log(1 - \theta),$$

which can be maximized in the M-step by

$$\widehat{\theta}_{(i+1)} = \frac{u(\widehat{\theta}_{(i)}, x)}{u(\widehat{\theta}_{(i)}, x) + v(\widehat{\theta}_{(i)}, x)}.$$ (1.13)

The E-step and the M-step are defined in (1.12) and (1.13), respectively.

1.6 Sample Size and Power

In the design of any medical study, sample size and power are calculated based on the scientific goals of the study. The basic purpose of sample size and power calculations is to avoid conducting an under-powered study. Here we give a brief introduction to power and sample size calculations. In Chap. 11, we discuss sample size and power calculations for single marker analysis, gene-gene interactions, and gene-environment interactions.

Suppose the null, H_0, and alternative, H_1, hypotheses are specified. A test statistic T to test the null hypothesis is given such that $T \sim N(0, 1)$ under H_0 and $T \sim N(\mu, \sigma^2)$ under H_1. The null hypothesis will be rejected if $|T| > z_{1-\alpha/2}$, where α is the significance level or the probability of Type I error (Sect. 1.2.2) and $z_{1-\alpha/2}$ is the upper $100(1 - \alpha/2)$th percentile of $N(0, 1)$. Statistical power is defined as the probability of rejecting H_0 when H_1 is true. Thus, the power is 1 minus the probability of Type II error (Sect. 1.2.2). Denote the probability of Type II error by β. Then the power is $1 - \beta$. The sample size n is the number of subjects enrolled in a study. The data from these n subjects are used in the test statistic T. The power $1 - \beta$ is increasing with the sample size n. However, a larger sample size means more cost of the study. To design a study, one needs to determine the sample size n such that, given T, α and H_0 and H_1, the power is greater than or equal to a pre-specified $1 - \beta$. On the other hand, when the sample size is constrained by cost, the power can also be calculated and compared to some prespecified values. In practice, $1 - \beta$ is at least 80%.

The test statistic T is a function of n, so that we can denote it by T_n. Similarly, we can denote (μ, σ) by (μ_n, σ_n). Then, to reach the prespecified power $1 - \beta$, we require

$$\Pr(|T_n| > z_{1-\alpha/2}|H_1) \geq 1 - \beta.$$

Note that $(T_n - \mu_n)/\sigma_n \sim N(0, 1)$ under H_1. The above expression can be further written as

$$1 - \beta \leq \Pr((T_n - \mu_n)/\sigma_n > (z_{1-\alpha/2} - \mu_n)/\sigma_n|H_1)$$
$$+ \Pr((T_n - \mu_n)/\sigma_n < -(z_{1-\alpha/2} + \mu_n)/\sigma_n|H_1)$$
$$= 1 - \Phi\left(\frac{z_{1-\alpha} - \mu_n}{\sigma_n}\right) + \Phi\left(-\frac{z_{1-\alpha} + \mu_n}{\sigma_n}\right).$$

Hence, given the sample size n, the power of T_n can be written as

$$\text{power} = 1 - \Phi\left(\frac{z_{1-\alpha} - \mu_n}{\sigma_n}\right) + \Phi\left(-\frac{z_{1-\alpha} + \mu_n}{\sigma_n}\right). \qquad (1.14)$$

On the other hand, the sample size can be obtained from (1.14), where the power is replaced by $1 - \beta$. The sample size n satisfying the above equation requires numerical calculation. Simplification can be obtained by noting that, under H_1, the probability that T_n is less (or greater) than $-z_{1-\alpha/2}$ is small when $T_n > z_{1-\alpha/2}$ (or $T_n < -z_{1-\alpha/2}$). Therefore, we can approximate the sample size n by

$$1 - \beta \approx \Pr((T_n - \mu_n)/\sigma_n > (z_{1-\alpha/2} - \mu_n)/\sigma_n | H_1),$$

from which we obtain that the sample size n satisfies

$$z_{1-\alpha/2} - z_\beta \sigma_n = \mu_n. \qquad (1.15)$$

For illustration, let us consider $X_1, \ldots, X_n \sim N(\mu, 1)$. We test $H_0 : \mu = 0$ against $H_1 : \mu \neq 0$. The test statistic $T_n = \sqrt{n}\bar{X} = \sqrt{n}\sum_{i=1}^{n} X_i/n$ is used. Under H_0, $T_n \sim N(0, 1)$. Assume the goal is to detect a difference in mean $\mu_0 \neq 0$, which is specified. Then $T_n \sim N(\sqrt{n}\mu_0, 1)$ under H_1, and so $\mu_n = \sqrt{n}\mu_0$ and $\sigma_n = 1$. The power can be calculated from the right hand side of (1.14) when the sample size n is given. To detect a mean difference of μ_0 with sample size n, the power is given by

$$\text{power} = 1 - \Phi(z_{1-\alpha/2} - \sqrt{n}\mu_0) + \Phi(-z_{1-\alpha/2} - \sqrt{n}\mu_0).$$

The power functions for $n = 50$, 100, and 500 are plotted in Fig. 1.4 for varying μ_0 (indicated as mu_0 in the figure). On the other hand, given α and $1 - \beta$, using (1.15), we obtain the sample size as

$$n = \left(\frac{z_{1-\alpha/2} - z_\beta}{\mu_0}\right)^2 = \left(\frac{z_{1-\alpha/2} + z_{1-\beta}}{\mu_0}\right)^2.$$

1.7 Asymptotic Relative Efficiency

A concept related to statistical power is efficiency. Suppose two consistent test statistics T_1 and T_2 are used respectively to test $H_0 : \mu = \mu_0$ against $H_1 : \mu > \mu_0$. A test for $H_0 : \mu = \mu_0$ is consistent if its power tends to one as the sample size goes to infinity for a fixed alternative $H_1 : \mu = \mu_1 > \mu_0$. One approach to compare the performance of T_1 and T_2 is to compare their asymptotic efficiencies under local alternatives $\mu_n = \mu_0 + cn^{-1/2}$ where $c > 0$ and n is the sample size. The alternative is local in the sense that $\mu_n \to \mu_0$ as $n \to \infty$. Denote the sample size for T_i under the local alternative by n_i. The asymptotic efficiency of using T_i is defined as

$$e_i = \lim_{n_i \to \infty} \frac{\mathrm{E}'_{\mu_0}(T_i)}{\sqrt{n_i}\,\mathrm{Var}_{\mu_0}(T_i)},$$

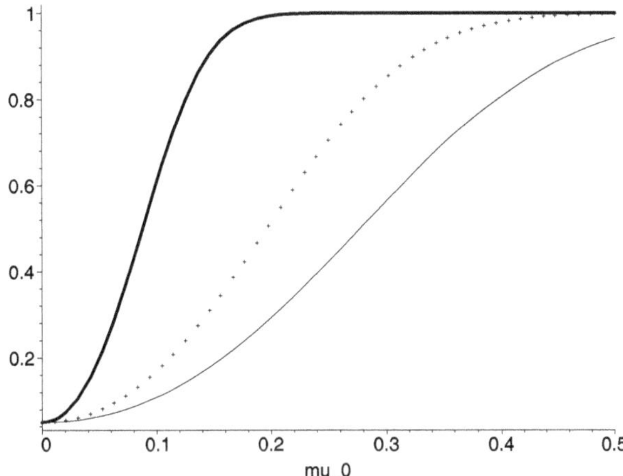

Fig. 1.4 Power functions given sample sizes 50 (the *solid curve*), 100 (the *dotted curve*) and 500 (the *thick curve*) and non-centrality parameter μ_0 (indicated as mu_0)

where $E'_{\mu_0}(T_i) = \partial E_\mu(T_i)/\partial\mu|_{\mu=\mu_0}$ is the partial derivative of $E_\mu(T_i)$ with respect to μ evaluated under H_0.

The asymptotic relative efficiency (ARE) of T_1 to T_2, also known as Pitman efficiency, is defined by

$$\text{ARE}(T_1, T_2) = \lim_{n_1,n_2\to\infty} \left(\frac{n_2}{n_1}\right) = \left(\frac{e_1}{e_2}\right)^2. \tag{1.16}$$

From (1.16),

$$\text{ARE}(T_1, T_2) = \left(\frac{e_1}{e_2}\right)^2 \approx \frac{n_2}{n_1}.$$

From the above expression, $\text{ARE}(T_1, T_2) \leq 1$ implies $n_2 \leq n_1$. Thus, when T_2 is more efficient than T_1, T_1 requires a larger sample size than T_2 in order to reach the same power. In other words, when T_2 is more efficient than T_1, it implies that T_2 is more powerful than T_1 given the same sample size. Note that, for a given alternative, if T_2 is asymptotically optimal, then $\text{ARE}(T_1, T_2) \leq 1$ for any consistent test T_1. Hence, the ARE can be used to measure the loss of efficiency of a test statistic relative to the optimal one. If $(T_1, T_2)^T$ asymptotically follows a bivariate normal distribution with the null correlation ρ_{12}, then $\text{ARE}(T_1, T_2) = \rho_{12}^2$, which can be used to evaluate the ARE. An example of finding the ARE is given in Problem 1.8.

1.8 Bibliographical Comments

Topics of statistical inference that are covered in this chapter can be found in many text books [27, 48, 279]. The book by Casella and Berger [27] provides basic statistical inference, while the books by Cox and Hinkley [48] and van der Vaart [279] are more advanced. More details of stochastic convergences can also be found in these references. Elston and Johnson [73] is an elementary introduction of biostatistics for geneticists and epidemiologists. A good resource for discrete and continuous distributions and their characteristics can be found in Evans et al. [79]. David and Nagaraja [57] is the classical text book for the theory and applications of order statistics. The distributions of order statistics are useful when studying the distributions of ordered p-values in genome-wide association studies or in meta-analysis to combine independent p-values.

In this chapter, we discussed multiple testing issues and three different approaches to correct for multiple testing. In particular, controlling the false discovery rate has been an active research area [14, 15, 260, 261]. More can be found in Dudoit and van der Laan [64]. The EM algorithm is a very useful tool which will be used in, e.g., Chap. 7. The concept of the EM algorithm was originally due to Ceppellini et al. [29], who studied estimations of ABO allele frequencies. The EM algorithm was later developed by Dempster et al. [58] (see also page 176 of Robert and Casella [218]).

The asymptotic relative efficiency was introduced by Pitman and was further developed by Noether [198]. See also [156]. The concept of ARE has been applied to derive robust test statistics [95, 96] with applications to genetic linkage studies [97], association studies using case-parents trios [333], and association studies using case-control data [91, 334]. Examples of calculations of the ARE and its applications can be found in Sect. 3.5 and Sects. 4.7, 4.8, 4.9 of Lachin [156].

1.9 Problems

1.1 Show that the joint density function of all n order statistics $X_{(1:n)}, \ldots, X_{(n:n)}$ is given by

$$f_{1\cdots n:n}(x_1, \ldots, x_n) = n! \prod_{i=1}^{n} f(x_i) \quad \text{for } x_1 < \cdots < x_n.$$

Prove that $\int \cdots \int_{x_1 < \cdots < x_n} f_{1\cdots n:n}(x_1, \ldots, x_n) dx_1 \cdots dx_n = 1$.

1.2 Show that, given $X_{(j-1:n)}$, the order statistics $(X_{(1:n)}, \ldots, X_{(j-2:n)})$ and $X_{(j:n)}$ are conditionally independent.

1.3 Let $X_{(1:n)} < \cdots < X_{(n:n)}$ be order statistics from a uniform distribution $F(x) = x$. Derive $f_{i:n}(x)$ and $f_{ij:n}(x_i, x_j)$ $(1 \le i < j \le n)$. In addition, find the mean and variance of $X_{(i:n)}$.

1.4 Let X_1 and X_2 be independent random variables, each having a $U(0, 1)$ distribution. Derive the PDF and CDF for $Y = -2\log(X_1) - 2\log(X_2)$.

1.5 Prove the following properties, given in (1.1) and (1.2),

$$E(X_2) = E\{E(X_2|X_1)\},$$

$$\mathrm{Var}(X_2) = \mathrm{Var}\{E(X_2|X_1)\} + E\{\mathrm{Var}(X_2|X_1)\}.$$

1.6 Let $(r_0, r_1, r_2) \sim Mul(r; p_0, p_1, p_2)$. Then the MLE of p_i is given by $\widehat{p}_i = r_i/r$. Consider the function $\Delta(p_1, p_2) = p_2 - (p_2 + p_1/2)^2$. Using the Delta method find the asymptotic variance of $\widehat{\Delta}(p_1, p_2) = \Delta(\widehat{p}_1, \widehat{p}_2)$.

1.7 Let $X_1, \ldots, X_n$ be independent, identically distributed random variables with the normal distribution $N(\mu, \sigma^2)$. Denote the median of the sample of size n by X_{med}. Using the result in Sect. 1.1.4, find the limiting distribution of $\sqrt{n}(X_{\mathrm{med}} - \mu)$.

1.8 Let X follow the location-scale distribution $F((x - \mu)/\sigma)$ with the continuous PDF $f((x - \mu)/\sigma)/\sigma$. Suppose $E(X) = \mu$ and $E(X^2) < \infty$. Let $X_1, \ldots, X_n$ be a random sample and X_{med} be its median. Both the sample mean $\bar{X}$ and the median X_{med} can be used to estimate μ, and both estimates are asymptotically unbiased, i.e., $E(\bar{X}) = \mu$ and $E(X_{\mathrm{med}}) \to \mu$ as $n \to \infty$. Let $T_1 = X_{\mathrm{med}}$ and $T_2 = \bar{X}$ be statistics testing $H_0 : \mu = 0$. Show that the asymptotic efficiencies of T_1 and T_2 are $e_1 = 2f(0)/\sigma$ and $e_2 = 1/\sigma$. Thus, the ARE is $\mathrm{ARE}(T_1, T_2) = 4f^2(0)$. When F is the normal distribution, $\mathrm{ARE}(T_1, T_2) = 2/\pi \approx 0.637$.

1.9 Let X_1 and X_2 follow a uniform distribution $U(0, 1)$. Denote $Y = \min(X_1, X_2)$. If X_1 and X_2 are positively correlated, show that $\Pr(Y < y) < y$.

1.10 Let p_1 and p_2 be two positively correlated p-values. Let $\mathrm{MIN2} = \min(p_1, p_2)$ be the minimum of the two p-values. Denote the p-value of MIN2 by p_{MIN2}. Then, using Problem 1.9, show that $p_{\mathrm{MIN2}} > \mathrm{MIN2}$.

1.11 Let $Z_i(X_n) = a_i(X_n)/b_i(X_n)$ $(i = 1, 2)$, where X_n is a random variable and $X_n \to \mu$ in probability as $n \to \infty$, a_i and b_i are both real-valued, non-random functions. Assume $a_i(X_n)$ is bounded for any X_n and $b_i(X_n)$ has finite second-order derivative for any X_n. Show that, without higher order terms,

$$\mathrm{Cov}(Z_1(X_n), Z_2(X_n)) = \mathrm{Cov}(a_1(X_n), a_2(X_n))/\{b_1(\mu)b_2(\mu)\}.$$

Chapter 2
Introduction to Genetic Epidemiology

Abstract Chapter 2 introduces a background to population genetics and genetic epidemiology. It starts with basic concepts of genetics and population genetics, including genes, alleles, genotypes, phenotypes, linkage disequilibrium, Hardy-Weinberg equilibrium, and population structure. Other terminology not covered in this chapter is discussed in later chapters. Designs of genetic association studies are then introduced, including population-based and family-based designs. Testing Hardy-Weinberg equilibrium proportions is covered. Goodness-of-fit, likelihood ratio and exact tests for deviation from Hardy-Weinberg equilibrium proportions are discussed. This chapter also discusses two types of risk measures: odds ratios and relative risks. Applying a logistic regression model for case-control data is presented.

This chapter introduces a background of population genetics and genetic epidemiology. It contains two parts. First, we start with basic concepts of population genetics, including alleles, genotypes, phenotypes, and linkage disequilibrium. Other terms that are not covered here will be discussed in later chapters. Designs of genetic association studies are then introduced, including case-control and family-based designs. We will focus here on case-control designs and family-based designs will be discussed in Chap. 13.

The Hardy-Weinberg law plays an important role in population genetics and the analysis of genetic data. Hardy-Weinberg equilibrium in a population is reviewed and the implications of departure from Hardy-Weinberg equilibrium are also demonstrated. Asymptotic and exact tests for Hardy-Weinberg proportions are given with examples. Calculation of the genotype frequencies in the population with or without Hardy-Weinberg proportions is given. The impact of departure from Hardy-Weinberg proportions is reviewed. It is well known that a case-control association study may be affected by hidden population substructure. Definitions of two common population substructures are given. Methods to correct for population substructure will be discussed in Chap. 9.

We discuss two measures of genotypic risks (odds ratio and relative risk) and their inference. The logistic regression models for case-control data are reviewed. Differences in the prospective and retrospective logistic regression models are briefly discussed. The conditional logistic regression model is often used for the

G. Zheng et al., *Analysis of Genetic Association Studies*,
Statistics for Biology and Health,
DOI 10.1007/978-1-4614-2245-7_2, © Springer Science+Business Media, LLC 2012

analysis of matched case-control data. A discussion of conditional logistic regression is given in Chap. 4.

2.1 Basic Genetic Terminology

With a few exceptions, human beings have in each cell nucleus 23 pairs of chromosomes, among which one pair comprises the sex chromosomes, also known as the X and Y chromosomes, and the other pairs are autosomal chromosomes. Within each chromosome is a molecule of DNA, which is made up of a long sequence of four different nucleotides labeled A, T, C, and G, with a structure that allows it to replicate itself. A gene is a series of DNA sequences that contain genetic information. For the purposes of this book we shall assume that along each chromosome pair hundreds or thousands of genes are arranged in a linear order (in the case of the sex chromosomes this occurs mostly along a single chromosome—from now on we shall restrict our discussion to autosomal chromosomes). This is perhaps not the case with the latest definition of a gene, but will suffice for our purposes. Similarly we shall define a locus to be the location of a gene or any DNA sequence on a chromosome pair. When the location of a DNA sequence on a chromosome pair is known, and that sequence varies in the population, it is also called a genetic marker. An allele is an alternative DNA sequence that can occur at a particular location on a single chromosome. Since chromosomes are present in pairs, at a given locus a person's gene or marker has two alleles, one on each chromosome. In the population, however, a gene or marker could have multiple (>2) alleles. We focus on diallelic markers, which have only two alleles in the population. A single nucleotide polymorphism (SNP) is a commonly used diallelic marker that varies in individuals owing to the difference of a single nucleotide (A, T, C, or G) in the DNA sequence. Although the location of a SNP is often referred to as a locus, it is more properly referred to as a site, a locus comprising more than one site.

We denote alleles by A and B for a single marker, where A is referred to as a wild type or a typical allele, and B is the complement of A, or the risk allele when a disease or trait is affected by this gene. For a multiallelic marker, it is possible that more than one allele may carry risks. (Other notation may also be used for alleles. In particular, when referring to two loci, we use a different notation: A and a for the alleles at one locus, and B and b for the alleles at the other locus.) Two alleles A and B at a locus form a genotype. There are four possible genotypes: AA, AB, BA and BB, but the two orders AB and BA are not distinguished. Hence only three genotypes are possible at a diallelic locus, denoted by AA, AB or BB. Genotypes AA and BB are said to be homozygous, and AB is heterozygous. For a multiallelic marker, more genotypes may be observed. For example, if a marker has three alleles, A, B and C, a total of six genotypes are possible: AA, AB, AC, BB, BC, and CC. Allele frequencies are usually the relative frequencies of the alleles in the population, denoted by $\Pr(B) = p$ and $\mathrm{pr}(A) = 1 - p$. Minor allele frequency (MAF) refers to the frequency of the allele with frequency no more than 0.5 in a population. Denote the three genotypes by $G_0 = AA$, $G_1 = AB$ and $G_2 = BB$.

Table 2.1 Joint distribution of marker and a functional locus

	B	b	
A	$(1-p)(1-q)+D$	$(1-p)q-D$	$1-p$
a	$p(1-q)-D$	$pq+D$	p
	$1-q$	q	1

The genotype frequencies are then the frequencies of the three genotypes in the population, denoted by $g_i = \Pr(G_i)$ for $i = 0$, 1 and 2, and $g_0 + g_1 + g_2 = 1$.

A phenotype is any observable characteristic or trait of an individual. It refers to a physical expression of genotypes at many loci and/or environmental factors. The trait can be continuous, e.g., blood pressure, weight, height etc., discrete, including binary such as diseased/case and normal/control, or ordinal categories related to different stages of a disease. A discrete trait can be defined based on a continuous trait. For example, cases and controls correspond to extremely high or low values of the trait, respectively. In some study designs, cases can be obtained from the extremely high values of the trait while controls are random samples from the population.

One of the goals of genetic association studies is to detect disease susceptibility genes (or functional loci). Suppose M_1 is a functional locus for a disease. The alleles at a functional locus are not observed. Suppose M_2 is an observed marker. Assume M_1 and M_2 have alleles A, a and B, b, respectively. Suppose the allele frequencies are given by $\Pr(a) = p$ and $\Pr(b) = q$. Thus, $\Pr(A) = 1 - p$ and $\Pr(B) = 1 - q$. The joint distribution of the alleles at the two loci (the marker and the functional locus) is given in Table 2.1, where

$$D = \Pr(AB) - \Pr(A)\Pr(B),$$

is the linkage disequilibrium coefficient. When $D = 0$, the two loci are independent, and we say the two loci are in gametic phase equilibrium. When $D \neq 0$, they are correlated and in gametic phase disequilibrium. When two loci are on the same chromosome pair and close enough to each other, their alleles are not transmitted independently to each offspring and the loci are said to be linked. Gametic phase disequilibrium between two linked loci is called linkage disequilibrium (LD). Most of the discussions in this book assume that a marker is also a functional locus and that they have the same allele frequencies. We refer to this model as a single-locus model, under which either $A = B$ and $a = b$ with $p = q$ or $A = b$ and $a = B$ with $p = 1 - q$. In the former case, $\Pr(AB) = \Pr(A) = 1 - p$ and $D = p(1 - p)$. In the latter case $\Pr(AB) = 0$ and $D = -p(1 - p)$. We also call the model with $D \neq 0$ a two-locus model. A common measure for LD is the standardized LD coefficient D', defined by

$$D' = \begin{cases} D/\min\{(1-q)p, (1-p)q\} & \text{if } D > 0, \\ D/\min\{(1-p)(1-q), pq\} & \text{if } D < 0. \end{cases} \tag{2.1}$$

Using D', complete LD refers to $|D'| = 1$; perfect LD refers to $|D'| = 1$ together with either $A = B$ and $a = b$ with $p = q$ ($D > 0$), or $A = b$ and $a = B$ with

$p = 1 - q$ ($D < 0$). Thus, the single-locus model refers to perfect LD, while the two-locus model refers to imperfect LD.

When $D \neq 0$, there are nine possible combinations of genotypes for the two loci:

$$(AA, BB), \quad (AA, Bb), \quad (AA, bb),$$
$$(Aa, BB), \quad (Aa, Bb), \quad (Aa, bb),$$
$$(aa, BB), \quad (aa, Bb), \quad (aa, bb).$$

Given genotypes (AA, BB), it is certain that alleles on both chromosomes are A and B. In this situation, phase is known. Given genotypes (Aa, Bb), however, it is not certain which two alleles are on the same chromosome; they can be AB and ab or Ab and aB. In this situation, phase is unknown. A different two-locus model is used in gene-gene interactions (Chap. 8), where the two loci refer to two disease susceptibility genes. It can also be modified to a two-marker model, in which both M_1 and M_2 are markers and both are in LD with a functional locus. It can be further extended to multiple markers. A disease can be affected by more than two markers in the form of a haplotype, which will be introduced and discussed in Chap. 7. Discussion of $D \neq 0$, when one locus is a marker and the other is a functional locus, will also be given for some topics in Chap. 11. Penetrance is defined as the probability of having a disease given a specific genotype at the marker, denoted by $f_i = \Pr(\text{case}\,|\,G_i)$ for genotype G_i, $i = 0, 1, 2$. Here we assume perfect LD. When there is no association, $f_0 = f_1 = f_2 = \Pr(\text{case})$. We denote $\Pr(\text{case}) = k$ as the prevalence of the disease.

2.2 Genetic Association Studies

In this section, we first show the relationship between LD and association under the imperfect LD model by varying the parameter D defined in Table 2.1, in which one locus is a marker with alleles A/a and the other is a functional locus with alleles B/b. We will discuss two types of designs: population based and family based. In the population-based design, we focus on the retrospective case-control study. We discuss case-control designs and analyses from the epidemiological perspective. Other relevant designs are also mentioned.

2.2.1 Linkage Disequilibrium and Association Studies

Because the functional locus (or disease locus) that has a causal relationship with a disease is unknown, a marker is genotyped and tested for association with the disease. If the marker is in LD with the disease locus, an association between the marker and the disease can be identified through testing for association. Figure 2.1 shows a diagram of the association between the marker and the disease, the causal

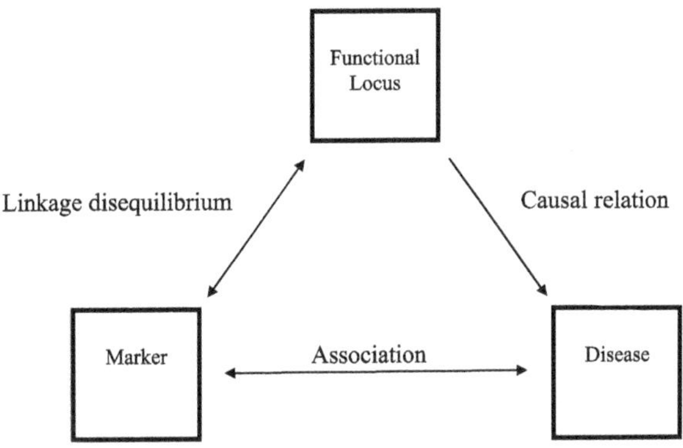

Fig. 2.1 Diagram of LD, association and causal relationship among the marker, functional locus and disease

relationship between the disease locus and the disease, and the LD between the two loci.

To demonstrate the relationship between the LD and association, we use the notation defined in Table 2.1. In addition, we assume the penetrances at the disease locus are $f_i^* = \Pr(\text{case}\,|G_i^*)$, where $(G_0^*, G_1^*, G_2^*) = (BB, Bb, bb)$. The penetrances at the marker are still denoted by $f_i = \Pr(\text{case}\,|G_i)$, where $(G_0, G_1, G_2) = (AA, Aa, aa)$. Denote

$$F_1 = 1 - q + D/(1 - p), \qquad F_2 = 1 - q - D/p,$$

$$F_3 = q - D/(1 - p), \qquad F_4 = q + D/p,$$

where p, q and D are given in Table 2.1. Denote $\lambda_1^* = f_1^*/f_0^*$ and $\lambda_2^* = f_2^*/f_0^*$, which are referred to as genotype relative risks (GRRs). More discussion of GRRs will be provided in Chap. 3. Then (Problem 2.2),

$$f_0 = f_0^*(F_1^2 + 2F_1 F_3 \lambda_1^* + F_3^2 \lambda_2^*), \tag{2.2}$$

$$f_1 = f_0^*(F_1 F_2 + F_1 F_4 \lambda_1^* + F_2 F_3 \lambda_1^* + F_3 F_4 \lambda_2^*), \tag{2.3}$$

$$f_2 = f_0^*(F_2^2 + 2F_2 F_4 \lambda_1^* + F_4^2 \lambda_2^*). \tag{2.4}$$

When $D = 0$, i.e., under linkage equilibrium, (2.2) to (2.4) reduce to

$$f_0 = f_1 = f_2 = f_0^*\{(1 - q)^2 + 2q(1 - q)\lambda_1^* + q^2 \lambda_2^*\} = k,$$

regardless of values of λ_1^* and λ_2^*. Hence, there is no association between the marker and the disease under linkage equilibrium. From Problem 2.3, when $D \neq 0$, the penetrances (f_0, f_1, f_2) are not equal, which leads to unequal distributions for genotype counts in cases and controls. Therefore, a standard chi-squared test can be applied to detect association between the genotypes of the marker and the disease. Association, however, can arise from other factors, e.g., population substructure (see Sect. 2.4). Associations not due to LD, or more generally to gametic phase disequilibrium, are called spurious associations. Table 2.2 reports the GRRs at the marker $\lambda_1 = f_1/f_0$ and $\lambda_2 = f_2/f_1$ given those at the disease locus $\lambda_1^* = f_1^*/f_0^*$, $\lambda_2^* = f_2^*/f_1^*$, and values of p, q, D' and disease prevalence k. Table 2.2 shows that the values of λ_2 are

Table 2.2 GRRs at the marker (λ_1, λ_2) given those at the disease locus $(\lambda_1^*, \lambda_2^*)$ with prevalence $k = 0.1$ and values of $p = \Pr(a)$ (marker allele frequency), $q = \Pr(b)$ (disease locus allele frequency) and LD parameter D'

λ_1^*	λ_2^*	p	q	D'	λ_1	λ_2
1.00	1.50	0.1	0.1	0.9	1.005	1.414
				0.8	1.008	1.336
			0.3	0.9	1.078	1.396
				0.8	1.072	1.332
1.30	1.60	0.3	0.1	0.9	1.268	1.567
				0.8	1.237	1.474
			0.3	0.9	1.185	1.369
				0.8	1.164	1.327
1.50	1.50	0.3	0.1	0.9	1.441	1.481
				0.8	1.384	1.455
			0.3	0.9	1.224	1.244
				0.8	1.196	1.232

smaller than those of λ_2^* when $|D'| < 1$, and λ_2 decreases with $|D'|$. This indicates that association becomes weaker with a weaker LD. A similar phenomenon is observed for λ_1 except for $\lambda_1^* = 1$, which corresponds to a recessive disease (for the definitions of genetic models, see Chap. 3).

2.2.2 Population-Based Designs

A typical population-based design is the case-control study. In this design, individuals are genetically unrelated. A retrospective case-control design is cost-effective and commonly used in genetic studies. In this book, we focus on the retrospective case-control design, in which a random sample of cases (controls) is drawn from the case (control) population. The numbers of cases and controls in practice are determined in the design stage based on considerations of power, cost, and the disease prevalence. Given the total sample size, a design with equal numbers of cases and controls is more powerful than one with unequal numbers. In epidemiology, the retrospective case-control design is particularly useful to study a rare disease. For each individual, the genotype of the marker of interest is obtained. The goal of this design is to test whether or not the disease is associated with the marker. The retrospective case-control design is also used in large-scale association studies, in particular for genome-wide association studies (GWAS) using 500,000 to more than a million SNPs.

Another type of population-based design is a prospective case-control (cohort) study. In this design, individuals entering the study are drawn randomly from the study population without the disease. Following a period of time after, say, a treatment or an intervention, individuals who develop the disease are called cases and those who do not are controls. This design, however, is not efficient for rare diseases. The outcome of this design is not restricted to a binary trait. It can be a quantitative trait, e.g., comparing the change of weight from baseline among three genotypes or between two alleles after a diet intervention.

In general, case-control designs are cost-effective for large-scale association studies. One potential concern of case-control studies is population substructure, which would lead to spurious association if not properly controlled.

2.2.3 Family-Based Designs

One simple family-based design for association studies is the case-parents trio design. In this design, an affected offspring is first ascertained and genotyped. The genotypes of the parents are also obtained. One approach to detect association in this design is based on a statistic comparing the number of marker alleles transmitted from parents to the offspring with the number not transmitted. In this case, only heterozygous parents are considered in the analysis. A typical method to analyze the trio data is called the transmission disequilibrium test (TDT). Because the untransmitted alleles can be regarded as controls for those transmitted, concern of population stratification, which can inflate the Type I error rate in population-based designs, is not relevant in the analysis of the trio design. This simple design has been extended to include multiple affected offspring (affected sibpairs), or disease-free siblings. For more details of this design and analysis, refer to Chap. 13.

More complicated family-based designs use data on large pedigrees with two or more generations. Some genotypes may not be available, especially for late onset diseases. Both binary traits and quantitative traits can be analyzed using family-based designs. Different kinds of family-based association tests can be used to analyze large family data in which correlations of traits among family members and their genetic relationships are incorporated into the analysis. A well-known example of this design is the Framingham Heart Study, which is a community-based family design. The original study began in 1948 and was designed to study cardiovascular disease and its risk factors in Framingham, Massachusetts. Now data from three generations have been obtained. Recent genetic studies, including linkage studies and GWAS, have been extensively reported.

Unlike population-based designs, family-based designs can eliminate the effects of population stratification using TDT statistics, without the need of the kinds of methods briefly described later. But these designs are typically not as efficient as population-based designs, especially for late onset diseases.

2.2.4 Other Designs

In addition to purely population-based and family-based designs, there are other designs for genetic studies. These designs use multi-stage samples. For example, in stage 1, family data are obtained for linkage studies, from which candidate-genes are identified. In the second stage, association studies (either population-based or family-based) are conducted. In another population-based design, controls may be shared by association studies for different diseases. In the Wellcome Trust Case-Control Consortium (WTCCC) study, 3,000 controls drawn from the British population were shared among association studies of seven diseases. Data from population-based and family-based designs can also be combined to enhance the power to detect true associations. The community-based Framingham Heart Study has been used to supply controls for association studies of diabetes. These designs arise because a genetic study often uses multi-stage samples and thousands of individuals to detect small to moderate genetic effects.

In testing gene-environment interaction for a rare disease when a genetic susceptibility and an environmental factor are independent in the population, a case-only design can be employed because the odds ratio relating the gene and environment to a disease is approximately the odds ratio relating the environmental factor to the genetic factor among cases. The case-only design is often more powerful to detect gene-environment interaction than a case-control design using a logistic regression model.

Many hybrid designs have been proposed for cost-effectiveness, including combining case-control and family-based designs to test for genetic associations, and combining case-control and case-only designs to test for gene-environment interactions. Many genetic studies have been conducted and data from various study designs are available. Thus, hybrid designs based on data sharing are becoming more important and popular.

2.3 Hardy-Weinberg Principle

The Hardy-Weinberg principle, also known as the Hardy-Weinberg law or Hardy-Weinberg equilibrium (HWE), is a well-known model in population genetics. It states that under random mating both allele and genotype frequencies in a population remain constant or stable if no disturbing factors are introduced. We first introduce HWE followed by testing for departure from Hardy-Weinberg proportions (usually erroneously called "testing for HWE"). Both asymptotic chi-squared tests and an exact test will be discussed. The impact of departure from Hardy-Weinberg proportions will also be discussed.

2.3.1 What Is Hardy-Weinberg Equilibrium?

Autosomal Chromosomes

Consider a diallelic locus with alleles A and B with population frequencies q and p, respectively. Assume males and females have the same allele frequencies.

Table 2.3 Genotype frequencies under random mating given male and female gametes

			Male gametes	
			A	B
			q	p
Female	A	q	g_0	$g_1/2$
gametes	B	p	$g_1/2$	g_2

Table 2.4 Mating types (MTs) with frequencies and conditional probabilities of zygotes given mating types

MTs	Freq.	Freq. of zygotes		
		AA	AB	BB
$\mathrm{MT}_1 : AA \times AA$	g_0^2	1	0	0
$\mathrm{MT}_2 : AA \times AB$	$2g_0g_1$	1/2	1/2	0
$\mathrm{MT}_3 : AA \times BB$	$2g_0g_2$	0	1	0
$\mathrm{MT}_4 : AB \times AB$	g_1^2	1/4	1/2	1/4
$\mathrm{MT}_5 : AB \times BB$	$2g_1g_2$	0	1/2	1/2
$\mathrm{MT}_6 : BB \times BB$	g_2^2	0	0	1

Then, under random mating, Table 2.3 gives the genotype frequencies $g_0 = \mathrm{Pr}(AA)$, $g_1 = \mathrm{Pr}(AB)$ and $g_2 = \mathrm{Pr}(BB)$ together with the male and female gametes and their frequencies.

When HWE holds in the population,

$$g_0 = q^2, \qquad g_1 = 2pq, \qquad g_2 = p^2. \tag{2.5}$$

Equations (2.5), known as HWE proportions or simply Hardy-Weinberg proportions, can be obtained assuming random mating, under which alleles of male and female gametes are independent. More assumptions, however, are required for HWE. In addition to random mating, it also requires that the population size is infinite, males and females have identical allele frequencies, there is no effect of migration or mutation, and there is no natural selection.

Assume that HWE does not hold at the current generation in the population. Under random mating, we will show that for one locus the proportions (2.5) hold in the population after one generation. The genotype frequencies are denoted by g_0, g_1, and g_2 as before. Then the allele frequencies of A and B in the population given the genotype frequencies can be written as $q = g_0 + g_1/2$ and $p = g_2 + g_1/2$, respectively. Table 2.4 shows six mating types MT_j for $j = 1, \ldots, 6$, their corresponding frequencies, and the conditional probabilities of their zygotes given the mating types.

In the next generation, the genotype frequencies can be obtained from

$$\Pr(G_i) = \sum_{j=1}^{6} \Pr(G_i|\mathrm{MT}_j)\,\Pr(\mathrm{MT}_j), \qquad (2.6)$$

where $(G_0, G_1, G_2) = (AA, AB, BB)$. It can be shown that (Problem 2.4), using (2.6) and Table 2.4,

$$\Pr(G_0) = (g_0 + g_1/2)^2 = q^2,$$
$$\Pr(G_1) = 2(g_0 + g_1/2)(g_2 + g_1/2) = 2pq,$$
$$\Pr(G_2) = (g_2 + g_1/2)^2 = p^2, \qquad (2.7)$$

where p and q are the frequencies of alleles B and A, respectively. Hence, at the next generation, the Hardy-Weinberg proportions hold. Note carefully that we have shown that one round of random mating results in these proportions, *not* that these proportions imply equilibrium. It is possible for these proportions to hold at every generation and yet the allele frequencies change from generation to generation.

The above results can be extended to multiallelic loci. In general, assume a locus has m alleles, denoted by A_j, $j = 1, \ldots, m$, with population frequencies $p_j = \Pr(A_j)$. Under HWE, the genotype frequencies are given by $\Pr(A_i A_j) = 2 p_i p_j$ for $i \neq j$ and $\Pr(A_j A_j) = p_j^2$.

The X Chromosome

For sex-linked loci, females have two copies of the X chromosome, while males have one copy of the X chromosome and one copy of the Y chromosome. We focus on the X chromosomes. Then the Hardy-Weinberg proportions, as defined for autosomal chromosomes, can be applied to females. For males, we assume that the allele frequency is identical to that of females. Hence, with Hardy-Weinberg proportions at the X chromosome, we have

$$\Pr(B|\text{male}) = \Pr(B|\text{female}) = p, \qquad \Pr(A|\text{male}) = \Pr(A|\text{female}) = q, \quad (2.8)$$
$$\Pr(G_0|\text{female}) = q^2, \qquad \Pr(G_1|\text{female}) = 2pq, \qquad \Pr(G_2|\text{female}) = p^2.$$
$$(2.9)$$

If (2.8) holds and (2.9) does not hold, it takes one generation to reach Hardy-Weinberg proportions. If (2.8) does not hold but (2.9) holds, it takes infinitely many generations to reach the proportions.

Table 2.5 Testing Hardy-Weinberg proportions: the observed genotype counts, the expected genotype counts under HWE, and estimates of the expected genotype counts

	AA	AB	BB
Observed	n_0	n_1	n_2
Expected	nq^2	$2npq$	np^2
Estimated	$n\widehat{q}^2$	$2n\widehat{p}\widehat{q}$	$n\widehat{p}^2$

2.3.2 Testing Hardy-Weinberg Equilibrium Proportions

We discuss asymptotic tests and an exact test for Hardy-Weinberg proportions in the population for autosomal chromosomes. Results for the X chromosome are given next.

A Simple Chi-Squared Test

Suppose a random sample of size n is drawn from the population and the genotype counts of the n individuals are obtained. Denote the genotype counts by (n_0, n_1, n_2) for $(G_0, G_1, G_2) = (AA, AB, BB)$, and $n_0 + n_1 + n_2 = n$. The allele counts are $2n_0 + n_1$ for A and $2n_2 + n_1$ for B among a total of $2n$ alleles. Let $p = \Pr(B)$. An estimate of p is given by $\widehat{p} = (2n_2 + n_1)/(2n)$. Likewise, an estimate of $q = \Pr(A)$ is given by $\widehat{q} = (2n_0 + n_1)/(2n)$. Table 2.5 shows the observed genotype counts, the expected genotype counts under Hardy-Weinberg proportions (the null hypothesis H_0), and estimates of the expected genotype counts under H_0.

A typical chi-squared test has the form

$$\chi^2 = \sum \frac{(\text{observed} - \text{expected})^2}{\text{expected}}.$$

Applying the above test to the data in Table 2.5 with the expected counts being replaced by the estimated ones, we have

$$\chi^2 = \frac{(n_0 - n\widehat{q}^2)^2}{n\widehat{q}^2} + \frac{(n_1 - 2n\widehat{p}\widehat{q})^2}{2n\widehat{p}\widehat{q}} + \frac{(n_2 - n\widehat{p}^2)^2}{n\widehat{p}^2}, \tag{2.10}$$

which has an asymptotic χ_1^2 distribution under H_0. Using a chi-squared distribution for the statistic based on discrete genotype data, a bias correction of $1/2$ may be used

$$\chi^2 = \sum \frac{(|\text{observed} - \text{expected}| - 1/2)^2}{\text{expected}}.$$

To apply the chi-squared test in (2.10) requires a large n and the expected counts in each of the three cells not too small. This may not be true for alleles with small MAFs, or a small sample size.

Test Based on Hardy-Weinberg Disequilibrium

An alternative derivation of the above chi-squared test is based on the Hardy-Weinberg disequilibrium (HWD) coefficient, defined by

$$\Delta = \Pr(BB) - \{\Pr(B)\}^2 = \Pr(BB) - \{\Pr(BB) + \Pr(AB)/2\}^2.$$

Under H_0, $\Delta = 0$. Hence, to test Hardy-Weinberg proportions, we can test $H_0 : \Delta = 0$. A test statistic can be constructed based on $\widehat{\Delta}$, given by

$$\widehat{\Delta} = \widehat{\Pr}(BB) - \{\widehat{\Pr}(BB) + \widehat{\Pr}(AB)/2\}^2 = \frac{n_2}{n} - \left(\frac{2n_2 + n_1}{2n}\right)^2.$$

Denote the mean and variance of $\widehat{\Delta}$ by $\mu = E(\widehat{\Delta})$ and $\sigma^2 = \text{Var}(\widehat{\Delta})$, where, ignoring terms with orders higher than $1/n$,

$$\mu = \Delta - \{p - 2p^2 + \Pr(BB)\}/(2n),$$
$$\sigma^2 = \{p^2(1 - p)^2 + (1 - 2p)^2\Delta - \Delta^2\}/n.$$

Under $H_0 : \Delta = 0$, after ignoring the terms with order $1/n$ in μ,

$$\mu = 0 \quad \text{and} \quad \sigma^2 = \frac{1}{n}p^2(1 - p)^2.$$

Hence, asymptotically,

$$\sqrt{n}\widehat{\Delta} \sim N(0, p^2(1 - p)^2) \quad \text{under } H_0,$$

which leads to an asymptotic chi-squared test

$$\chi^2 = \frac{n\widehat{\Delta}^2}{\widehat{p}^2(1 - \widehat{p})^2} \sim \chi_1^2, \tag{2.11}$$

where $\widehat{p} = n_2/n + n_1/(2n)$ is same as in (2.10).

Using data on the MN blood groups in a British population, $n = 1000$ with $n_0 = 298$, $n_1 = 489$ and $n_2 = 213$, the estimate of p is $\widehat{p} = (2 \times 213 + 489)/(2000) = 0.4575$, and the estimate of Δ is $\widehat{\Delta} = 213/1000 - \widehat{p}^2 = 0.003694$. From (2.11),

$$\chi^2 = \frac{1000 \times 0.003694^2}{0.4575^2(1 - 0.4575)^2} \approx 0.22152.$$

If we use (2.10), the estimates of the expected genotype counts corresponding to (n_0, n_1, n_2) are (294.306, 496.388, 209.306). Hence,

$$\chi^2 = \frac{(298 - 294.306)^2}{294.306} + \frac{(489 - 496.388)^2}{496.388} + \frac{(213 - 209.306)^2}{209.306} \approx 0.22152,$$

which is identical to the previous chi-squared statistic (Problem 2.5). The p-value for $\chi^2 = 0.222$ is 0.67, so there is no strong evidence to indicate deviation from Hardy-Weinberg proportions.

Likelihood Ratio Test

The LRT can be used to test Hardy-Weinberg proportions. The genotype counts (n_0, n_1, n_2) follow the multinomial distribution $Mul(n; p_0, p_1, p_2)$, where $p_i = \Pr(G_i)$ for $i = 0, 1, 2$. Then the likelihood function can be written as

$$L(p_0, p_1, p_2) = \frac{n!}{n_0! n_2! n_2!} p_0^{n_0} p_1^{n_1} p_2^{n_2}.$$

The MLE for p_i is $\widehat{p}_i = n_i / n$. Thus, the maximum of the likelihood function is

$$L(\widehat{p}_0, \widehat{p}_1, \widehat{p}_2) = \frac{n!}{n_0! n_2! n_2!} \frac{n_0^{n_0} n_1^{n_1} n_2^{n_2}}{n^n}.$$

Under the null hypothesis H_0, the likelihood function is

$$L_0(p, q) = \frac{n!}{n_0! n_2! n_2!} 2^{n_1} p^{n_1 + 2n_2} q^{n_1 + 2n_0}.$$

The MLEs are $\widehat{p} = (2n_2 + n_1)/(2n)$ and $\widehat{q} = (2n_0 + n_1)/(2n)$. Thus,

$$L_0(\widehat{p}, \widehat{q}) = \frac{n!}{n_0! n_2! n_2!} \frac{2^{n_1} (n_1 + 2n_2)^{n_1 + 2n_2} (n_1 + 2n_0)^{n_1 + 2n_0}}{(2n)^{2n}}.$$

Hence, the LRT can be written as

$$\text{LRT} = 2 \log \frac{L(\widehat{p}_0, \widehat{p}_1, \widehat{p}_2)}{L_0(\widehat{p}, \widehat{q})}$$

$$= 2 \log \frac{(2n)^{2n} n_0^{n_0} n_1^{n_1} n_2^{n_2}}{2^{n_1} n^n (n + 1 + 2n_2)^{n_1 + 2n_2} (n_1 + 2n_0)^{n_1 + 2n_0}} \sim \chi_1^2 \quad \text{under } H_0.$$

Applying the LRT to the above data, we obtain

$$\text{LRT} = 2 \sum_{i=0}^{2} n_i \log n_i + 4n \log(2n) - 2n \log n - 2n_1 \log 2$$

$$-2(n_1 + 2n_2) \log(n_1 + 2n_2) - 2(n_1 + 2n_0) \log(n_1 + 2n_2) \approx 0.22147,$$

which is essentially the same p-value as we obtained before.

The asymptotic test given in (2.10) can be easily modified for testing Hardy-Weinberg proportions for a multiallelic locus. Suppose the following genotype counts are observed for $m(m - 1)/2$ genotypes with m alleles:

$$\{n_{ij} : i, j = 1, \dots, m, \ i \le j\}.$$

Let $n = \sum_{i \le j} n_{ij}$ and $\widehat{p}_j = (2n_{jj} + \sum_{i<j} n_{ij} + \sum_{k>j} n_{jk})/(2n)$. Then

$$\chi^2 = \sum_{j=1}^{m} \frac{(n_{jj} - n\widehat{p}_j^2)^2}{n\widehat{p}_j^2} + \sum_{j=1}^{m} \sum_{i<j} \frac{(n_{ij} - 2n\widehat{p}_i \widehat{p}_j)^2}{2n\widehat{p}_i \widehat{p}_j} + \sum_{j=1}^{m} \sum_{k>j} \frac{(n_{jk} - 2n\widehat{p}_k \widehat{p}_j)^2}{2n\widehat{p}_k \widehat{p}_j}.$$

Under H_0, $\chi^2 \sim \chi^2_{m(m-1)/2}$. However, a more powerful test, based on χ^2_1, is obtained by modeling the genotype frequencies as

$$\Pr(A_i A_j) = 2(1 - F) p_i p_j \quad \text{for } i \neq j,$$

$$\Pr(A_i A_i) = (1 - F) p_i^2 + F p_i,$$

and testing the null hypothesis $H_0 : F = 0$, where F is Wright's inbreeding coefficient.

Exact Test

The performance of asymptotic chi-squared tests depends on approximations of the distributions of test statistics under H_0. Because the genotype counts are discrete data, the approximations are not always accurate. In this case, an exact test may be preferred. Note that HWE is a model for calculating genotype frequencies using allele frequencies. Therefore, the exact test for Hardy-Weinberg proportions is based on the probability distribution of all possible genotype counts under HWE conditional on the observed allele counts.

Let (n_0, n_1, n_2) be the genotype counts for (AA, AB, BB) and (n_A, n_B) be the allele counts for (A, B). Then $n_A = 2n_0 + n_1$, $n_B = 2n_2 + n_1$, and $n_A + n_B = 2n$. The genotype counts follow the multinomial distribution: $(n_0, n_1, n_2) \sim Mul(n; q^2, 2pq, p^2)$ under HWE, where $p = \Pr(B)$, i.e.,

$$\Pr(n_0, n_1, n_2) = \frac{n!}{n_0! n_1! n_2!} (q^2)^{n_0} (2pq)^{n_1} (p^2)^{n_2} = \frac{n!}{n_0! n_1! n_2!} 2^{n_1} p^{n_B} q^{n_A}.$$

The allele counts (n_A, n_B) have the binomial distribution given by

$$\Pr(n_A, n_B) = \frac{(2n)!}{n_A! n_B!} p^{n_B} q^{n_A}.$$

Since the allele counts are determined by the genotype counts, we have

$$\Pr(n_0, n_1, n_2, n_A, n_B) = \Pr(n_0, n_1, n_2).$$

Hence,

$$\Pr(n_0, n_1, n_2 | n_A, n_B) = \frac{\Pr(n_0, n_1, n_2)}{\Pr(n_A, n_B)} = \frac{n! n_A! n_B! 2^{n_1}}{n_0! n_1! n_2! (2n)!}. \tag{2.12}$$

Substituting $n_A = 2n - n_B$, $n_0 = (n_A - n_1)/2 = n - (n_B + n_1)/2$ and $n_2 = (n_B - n_1)/2$ into (2.12), we obtain

$$\Pr(n_1 | n_B) = \frac{n! (2n - n_B)! n_B! 2^{n_1}}{[n - (n_B + n_1)/2]! n_1! [(n_B - n_1)/2]! (2n)!}, \tag{2.13}$$

which only depends on n_1 given n_B and n (n_A is determined by n_B and n).

Table 2.6 Conditional probabilities of n_1 given $n_B = 8$ and $n = 30$

n_1	$n - \frac{n_B + n_1}{2}$	$\frac{n_B - n_1}{2}$	$\Pr(n_1 \mid n_B)$
0	26	4	0.000011
2	25	3	0.0022
4	24	2	0.0557
6	23	1	0.3565
8	22	0	0.5856

Choose all valid values of n_1 given n_B and n, including the observed number with genotype AB. The valid value of n_1 has to be bounded by $0 \le n_1 \le \min(n_B, 2n - n_B)$, and $(n_B - n_1)/2$ is an integer. This implies that n_1 is even (odd) if n_B is. Calculate the probability in (2.13) for each valid n_1. The exact p-value is the sum of probabilities with valid n_1 smaller than or equal to the observed number with genotype AB. In practice, to apply (2.13), the allele with smaller allele count is denoted by B and its corresponding allele count by n_1, which will reduce the computation burden of (2.13).

Applying the exact test for Hardy-Weinberg proportions to the genotype counts $(n_0, n_1, n_2) = (24, 4, 2)$ with $n = 30$, the allele counts are $(n_A, n_B) = (52, 8)$. Note that $n_B < n_A$ and n_B is even. Hence, the only valid values for n_1 are 0, 2, 4, 6 and 8. The corresponding probabilities of (2.13) are reported in Table 2.6. Then the sum of probabilities that are smaller than or equal to 4 is the exact p-value. Using Table 2.6, we have $p = 0.000011 + 0.0022 + 0.0557 = 0.0579$, not significant at the 5% level.

Test Hardy-Weinberg Proportions for the X Chromosome

If the allele frequency in males is identical to that in females, Hardy-Weinberg proportions can be tested among females using χ^2 as given in (2.10) or (2.11) and the exact test. The male allele frequency may not be equal to that of females owing to many reasons, including genotyping errors. Therefore one may also test whether or not the male allele frequency is equal to that of females.

Let $p_m = \Pr(B \mid \text{male})$ and $p_f = \Pr(B \mid \text{female})$. Let (n_0^f, n_1^f, n_2^f) be the genotype counts in females and (n_A^m, n_B^m) be the allele counts in males. Let Δ_f be the HWD coefficient for females. The null hypothesis consists of $H_{0a} : p_M = p_F$ and $H_{0b} : \Delta_f = 0$, i.e., Hardy-Weinberg proportions hold in females. Let $n^m = n_A^m + n_B^m$ and $n^f = n_0^f + n_1^f + n_2^f$. Using the data, estimates of p_m and p_f are given by $\widehat{p}_m = n_B^m / n^m$ and $\widehat{p}_f = (2n_2^f + n_1^f)/(2n^f)$. Note that $\mathrm{Var}(\widehat{p}_m) = p_m(1 - p_m)/n^m$ and $\mathrm{Var}(\widehat{p}_f) = p_f(1 - p_f)/(2n^f)$, which can be estimated by $\widehat{\mathrm{Var}}(\widehat{p}_m) = \widehat{p}_m(1 - \widehat{p}_m)/n^m$ and $\widehat{\mathrm{Var}}(\widehat{p}_f) = \widehat{p}_f(1 - \widehat{p}_f)/(2n^f)$. A test statistic for H_{0a} can be written as

$$Z = \frac{\widehat{p}_m - \widehat{p}_f}{\sqrt{\widehat{\mathrm{Var}}(\widehat{p}_m) + \widehat{\mathrm{Var}}(\widehat{p}_f)}} \sim N(0, 1) \quad \text{under } H_{0a}.$$

In Problem 2.6, it is shown that Z and χ^2 are asymptotically uncorrelated under H_{0a} and H_{0b}. Thus, each test can be applied at the $\alpha/2$ level to control for multiple testing.

2.3.3 Impact of Hardy-Weinberg Equilibrium or Disequilibrium

In population genetics, HWE is used as a reference model to compare with other models. It is built on many assumptions which may not hold true. On the other hand, for genetic association studies, testing Hardy-Weinberg proportions has been used as a tool to detect genotyping errors. In research articles, p-values from testing Hardy-Weinberg proportions are often reported together with p-values of the association tests. Others, however, argue that a typical chi-squared test is not sensitive to departure from Hardy-Weinberg proportions (see Bibliographical Comments in Sect. 2.7). Hence the power to detect genotyping errors is low. Random mating is a necessary condition for HWE, which is also a requirement for applying the allele-based association test (Chap. 3). But failure to reject the null hypothesis that Hardy-Weinberg proportions hold does not mean the null hypothesis is true. Deviation from Hardy-Weinberg proportions in case-control data may also imply inbreeding or population stratification.

Testing Hardy-Weinberg proportions is based on samples drawn from the population. When case-control data are used, testing Hardy-Weinberg proportions is usually based on controls when studying a rare disease, because then the population and control genotypic distributions are similar. On the other hand, deviation from Hardy-Weinberg proportions in cases may indicate association when it holds in the population (or, for a rare disease, controls). Association tests incorporating HWD have been proposed to improve efficiency and power to detect true associations.

When Hardy-Weinberg proportions do not hold, the inbreeding coefficient, F, has been used above. Using F, given the allele frequencies, the genotype frequencies can be written as

$$g_0 = q^2 + pqF, \qquad g_1 = 2pq(1-F), \qquad g_2 = p^2 + pqF.$$

Hence, Hardy-Weinberg proportions hold if and only if $F = 0$.

2.4 Population Substructure

The case-control design for genetic association studies may be affected by population substructure. Two types of substructure are considered in the literature. One is population stratification (PS) and the other is cryptic relatedness (CR). Case-control samples may be affected by PS or CR or both. We given brief introductions to PS and CR in this section. More details and corrections for these two substructures will be deferred to Chap. 9.

2.4.1 Population Stratification

Population stratification often refers to the situation that the allele (or genotype) frequency of the marker changes across the subpopulations. However, when testing association between a marker and a disease, the hidden PS influences the test result only if the following two conditions are both satisfied:

I. *The allele (or genotype) frequency of the marker varies across the subpopulations,*
II. *The disease prevalence varies across the subpopulations.*

Suppose there are two subpopulations, denoted by Z_1 and Z_2, with allele frequencies of a marker of interest $P_j = \Pr(B|Z_j)$ for $j = 1, 2$. In each subpopulation, penetrances are all equal to the disease prevalence $f_{0j} = f_{1j} = f_{2j} = k_j = \Pr(\text{case} \,|Z_j)$, $j = 1, 2$. Hence, there is no association between the marker and the disease in each subpopulation.

Suppose the subpopulations are known so that r_j cases and s_j controls can be drawn from the jth subpopulation. One example is that the subpopulations are defined by geographical regions or ethnicities. The total numbers of cases and controls are $r = r_1 + r_2$ and $s = s_1 + s_2$, respectively. Denote the estimates of allele frequencies using cases and controls from the jth subpopulation by $\widehat{p}_{1j} = n_{Aj}/r_j$ and $\widehat{p}_{0j} = m_{Aj}/s_j$, respectively, where n_{Aj} and m_{Aj} are the numbers of A alleles among cases and controls in the jth subpopulation. Then,

$$\mathrm{E}(\widehat{p}_{1j}) = \mathrm{E}(\widehat{p}_{0j}) = p_j, \quad j = 1, 2.$$

That is, the estimates using cases and controls have the same expectation in each subpopulation. When cases and controls from the two subpopulations are pooled (ignoring the existence of subpopulations), we have r cases and s controls. We estimate allele frequency from the r cases, denoted by $\widehat{p}_1 = (n_{A1} + n_{A2})/r$, and from the s controls, denoted by $\widehat{p}_0 = (m_{A1} + m_{A2})/s$. Their expectations, conditional on $\{r_i, s_i; i = 1, 2\}$, are given by

$$\mathrm{E}(\widehat{p}_1) = (r_1 p_1 + r_2 p_2)/r,$$
$$\mathrm{E}(\widehat{p}_0) = (s_1 p_1 + s_2 p_2)/s.$$

If $\mathrm{E}(\widehat{p}_1) \neq \mathrm{E}(\widehat{p}_0)$, then there is association between the disease and the marker at the total population level, even though there is no association in each subpopulation. This is spurious association caused by PS, which is ignored in the above calculations.

A sufficient condition for $\mathrm{E}(\widehat{p}_1) = \mathrm{E}(\widehat{p}_0)$ is $s_j = mr_j$ for all j, where m does not change with j. This condition is satisfied under the matched case-control design (Chap. 4). When $m = 1$, the design is called a matched-pair design, in which equal numbers of cases and controls are drawn from each subpopulation. Another sufficient condition for $\mathrm{E}(\widehat{p}_1) = \mathrm{E}(\widehat{p}_0)$ is $p_1 = p_2$, i.e., the allele frequency does not change across the subpopulations.

To take account of the known subpopulations, stratified estimates should be used, which are given by

$$\widehat{p}_1 = \sum_{j=1}^{2} w_j \frac{n_{Aj}}{r_j}, \qquad \widehat{p}_0 = \sum_{j=1}^{2} w_j \frac{m_{Aj}}{s_j},$$

with weights $w_j = (r_j + s_j)/\sum_j (r_j + s_j)$, proportional to the size of the jth subpopulation. It follows that

$$\mathrm{E}(\widehat{p}_1) = \mathrm{E}(\widehat{p}_0) = \sum_j w_j p_j.$$

For PS to have an effect, it is necessary that the disease prevalence k_j varies across the subpopulations. The disease prevalence is not used in the above arguments because the subpopulations are known, so that cases and controls can be drawn separately from each subpopulation and then pooled. In practice, PS is latent (i.e., the subpopulations are not known), and definitions of subpopulations by geographical regions are not perfect (see discussion in Chap. 9). In this case, suppose r cases and s controls are drawn from the case population and control population, respectively. Then r_j cases (s_j controls) belong to the jth subpopulation for $j = 1, 2$, which are random and unknown. Note that

$$\mathrm{E}(r_j/r) = \mathrm{Pr}(Z_j \mid \mathrm{case}) = \frac{\mathrm{Pr}(Z_j)k_j}{\mathrm{Pr}(\mathrm{case})},$$

$$\mathrm{E}(s_j/s) = \mathrm{Pr}(Z_j \mid \mathrm{control}) = \frac{\mathrm{Pr}(Z_j)(1 - k_j)}{1 - \mathrm{Pr}(\mathrm{case})}.$$

If $k_1 = k_2$, there is no change in disease prevalence across the subpopulations, and $k_1 = k_2 = \mathrm{Pr}(\mathrm{case})$. Hence, $\mathrm{E}(r_j/r) = \mathrm{E}(s_j/s)$, equivalent to a matched case-control design. Under this sampling design,

$$\mathrm{E}(\widehat{p}_1) = \mathrm{E}\{\mathrm{E}(\widehat{p}_1 \mid r_1, r_2)\} = \mathrm{E}(r_1/r)p_1 + \mathrm{E}(r_2/r)p_2,$$

$$\mathrm{E}(\widehat{p}_0) = \mathrm{E}\{\mathrm{E}(\widehat{p}_0 \mid s_1, s_2)\} = \mathrm{E}(s_1/s)p_1 + \mathrm{E}(s_2/s)p_2.$$

Hence $\mathrm{E}(\widehat{p}_1) = \mathrm{E}(\widehat{p}_0)$ if either $k_1 = k_2$ or $p_1 = p_2$.

2.4.2 Cryptic Relatedness

A simple model for cryptic relatedness in a population is that HWE does not hold due to unknown relatedness among individuals in the population. For this simple CR model, we assume the population does not contain subpopulations with varying allele frequencies. However, HWE does not hold because of unknown relatedness among individuals. This CR model is also studied in Chap. 9. In Sect. 2.4.1, we considered the bias of estimates of allele frequencies using cases and controls in the presence of PS. The variance of the estimates would be affected in the presence of CR, which will be also discussed in Chap. 9.

One can also consider a more general model of CR with several subpopulations. In each subpopulation, HWE does not hold, but individuals across the subpopulations are not genetically related. In this generalized model, how the allele frequencies and disease prevalences change across the subpopulations is not specified. If, in addition to relatedness among individuals in each subpopulation, the allele frequencies and disease prevalences also change across the subpopulations, then the PS and CR can be studied simultaneously.

2.5 Odds Ratio and Relative Risk

2.5.1 Odds Ratios

Definitions

The odds ratio (OR) is commonly used to measure association in epidemiology. For a prospective case-control study, the odds of being a case versus a control for a given risk factor $R = E+$ (exposed) or $R = E-$ (not exposed) is defined as

$$\frac{\Pr(d = 1|R)}{\Pr(d = 0|R)}, \tag{2.14}$$

where $d = 1$ is for a case and $d = 0$ is for a control. The OR with respect to two levels of R is defined as

$$\mathrm{OR}_{d=1:d=0} = \frac{\Pr(d = 1|E+)}{\Pr(d = 0|E+)} \Big/ \frac{\Pr(d = 1|E-)}{\Pr(d = 0|E-)}.$$

For a retrospective case-control study, the odds of being $E+$ versus being $E-$ in cases ($d = 1$) or controls ($d = 0$) is defined as

$$\frac{\Pr(E + |d)}{\Pr(E - |d)}. \tag{2.15}$$

The OR with respect to case and control groups is

$$\mathrm{OR}_{R=E+:R=E-} = \frac{\Pr(E + |d = 1)}{\Pr(E - |d = 1)} \Big/ \frac{\Pr(E + |d = 0)}{\Pr(E - |d = 0)}.$$

It can be shown that

$$\frac{\Pr(E + |d = 1)\Pr(E - |d = 0)}{\Pr(E - |d = 1)\Pr(E + |d = 0)} = \frac{\Pr(d = 1|E+)\Pr(d = 0|E-)}{\Pr(d = 1|E-)\Pr(d = 0|E+)}.$$

Thus, the ORs for the retrospective and prospective case-control studies are identical. This property, along with its close relation with relative risk as mentioned below, makes the OR a widely used measure of association in epidemiology.

Table 2.7 A 2 × 2 table with case and control status and levels of a risk factor for n subjects

	$E+$	$E-$	
Case	a	b	$a+b$
Control	c	d	$c+d$
	$a+c$	$b+d$	n

Inference

For a general 2 × 2 table as given in Table 2.7, the estimate of the OR is given by

$$\widehat{\text{OR}} = \frac{ad}{bc}, \quad \text{or} \quad \log \widehat{\text{OR}} = \log\left(\frac{ad}{bc}\right).$$

Note that if any entry in Table 2.7 is 0, a constant $1/2$ is often added to each cell in the table. When there is no association in the 2 × 2 table, $\widehat{\text{OR}} \approx 1$. If the exposure to the risk factor ($E+$) increases the risk of having the disease, $\widehat{\text{OR}} > 1$.

A consistent estimate of the variance of the log OR can be written as (Problem 2.7)

$$\widehat{\text{Var}}(\log \widehat{\text{OR}}) = \frac{1}{a} + \frac{1}{b} + \frac{1}{c} + \frac{1}{d}, \tag{2.16}$$

which is referred to as Woolf's estimate of the variance of the log OR. The confidence interval for the log OR can be obtained from

$$\frac{\log \widehat{\text{OR}} - \log \text{OR}}{\sqrt{\widehat{\text{Var}}(\log \widehat{\text{OR}})}} \to N(0, 1). \tag{2.17}$$

That is, $\log \widehat{\text{OR}} \pm z_{1-\alpha/2}\sqrt{\widehat{\text{Var}}(\log \text{OR})}$. Denote $z = z_{1-\alpha/2}\sqrt{\widehat{\text{Var}}(\log \text{OR})}$. Then, the $100(1 - \alpha)\%$ confidence interval for the OR is $(\widehat{\text{OR}}/e^z, \widehat{\text{OR}}e^z)$. Under the null hypothesis of no association H_0, $\log \text{OR} = 0$. Thus, after substituting $\log \text{OR} = 0$, the left hand side of (2.17) can be used as a test statistic for association.

Odds Ratios for Genetic Associations

For a diallelic marker with alleles A and B, and three genotypes $(G_0, G_1, G_2) = (AA, AB, BB)$, case-control data can be displayed in a 2 × 3 table. For Table 2.8, two ORs can be used to measure association. One is between AB and AA, denoted as OR_1. The other is between BB and AA, denoted as OR_2. In both ORs, genotype $G_0 = AA$ is used as the reference.

The formulas for the estimates of the two log ORs and their asymptotic variances are given by

$$\log \widehat{\text{OR}}_1 = \log\left(\frac{r_1 s_0}{r_0 s_1}\right), \quad \widehat{\text{Var}}(\log \widehat{\text{OR}}_1) = \frac{1}{r_0} + \frac{1}{r_1} + \frac{1}{s_0} + \frac{1}{s_1}, \tag{2.18}$$

Table 2.8 A 2×3 table with case and control status and three genotypes

	AA	AB	BB
Case	r_0	r_1	r_2
Control	s_0	s_1	s_2

$$\log \widehat{OR}_2 = \log\left(\frac{r_2 s_0}{r_0 s_2}\right), \qquad \widehat{Var}(\log \widehat{OR}_2) = \frac{1}{r_0} + \frac{1}{r_2} + \frac{1}{s_0} + \frac{1}{s_2}. \qquad (2.19)$$

The estimates $\log \widehat{OR}_1$ and $\log \widehat{OR}_2$ are negatively correlated with covariance (Problem 2.8)

$$\widehat{Cov}(\log \widehat{OR}_1, \log \widehat{OR}_2) = -\frac{1}{r_0} - \frac{1}{s_0}. \qquad (2.20)$$

If one is interested in the OR between AA versus genotypes with at least one allele B (i.e., AB and BB), the estimate of the log OR can be written as

$$\log \widehat{OR} = \log\left(\frac{s_0(r_1 + r_2)}{r_0(s_1 + s_2)}\right),$$

with an estimated asymptotic variance

$$\widehat{Var}(\log \widehat{OR}) = \frac{1}{r_0} + \frac{1}{r_1 + r_2} + \frac{1}{s_0} + \frac{1}{s_1 + s_2}.$$

On the other hand, to calculate the OR between BB versus genotypes with at least one allele A (i.e., AA and AB), one has

$$\log \widehat{OR} = \log\left(\frac{r_2(s_0 + s_1)}{s_2(r_0 + r_1)}\right),$$

$$\widehat{Var}(\log \widehat{OR}) = \frac{1}{r_0 + r_1} + \frac{1}{r_2} + \frac{1}{s_0 + s_1} + \frac{1}{s_2}.$$

As before, infinite estimates and variances can be avoided by adding $1/2$ to each cell in Table 2.8.

2.5.2 Relative Risks

Definition and Relation with Odds Ratio

Define $f_1 = \Pr(d = 1 | E+)$ and $f_0 = \Pr(d = 1 | E-)$. Then the relative risk (RR) of the disease on being exposed versus not being exposed is

$$RR = \frac{f_1}{f_0}.$$

If the data in Table 2.7 are collected in a prospective case-control design, the estimate of the RR is given by

$$\widehat{RR} = \frac{\widehat{f_1}}{\widehat{f_0}} = \frac{a(b+d)}{b(a+c)},$$

where $\widehat{f_0} = b/(b+d)$ and $\widehat{f_1} = a/(a+c)$. To obtain the asymptotic variance of $\widehat{RR}$, it is easier to work with the log RR. Note that, in a prospective study, $\widehat{f_0}$ and $\widehat{f_1}$ are independent. Thus, $\mathrm{Var}\{\log(\widehat{f_1}/\widehat{f_0})\} = \mathrm{Var}(\log \widehat{f_1}) + \mathrm{Var}(\log \widehat{f_0})$. Denote $n_0 = b+d$ and $n_1 = a+c$. Then both a and b follow binomial distributions, $a \sim B(n_1; f_1)$ and $b \sim B(n_0; f_0)$. Thus, by the Delta method,

$$\mathrm{Var}(\log \widehat{f_i}) \approx \frac{1}{f_i^2} \frac{f_i(1 - f_i)}{n_i} = \frac{1 - f_i}{f_i n_i}.$$

Hence,

$$\widehat{\mathrm{Var}}\left\{\log\left(\frac{\widehat{f_1}}{\widehat{f_0}}\right)\right\} = \frac{c}{a(a+c)} + \frac{d}{b(b+d)}.$$

From the expression for the OR, we have

$$OR_{d=1:d=0} = OR_{R=E+:R=E-} = \frac{f_1(1 - f_0)}{f_0(1 - f_1)} = \frac{f_1}{f_0}\left(1 + \frac{f_1 - f_0}{1 - f_1}\right).$$

Thus, for a rare disease ($f_1 - f_0 \approx 0$ and $f_1 \approx 0$),

$$OR_{d=1:d=0} = OR_{R=E+:R=E-} \approx RR.$$

Genotype Relative Risks

For the data presented in Table 2.8, two GRRs can be defined,

$$GRR_1 = \Pr(d = 1|AB)/\Pr(d = 1|AA),$$

$$GRR_2 = \Pr(d = 1|BB)/\Pr(d = 1|AA).$$

When there is no association between the case-control status and the marker, $GRR_1 = GRR_2 = 1$. In general, unbiased estimates for GRRs are not available using retrospective case-control data.

2.6 Logistic Regression for Case-Control Studies

2.6.1 Prospective Case-Control Design

Likelihood Function

A logistic regression model is often used for the analysis of prospective case-control data. Let $d = 1$ denote a case and $d = 0$ a control. Denote $\mathbf{X} = (X_1, \ldots, X_p)^T$ a vector of covariates and $H(\mathbf{X}) = (h_1(\mathbf{X}), \ldots, h_p(\mathbf{X}))^T$, where h_i is a coding function or transformation of covariates. Then using logistic regression, one has

$$P(\mathbf{x}) = \Pr(d = 1 | \mathbf{X} = \mathbf{x}) = \frac{\exp\{\beta_0 + \beta_1^T H(\mathbf{x})\}}{1 + \exp\{\beta_0 + \beta_1^T H(\mathbf{x})\}}$$

and $\Pr(d = 0 | \mathbf{X} = \mathbf{x}) = 1 - \Pr(d = 1 | \mathbf{X} = \mathbf{x})$. The prospective likelihood function can be written as

$$
\begin{aligned}
L_{\mathrm{pros}}(\beta_0, \beta_1) &= \prod_{j=1}^{n} \{p(\mathbf{x_j})\}^{d_j} \{1 - p(\mathbf{x_j})\}^{1 - d_j} \\
&= \prod_{j=1}^{n} \frac{\exp\{\beta_0 d_j + \beta_1^T H(\mathbf{x_j}) d_j\}}{1 + \exp\{\beta_0 + \beta_1^T H(\mathbf{x})\}}.
\end{aligned}
\tag{2.21}
$$

Inference for β_1 can be made using (2.21).

Examples

For the first example, consider a single binary covariate in the logistic regression model. Hence, $H(\mathbf{X}) = H(X) = 0$ for not exposed ($E-$) and 1 for exposed ($E+$). For the second example, consider a single genetic marker G as a covariate. Denote the three genotypes as $(G_0, G_1, G_2) = (AA, AB, BB)$. There are several ways to code (or score) the genotype G. For examples, a two-dimensional scoring function is $H(G) = (h_1(G), h_2(G))^T$, where $h_1(G) = 0, 0, 1$ and $h_2(G) = 0, 1, 1$ if $G = G_0, G_1, G_2$, respectively, and a one-dimensional scoring function is $H(G) = i$ if $G = G_i$ for $i = 0, 1, 2$.

2.6.2 Retrospective Case-Control Design

The retrospective case-control design differs from the prospective case-control design. The data in the retrospective design are not drawn from the general population. They are sampled from a population with selected samples ($S = 1$) of cases and controls. The proportion of cases in the selected population is often different from the disease prevalence in the general population. In fact, this is an important difference between the retrospective and prospective designs.

In a retrospective case-control study, the covariates $\mathbf{X}$ of a case $d = 1$ or a control $d = 0$ in the selected population $S = 1$ are obtained. Thus, the likelihood of observing $\mathbf{X} = \mathbf{x}$ is

$$\Pr(\mathbf{X} = \mathbf{x}|d, S = 1),$$

where $d = 0$ or 1. The likelihood function can be written as

$$L_{\text{retro}}(\beta_0, \beta_1) = \prod_{j=1}^{n} \{\Pr(\mathbf{X_j} = \mathbf{x_j}|d_j = 1, S_j = 1)\}^{d_j}$$

$$\times \{1 - \Pr(\mathbf{X_j} = \mathbf{x_j}|d_j = 0, S_j = 1)\}^{1-d_j}. \tag{2.22}$$

Denote $\widetilde{p}(\mathbf{x_j}) = \Pr(d_j = 1|S_j = 1, \mathbf{X_j} = \mathbf{x_j})$ and $\pi_i = \Pr(S_j = 1|d_j = i, \mathbf{X_j} = \mathbf{x_j})$, $i = 0, 1$. Then it can be shown that

$$\text{logit}\,\widetilde{p}(\mathbf{x_j}) = \frac{\widetilde{p}(\mathbf{x_j})}{1 - \widetilde{p}(\mathbf{x_j})} = \frac{\pi_1}{\pi_0} \frac{p(\mathbf{x_j})}{1 - p(\mathbf{x_j})} = \exp\{\widetilde{\beta}_0 + \beta_1^T H(\mathbf{x_j})\},$$

where $\widetilde{\beta}_0 = \beta_0 + \log(\pi_1/\pi_0)$. Thus, the odds of observing $\mathbf{x}$ in the selected case-control samples is proportional to the odds of observing $\mathbf{x}$ in the population. Therefore, the OR in the selected population equals that in the population. The proportion

$$\pi_1/\pi_0 = \frac{\Pr(d_j = 1|S_j = 1, \mathbf{x_j})}{\Pr(d_j = 0|S_j = 1, \mathbf{x_j})} \bigg/ \frac{\Pr(d_j = 1|\mathbf{x_j})}{\Pr(d_j = 0|\mathbf{x_j})}$$

is the ratio of probabilities of cases to controls in the selected samples with respect to that in the population.

The likelihood (2.22) can be further written as

$$L_{\text{retro}}(\beta_0, \beta_1) = \prod_{j=1}^{n} \{\widetilde{p}(\mathbf{x_j})\}^{d_i} \{1 - \widetilde{p}(\mathbf{x_j})\}^{1-d_i} \tag{2.23}$$

$$\times \prod_{j=1}^{n} \left\{ \frac{\Pr(\mathbf{x_j}|S_j = 1)}{\Pr(d_j = 1|S_j = 1)} \right\}^{d_j} \left\{ \frac{\Pr(\mathbf{x_j}|S_j = 1)}{\Pr(d_j = 0|S_j = 1)} \right\}^{1-d_j}.$$

$$\tag{2.24}$$

If (2.24) does not depend on the coefficient β_1 which appears in (2.23), then (2.23) can be used for the analysis of the retrospective data. Thus, the prospective likelihood function L_{pros} can be used for the retrospective case-control data for inference of β_1.

2.7 Bibliographical Comments

This book focuses on the analysis of genetic case-control association studies. Therefore, only the background in population genetics needed for case-control association studies is introduced in this chapter. More about population genetics can be found in other textbooks or Refs. [49, 71], and [117]. In Chap. 13, we will discuss linkage and association studies using family data. Some background related to the analysis of family data will be given there. Basic statistical methods for testing association and other genetic studies, including linkage analysis and family-based association studies, can be found in [12, 165, 240, 245], and [299]. Elston et al. [74] reviewed multi-stage sampling for various genetic studies, including family and/or case-control data. The TDT was proposed by Spielman et al. [255]. For the GWAS design with 3,000 common controls shared with seven different diseases, refer to the WTCCC [301].

The Hardy-Weinberg principle was independently introduced by Hardy [115] and Weinberg [297] in 1908. A triangle diagram for Hardy-Weinberg proportions was given by Edwards [67]. Testing Hardy-Weinberg proportions and interpretation of deviation from Hardy-Weinberg proportions can be found in Weir [299] and Sham [240]. The example used to test Hardy-Weinberg proportions in Sect. 2.3.2 comes from Hartl and Clark [117]. Comparison of various asymptotic tests for Hardy-Weinberg proportions can be found in Emigh [76]. The exact test for Hardy-Weinberg proportions was first proposed by Haldane [112]. Guo and Thompson [109] studied exact tests for Hardy-Weinberg proportions for multiallelic loci. A definition of HWE on the X chromosome and its properties were given in Li [165]. Testing Hardy-Weinberg proportions on the X chromosome was studied by Zheng et al. [339]. Nielsen et al. [193] and Song and Elston [251] studied the departure from Hardy-Weinberg proportions in cases and/or case-control association studies. Li [164] showed that one can have Hardy-Weinberg proportions and yet the population is not in equilibrium.

The concept of LD between two loci and the use of D' can be found in Lewontin [162] and Weir [299]. The formulas (2.2) to (2.4) are studied by Zheng et al. [340]. Similar formulas were also given in Nielsen and Weir [195]. Lewontin did not mean his coefficient D' to refer solely to linked loci (personal communication) but rather to any two loci, and hence intended D' to be the more general measure of genetic phase disequilibrium. See also discussion of this in Wang et al. [293].

Population substructure is an important issue for genetic case-control association studies [66, 283]. The definition of PS can be also found in Crow and Kimura [49] (p. 54) and Elandt-Johnson [71] (p. 228). The simple definition of CR was given by Voight and Pritchard [282]. The more general definition of CR given in Sect. 2.4.2 was used by Crow and Kimura [49] (p. 64), Elandt-Johnson [71] (p. 213), Devlin and Roeder [60], and Whittemore [302]. Recent discussions can be found in Astle and Balding [10] and Zheng et al. [341].

Measures of risks and their inference can be found in many epidemiological or biostatistics textbooks, e.g., Fleiss et al. (Chaps. 7, 11 and 13) [86] and Sahai and Khurshid [222]. Using the prospective logistic regression model for the retrospective case-control data was studied by Prentice and Pyke [204]. Their results hold for both the unmatched case-control design discussed here and for the matched case-control design discussed in Chap. 4. The derivation of the likelihood functions for the retrospective data presented here can be found in Sahai and Khurshid [222].

2.8 Problems

2.1 Let F_1, F_2, F_3 and F_4 be defined as in Sect. 2.2.1. Show that $F_1 F_4 = F_2 F_3$ if and only if $D = 0$.

2.2 Using the notation defined in Sect. 2.2.1, show that

$$f_0 = f_0^*(F_1^2 + 2F_1 F_3 \lambda_1^* + F_3^2 \lambda_2^*),$$
$$f_1 = f_0^*(F_1 F_2 + F_1 F_4 \lambda_1^* + F_2 F_3 \lambda_1^* + F_3 F_4 \lambda_2^*),$$
$$f_2 = f_0^*(F_2^2 + 2F_2 F_4 \lambda_1^* + F_4^2 \lambda_2^*).$$

2.3 Using (2.2) to (2.4), show that

$$f_1 - f_0 = \frac{D f_0^*}{p(1-p)}\{F_1(\lambda_1^* - 1) + F_3(\lambda_2^* - \lambda_1^*)\},$$
$$f_2 - f_1 = \frac{D f_0^*}{p(1-p)}\{F_2(\lambda_1^* - 1) + F_4(\lambda_2^* - \lambda_1^*)\}.$$

Further, when $D \neq 0$, $f_0 = f_1 = f_2$ holds if and only of $\lambda_1^* = \lambda_2^* = 1$ holds.

2.4 Using (2.6) and Table 2.4, derive (2.7).

2.5 Show that the chi-squared tests for Hardy-Weinberg proportions in (2.10) and (2.11) are identical.

2.6 Show that, ignoring higher order terms, the test for equal allele frequencies in males and females and the test for Hardy-Weinberg proportions in females are uncorrelated under H_{0a} and H_{0b}.

2.7 Under a prospective case-control design, $a \sim B(a+c;\, f_1)$ and $b \sim B(b+d;\, f_0)$ (binomial distributions). The OR is given by OR $= f_1(1 - f_0)/\{f_0(1 - f_1)\}$. Derive the variance of the estimate of log OR and show its estimate can be written as (2.16).

2.8 Derive the covariance of the estimates of ORs given in (2.18) and (2.19) using multinomial distributions for the genotype counts of cases and controls and the fact that the genotype counts of cases and controls are independent.

Part II
Single-Marker Analysis for Case-Control Data

Chapter 3
Single-Marker Analysis for Unmatched Case-Control Data

Abstract   Chapter 3 begins with an introduction to the notation for penetrance and genotype relative risk. Since many statistical analyses of a case-control association study depend on the underlying genetic model, the genetic models are introduced in terms of genotype relative risks. Test statistics for genetic association covered in this chapter include genotype-based tests (Pearson's chi-squared test, the Cochran-Armitage trend test, and the likelihood-ratio test), the allelic test, exact tests, and the Hardy-Weinberg disequilibrium trend test. Combining the Hardy-Weinberg disequilibrium trend test with the Cochran-Armitage trend test is also discussed. Numerical and analytical comparisons between the allelic and genotype-based tests are given. This chapter also discusses how to obtain the trend test and Pearson's chi-squared test as the Score tests from logistic regression models. Estimates of odds ratios and their confidence intervals are given. Results from simulation studies are presented. Common approaches to simulate case-control data with or without covariates are given. Examples and case studies are presented.

In single-marker analysis, a diallelic marker is genotyped for cases and controls. The cases and controls are retrospectively sampled from the study population. The case-control data can be presented in a contingency table, either in a 2×2 table when alleles are counted or a 2×3 table when genotypes are counted. When the genetic marker is in LD with a disease locus, the association between the genetic marker and the disease can be detected by independence tests of the contingency table data. Single-marker analysis is one of the most important analyses in case-control genetic association studies. It is often the first analysis carried out in GWAS. Other analyses involving multiple markers will be discussed in Chap. 7 (haplotype analysis) and Chap. 8 (gene-gene interaction).

This chapter begins with an introduction of notation for penetrance and GRRs. Since many statistical analyses of a case-control association study depend on the underlying genetic model, we introduce in detail the concept of genetic models in terms of the GRRs. Test statistics covered in this chapter include genotype-based tests (Pearson's chi-squared test, the Cochran-Armitage trend test (CATT) and the LRT), the allelic test, exact tests, and the HWD trend test. Combination of the HWD trend test with the CATT is discussed. Estimates of ORs and their CIs are studied. To evaluate the performance of the various tests, simulation studies are often

G. Zheng et al., *Analysis of Genetic Association Studies*,
Statistics for Biology and Health,
DOI 10.1007/978-1-4614-2245-7_3, © Springer Science+Business Media, LLC 2012

conducted. Simple approaches to simulate case-control data are presented in this chapter. Examples and case studies are presented.

3.1 Penetrance and Genotype Relative Risks

Consider a diallelic marker M, typically a SNP, with alleles A and B. Let the three genotypes of M be $G_0 = AA$, $G_1 = AB$, and $G_2 = BB$. The allele frequencies in the population are denoted by $p = \Pr(B)$ and $q = \Pr(A) = 1 - p$. The genotype frequencies of G_j in the population are denoted by $g_j = \Pr(G_j)$ for $j = 0, 1, 2$, which are given by (Sect. 2.3)

$$g_0 = q^2 + pqF, \quad g_1 = 2pq(1 - F), \quad \text{and} \quad g_2 = p^2 + pqF, \tag{3.1}$$

where F is Wright's coefficient of inbreeding. For humans, F is usually between 0 and 0.05. If Hardy-Weinberg proportions hold in the population, $F = 0$. Then $g_0 = q^2$, $g_1 = 2pq$, and $g_2 = p^2$.

The disease prevalence in the population is denoted by $k = \Pr(\text{case})$. The penetrance of a disease given a genotype is denoted by $f_j = \Pr(\text{case}\,|G_j)$ for $j = 0, 1, 2$. Then,

$$k = \sum_{j=0}^{2} \Pr(G_j)\Pr(\text{case}\,|G_j) = f_0 g_0 + f_1 g_1 + f_2 g_2.$$

In case-control studies, cases and controls are retrospectively sampled from case and control populations (Sect. 2.2.2). Their genotypes at marker M are obtained and the genotype counts are presented in Table 3.1, in which (r_0, r_1, r_2) and (s_0, s_1, s_2) are genotype counts for (G_0, G_1, G_2) in cases and controls, respectively. The total numbers of cases and controls are respectively $r = r_0 + r_1 + r_2$ and $s = s_0 + s_1 + s_2$. The total number with genotype G_j is denoted by $n_j = r_j + s_j$. Let $n = r + s = n_0 + n_1 + n_2$ be the total number of individuals. The genotype counts (r_0, r_1, r_2) and (s_0, s_1, s_2) follow multinomial distributions $Mul(r; p_0, p_1, p_2)$ and $Mul(s; q_0, q_1, q_2)$, respectively, where $p_j = \Pr(G_j\,|\text{case})$ and $q_j = \Pr(G_j\,|\text{control})$ for $j = 0, 1, 2$. Let d denote the disease status (case with $d = 1$ or control with $d = 0$). From

$$\Pr(G_j\,|d) = \frac{\Pr(G_j)\Pr(d|G_j)}{\Pr(d)},$$

we obtain

$$p_j = \frac{g_j f_j}{k} \quad \text{and} \quad q_j = \frac{g_j(1 - f_j)}{(1 - k)}. \tag{3.2}$$

These two formulas are often used to calculate the genotype probabilities in the case and control groups in simulation studies.

Table 3.1 Genotype counts of case-control samples for a single marker with alleles A and B

	AA	AB	BB	Total
Cases	r_0	r_1	r_2	r
Controls	s_0	s_1	s_2	s
Total	n_0	n_1	n_2	n

Denote GRR by $\lambda_i = f_i/f_0$ for $i = 1, 2$, where $f_0 > 0$ is used as the reference penetrance. Using the GRRs, $k = f_0(g_0 + \lambda_1 g_1 + \lambda_2 g_2)$. Under the null hypothesis of no association between the disease status d and the genotype, the penetrances are equal to the prevalence, i.e., $f_0 = f_1 = f_2 = k$. That is, $\lambda_1 = \lambda_2 = 1$.

3.2 Genetic Models

A genetic model refers to a specific mode of inheritance. Four common genetic models are discussed in the literature: the recessive (REC), additive (ADD), multiplicative (MUL), and dominant (DOM) models. Assume that marker M described in Sect. 3.1 is associated with a disease and that allele B is the risk allele in the sense that

$$\Pr(\text{case} \,|\, G_2) \geq \Pr(\text{case} \,|\, G_1) \geq \Pr(\text{case} \,|\, G_0)$$

$$\text{and} \quad \Pr(\text{case} \,|\, G_2) > \Pr(\text{case} \,|\, G_0). \tag{3.3}$$

That is, the probability of developing the disease increases with the number of risk alleles carried. Then, (3.3) implies $f_2 \geq f_1 \geq f_0$ and $f_2 > f_0$. Throughout this chapter we assume B is the risk allele. The alternative hypothesis H_1 of association can be stated as H_1: $\lambda_2 \geq \lambda_1 \geq 1$ and $\lambda_2 > 1$. Hence, two GRRs, (λ_1, λ_2), are required to define an alternative hypothesis. A genetic model specifies a relationship among the three penetrances, and hence between the two GRRs.

A genetic model is called REC, ADD, MUL, and DOM if

$$f_1 = f_0,$$
$$f_1 = (f_0 + f_2)/2,$$
$$f_1 = \sqrt{f_0 f_2},$$
$$f_1 = f_2,$$

respectively. Using the GRRs, the above four equations can be also written as

$$\lambda_1 = 1, \quad \lambda_1 = (1 + \lambda_2)/2, \quad \lambda_1 = \lambda_2^{1/2}, \quad \text{and} \quad \lambda_1 = \lambda_2.$$

Hence, given $\lambda_2 = \lambda$ and one of the four genetic models, λ_1 can be calculated using λ. Note that the definitions of the REC and DOM models depend on which allele is

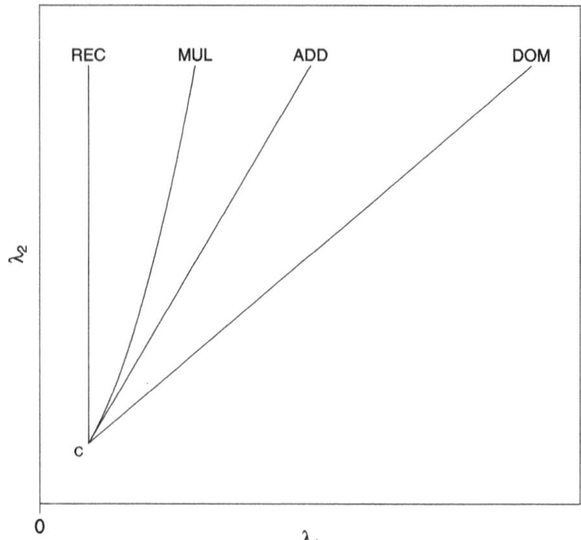

Fig. 3.1 Plot of the four common genetic models in the genetic model space Λ constrained by the *rays*, from the *point* $C(1, 1)$, corresponding to the REC and DOM models

the risk allele. If the same GRRs $\lambda_i = f_i/f_0$, $i = 1, 2$ are used but allele A is the risk allele, then the REC and DOM models refer to $\lambda_1 = \lambda_2$ and $\lambda_1 = 1$, respectively. When the GRRs are weak (i.e. $\lambda_1 \approx 1$ and $\lambda_2 \approx 1$), the ADD model is a good approximation for the MUL model. This can be shown by expressing the ADD model as $\lambda_2 = 2\lambda_1 - 1$ and using the Taylor expansion about $\lambda_2 - 1 \approx 0$,

$$\lambda_2^{1/2} = (1 + \lambda_2 - 1)^{1/2} \approx 1 + (\lambda_2 - 1)/2 = 1 + (2\lambda_1 - 1 - 1)/2 = \lambda_1,$$

which is the MUL model.

In Fig. 3.1, the four common genetic models are plotted in the GRR space $\Lambda = \{(\lambda_1, \lambda_2) : \lambda_2 \geq \lambda_1 \geq 1\}$. The line corresponding to the ADD model is the tangent line at $C = (1, 1)$ for the curve corresponding to the MUL model. The REC and DOM models form the boundaries for Λ. In addition to the four common genetic models, the space Λ in Fig. 3.1 defines a family of genetic models indexed by $\theta \in [0, 1]$ as

$$\Lambda = \{(\lambda_1, \lambda_2) : \lambda_1 = (1 - \theta) + \theta\lambda_2,\ 0 \leq \theta \leq 1\}. \tag{3.4}$$

The REC, ADD, and DOM models correspond to $\theta = 0$, $1/2$, and 1, respectively. In practice, the true genetic model is usually unknown. It could correspond to Λ with any $\theta \in [0, 1]$, or not even constrained in Λ. For example, the overdominant model has $(\lambda_1, \lambda_2) \notin \Lambda$, because, under the overdominant model, the risk of the disease is higher for genotype AB than for genotype BB, even though B is the risk allele. We focus on the constrained genetic model space Λ given in (3.4). Discussion of results for genetic models outside of Λ will be briefly mentioned if such models are used.

3.3 Genotype-Based Tests

To test for genetic association using a case-control design, the CATT (the trend test, for short) and Pearson's chi-squared test (Pearson's test, for short) are two commonly used test statistics. The trend test relies on the assumptions that one of the alleles is the risk allele and that the risk of developing the disease increases with the number of the risk alleles in the genotype. Different trend tests are used for the four different genetic models discussed in Sect. 3.2. The trend test may not be robust when the genetic model is misspecified. Pearson's test, on the other hand, is robust to the underlying genetic model, because it does not require the genetic model. Both tests asymptotically follow chi-squared distributions even when Hardy-Weinberg proportions do not hold in the population.

3.3.1 Cochran-Armitage Trend Tests

In the literature, the CATT may only refer to the trend test that we describe below under the ADD model. We treat all trend tests as CATTs with different scores. The trend test is used to test for association in ordered categorical data. The case-control data presented in Table 3.1 is ordered if the risk of the disease increases with the number of the risk allele in the three genotypes. The trend test utilizes the order of the risks for the genotypes by assigning a set of increasing scores to the three genotypes. Let the scores be (x_0, x_1, x_2) for the three genotypes (G_0, G_1, G_2). Then the scores are increasing: $x_0 \leq x_1 \leq x_2$ and $x_0 < x_2$. The trend test is based on the differences between the estimates of the genotype frequencies in cases (r_j/r) and in the combined case-control samples (n_j/n) weighted by the increasing scores:

$$U = \sum_{j=0}^{2} x_j \left(\frac{r_j}{r} - \frac{n_j}{n} \right) = \frac{1}{nr} \sum_{j=0}^{2} x_j (sr_j - rs_j)$$

$$= \frac{1}{r} \sum_{j=0}^{2} x_j \{(1 - \phi)r_j - \phi s_j\}, \tag{3.5}$$

where $\phi = r/n$ is the proportion of cases. The variance of the statistic U can be written as (Problem 3.2)

$$\mathrm{Var}(U) = \frac{n}{r^2} \phi (1 - \phi)^2 \left\{ \sum_{j=0}^{2} x_j^2 p_j - \left(\sum_{j=0}^{2} x_j p_j \right)^2 \right\}$$

$$+ \frac{n}{r^2} \phi^2 (1 - \phi) \left\{ \sum_{j=0}^{2} x_j^2 q_j - \left(\sum_{j=0}^{2} x_j q_j \right)^2 \right\}. \tag{3.6}$$

Then the trend test can be written as

$$Z_{CATT} = \frac{U}{\sqrt{\widehat{Var}(U)}}, \tag{3.7}$$

where, in (3.6), the genotype frequencies in cases and controls, p_j and q_j, are estimated using the combined case-control samples under $H_0 : p_j = q_j$, i.e. $\widehat{p}_j = \widehat{q}_j = n_j/n$ for $j = 0, 1, 2$. This leads to

$$Z_{CATT} = \frac{\sum_{j=0}^{2} x_j((1 - \phi)r_j - \phi s_j)}{\sqrt{n\phi(1 - \phi)\{\sum_{j=0}^{2} x_j^2 n_j/n - (\sum_{j=0}^{2} x_j n_j/n)^2\}}}. \tag{3.8}$$

An alternative approach is to estimate p_j and q_j in (3.6) using cases and controls separately, i.e.

$$\widehat{p}_j = r_j/r \quad \text{and} \quad \widehat{q}_j = s_j/s.$$

Both estimates of the variance, using either the combined or separate case-control samples, are consistent under H_0. Thus, Z_{CATT}, with either estimate of the variance, asymptotically follows $N(0, 1)$ under H_0. Under the alternative hypothesis, however, only the estimate using the separate case-control samples is consistent. Thus, the trend test using the estimate with the separate case-control samples is more powerful than that using the estimate with the combined case-control samples. The cost of this improved power is that using the combined case-control samples has better control of Type I error than using the separated case-control samples under the null hypothesis (see Problem 3.8). Because the risk allele is unknown, a two-sided test is used. The null hypothesis of no association is rejected at the significance level α if $|Z_{CATT}| > z_{1-\alpha/2}$, where $z_{1-\alpha/2}$ is the $100(1 - \alpha/2)$th percentile of $N(0, 1)$.

The trend test depends on the choice of scores, but it is invariant under a linear transformation of the scores. That is, the trend tests are identical if the following two sets of scores are used: (x_0, x_1, x_2) where $x_0 \leq x_1 \leq x_2$, $x_0 < x_2$ and $(0, (x_1 - x_0)/(x_2 - x_0), 1)$ where $0 \leq (x_1 - x)/(x_2 - x_0) \leq 1$. Thus, without loss of generality, we consider a set of scores $(0, x, 1)$, where $0 \leq x \leq 1$, and denote the corresponding trend test as $Z_{CATT}(x)$. The optimal score x depends on the underlying genetic model. For the REC model, genotypes AA and AB have the same risk. Therefore, $x = 0$ is used (both genotypes have the same score). On the other hand, for the DOM model, AB and BB have the same risk. Hence, $x = 1$ is used (both genotypes have the same score). For the ADD and MUL models, $x = 1/2$ is used. The scores $(0, 1/2, 1)$ is equivalent to using the proportion of risk alleles in the three genotypes. In practice, when the true genetic model is unknown, $x = 1/2$ is used, because it is the most robust among all trend tests with $0 \leq x \leq 1$ (Problem 3.9). The robustness of the trend tests will be further discussed in Chap. 6, where several other robust tests will also be studied.

Table 3.2 presents simulated case-control samples for a single marker, where $(r_0, r_1, r_2) = (317, 171, 12)$ and $(s_0, s_1, s_2) = (264, 208, 28)$. Thus, $(n_0, n_1, n_2) = (581, 379, 40)$ and $n = 1000$. The proportion of cases $\phi = 0.5$. The risk allele is

Table 3.2 Simulated case-control samples for a single marker with 500 cases and 500 controls: the allele frequency of B is 0.25 under the ADD model with an OR of 0.5		*AA*	*AB*	*BB*	Total
	Cases	317	171	12	500
	Controls	264	208	28	500
	Total	581	379	40	1000

unknown. If we estimate $\widehat{\Pr}(B|\text{case}) = (r_1 + 2r_2)/(2r) = \{171 + 2(12)\}/1000 = 0.195$ and $\widehat{\Pr}(B|\text{control}) = (s_1 + 2s_2)/(2s) = \{208 + 2(28)\}/1000 = 0.264$, it shows $\Pr(B|\text{case}) < \Pr(B|\text{control})$. Thus, B is not likely the risk allele. However, we can still use (3.8) to compute the CATT and report a two-sided p-value when the risk allele is unknown. Using estimates of $\widehat{p}_j = \widehat{q}_j = n_j/n$,

$$Z_{\text{CATT}}\left(\frac{1}{2}\right) = \frac{\frac{1}{2}(171/2 - 208/2) + (12/2 - 28/2)}{\sqrt{1000 \times \frac{1}{2} \times \frac{1}{2} \times \{(\frac{1}{2})^2 \times \frac{379}{1000} + \frac{40}{1000} - (\frac{1}{2} \times \frac{379}{1000} + \frac{40}{1000})^2\}}}$$

$$\approx -3.808.$$

The two-sided p-value using the standard normal distribution is $p = 0.00014$. The trend test is negative because we treat allele B as the risk allele even though A is the risk allele. Using the alternative variance estimates $\widehat{p}_j = r_j/r$ and $\widehat{q}_j = s_j/s$, $\sum_{j=0}^{2} x_j^2 r_j/r - (\sum_{j=0}^{2} x_j r_j/r)^2 = 0.071475$ and $\sum_{j=0}^{2} x_j^2 s_j/s - (\sum_{j=0}^{2} x_j s_j/s)^2 = 0.090304$. The denominator of (3.7) is

$$\sqrt{\widehat{\text{VAR}}(U)} = \sqrt{\{1000/(8 \times 500^2)\}(0.071475 + 0.090304)} = 0.008994.$$

Hence,

$$Z_{\text{CATT}}\left(\frac{1}{2}\right) = \frac{(\frac{1}{2}(171/2 - 208/2) + (12/2 - 28/2))/500}{0.008994} \approx -3.836.$$

The two-sided p-value is $p = 0.000125$. The p-value of the trend test with the variance estimated using the separate case-control samples is smaller than that with the variance estimated using the combined case-control samples.

3.3.2 Trend Test Obtained from the Logistic Regression Model

The trend test $Z_{\text{CATT}}(x)$ in (3.8) can be obtained as a Score statistic from a logistic regression model. Define an indicator function of genotype as $I(G) = 0$ if $G = AA$, x if $G = AB$, and 1 if $G = BB$. The prospective logistic regression model is often used for retrospective case-control data (Sect. 2.6). Thus,

$$\Pr(\text{case}|G) = \frac{\exp\{\beta_0 + \beta_1 I(G)\}}{1 + \exp\{\beta_0 + \beta_1 I(G)\}}. \tag{3.9}$$

Let $d_i = 1$ for case and 0 for control for $i = 1, \ldots, n$. The likelihood function for the case-control data in Table 3.1 is

$$L(\beta_0, \beta_1) = \prod_{i=1}^{n} \{\Pr(\text{case}\,|G_i)\}^{d_i} \{1 - \Pr(\text{case}\,|G_i)\}^{1-d_i}$$

$$= \frac{\exp\{r\beta_0 + (xr_1 + r_2)\beta_1\}}{\{1 + \exp(\beta_0)\}^{n_0}\{1 + \exp(\beta_0 + x\beta_1)\}^{n_1}\{1 + \exp(\beta_0 + \beta_1)\}^{n_2}}.$$

We test $H_0 : \beta_1 = 0$ and β_0 is a nuisance parameter. The Score test given in (1.9) can be directly applied after we replace $\theta = (\psi, \eta)^T$ in (1.9) by $\beta = (\beta_1, \beta_0)^T$. Denote the log-likelihood function by $l(\beta)$. Then, from

$$\frac{\partial l(\beta)}{\partial \beta_0}\Big|_{H_0} = r - n\exp(\beta_0)/(1 + \exp(\beta_0)) = 0,$$

we obtain the MLE for β_0 restricted under H_0 as $\widetilde{\beta}_0 = \log(r/s)$. Thus, $\widetilde{\beta} = (0, \widetilde{\beta}_0)^T$. The Score function, evaluated with $\beta = \widetilde{\beta}$, can be written as

$$U(\widetilde{\beta}) = \frac{\partial l(\beta)}{\partial \beta_1}\Big|_{\beta=\widetilde{\beta}} = (xr_1 + r_2) - (xn_1 + n_2)\frac{r}{n}$$

$$= rU = \sum_{j=0}^{2} x_j\{(1 - \phi)r_j - \phi s_j\}, \tag{3.10}$$

where U is the statistic given in (3.5) with scores $(x_0, x_1, x_2) = (0, x, 1)$. The observed Fisher information matrix can be written as (Problem 3.3)

$$i_n(\widetilde{\beta}) = -\begin{bmatrix} \frac{\partial^2 l}{\partial \beta_1^2} & \frac{\partial^2 l}{\partial \beta_1 \beta_0} \\ \frac{\partial^2 l}{\partial \beta_0 \beta_1} & \frac{\partial^2 l}{\partial \beta_0^2} \end{bmatrix}\Big|_{\beta=\widetilde{\beta}} = \frac{rs}{n^2}\begin{bmatrix} \sum_{j=0}^{2} x_j^2 n_j & \sum_{j=0}^{2} x_j n_j \\ \sum_{j=0}^{2} x_j n_j & n \end{bmatrix}.$$

The element corresponding to the parameter β_1, the $(1, 1)$th element, in the inverse of the above matrix, $i_n^{-1}(\widetilde{\beta})$, is

$$i^{\beta_1\beta_1}(\widetilde{\beta}) = \frac{n^3}{rs\{n\sum_{j=0}^{2} x_j^2 n_j - (\sum_{j=0}^{2} x_j n_j)^2\}},$$

whose inverse, $n\phi(1 - \phi)\{\sum_j x_j^2 n_j/n - (\sum_j x_j n_j/n)^2\}$, is also a consistent estimate of the variance for the Score function (3.10). The Score statistic of (1.9) is

$$\text{ST} = U^2(\widetilde{\beta})i^{\beta_1\beta_1}(\widetilde{\beta}) = Z^2_{\text{CATT}},$$

where Z_{CATT} is given in (3.8).

3.3.3 Pearson's Chi-Squared Test

Pearson's test compares the observed genotype counts in cases (r_0, r_1, r_2) and controls (s_0, s_1, s_2) with their expected values under the null hypothesis that the disease status and genotypes are independent. Under H_0, the expected counts for r_j and s_j are $n_j r / n$ and $n_j s / n$, respectively. Therefore, Pearson's test can be written as

$$T_{\chi_2^2} = \sum_{j=0}^{2} \frac{(r_j - n_i r / n)^2}{n_i r / n} + \sum_{j=0}^{2} \frac{(s_j - n_j s / n)^2}{n_j s / n}. \tag{3.11}$$

Under H_0, $T_{\chi_2^2}$ asymptotically follows χ_2^2. H_0 is rejected at the level α if $T_{\chi_2^2} > \chi_2^2(1 - \alpha)$, where $\chi_2^2(1 - \alpha)$ is the $100(1 - \alpha)$th percentile of χ_2^2.

Applying $T_{\chi_2^2}$ to the simulated data in Table 3.2 with $(r_0, r_1, r_2) = (317, 171, 12)$ and $(s_0, s_1, s_2) = (264, 208, 28)$, the expected genotype counts of AA, AB and BB for both cases and controls are 290.5, 189.5 and 20. Hence, $T_{\chi_2^2} = 14.8469$ with p-value $p = 0.000597$.

3.3.4 Pearson's Test Obtained from the Logistic Regression Model

Like the trend test, Pearson's test can also be obtained from the prospective logistic regression model. Define two indicator functions $I_1(G)$ and $I_2(G)$ as follows: $I_1(G) = I_2(G) = 0$ if $G = AA$, $I_1(G) = 0$ and $I_2(G) = 1$ if $G = AB$, and $I_1(G) = I_2(G) = 1$ if $G = BB$. Applying

$$\Pr(\text{case} \,|\, I_1(G), I_2(G)) = \frac{\exp\{\beta_0 + \beta_1 I_1(G) + \beta_2 I_2(G)\}}{1 + \exp\{\beta_0 + \beta_1 I_1(G) + \beta_2 I_2(G)\}}, \tag{3.12}$$

the likelihood function is proportional to

$$L(\beta_0, \beta_1, \beta_2) = \prod_{i=1}^{n} \{\Pr(\text{case} \,|\, I_1(G_i), I_2(G_i))\}^{d_i} \{1 - \Pr(\text{case} \,|\, I_1(G_i), I_2(G_i))\}^{1 - d_i}$$

$$= \frac{\exp\{r\beta_0 + r_2\beta_1 + (r_1 + r_2)\beta_2\}}{\{1 + \exp(\beta_0)\}^{n_0} \{1 + \exp(\beta_0 + \beta_2)\}^{n_1} \{1 + \exp(\beta_0 + \beta_1 + \beta_2)\}^{n_2}},$$

where $d_i = 1$ $(d_i = 0)$ when the ith individual is a case (a control).

We test $H_0 : \beta_1 = \beta_2 = 0$ and β_0 is the nuisance parameter. Let $\beta = (\beta_1, \beta_2, \beta_0)^T$. Under H_0, $\tilde{\beta} = (0, 0, \tilde{\beta}_0)$, where $\tilde{\beta}_0 = \log(r/s)$. Let the log-likelihood function be $l(\beta)$. From Problem 3.4, the Score function is $U(\tilde{\beta}) = (U_1(\tilde{\beta}), U_2(\tilde{\beta}))^T$, where

$$U_1(\tilde{\beta}) = \frac{\partial l(\beta)}{\partial \beta_1} \Big|_{\beta=\tilde{\beta}} = \frac{1}{n}(sr_2 - rs_2),$$

$$U_2(\tilde{\beta}) = \frac{\partial l(\beta)}{\partial \beta_2}\big|_{\beta=\tilde{\beta}} = \frac{1}{n}\{s(r_1 + r_2) - r(s_1 + s_2)\}.$$

Then $i^{\psi\psi}(\tilde{\beta})$, $\psi = (\beta_1, \beta_2)^T$, given in (1.9) can be written as (Problem 3.4)

$$i^{\psi\psi}(\tilde{\beta}) = \frac{1}{\phi(1-\phi)}\begin{bmatrix} \frac{n_1+n_2}{n_1 n_2} & -\frac{1}{n_1} \\ -\frac{1}{n_1} & \frac{n_0+n_1}{n_0 n_1} \end{bmatrix}.$$

Thus, the Score statistic can be written as

$$\tilde{T}_{\chi_2^2} = U(\tilde{\beta})^T i^{\psi\psi}(\tilde{\beta}) U(\tilde{\beta})$$

$$= \frac{1}{1-\rho^2}\{Z_{\mathrm{CATT}}^2(0) - 2\rho Z_{\mathrm{CATT}}(0) Z_{\mathrm{CATT}}(1) + Z_{\mathrm{CATT}}^2(1)\}, \qquad (3.13)$$

where

$$\rho = \sqrt{\frac{n_0 n_2}{(n_1 + n_2)(n_0 + n_1)}}.$$

It can be shown that $T_{\chi_2^2}$ and $\tilde{T}_{\chi_2^2}$ are equivalent (Problem 3.5). Note that in (3.13), Pearson's test is written as a function of the two trend tests with scores $(0, 0, 1)$ for the REC model and scores $(0, 1, 1)$ for the DOM model.

3.3.5 Other Likelihood-Based Tests

Using the likelihood functions given in Sect. 3.3.2 and Sect. 3.3.4, the Score statistics were derived. Using these likelihood functions, the standard LRT and Wald test can also be derived following Sect. 1.2.4, which can also be found in many statistical inference books. We illustrate the LRT here.

The likelihood function is given by

$$L(\beta) = L(\beta_0, \beta_1, \ldots, \beta_l) = \frac{\exp(r\beta_0 + \sum_{i=1}^{n} d_i \sum_{j=1}^{l} \beta_j X_{ij})}{\prod_{i=1}^{n}\{1 + \exp(\beta_0 + \sum_{j=1}^{l} \beta_j X_{ij})\}},$$

where $(X_{i1}, \ldots, X_{il})$ are the covariates for the ith individual (e.g., indicators for genotypes). Under a global null hypothesis $H_0 : \beta_1 = \cdots = \beta_l = 0$, the likelihood function is $L_0(\beta_0) = L(\beta_0, 0, \ldots, 0)$, which is maximized by $\tilde{\beta}_0 = \log(r/s)$. Thus, $\tilde{\beta} = (\tilde{\beta}_0, 0, \ldots, 0)^T$. Denote $l_0(\tilde{\beta}) = \log L_0(\tilde{\beta}_0)$. Without any restriction, the MLE $\hat{\beta}$ can be solved from $\partial \log L(\beta)/\partial \beta = 0$, i.e.,

$$r - \sum_{i=1}^{n} \frac{\exp(\beta_0 + \sum_{j=1}^{l} \beta_j X_{ij})}{1 + \exp(\beta_0 + \sum_{j=1}^{l} \beta_j X_{ij})} = 0,$$

Table 3.3 Allele counts of case-control samples for a single marker

	A	B	Total
Cases	$2r_0 + r_1$	$2r_2 + r_1$	$2r$
Controls	$2s_0 + s_1$	$2s_2 + s_2$	$2s$
Total	$2n_0 + n_1$	$2n_2 + n_1$	$2n$

$$\sum_{i=1}^{n} X_{ij} d_i - \sum_{i=1}^{n} \frac{X_{ij}\exp(\beta_0 + \sum_{j=1}^{l}\beta_j X_{ij})}{1+\exp(\beta_0 + \sum_{j=1}^{l}\beta_j X_{ij})} = 0, \quad \text{for } j = 1,\ldots,l.$$

The solutions have no closed forms and can be found numerically. Denote $l(\widehat{\beta}) = \log L(\widehat{\beta})$. Then, from (1.11), the LRT can be written as

$$\text{LRT} = 2l(\widehat{\beta}) - 2l_0(\widetilde{\beta}) \sim \chi_l^2 \quad \text{under } H_0.$$

3.4 Allele-Based Test

3.4.1 Test Statistics

The allele-based test (ABT) or allelic test is another commonly used test for genetic association using case-control data. It compares the allele frequencies between cases and controls. Instead of presenting genotype counts as in Table 3.1, the data for the ABT, displayed in Table 3.3, comprise the number of alleles A and B in cases and controls. Because each individual has two alleles, the total number of alleles is $2n$.

Let p and q be the frequencies of B in cases and controls, respectively. Then, under the null hypothesis of no association H_0, $p = q$. The MLEs of p and q are given by

$$\widehat{p} = (2r_2 + r_1)/(2r) = r_2/r + r_1/(2r),$$

$$\widehat{q} = (2s_2 + s_1)/(2s) = s_2/s + s_2/(2s). \tag{3.14}$$

By the property of MLEs (Sect. 1.2.1), we have

$$\widehat{p} \sim N(p, \text{Var}(\widehat{p})) \quad \text{and} \quad \widehat{q} \sim N(q, \text{Var}(\widehat{q}))$$

asymptotically, where

$$\text{Var}(\widehat{p}) = p(1-p)/(2r) \quad \text{and} \quad \text{Var}(\widehat{q}) = q(1-q)/(2s).$$

The ABT for association of Table 3.3 can be written as

$$Z_{\text{ABT}} = \frac{\widehat{p} - \widehat{q}}{\sqrt{\text{Var}(\widehat{p} - \widehat{q})}} \tag{3.15}$$

where $\widehat{\mathrm{Var}}(\widehat{p} - \widehat{q})$ can be written as

$$\widehat{\mathrm{Var}}(\widehat{p} - \widehat{q}) = \left(\frac{1}{2r} + \frac{1}{2s}\right)\bar{p}(1 - \bar{p}), \tag{3.16}$$

where $\bar{p} = (2n_2 + n_1)/(2n)$; or

$$\widehat{\mathrm{Var}}(\widehat{p} - \widehat{q}) = \widehat{p}(1 - \widehat{p})/(2r) + \widehat{q}(1 - \widehat{q})/(2s), \tag{3.17}$$

where $\widehat{p}$ and $\widehat{q}$ are given in (3.14). Both estimates of variances in (3.16) and (3.17) are asymptotically equivalent under H_0. Thus, Z_{ABT} asymptotically follows $N(0, 1)$ under H_0. Under the alternative hypothesis H_1, however, the estimate in (3.16) is not consistent while the estimate of (3.17) is still consistent. Therefore, the ABT using (3.17) is expected to be more powerful than that using (3.16) under H_1, but with the cost that using the estimate (3.16) has better control of Type I error than using (3.17) under H_0 (Problem 3.8).

Using the simulated data in Table 3.2, $2r_0 + r_1 = 805$, $2r_2 + r_1 = 195$, $2s_0 + s_1 = 736$, $2s_2 + s_1 = 264$, $2n_0 + n_1 = 1541$, and $2n_2 + n_1 = 459$. Thus, $\widehat{p} = 0.195$ and $\widehat{q} = 0.264$. The estimate of variance using (3.16) is

$$\widehat{\mathrm{Var}}(\widehat{p} - \widehat{q}) = (1/1000 + 1/1000)(459/2000)(1 - 459/2000) = 0.000354,$$

which yields $Z_{\mathrm{ABT}} = -3.6673$ with two-sided p-value $p = 0.000245$; and the estimate of variance using (3.17) is

$$\widehat{\mathrm{Var}}(\widehat{p} - \widehat{q}) = 0.195(1 - 0.195)/1000 + 0.264(1 - 0.264)/1000 = 0.000351,$$

which yields $Z_{\mathrm{ABT}} = -3.6829$ with two-sided p-value $p = 0.000231$. Note that both p-values are larger than those of the trend tests with scores $(0, 1/2, 1)$.

3.4.2 Comparison of the Allele-Based Test with the Trend Test

The numerator of Z_{ABT} in (3.15) can be written as

$$\left(\frac{r_2}{r} - \frac{s_2}{s}\right) + \frac{1}{2}\left(\frac{r_1}{r} - \frac{s_1}{s}\right) = \sum_{j=0}^{2} x_j \left(\frac{r_j}{r} - \frac{s_j}{s}\right),$$

where $(x_0, x_1, x_2) = (0, 1/2, 1)$. Therefore, the numerator of Z_{ABT} is identical to that of the trend test for the ADD model $Z_{\mathrm{CATT}}(1/2)$. The difference between them is the estimates of their variances. Two algebraic relationships between the ABT and the trend test for the ADD model have been obtained in the literature, both using the variance estimates based on the combined case-control samples.

First, it can be shown that

$$Z_{\mathrm{ABT}}^2 = Z_{\mathrm{CATT}}^2\left(\frac{1}{2}\right)\left\{1 + \frac{4n_0 n_2 - n_1^2}{(n_1 + 2n_2)(n_1 + 2n_0)}\right\}. \tag{3.18}$$

Denote the estimate of genotype frequency using the combined case-control samples by $\bar{p}_j = n_j/n$ for $j = 0, 1, 2$. Then, it can be shown that

$$4n_0 n_2 - n_1^2 = 0 \quad \text{and} \quad \bar{p}_2 = (\bar{p}_2 + \bar{p}_1/2)^2$$

are equivalent (Problem 3.6), where the latter indicates that Hardy-Weinberg proportions hold in the combined case-control samples, under which $4n_0 n_2 - n_1^2$ should be asymptotically equal to 0. Hence, Z_{ABT} and Z_{CATT} are asymptotically equivalent. Although Eq. (3.18) is derived for studying the validity of the ABT under the null hypothesis, the asymptotic equivalence of Z_{ABT} and Z_{CATT} holds under both null and alternative hypotheses when Hardy-Weinberg proportions hold in the combined case-control samples.

In practice, however, we do not test whether or not Hardy-Weinberg proportions hold in the combined case-control samples. In particular, when the marker is associated with the disease, departure from Hardy-Weinberg proportions in the combined samples may occur. A more useful assumption is that Hardy-Weinberg proportions hold in the population, although this assumption cannot be tested using case-control samples unless the disease prevalence is known (see Sect. 2.3).

Rewriting (3.18), the second algebraic relationship is given by

$$Z_{ABT}^2 = Z_{CATT}^2 \left(\frac{1}{2}\right)\left\{1 + \frac{\bar{p}_2 - \bar{p}^2}{\bar{p}(1 - \bar{p})}\right\}, \tag{3.19}$$

where $\bar{p}_2 = n_2/n$ and $\bar{p} = (2n_2 + n_1)/(2n)$. It can be shown that, as $n \to \infty$,

$$\bar{p}_2 - (\bar{p})^2 \to p_2 - p^2 \quad \text{in probability}$$

under H_0, where p_2 is the population frequency of genotype BB and p is the population frequency of allele B. Hence, when Hardy-Weinberg proportions hold in the population, $\bar{p}_2 - (\bar{p})^2$ converges to 0 in probability, which implies that Z_{ABT} and Z_{CATT} are asymptotically equivalent under H_0. Thus, the ABT is then valid. On the other hand, when Hardy-Weinberg proportions do not hold in the population (e.g., due to allelic correlation), the ABT is not valid, because in Table 3.3 the columns are not independent. Under the alternative hypothesis H_1, however, $\bar{p}_2 - (\bar{p})^2 \to p_2 - p^2$ does not usually hold even when Hardy-Weinberg proportions hold in the population (Problem 3.7). Therefore, under H_1, Z_{ABT} and Z_{CATT} may have different power.

Table 3.4 reports the simulated Type I error rates of Z_{ABT} and Z_{CATT} under H_0 given the allele frequency of B is $p = 0.10, 0.30$ and 0.50, the prevalence $k = 0.10$, and $F = 0$ (under Hardy-Weinberg proportions), 0.05 and 0.10 with 500 cases and 500 controls. The Type I error rates were estimated using 10,000 replicates. Both tests use the variance estimates of the combined case-control samples. Results in Table 3.4 show that both tests have good control of Type I error rates when Hardy-Weinberg proportions hold ($F = 0$). When F becomes larger than 0, the size of the trend test is still close to the nominal level while that of the ABT increases with F and is much larger than $\alpha = 0.05$ when $F = 0.05$ and 0.10.

Table 3.4 Simulated Type I error rates of Z_{ABT} and $Z_{CATT}(1/2)$ with 500 cases and 500 controls based on 10,000 replicates ($F = 0$ under Hardy-Weinberg proportions). The nominal level is $\alpha = 0.05$

F	$p = 0.1$		$p = 0.3$		$p = 0.5$	
	Z_{ABT}	Z_{CATT}	Z_{ABT}	Z_{CATT}	Z_{ABT}	Z_{CATT}
0	0.0452	0.0453	0.0519	0.0517	0.0524	0.0512
0.05	0.0560	0.0497	0.0539	0.0488	0.0580	0.0520
0.10	0.0620	0.0502	0.0638	0.0502	0.0627	0.0498

Table 3.5 Simulated power of Z_{ABT} and $Z_{CATT}(1/2)$ under Hardy-Weinberg proportions in the population with 500 cases and 500 controls based on 10,000 replicates (GRR $\lambda_2 = 1.5$). The nominal level is $\alpha = 0.05$

p	REC		ADD		MUL		DOM	
	Z_{ABT}	Z_{CATT}	Z_{ABT}	Z_{CATT}	Z_{ABT}	Z_{CATT}	Z_{ABT}	Z_{CATT}
0.10	0.0631	0.0603	0.3936	0.3948	0.3404	0.3402	0.8065	0.8106
0.30	0.3732	0.3574	0.6779	0.6783	0.6511	0.6514	0.8825	0.8895
0.50	0.7892	0.7711	0.7035	0.7012	0.7082	0.7042	0.6324	0.6460

Assuming Hardy-Weinberg proportions hold in the population, we compare the simulated power of Z_{ABT} and $Z_{CATT}(1/2)$ (both variances are estimated using the combined case-control samples) under the four common genetic models: REC, ADD, MUL and DOM models. In the simulation, p and k are equal to those used in Table 3.4 and the GRR $\lambda_2 = 1.5$. Based on the results in Table 3.5, the power of the ABT and the trend test are similar under the MUL model. But under the REC model the ABT is slightly more powerful, while under the DOM model the trend test is slightly more powerful. Under the ADD and MUL models, their power is similar. Although these conclusions may change when other parameter values are used, the results in Table 3.5 demonstrate that the ABT and the trend test could have different performance under H_1, although the power difference is usually less than 1%.

3.5 Exact Tests

Two types of exact tests are used in the analysis of case-control association studies. In the first type, all possible 2×3 tables (Table 3.1) or all possible 2×2 tables (Table 3.3) are formed with the margins fixed at their values in the observed 2×3 or 2×2 table. The probabilities for all possible tables under the null hypothesis are obtained, from which the p-value for the observed table can be calculated. Fisher's exact test is one such test for testing association in 2×2 tables. The second type is a Monte-Carlo based-test, which generates a large number of replicates of the case-control samples under the null hypothesis based on the observed data. This approach includes permutation and parametric bootstrap methods. Typically, an exact test refers to the first type. The Monte-Carlo based-tests are also called exact tests here because they give accurate p-values provided the number of replicates used is large enough.

These exact tests are often used for sparse contingency tables where the MAF is small, because the asymptotic normal distribution does not then provide a good approximation of the null distribution of the test statistic. For example, in Table 3.1, if the population allele frequency for B is $p = 0.1$, the disease prevalence is $k = 0.1$, and the GRRs $(\lambda_1, \lambda_2) = (1, 2)$ (the REC model), then the genotype frequency for BB in cases is $p_2 = 0.0198$ under Hardy-Weinberg proportions. Therefore, the expected genotype count for BB is $r_2 = rp_2 < 2$ even if $r = 100$ cases are sampled. The Monte-Carlo approach is also useful when the null distribution of a test statistic is not available. Hence, the Monte-Carlo method is used to simulate the null distribution. Some of these test statistics will be discussed later in Chap. 6.

The first type of exact tests can be computationally intensive because it involves computing probabilities from the central hypergeometric distribution and has been criticized as being too conservative. Monte-Carlo based-tests, however, can be efficiently applied. On the other hand, Monte-Carlo tests may also be computationally prohibitive when the significance level is extremely small. For example, the significance level is $\alpha = 5 \times 10^{-7}$ for testing each genetic marker in a GWAS in which 500,000 to more than a million genetic markers are tested. Hence, the number of replicates, in applying the parametric bootstrap method, should be at least 10 million per marker in order to obtain an accurate estimate of the p-value.

3.5.1 Exact Tests

For the case-control samples presented in Table 3.1, the exact test relies on generating all possible 2×3 tables fixing the margins. Given the five margins (r, s, n_0, n_1, n_2), two of the six cells in the 2×3 table are free, which determine the other four cells. Let r_0 and r_1 be free. Note that $r_0 \leq r$ and $r_0 \leq n_0$. Thus, $r_0 \leq \min(r, n_0)$. On the other hand, $r_0 = n_0 - s_0 \geq n_0 - s$ and $r_0 = r - r_1 - r_2 \geq r - n_1 - n_2$. Given that $n_0 - s = r - n_1 - n_2$ and $r_0 \geq 0$, we have $r_0 \geq \max(n_0 - s, 0)$. Likewise, given the margins and r_0, r_1 is between $\max(n_1 - s + s_0, 0)$ and $\min(r - r_0, n_1)$. Hence, the following algorithm can be used to generate all possible tables with the same fixed margins:

1. Let r_0 run from $\max(n_0 - s, 0)$ to $\min(r, n_0)$, and set $s_0 = n_0 - r_0$;
2. Let r_1 run from $\max(n_1 - s + s_0, 0)$ to $\min(r - r_0, n_1)$, and set $s_1 = n_1 - r_1$;
3. Set $r_2 = r - r_0 - r_1$ and $s_2 = n_2 - r_2$.

For each such table, the probability of obtaining it under H_0 can be calculated from the central hypergeometric distribution as

$$\Pr_{H_0}(r_j, s_j; j = 0, 1, 2 | r, s, n_j, j = 0, 1, 2) = \frac{r! s! n_0! n_1! n_2!}{n! r_0! r_1! r_2! s_0! s_1! s_2!}.$$

All the null probabilities are sorted, including the one corresponding to the observed 2×3 table. The p-value for the observed table is then the sum of the null probabilities of all the tables whose probabilities are at least as small as that of the observed table.

The same idea for the 2×3 table can be applied to the 2×2 table (Table 3.3). For simplicity, let $a = 2r_0 + r_1$, $b = 2r_2 + r_1$, $c = 2s_2 + s_1$, and $d = 2s_2 + s_1$. The above algorithm for the 2×3 table is modified to:

1. Let a run from $\max(2n_0 + n_1 - 2s, 0)$ to $\min(2n_0 + n_1, 2r)$;
2. Set $b = 2r - a$, $c = 2n_0 + n_1 - a$, and $d = 2s - c$.

For each table, the probability of obtaining it under H_0 can also be calculated from the central hypergeometric distribution as

$$\mathrm{Pr}_{H_0}(a, b, c, d \mid r, s, n_0, n_1, n_2) = \frac{(2n_0 + n_1)!(2n_2 + n_1)!(2r)!(2s)!}{(2n)!a!b!c!d!}.$$

The p-value for the observed 2×2 table can then be calculated in the same manner as that for the 2×3 table.

Using the data presented in Table 3.2, $\max(n_0 - s, 0) = 81$, $\min(r, n_0) = 500$, $\max(n_1 - s + s_0, 0) = 143$, and $\min(r - r_0, n_1) = 183$. Thus, r_0 runs from 81 to 500 and r_1 runs from 143 to 183. A total of 17,220 genotype-based tables will be formed whose probabilities need to be calculated. For the allele-based table, $\max(2n_0 + n_1 - 2s, 0) = 541$ and $\min(2n_0 + n_1, 2r) = 1000$. Thus, only 460 tables will be formed. Many software packages conduct the above exact tests.

Other algorithms to simplify the computation are available. For example, a short cut calculation for a 2×2 table is given as follows: (i) Let a be the smallest value among the four values in the 2×2 table. (ii) At step k ($k = 1, \ldots, a$), consider a new 2×2 table with the counts (a, b, c, d) replaced by $(a - k, b + k, c + k, d - k)$. The four margins of the new table do not change. Denote the probability of the central hypergeometric distribution for this table as p_k. (iii) Then

$$p_k = \frac{(a - (k - 1))(d - (k - 1))}{(c + (k + 1))(b + (k + 1))} p_{k-1}.$$

(iv) The exact p-value for the 2×2 table is given by $\sum_{k=0}^{a} p_k$, where p_0 is the probability of the central hypergeometric distribution for the observed 2×2 table.

3.5.2 Permutation Approach

To apply the permutation approach to the 2×3 table, we fix the genotype of each individual and permute the case and control status among them. This generates a new 2×3 table under H_0 with fixed margins. For each generated table, the p-value of the test statistic can be calculated. After a large number of permutations, all the p-values can be sorted and the p-value of the observed table can be estimated by

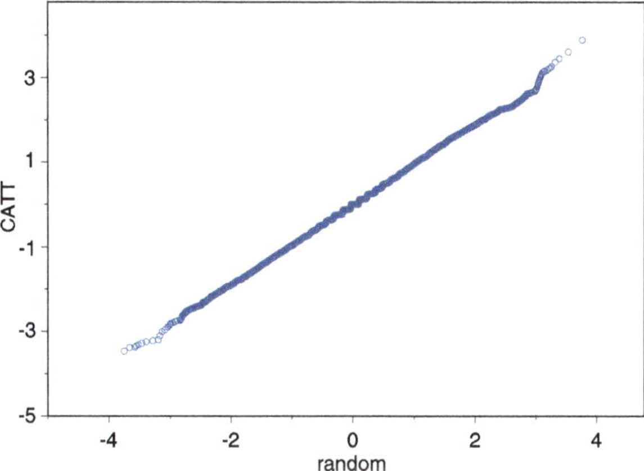

Fig. 3.2 Plot of 10,000 random variates $N(0, 1)$ and 10,000 bootstrapped trend tests using the data in Table 3.2

the proportion of tables whose p-values are at least as small as that of the observed table. The permutation for the 2×2 table can be done in the same manner as for the 2×3 table.

3.5.3 Parametric Bootstrap Approach

Both exact tests and the permutation procedure fix the margins. The parametric bootstrap method only fixes the numbers of cases (r) and controls (s), but not the numbers of genotypes. For each replicate, case genotype counts (r_0, r_1, r_2) are simulated from $Mul(r; n_0/n, n_1/n, n_2/n)$ and control genotype counts are simulated from $Mul(s; n_0/n, n_1/n, n_2/n)$, where n_0, n_1, n_2 are the observed genotype counts in the combined case-control samples. Each replicate simulates a case-control dataset under H_0, from which the test statistic can be calculated. After a large number of replicates, the simulated test statistics form an approximation to the empirical distribution under the null hypothesis, from which the approximate p-value or the critical value can be obtained. The parametric bootstrap method will be further discussed in Chap. 6.

Using the simulated case-control samples in Table 3.2, we apply the parametric bootstrap with 10,000 replicates. In each replicate $Z_{\mathrm{CATT}}(1/2)$ is calculated. A random sample of size 10,000 is also drawn from $N(0, 1)$. Figure 3.2 displays the plot for the bootstrapped $Z_{\mathrm{CATT}}(1/2)$ and the random normal samples, in which the ranked values of the bootstrapped $Z_{\mathrm{CATT}}(1/2)$ sample are plotted against the ranked values of the random normal sample. The plot shows that the bootstrapped test statistics are close to the normal random samples. The bootstrapped p-values using the data in Table 3.2 with various numbers of replicates are reported in Table 3.6 together with the asymptotic p-value reported in Sect. 3.3.1. From Table 3.6, we see that using 10,000 replicates may not be sufficient to provide an accurate estimate of the p-value when the true (asymptotic) p-value is about 10^{-4}. It takes 6 minutes to simulate 10 million replicates using a personal computer (Pentium(R)

Table 3.6 Asymptotic and bootstrapped p-values for the trend test $Z_{\text{CATT}}(1/2)$ using the data in Table 3.2

Asymptotic	Number of replicates			
	10,000	100,000	1,000,000	10,000,000
0.00014	0	0.00009	0.000084	0.0000891

4 CPU 3.40 GHz, 3.39 GHz, 0.99 GB of RAM). Although computing the asymptotic p-value from the trend test is convenient, this example shows that it appears to be more conservative than the parametric bootstrap method with a large number of replicates.

3.6 Hardy-Weinberg Disequilibrium Trend Test

It is known that when the marker is associated with the disease, departure from Hardy-Weinberg proportions in cases can be used to test for association. Departure from Hardy-Weinberg proportions is measured by the Hardy-Weinberg disequilibrium (HWD) coefficient, denoted in a given population by

$$\Delta = \Pr(BB) - \{\Pr(BB) + \Pr(AB)/2\}^2.$$

When Hardy-Weinberg proportions hold in the population, $\Delta = 0$. Denote HWD coefficients in cases and in controls by Δ_p and Δ_q, respectively, which are given by

$$\Delta_p = p_2 - p_M^2 \quad \text{and} \quad \Delta_q = q_2 - q_M^2,$$

where $p_M = p_2 + p_1/2$ and $q_M = q_2 + q_1/2$. When Hardy-Weinberg proportions hold in the case (control) population, $\Delta_p = 0$ ($\Delta_q = 0$). Under the null hypothesis of no association, $H_0 : \Delta = \Delta_p = \Delta_q$. Hence, when $\Delta = 0$, the null hypothesis of no association can be tested by $H_0 : \Delta_p = \Delta_q$ against the alternative hypothesis $H_1 : \Delta_p \neq \Delta_q$. The HWD trend test (HWDTT) is based on the difference of HWD in cases and controls to test for association. For a rare disease, the HWDTT can be based only on the HWD in cases because $\Delta_q \approx 0$ when Hardy-Weinberg proportions hold in the population (see Problem 3.13).

The estimates of HWD coefficients in cases and controls are given by

$$\widehat{\Delta}_p = \widehat{p}_2 - (\widehat{p}_2 + \widehat{p}_1/2)^2 \quad \text{and} \quad \widehat{\Delta}_q = \widehat{q}_2 - (\widehat{q}_2 + \widehat{q}_1/2)^2,$$

where $\widehat{p}_j = r_j/r$ and $\widehat{q}_j = s_j/s$ for $j = 0, 1, 2$. Note that

$$\mathrm{E}(\widehat{\Delta}_p) = \Delta_p - (p_M(1 - p_M) + \Delta_p)/(2r) \approx \Delta_p,$$

$$\mathrm{Var}(\widehat{\Delta}_p) \approx \{p_M^2(1 - p_M)^2 + (1 - 2p_M)^2 \Delta_p - \Delta_p^2\}/r,$$

which hold under both H_0 and H_1, and asymptotically,

$$\widehat{\Delta}_p \sim N(\mathrm{E}(\widehat{\Delta}_p), \mathrm{Var}(\widehat{\Delta}_p)).$$

Similar expressions can be obtained for $\widehat{\Delta}_q$. The HWDTT can therefore be written as

$$Z_{\mathrm{HWDTT}} = \frac{\widehat{\Delta}_p - \widehat{\Delta}_q}{\sqrt{\widehat{\mathrm{Var}}(\widehat{\Delta}_p) + \widehat{\mathrm{Var}}(\widehat{\Delta}_q)}},$$

where, under $H_0 : \Delta_p = \Delta_q$,

$$\widehat{\mathrm{Var}}(\widehat{\Delta}_p) + \widehat{\mathrm{Var}}(\widehat{\Delta}_q) = (1/r + 1/s)\{\bar{p}_M^2(1 - \bar{p}_M)^2 + (1 - 2\bar{p}_M)^2\bar{\Delta}_p - \bar{\Delta}_p^2\},$$

in which $\bar{p}_M = (2n_2 + n_1)/(2n)$ and $\bar{\Delta}_p = n_2/n - \{n_2/n + n_1/(2n)\}^2$. Further simplifying the denominator of Z_{HWDTT} and assuming Hardy-Weinberg proportions in the population, we obtain

$$Z_{\mathrm{HWDTT}} = \frac{\sqrt{rs/n}(\widehat{\Delta}_p - \widehat{\Delta}_q)}{\{1 - n_2/n - n_1/(2n)\}\{n_2/n + n_1/(2n)\}}. \tag{3.20}$$

Under H_0, $Z_{\mathrm{HWDTT}} \sim N(0, 1)$ asymptotically.

From Problem 3.10, the expected value of Z_{HWDTT} under the MUL model is asymptotically 0. Thus, Z_{HWDTT} has no power to test for association under this model. From Sect. 3.2, the ADD model approximates the MUL model near the null hypothesis. Thus, the power of Z_{HWDTT} for the ADD model is also low unless the GRRs are large. For example, using the simulated data of Table 3.2, $Z_{\mathrm{HWDTT}} = -0.0294$ with p-value $= 0.9765$.

3.7 Combining the HWDTT and the CATT

A simulation study is conducted to compare the empirical power of $Z_{\mathrm{CATT}}(1/2)$ and Z_{HWDTT} under the four common genetic models and various settings. The empirical power is estimated using 10,000 replicates. The results are presented in Table 3.7. The results indicate that Z_{HWDTT} is slightly more powerful than $Z_{\mathrm{CATT}}(1/2)$ under the REC model with small to moderate MAFs. On the other hand, Z_{HWDTT} has moderate power under the DOM model with moderate to common MAFs, though it has substantially less power than $Z_{\mathrm{CATT}}(1/2)$. Under the ADD model, however, the power of Z_{HWDTT} is close to the significance level unless the genetic effect is much larger than $\lambda_2 = 2.0$. The performance of Z_{HWDTT} under the ADD model provides insight into the result of applying Z_{HWDTT} to the simulated data in Sect. 3.6.

Although $Z_{\mathrm{CATT}}(1/2)$ outperforms Z_{HWDTT} in many practical situations, we will show that Z_{HWDTT} actually provides useful information in addition to $Z_{\mathrm{CATT}}(1/2)$ that can be incorporated into an analysis together with $Z_{\mathrm{CATT}}(1/2)$ and may result in more powerful approaches than using $Z_{\mathrm{CATT}}(1/2)$ alone.

Table 3.7 Empirical power of $Z_{\text{CATT}}(1/2)$ and Z_{HWDTT} under Hardy-Weinberg proportions in the population with 500 cases and 500 controls, and $k = 0.1$. The significance level is $\alpha = 0.05$

GRR λ_2	p	REC		ADD		DOM	
		CATT	HWDTT	CATT	HWDTT	CATT	HWDTT
1.2	0.1	0.0487	0.0681	0.1099	0.0513	0.2417	0.0555
	0.3	0.0992	0.1128	0.1862	0.0472	0.3100	0.1071
	0.5	0.2173	0.1284	0.2067	0.0518	0.1956	0.1264
1.5	0.1	0.0663	0.1351	0.3977	0.0510	0.8266	0.1098
	0.3	0.3496	0.3796	0.6811	0.0512	0.8842	0.3673
	0.5	0.7741	0.4205	0.7040	0.0516	0.6449	0.4088
2.0	0.1	0.1053	0.3316	0.8885	0.0555	0.9994	0.3891
	0.3	0.8306	0.8556	0.9897	0.0733	0.9994	0.8471
	0.5	0.9986	0.8348	0.9879	0.0661	0.9625	0.8132

From Problem 3.11, the two trend tests $Z_{\text{CATT}}(1/2)$ and Z_{HWDTT} are asymptotically uncorrelated under the null hypothesis of no association when Hardy-Weinberg proportions hold in the population, i.e.

$$\text{Corr}_{H_0}(Z_{\text{CATT}}(1/2), Z_{\text{HWDTT}}) = 0 \quad \text{as } n \to \infty. \tag{3.21}$$

By the joint normality of the two trend tests, the above property indicates that the two trend tests are asymptotically independent when Hardy-Weinberg proportions hold in the population. This property can be incorporated in the analysis of case-control association studies using the trend test.

We first consider Fisher's combination of the p-values of the two trend tests. Let p_{CATT} and p_{HWDTT} be p-values of $Z_{\text{CATT}}(1/2)$ and Z_{HWDTT}. Then Fisher's combination test is written as

$$T_F = -2\log(p_{\text{CATT}}) - 2\log(p_{\text{HWDTT}}),$$

which asymptotically follows χ_4^2 under H_0. Thus, H_0 is rejected at the level α if $T_F > \chi_4^2(1-\alpha)$, where $\chi_4^2(1-\alpha)$ is the $100(1-\alpha)$th percentile of χ_4^2. The p-value of T_F is given in Problem 3.12. An alternative simple approach is to combine the two test statistics directly as given by

$$T_{\text{SUM}} = Z_{\text{HWDTT}}^2 + Z_{\text{CATT}}^2(1/2),$$

which has an asymptotic χ_2^2 distribution under H_0.

Tables 3.8, 3.9 report the results from simulation studies comparing $Z_{\text{CATT}}(1/2)$ with T_F, Pearson's test and T_{SUM} under the null hypothesis and under alternative hypotheses with various genetic models. The Type I error and power are estimated based on 100,000 replicates. The results for all four test statistics are not sensitive

Table 3.8 Empirical power of $Z_{CATT}(1/2)$, Fisher's combination test T_F, Pearson's test $T_{\chi_2^2}$, and the sum of the two trend tests T_{SUM} with 500 cases and 500 controls (GRR is 1.5), and 250 cases and 250 controls (GRR is 2.0), $k = 0.1$ and 100,000 replicates. The nominal level is $\alpha = 0.05$ and $F = 0$ (Hardy-Weinberg proportions hold)

Model	λ_2	p	CATT	T_F	$T_{\chi_2^2}$	T_{SUM}
NULL	1	0.1	0.0493	0.0489	0.0466	0.0485
		0.3	0.0499	0.0490	0.0486	0.0486
		0.5	0.0501	0.0493	0.0497	0.0497
REC	1.5	0.1	0.0658	0.0974	0.0913	0.0968
		0.3	0.3507	0.5228	0.4995	0.5154
		0.5	0.7742	0.8402	0.8370	0.8355
	2.0	0.1	0.0755	0.1231	0.1031	0.1211
		0.3	0.5543	0.7600	0.7290	0.7510
		0.5	0.9263	0.9596	0.9596	0.9580
ADD	1.5	0.1	0.4025	0.3064	0.3099	0.3132
		0.3	0.6851	0.5689	0.5811	0.5817
		0.5	0.7013	0.5861	0.5995	0.5995
	2.0	0.1	0.6108	0.4923	0.4936	0.5043
		0.3	0.8553	0.7696	0.7802	0.7811
		0.5	0.8422	0.7508	0.7636	0.7635
MUL	1.5	0.1	0.3541	0.2671	0.2704	0.2725
		0.3	0.6540	0.5351	0.5459	0.5464
		0.5	0.7095	0.5958	0.6083	0.6083
	2.0	0.1	0.5000	0.3842	0.3838	0.3949
		0.3	0.8245	0.7233	0.7364	0.7373
		0.5	0.8595	0.7676	0.7799	0.7799
DOM	1.5	0.1	0.8253	0.7672	0.7641	0.7741
		0.3	0.8871	0.9011	0.8944	0.9005
		0.5	0.6337	0.7443	0.7387	0.7374
	2.0	0.1	0.9545	0.9338	0.9294	0.9376
		0.3	0.9638	0.9753	0.9718	0.9750
		0.5	0.7448	0.8605	0.8579	0.8544

to departure from Hardy-Weinberg proportions. The power of Fisher's combination test T_F and T_{SUM} are much higher than using Z_{HWDTT} alone, in particular under the ADD and MUL models. Results show that T_F and T_{SUM} are more powerful than $Z_{CATT}(1/2)$ under the REC model but less powerful under the ADD and MUL models. Under the DOM model, $Z_{CATT}(1/2)$, T_F and T_{SUM} have similar performance, although T_F and T_{SUM} are slightly more powerful than $Z_{CATT}(1/2)$. T_F also out-

Table 3.9 Empirical power of $Z_{CATT}(1/2)$, Fisher's combination test T_F, Pearson's test $T_{\chi_2^2}$, and the sum of the two trend tests T_{SUM} with 500 cases and 500 controls (GRR is 1.5), and 250 cases and 250 controls (GRR is 2.0), $k = 0.1$, based on 100,000 replicates. The significance level is $\alpha = 0.05$ and $F = 0.05$ (Hardy-Weinberg proportions do not hold)

Model	λ_2	p	CATT	T_F	$T_{\chi_2^2}$	T_{SUM}
NULL	1	0.1	0.0498	0.0493	0.0477	0.0491
		0.3	0.0507	0.0501	0.0497	0.0498
		0.5	0.0509	0.0500	0.0500	0.0500
REC	1.5	0.1	0.0794	0.1372	0.1158	0.1354
		0.3	0.4010	0.5797	0.5406	0.5716
		0.5	0.7899	0.8456	0.8447	0.8420
	2.0	0.1	0.1047	0.2034	0.1598	0.1978
		0.3	0.6161	0.8097	0.7699	0.8013
		0.5	0.9352	0.9614	0.9626	0.9604
ADD	1.5	0.1	0.4142	0.3215	0.3228	0.3273
		0.3	0.7028	0.5852	0.5991	0.5979
		0.5	0.7236	0.6121	0.6237	0.6239
	2.0	0.1	0.6252	0.5053	0.5137	0.5165
		0.3	0.8695	0.7854	0.7946	0.7970
		0.5	0.8578	0.7731	0.7846	0.7851
MUL	1.5	0.1	0.3673	0.2835	0.2821	0.2885
		0.3	0.6772	0.5616	0.5733	0.5748
		0.5	0.7311	0.6158	0.6288	0.6288
	2.0	0.1	0.5283	0.4223	0.4180	0.4301
		0.3	0.8426	0.7471	0.7581	0.7597
		0.5	0.8733	0.7861	0.7977	0.7978
DOM	1.5	0.1	0.8136	0.7347	0.7591	0.7458
		0.3	0.8879	0.8944	0.8961	0.8946
		0.5	0.6633	0.7656	0.7585	0.7588
	2.0	0.1	0.9493	0.9185	0.9267	0.9242
		0.3	0.9640	0.9739	0.9727	0.9737
		0.5	0.7700	0.8773	0.8732	0.8720

performs both Pearson's test and T_{SUM} under the REC model, but is slightly less powerful under the ADD and MUL models. Under the DOM model, T_F, $T_{\chi_2^2}$ and T_{SUM} have comparable power.

Applying Fisher's combination test to the simulated data of Table 3.2, we have $p_{CATT} = 0.00014$ and $p_{HWDTT} = 0.9765$. Thus, Fisher's combination test is

$T_F = -2\log(0.00014) - 2\log(0.9765) = 17.7953$ with p-value $= 0.00135$. However, when T_{SUM} is applied, the p-value is 0.00071.

3.8 Estimates of Odds Ratios

Using the notation given in Sect. 2.5 and the case-control data in Table 3.1, two ORs, $\text{OR}_{G_1:G_0} = \text{OR}_1$ and $\text{OR}_{G_2:G_0} = \text{OR}_2$, are given by

$$\text{OR}_{G_1:G_0} = \frac{f_1(1-f_0)}{f_0(1-f_1)}, \tag{3.22}$$

$$\text{OR}_{G_2:G_0} = \frac{f_2(1-f_0)}{f_0(1-f_2)}. \tag{3.23}$$

Dividing (3.23) by (3.22), we also have

$$\text{OR}_{G_2:G_1} = \frac{\text{OR}_{G_2:G_0}}{\text{OR}_{G_1:G_0}} = \frac{f_2(1-f_1)}{f_1(1-f_2)}.$$

OR_i, $i = 1, 2$ compares the risk of the heterozygous genotype $G_1 = AB$ or homozygous genotype $G_2 = BB$ with the reference genotype $G_0 = AA$.

The genetic models can be defined using GRRs. Note that the REC ($f_1 = f_0$) and DOM ($f_1 = f_2$) models are equivalent to $\text{OR}_{G_1:G_0} = 1$ and $\text{OR}_{G_2:G_1} = 1$, respectively. However, the ADD or MUL model cannot be represented in a simple form by ORs. Assuming $0 < f_j < 1$ for $j = 0, 1, 2$, under the ADD model,

$$1 + \text{OR}_{G_2:G_0} - 2\text{OR}_{G_1:G_0} = \frac{(f_2 - f_1)(2 - f_0 - f_2)}{f_0(1-f_1)(1-f_2)} > 0, \tag{3.24}$$

and under the MUL model,

$$\text{OR}_{G_2:G_0} - \text{OR}_{G_1:G_0}^2 = \frac{(1-f_0)f_2(f_0 + f_2 - 2f_1)}{f_0(1-f_1)^2(1-f_2)} > 0. \tag{3.25}$$

Note that (3.24) and (3.25) can be directly verified (see Problem 3.1).

Using the data in Table 3.1, the estimates of OR_1 and OR_2 are

$$\widehat{\text{OR}}_1 = \frac{r_0 s_1}{r_1 s_0} \quad \text{and} \quad \widehat{\text{OR}}_2 = \frac{r_0 s_2}{r_2 s_0}.$$

Consistent estimates of the variances of $\widehat{\text{OR}}_1$ and $\widehat{\text{OR}}_2$ can be obtained from Sect. 2.5.

Applying the results to the simulated data in Table 3.2,

$$\widehat{\text{OR}}_1 = 1.46 \quad \text{and} \quad \widehat{\text{Var}}(\log \widehat{\text{OR}}_1) = 0.01760.$$

Hence, the 95% CI for OR_1 is $(1.13, 1.89)$, which indicates the odds of having the disease in the genotype AB group is significantly higher than that in the genotype

AA group. Likewise, we obtain $\widehat{OR}_2 = 2.80$ and $\widehat{Var}(\log \widehat{OR}_2) = 0.1260$. Thus, the 95% CI for OR_2 is $(1.40, 5.61)$. This also indicates a significant association between case/control and genotypes *AA/BB*.

An OR for these data can also be computed for the allelic data given in Table 3.3. Then $a = 805$, $b = 195$, $c = 736$, and $d = 264$. The estimate of the OR is $\widehat{OR} = 1.48$ with 95% CI $(1.20, 1.83)$. When the underlying genetic model is REC or DOM, the genotype data can be reduced to a 2×2 table. For the REC model, $a = r_0 + r_1$, $b = r_2$, $c = s_0 + s_1$, and $d = s_2$. For the DOM model, $a = r_0$, $b = r_1 + r_2$, $c = s_0$, and $d = s_1 + s_2$. For the ADD model, however, the estimate of the OR and its variance estimate can be obtained from the prospective logistic regression model in Sect. 3.3.2 with the score $I(G) = 1/2$ for $G = AB$. Then, $\widehat{OR} = \exp(\widehat{\beta}_1)$. See the real data analysis in Sect. 3.11.

3.9 Simulating Case-Control Samples

Cases and controls can be simulated independently from multinomial distributions with fixed r and s using the parametric bootstrap method described in Sect. 3.5.3. In the following, we discuss two approaches using logistic regression models, in which covariates can be adjusted out.

3.9.1 Without Covariates

To simulate case-control samples without covariates for genetic marker M given a specific genetic model, the following algorithm can be used:

1. Specify the numbers of cases (r) and controls (s), the disease prevalence k, the allele frequency p for the risk allele B (the minor allele if the risk allele is unknown), and the GRR $\lambda_2 = \lambda$;
2. Calculate the GRR λ_1 based on the given genetic model and population genotype frequencies g_0, g_1 and g_2 using (3.1) (where $F = 0$ under Hardy-Weinberg proportions in the population);
3. Calculate $f_0 = k/(g_0 + \lambda_1 g_1 + \lambda_2 g_2)$, $f_1 = \lambda_1 f_0$, and $f_2 = \lambda_2 f_0$;
4. Calculate $p_j = g_j f_j / k$ and $q_j = g_j (1 - f_j)/(1 - k)$ for $j = 0, 1, 2$;
5. Generate random samples (r_0, r_1, s_2) and (s_0, s_1, s_2) independently from the multinomial distributions $Mul(r; p_0, p_1, p_2)$ and $Mul(s; q_0, q_1, q_2)$, respectively.

The above procedure can be used to generate case-control samples under the null and alternative hypotheses, where $\lambda = 1$ for H_0 (regardless of the genetic model specified) and $\lambda > 1$ for H_1. When the genetic model is unknown, both GRRs (λ_1, λ_2) need to be specified. The following is an example to generate a case-control dataset for $r = s = 500$, $p = 0.25$, $k = 0.10$, and $\lambda = 1.5$ under the ADD model:

	AA	AB	BB
case	251	213	36
control	270	195	35

When the ORs, $\mathrm{OR}_{G_1:G_0} = \mathrm{OR}_1$ and $\mathrm{OR}_{G_2:G_0} = \mathrm{OR}_2$, are given instead of the GRRs, we can specify the reference penetrance f_0, and use the prospective logistic regression model to calculate f_i as

$$f_i = \Pr(\text{case}\,|\,G_i) = \frac{\exp(\beta_0 + \beta_i)}{1 + \exp(\beta_0 + \beta_i)}, \quad \text{for } i = 1, 2,$$

where $\beta_0 = \log(f_0/(1 - f_0))$ and $\beta_i = \log(\mathrm{OR}_i)$ for $i = 1, 2$. Then, k is calculated by $k = \sum_{j=0}^{2} g_j f_j$. When the underlying genetic model defined in (3.4) is known, we only need to specify f_0 and OR_2. Then f_2 can be calculated from OR_2 and f_1 can be calculated from f_0 and f_2 from (3.4). After the penetrances f_0, f_1, and f_2 are calculated, the above algorithm can be used to generate genotype counts in cases and controls. To generate data with ORs, the previous example for the ADD model is modified with $r = s = 500$, $p = 0.25$, $f_0 = 0.01$, and $\mathrm{OR}_2 = 0.5$ (here A is the risk allele) as follows:

	AA	AB	BB
case	317	171	12
control	264	208	28

The above data are also presented in Table 3.2.

3.9.2 With Covariates

We can generate case-control samples incorporating covariates for each individual, e.g., age and sex. Let X_{it} be the tth covariate value for the ith individual $i = 1, \ldots, n$ and $t = 1, \ldots, T$. Define

$$f_{0i} = \frac{\exp(\beta_0 + \sum_{t=1}^{T} \beta_{0t} x_{it})}{1 + \exp(\beta_0 + \sum_{t=1}^{T} \beta_{0j} x_{it})}$$

and

$$f_{2i} = \frac{\exp(\beta_0 + \sum_{t=1}^{T} \beta_{0t} x_{it} + \beta_2)}{1 + \exp(\beta_0 + \sum_{t=1}^{T} \beta_{0t} x_{it} + \beta_2)},$$

where β_0 and β_{0t} $(t = 1, \ldots, T)$ are prespecified effects, $\beta_2 = \log(\mathrm{OR}_2)$ for genotype BB, and x_{it} are observed covariates for the ith individual, which can be simulated from the distribution of X_{it}. A real example is given later in which case-control samples are generated with individual age and sex and the distributions of age and sex are fitted based on a real dataset. Given the underlying genetic model, f_{0i} and f_{2i}, f_{1i} can be calculated for the ith individual. Then, for each $i = 1, \ldots, n$, calculate

$$k_i = \sum_{j=0}^{2} g_j f_{ji}, \quad p_{ji} = \frac{g_j f_{ji}}{k_i}, \quad \text{and} \quad q_{ji} = \frac{g_j(1 - f_{ji})}{(1 - k_i)}, \quad \text{for } j = 0, 1, 2.$$

The genotype of a case (or a control) with covariates $X_{it} = x_{it}$ ($t = 1, \ldots, T$) can be simulated from $Mul(1; p_{0i}, p_{1i}, p_{2i})$ (or $Mul(1; q_{0i}, q_{1i}, q_{2i})$). This can be repeated until all r cases and s controls are generated.

For example, consider a GWAS for age-related macular degeneration (AMD). The data contains 46 cases and 50 controls with the covariates age and sex. The following logistic regression model for the reference penetrance is used

$$f_0 = \Pr(\text{case}|\text{sex}, \text{age}) = \frac{\exp(\beta_0 + \beta_1 \text{sex} + \beta_2 \text{age})}{1 + \exp(\beta_0 + \beta_1 \text{sex} + \beta_2 \text{age})}. \tag{3.26}$$

Fitting the above model using the real data, the estimates of β_0, β_1 and β_2 are -18.99 (p-value $= 0.0000186$), 0.45 (p-value $= 0.239$), and 0.22 (p-value $= 0.0000356$). Then, for the ith individual, (3.26) is modified to

$$f_{0i} = \frac{\exp(\widehat{\beta}_0 + \widehat{\beta}_1 \text{sex} + \widehat{\beta}_2 \text{age})}{1 + \exp(\widehat{\beta}_0 + \widehat{\beta}_1 \text{sex} + \widehat{\beta}_2 \text{age})},$$

where the age and sex for the ith individual are generated from the normal and binomial distributions whose parameters are estimated based on the observed AMD data. For a given GRR λ_2, $f_{2i} = \lambda_2 f_{0i}$ is calculated. If a genetic model is assumed, λ_{1i} can be obtained based on the underlying genetic model. Then, the procedures in Sect. 3.9.2 can be followed.

3.10 Adjusting out Covariates

The statistical methods to test for association introduced in this chapter use either the genotype data or the allele data (Tables 3.1 and 3.3). In practice, measured covariates are also available, including age, sex, and race. If a covariate is associated with the disease, it may be a confounder for association between the genetic marker and the disease. Adjusting out and correcting for such confounding effects is important in a genetic association study. Not all procedures that are covered in this chapter can allow adjusting out covariates. The genotype-based and allele-based analyses, however, can allow for covariates using the prospective logistic regression model.

As shown in Sect. 3.3.2 and Sect. 3.3.4, the trend test and Pearson's chi-squared test can be obtained from the logistic regression models. To adjust out covariates X, we modify the logistic regression models in (3.9) and (3.12) as

$$\Pr(\text{case} \,|\, G, X) = \frac{\exp(\beta_0 + \beta_1 I(G) + \beta_X X)}{1 + \exp(\beta_0 + \beta_1 I(G) + \beta_X X)},$$

$$\Pr(\text{case} \,|\, I_1(G), I_2(G), X) = \frac{\exp(\beta_0 + \beta_1 I_1(G) + \beta_2 I_2(G) + \beta_X X)}{1 + \exp(\beta_0 + \beta_1 I_1(G) + \beta_2 I_2(G) + \beta_X X)},$$

respectively. The null hypotheses of no association between the genetic marker and the disease are stated as $H_0 : \beta_1 = 0$ and $H_0 : \beta_1 = \beta_2 = 0$, respectively. The Score test, LRT and Wald test given in Sect. 1.2.4 can be applied.

3.11 Examples and Case Studies

3.11.1 Data from Genome-Wide Association Studies

Seventeen SNPs were chosen from four GWAS: AMD, prostate cancer, breast cancer, and hypertension. These SNPs were reported to have true association with the diseases (see Sect. 3.12). Table 3.10 reports the genotype counts for each SNP with a unique SNP ID. The minor alleles are defined using the controls, that is, an allele is minor if its allele frequency is equal to $\min\{(2s_0 + s_1)/(2s_0 + 2s_1 + 2s_2), (2s_2 + s_1)/(2s_0 + 2s_1 + 2s_2)\}$. Then the frequency of that allele in cases is estimated. Using SNP rs380390 as an example, the allele frequencies for A and B are $(2 \times 6 + 25)/\{2(6 + 25 + 19)\} = 0.37$ and $(2 \times 19 + 25)/\{2(6 + 25 + 19)\} = 0.63$, respectively. Thus, allele A is minor. The frequency of allele A in cases is $(2 \times 50 + 35)/\{2(50 + 35 + 11)\} \approx 0.7031$, which appears in the first row of Table 3.10.

3.11.2 Association Tests

Using the data in Table 3.10, four test statistics (the ABT, the trend test for the ADD model, Pearson's test and Fisher's combination of the trend test and the HWDTT) and their corresponding p-values are calculated. The p-values were obtained from the asymptotic distributions of the test statistics without assuming which is the risk allele. The results are reported in Table 3.11. Overall, the ABT and CATT with the score $x = 1/2$ have comparable p-values, but Pearson's test and Fisher's combination test are more robust. For example, there are three SNPs (rs12505080, rs7696175, and rs2398162) associated with breast cancer that have p-values greater than 0.05 using Z_{ABT} and Z_{CATT} but have much stronger evidence of association when $T_{\chi_2^2}$ and T_F are used.

To illustrate the exact tests, we only consider the first two SNPs in Table 3.10. The exact tests for the genotype and allelic data are considered. The p-values for

Table 3.10 The genotype distributions and MAFs for the 17 SNPs with true associations in four genetic studies

SNP ID	MAFs		Cases			Controls		
	cases	controls	r_0	r_1	r_2	s_0	s_1	s_2
AMD								
rs380390	0.7031	0.3700	50	35	11	6	25	19
rs1329428	0.1489	0.4063	2	24	68	5	29	14
Prostate cancer								
rs1447295	0.1421	0.1029	25	283	864	10	218	929
rs6983267	0.5546	0.4896	223	598	351	301	579	277
rs7837688	0.1439	0.0986	27	283	861	11	206	939
Breast cancer								
rs10510126	0.0873	0.1316	10	180	955	14	272	854
rs12505080	0.2542	0.2670	50	477	608	99	408	628
rs17157903	0.1584	0.1227	18	316	777	26	220	862
rs1219648	0.4555	0.3848	250	543	352	170	538	433
rs7696175	0.4275	0.4356	187	605	353	249	496	396
rs2420946	0.4498	0.3796	242	546	357	165	537	440
Hypertension								
rs2820037	0.1709	0.1410	40	587	1325	72	684	2180
rs6997709	0.2441	0.2851	118	716	1116	237	1201	1500
rs7961152	0.4605	0.4147	416	963	570	492	1448	992
rs11110912	0.2002	0.1652	67	647	1237	83	804	2049
rs1937506	0.2480	0.2886	113	742	1097	244	1205	1484
rs2398162	0.2180	0.2581	111	624	1205	194	1121	1608

the first SNP (rs380390) are 4.56e$-$7 (genotype-based) and 2.30e$-$8 (allele-based). The p-values for the second SNP (rs1329428) are 1.28e$-$6 (genotype-based) and 1.42e$-$6 (allele-based). Two types of notation are used for p-values. Here 4.56e$-$7 (or 4.56E$-$7) is equivalent to 4.56×10^{-7}.

3.11.3 Estimates of Odds Ratios

Finally we calculate ORs and their 95% CIs (Sect. 3.8). Three ORs are considered. The first one is based on the linear trend or the ADD model. The estimate of the OR (or the log OR) under the ADD model is evaluated numerically. Standard software reports the OR and its 95% CI under the ADD model once scores $(0, 1/2, 1)$ are chosen. When the OR is greater (less) than 1, it indicates that the logit of the probability of having the disease increases linearly with the number of the risk allele B

Table 3.11 Test statistics and p-values for the 17 SNPs in Table 3.10. The trend test has the scores $(0, 1/2, 1)$ indicating the proportion of B alleles in the genotype

SNP ID	ABT		CATT(1/2)		χ_2^2		Fisher's	
	Z_{ABT}	p-value	Z_{CATT}	p-value	$T_{\chi_2^2}$	p-value	T_F	p-value
rs380390	-5.49	4.01e-8	-5.12	3.10e-7	26.51	1.75e-6	32.35	1.62e-6
rs1329428	4.83	1.36e-6	4.92	8.70e-7	25.05	3.64e-6	33.51	9.39e-7
rs1447295	-4.08	4.50e-5	-4.08	4.50e-5	17.12	1.91e-4	21.45	2.58e-4
rs6983267	4.44	9.03e-6	4.47	7.91e-6	20.54	3.46e-5	25.08	4.84e-5
rs7837688	-4.73	2.26e-6	-4.69	2.68e-6	22.15	1.55e-5	26.81	2.17e-5
rs10510126	4.79	1.66e-6	4.83	1.38e-6	25.02	3.69e-6	26.19	3.02e-6
rs12505080	0.98	3.27e-1	0.99	3.24e-1	21.82	1.83e-5	29.13	2.90e-5
rs17157903	-3.41	6.30e-4	-3.42	6.32e-4	23.05	9.87e-6	28.66	7.37e-6
rs1219648	-4.84	1.28e-6	-4.77	1.81e-6	26.61	7.46e-6	26.52	9.15e-6
rs7696175	0.55	5.82e-1	0.55	5.85e-1	22.07	1.61e-5	28.17	2.49e-5
rs2420946	-4.82	1.46e-6	-4.76	1.94e-6	23.28	8.80e-6	35.06	1.15e-5
rs2820037	-4.02	5.94e-5	-4.02	5.76e-5	28.17	7.66e-7	23.97	4.51e-7
rs6997709	4.47	7.71e-6	4.47	7.88e-6	20.08	4.36e-5	25.29	8.10e-5
rs7961152	-4.47	7.87e-6	-4.48	7.39e-6	20.81	3.03e-5	27.46	4.40e-5
rs11110912	-4.41	1.01e-5	-4.44	9.18e-6	21.70	1.94e-5	44.89	1.61e-5
rs1937506	4.42	9.77e-6	4.43	9.23e-6	20.00	4.53e-5	43.19	6.67e-5
rs2398162	4.52	6.22e-6	4.47	7.85e-6	24.16	5.67e-6	28.99	7.85e-6

(A) in the genotype. This association is significant at the 0.05 level if the 95% CI does not contain 1.

The other two types of ORs compare $AB + BB$ versus AA and $AB + AA$ versus BB. When B is the risk allele, the first type assumes a DOM model while the second type assumes a REC model. However, when A is the risk allele, the DOM and REC models are switched. For the REC and DOM models, ORs and their confidence intervals can be obtained explicitly (Sect. 3.8). However, they can also be obtained from the standard logistic regression model by scoring the three genotypes by $(0, 0, 1)$ for the REC model and $(0, 1, 1)$ for the DOM model when B is the risk allele.

All three types of ORs and their CIs are reported in Table 3.12. The results in Table 3.12 show that whether the CIs contain 1 may depend on the underlying genetic model. For example, for SNP rs12505080, when B is the risk allele, the OR for comparing $AB + BB$ versus AA is significant at the 0.05 level, which indicates a strong DOM effect. But the other two ORs are not significant. On the other hand, some SNPs are significant regardless of the underlying genetic model. Therefore, reporting ORs along with their corresponding genetic models is important. A genetic model could be determined *a priori*; otherwise ORs for all genetic models need to be reported, not just choosing a genetic model with the significant OR.

Table 3.12 The ORs and their 95% CIs for the 17 SNPs with true associations in four genetic studies

SNP ID	ADD model		$AB+BB$ vs AA		$AB+AA$ vs BB	
	OR	CI	OR	CI	OR	CI
rs380390	0.27	(0.16, 0.46)	0.13	(0.05, 0.32)	0.21	(0.09, 0.49)
rs1329428	4.80	(2.44, 9.46)	5.35	(1.00, 28.7)	6.35	(2.94, 13.7)
rs1447295	0.69	(0.58, 0.83)	0.40	(0.19, 0.84)	0.69	(0.58, 0.84)
rs6983267	1.30	(1.16, 1.47)	1.50	(1.23, 1.82)	1.36	(1.13, 1.63)
rs7837688	0.65	(0.55, 0.78)	0.41	(0.20, 0.83)	0.64	(0.53, 0.78)
rs10510126	1.60	(1.32, 1.94)	1.41	(0.62, 3.19)	1.68	(1.37, 2.07)
rs12505080	1.07	(0.94, 1.22)	2.07	(1.46, 2.94)	0.93	(0.79, 1.10)
rs17157903	0.74	(0.63, 0.88)	1.46	(0.80, 2.68)	0.66	(0.55, 0.80)
rs1219648	0.75	(0.67, 0.85)	0.63	(0.51, 0.78)	0.73	(0.61, 0.86)
rs7696175	1.03	(0.92, 1.16)	1.43	(1.16, 1.77)	0.84	(0.70, 1.00)
rs2420946	0.75	(0.67, 0.85)	0.63	(0.51, 0.78)	0.72	(0.61, 0.86)
rs2820037	0.80	(0.71, 0.89)	1.20	(0.81, 1.78)	0.73	(0.65, 0.83)
rs6997709	1.24	(1.13, 1.35)	1.36	(1.08, 1.71)	1.28	(1.14, 1.44)
rs7961152	0.83	(0.76, 0.90)	0.74	(0.64, 0.86)	0.81	(0.71, 0.92)
rs11110912	0.79	(0.71, 0.88)	0.82	(0.59, 1.14)	0.75	(0.66, 0.85)
rs1937506	1.23	(1.12, 1.35)	1.48	(1.17, 1.86)	1.25	(1.12, 1.41)
rs2398162	1.24	(1.13, 1.37)	1.17	(0.92, 1.49)	1.34	(1.19, 1.51)

3.12 Bibliographical Comments

Several test statistics for association are discussed. The CATT, the ABT and Pearson's chi-squared test are most commonly used in analysis for case-control genetic associations. Sham [240], Thomas [270], Ziegler and Köenig [351], and Siegmund and Yakir [245] also contain some of these association test statistics. Two reviews also discussed basic statistical tests for the analysis of case-control data (Balding [12] and Li [171]).

Armitage [9] and Cochran [40] proposed the trend test to analyze a linear trend in ordered categorical data (Agresti [4]). Sasieni [223] compared the trend test and the ABT for testing genetic association using case-control samples. In particular, he studied some conditions under which the two tests are asymptotically equivalent under the null hypothesis. The choice of scores in the trend test has been extensively discussed in the context of the analysis of ordered categorical data (e.g., Graubard and Korn [106]) and case-control genetic association studies (Sasieni [223], Devlin and Roeder [60], Slager and Schaid [248], Freidlin et al. [91], and Zheng et al. [336]). Kim et al. [143] show that the association model becomes the ADD as the distance between two loci increases regardless of the true genetic model. Zheng et al. [340] show that, when the marker and the functional locus have imperfect LD, the genetic model space defined at the functional locus tends to shrink towards the ADD model at the marker. That means that there are no pure REC or DOM models at the marker locus unless the linkage disequilibrium is perfect, a justification for using the ADD model as a robust model under model uncertainty. More discussion of robust tests will be provided in Chap. 6.

Zheng and Gastwirth [345] discussed the two different estimates of the variance in the trend test obtained by using the combined case-control samples or the separate case-control samples. Skol et al. [246] estimated the variance of the ABT using the separate case-control samples. Expressing Pearson's chi-squared test in terms of the trend tests or the logistic regression model was used by Zheng et al. [335] to correct for population substructure for tests with two degrees of freedom, and by Zheng et al. [343] to prove that the ratio of the trend test to Pearson's test and Pearson's test are asymptotically independent under the null hypothesis of no association.

The asymptotic equivalence of the trend test (for the ADD model) and the ABT under the null hypothesis has been studied by Sasieni [223], Guedj et al. [108], and Knapp [146]. Sasieni [223] studied Hardy-Weinberg proportions in the combined samples while Guedj et al. [108] and Knapp [146] considered Hardy-Weinberg proportions in the population. The condition for the asymptotic equivalence between these two tests under the alternative hypothesis has been studied by Zheng [329], who related the condition to the sampling scheme in the retrospective case-control design. Schaid and Jacobsen [233] and Knapp [145] studied the impact of departure from Hardy-Weinberg proportions on the ABT and provided some corrections. Issues of testing Hardy-Weinberg proportions can be found in Zou and Donner [355]. See Nielsen et al. [193] and Song and Elston [250] for using departure from HWD (Weir [299]) to detect association. Song and Elston [251] further studied the HWDTT and proposed to combine it with the trend test for the ADD model in a linear combination. Other combinations have been studied by Li [163], Zheng et al. [345] and Zheng et al. [343].

Exact tests are covered in many biostatistics textbooks, e.g., Lachin [156]. Many algorithms for calculating the exact p-value for a 2×2 or 2×3 tables are available. See [5, 181] and [212]. Applications of exact tests in case-control studies can be found in Neuhauser [192] and Guedj et al. [107]. In the case of the trend test for association using case-control data with a multiallelic marker, Czika and Weir [52] proposed a linear trend test. Exploring Hardy-Weinberg proportions, Chen and Chatterjee [32] studied a new class of tests for association, which may be more powerful than the linear combination of the trend test and the HWDTT of Song and Elston [251].

The data for the four GWAS were used by Li et al. [170]. Klein et al. [144] studied 100,000 SNPs for AMD. The prostate cancer, breast cancer, and hypertension data were studied by Yeager et al. [313], Hunter et al. [127], and the Wellcome Trust Case-Control Consortium [301], respectively. For the last three studies, about 300,000 to 500,000 SNPs were used.

3.13 Problems

3.1 Prove the equations and inequalities for the ADD and MUL models given in (3.24) and (3.25).

3.2 Derive the variance of the statistic U for the trend test given in (3.6).

3.3 Using the prospective log-likelihood function for case-control samples, show that the observed Fisher information matrix can be written as

$$
-\begin{bmatrix}
\dfrac{\partial^2 l}{\partial \beta_1^2} & \dfrac{\partial^2 l}{\partial \beta_1 \beta_0} \\[2ex]
\dfrac{\partial^2 l}{\partial \beta_0 \beta_1} & \dfrac{\partial^2 l}{\partial \beta_0^2}
\end{bmatrix}_{\beta=\tilde{\beta}}
= \frac{rs}{n^2}
\begin{bmatrix}
\displaystyle\sum_{j=0}^{2} x_j^2 n_j & \displaystyle\sum_{j=0}^{2} x_j n_j \\[2ex]
\displaystyle\sum_{j=0}^{2} x_j n_j & n
\end{bmatrix}.
$$

3.4 Derive Pearson's test as a Score test.

(a) Show the Score functions can be written as

$$
U_1(\tilde{\beta}) = \frac{\partial l}{\partial \beta_1}\Big|_{\beta=\tilde{\beta}} = \frac{1}{n}(sr_2 - rs_2),
$$

$$
U_2(\tilde{\beta}) = \frac{\partial l}{\partial \beta_2}\Big|_{\beta=\tilde{\beta}} = \frac{1}{n}\{s(r_1 + r_2) - r(s_1 + s_2)\}.
$$

(b) Find the observed Fisher information matrix evaluated under H_0 where β_0 is replaced with $\tilde{\beta}_0$.
(c) Find the inverse of the observed Fisher information matrix.
(d) Show that the Score statistic obtained from the logistic regression model can be written as (3.13).

3.5 Show that $T_{\chi_2^2}$ in (3.11) and $\tilde{T}_{\chi_2^2}$ in (3.13) are equivalent.

3.6 Show that the conditions $4n_0 n_2 - n_1^2 = 0$ and $\bar{p}_2 = (\bar{p}_2 + \bar{p}_1/2)^2$ are equivalent.

3.7 Assume $r/n \to \phi \in (0, 1)$ as $n \to \infty$. Find the limit of $\widehat{p}_2 - \widehat{p}^2$ under the alternative hypothesis of association H_1, where $\widehat{p}_2 = n_2/n$ and $\widehat{p}^2 = (2n_2 + n_1)/(2n)$. Discuss when the above limit is zero under H_1 if HWE proportions hold in the population (Hint: $\phi = k = \Pr(\text{case})$).

3.8 Comparison of the variance estimates for the trend test and the ABT.

(a) Write an R program (or other program) to simulate 1,000 replicates of case-control samples without covariates under the null hypothesis (GRRs $\lambda_1 = \lambda_2 = 1$), each with $p = \Pr(B) = 0.2$, Hardy-Weinberg proportions in the population, equal numbers of cases and controls with total sample size $n = 100$, and the disease prevalence $k = 0.10$.

(b) Apply the trend tests to the 1,000 simulated datasets with three different scores $(0,0,0)$, $(0,1/2,1)$, and $(0,1,1)$, each with the variances estimated from the separate case-control samples and the combined case-control samples. Using the significance level $\alpha = 0.05$, estimate the probability of Type I error for each of the six trend tests from the 1,000 replicates (combinations of three sets of scores and two variance estimates). Keep other parameters the same, and repeat this for $n = 500$ and $n = 2{,}000$. Summarize your results of the estimated Type I error rates.

(c) Apply the ABT to the same 1,000 simulated datasets with the two different variance estimates. Repeat problem (b) for the ABT with different variance estimates.

3.9 Choices of scores for the trend and genetic models.

Write an R program (or other program) to conduct simulation studies to examine how the power of the trend test depends on the choices of scores when the underlying genetic models are REC, ADD, MUL and DOM.

3.10 Show that $E(\widehat{\Delta}_p - \widehat{\Delta}_q) = 0$ under the MUL model (Sect. 3.6). Hence, Z_{HWDTT} cannot be applied to test for association under the MUL model.

3.11 Asymptotic null correlations between $Z_{\text{CATT}}(x)$ and Z_{HWDTT}.

Using the results of Problem 1.11 show that, when Hardy-Weinberg proportions hold in the population and under H_0,

$$\text{Corr}(Z_{\text{CATT}}(0), Z_{\text{HWDTT}}) = \sqrt{\frac{1-p}{1+p}} + o(n^{-1}),$$

$$\text{Corr}(Z_{\text{CATT}}(1/2), Z_{\text{HWDTT}}) = o(n^{-1}),$$

$$\text{Corr}(Z_{\text{CATT}}(1), Z_{\text{HWDTT}}) = -\sqrt{\frac{p}{2-p}} + o(n^{-1}),$$

where p is the frequency of allele B (see Zheng and Ng [344]).

3.12 Let p_1 and p_2 be p-values of two asymptotically independent test statistics. Fisher's combination test $T_F = -2\log(p_1) - 2\log(p_2)$ asymptotically follows a chi-squared distribution with 4 degrees of freedom. Show that the p-value of Fisher's combination test is given by $p = p_1 p_2 \{1 - \log(p_1 p_2)\}$. [Note that the CDF for T_F is $F(x) = 1 - (1 + x/2)\exp(-x/2)$.]

3.13 The HWDTT is based on the estimate of the difference in HWD between cases and controls. Modify the HWDTT to be based only on the estimate of HWD using cases. Conduct a simulation study to compare the power of the original HWDTT with the modified one on changing the disease prevalence.

Chapter 4
Single-Marker Analysis for Matched Case-Control Data

Abstract Chapter 4 studies a matched case-control design. Matching is often used to control for confounding variables and a known population stratification. The typical method for the analysis of a matched case-control study is the conditional logistic regression model. This chapter focuses on a matched retrospective case-control study using the conditional approach with a prospective likelihood. It discusses $1 : m$ ($m = 1$) matching and a more flexible matching such that m is not fixed but changes over the different matched sets. The matched trend test, the matched disequilibrium test, and a model-free test are derived. Methods to simulate matched case-control data are discussed. Results of simulation studies are reported.

Matching is a technique that is often used in epidemiological studies to control for confounding variables and known population stratification. Common confounding variables for genetic case-control association studies include race, sex, and age. Unlike an unmatched case-control study, which is usually analyzed based on the unconditional logistic regression model (e.g., the CATT and Pearson's chi-squared test in Chap. 3), the typical method for the analysis of a matched case-control study is the conditional logistic regression model. We focus on analyses of a matched retrospective case-control study using the conditional approach with a prospective likelihood.

For a matched design, the values of the confounding variables are used to define strata from which matched sets are sampled. A matched set contains one case and one or more controls so that the case and controls share the same confounding variable values. In each stratum, previous concepts for unmatched designs (e.g., penetrance, prevalence, GRRs and genetic models) can be directly used. The matched trend tests (MTTs) are first introduced with score specifications corresponding to various underlying genetic models. The MTT is an extension of McNemar's test, and can be used to test association of a marker with the disease under study. Asymptotically, the test statistic follows a chi-squared distribution with one degree of freedom. Matched disequilibrium tests (MDTs) also have an asymptotic chi-squared distribution with one degree of freedom. They compare the average scores of genotypes in cases and controls within each matched set. Both tests depend on the underlying genetic model. The model-free two-degree-of-freedom chi-squared test, analogous to Pearson's test, is also known as the Cochran-Mantel-Haenszel test and

G. Zheng et al., *Analysis of Genetic Association Studies*,
Statistics for Biology and Health,
DOI 10.1007/978-1-4614-2245-7_4, © Springer Science+Business Media, LLC 2012

Table 4.1 Genotype counts for a single marker with alleles A and B in a matched pair design with n matched sets

Cases	Controls			Total
	AA	AB	BB	
AA	m_{00}	m_{01}	m_{02}	r_0
AB	m_{10}	m_{11}	m_{12}	r_1
BB	m_{20}	m_{21}	m_{22}	r_2
Total	s_0	s_1	s_2	n

can be expressed in terms of matched trend tests. We focus on the above three tests for a $1 : m$ matched design, in which each matched set contains one case and $m \geq 1$ controls (including the $1 : 1$ and $1 : 2$ matched designs). Statistics for more general situations with a variable number of controls matched to each case will also be discussed. Robust statistics for a matched case-control design will be discussed in Chap. 6.

Using simulation studies, we compare the performance of the above three test statistics under the null and alternative hypotheses for various genetic models. Estimates of RRs and ORs for a matched design are studied. Their large sample properties and confidence intervals are provided. We focus on analyses based on genotypes of cases and controls. Finally, technical comments are given.

4.1 Notation and Models

Suppose the values of confounding variables z are used to define J strata, denoted by $\{z_1, \ldots, z_J\}$. For example, if sex (male and female) and race (African American and Caucasian) are the only confounding variables, four strata can be formed ($J = 4$). Then n matched sets are sampled. Each matched set contains one case and m controls, all belonging to the same stratum. This matching is referred to as $1 : m$ matching. In practice, owing to the cost of matching, m is often taken to be 1 or 2 and is rarely larger than 5. The $1 : 1$ matched design is also called a matched pair design. When a continuous confounding variable, such as age, is taken into account, a discretization technique is often employed. For example, a five-year window can be used to stratify on age. Then, race, sex and discretized age can be used to define strata, from which we sample matched sets with one case and m controls having the same race, same sex and age within five years. In a matched set, if the case or all the controls are missing, then this matched set does not contain information about the association between the disease status and the genetic marker. Hence, we assume a matched set contains one case and at least one control.

The genotype counts for a matched pair design with n matched sets are given in Table 4.1. A total of $2n$ genotypes are observed for the n matched sets. In Table 4.1, there are m_{00} matched sets in which both case and control have genotype AA, and m_{01} matched sets in which the case has genotype AA and the control has

Table 4.2 Genotype counts of a single marker with alleles A and B in a $1 : 2$ matched design with n matched sets

Cases	Controls						Total
	AA, AA	AA, AB	AA, BB	AB, AB	AB, BB	BB, BB	
AA	$m_{0,00}$	$m_{0,01}$	$m_{0,02}$	$m_{0,11}$	$m_{0,12}$	$m_{0,22}$	r_0
AB	$m_{1,00}$	$m_{1,01}$	$m_{1,02}$	$m_{1,11}$	$m_{1,12}$	$m_{1,22}$	r_1
BB	$m_{2,00}$	$m_{2,01}$	$m_{2,02}$	$m_{2,11}$	$m_{2,12}$	$m_{2,22}$	r_2
Total	s_{00}	s_{01}	s_{02}	s_{11}	s_{12}	s_{22}	n

Table 4.3 Example (ACCESS): genotype counts for the $KM(1,3)$ polymorphism in a matched pair design

Cases	Controls			Total
	AA	AB	BB	
AA	35	45	5	85
AB	57	40	9	106
BB	13	13	2	28
Total	105	98	16	219

genotype AB. Table 4.2 displays the genotype counts for a $1 : 2$ matched design with n matched sets and a total of $3n$ genotypes.

Table 4.3 is a subset of the matched pair data from a case-control etiologic study of sarcoidosis (ACCESS). There are 219 African-American matched pairs presented in the table, who were matched based on age (within 5 years) and sex. The candidate gene presented in Table 4.3 is the $KM(1,3)$ polymorphism, whose alleles are denoted by A and B. Age is not shown in Table 4.3. If we define six categories based on male and female and three categories for ages: age group $= 1$ if age ≤ 40; age group $= 2$ if age is > 40 and ≤ 60, and age group $= 3$ if age > 60, then the matched pairs in Table 4.3 can be displayed as in Table 4.4, where the information on matching is retained.

We have focused on $1 : m$ matching, but the general situation is that a case and a variable number of controls are matched in the various matched sets. In the latter case, we divide the n matched sets into $n_1, \ldots, n_m$ sets such that $n = \sum_{j=1}^{m} n_j$, where n_j is the number of matched sets in which j controls are matched to a case for $j = 1, \ldots, m$. The total number of matched sets is still n. Hence, each matched set contains one case and at least one control. A matched pair design and a $1 : m$ matched design can be obtained as special cases.

The following notation is used in this chapter. Assume cases and controls are matched based on the values of confounding variables z with a total of J strata $\{z_1, \ldots, z_J\}$. The notation and definitions of the penetrances and the disease prevalence for an unmatched case-control study can be used in each stratum for the matched design. In the jth stratum (note that the index j was used before to indicate

Table 4.4 Stratifying the matched pair data in Table 4.3 into six strata

Female age group	Cases	Controls		
		AA	AB	BB
	AA	9	10	0
1	AB	21	15	6
	BB	6	5	0
	AA	12	20	4
2	AB	17	10	1
	BB	2	6	1
	AA	3	4	0
3	AB	2	1	1
	BB	0	0	0

Male age group	Cases	Controls		
		AA	AB	BB
	AA	8	5	1
1	AB	8	8	1
	BB	2	1	1
	AA	3	6	0
2	AB	8	5	0
	BB	3	1	0
	AA	0	0	0
3	AB	1	1	0
	BB	0	0	0

the jth control in a matched set), denote $k_j = \Pr(\text{case}\,|z_j)$, $p_{ij} = \Pr(G_i\,|\,\text{case}, z_j)$, $q_{ij} = \Pr(G_i\,|\,\text{control}, z_j)$, $g_{ij} = \Pr(G_i\,|z_j)$, and $f_{ij} = \Pr(\text{case}\,|G_i, z_j)$ for $i = 0, 1, 2$ and $j = 1, \ldots, J$. Then, for $j = 1, \ldots, J$,

$$p_{ij} = g_{ij} f_{ij}/k_j \quad \text{and} \quad q_{ij} = g_{ij}(1 - f_{ij})/(1 - k_j).$$

The GRRs are given by $\lambda_{1j} = f_{1j}/f_{0j}$ and $\lambda_{2j} = f_{2j}/f_{0j}$. Given λ_{2j} and λ_{1j}, the REC, ADD, MUL and DOM models in each stratum are defined as before (see Sect. 3.2):

$$\lambda_{1j} = 1, \quad \lambda_{1j} = (1 + \lambda_{2j})/2, \quad \lambda_{1j} = \lambda_{2j}^{1/2}, \quad \text{and} \quad \lambda_{1j} = \lambda_{2j}$$

for all $j = 1, \ldots, J$. To pool information across strata, we need the following homogeneity assumption

$$\lambda_{1j} \equiv \lambda_1, \quad \lambda_{2j} \equiv \lambda_2.$$

4.2 Conditional Likelihoods for Matched Case-Control Data

Suppose the jth matched set has 1 case and m_j controls and $n_j = 1 + m_j$. The score for an individual is 0, x or 1 if his genotype is $G_0 = AA$, $G_1 = AB$ or $G_2 = BB$, where $x = 0$, $1/2$ and 1 for the REC, ADD/MUL, and DOM models. For a general set-up of a conditional likelihood, the score is denoted as X, which takes value of 0, x, or 1. The probabilities of a case or a control given any score X can be written as

$$\pi_1(X) = \Pr(\text{case}\,|X) = \frac{\exp(\alpha_j + X\beta)}{1 + \exp(\alpha_j + X\beta)},$$

$$\pi_0(X) = \Pr(\text{control}\,|X) = \frac{1}{1 + \exp(\alpha_j + X\beta)}.$$

Note that a common (homogeneous) β is assumed but we allow α_j vary across the matched sets, characterizing the stratum-specific properties. In the jth matched set, the n_j genotypes are conditionally independent. Denote the event that a randomly sampled individual from all n_j samples is a case by $(1, m_j)$. Let x_{ij} be the score for the ith individual, $i = 1, \ldots, n_j$. Like the analysis of unmatched data, the prospective conditional logistic regression model can be used for the matched retrospective case-control data. The conditional likelihood for the jth matched set can be written as

$$L_j(\beta|z) = \Pr(1 \text{ case with score } x_{1j} \text{ and } m_j \text{ controls with other scores}|(1, m_j))$$

$$= \frac{\pi_1(x_{1j}) \prod_{i=2}^{n_j} \pi_0(x_{ij})}{\sum_{l=1}^{n_j} \pi_1(x_{lj}) \prod_{l*\neq l} \pi_0(x_{l*j})} = \frac{\exp(\beta x_{1j})}{\sum_{l=1}^{n_j} \exp(\beta x_{lj})}. \tag{4.1}$$

For a $1 : m$ matched design, (4.1) can be used with n_j replaced by $m + 1$. In the conditional likelihood function (4.1), the nuisance parameter α_j is eliminated. The full conditional likelihood can be written as

$$L(\beta|z) = \prod_j L_j(\beta|z).$$

The above conditional likelihood function can also incorporate other covariates by changing βx_{ij} to $\beta^T x_{ij}$, where β and x_{ij} are both vectors.

4.3 Matched Trend Tests

We first consider the case that each matched set contains one case and m controls. The situation that a variable number of controls are matched to a case in some matched sets will be discussed later. For each individual, only the genotype score is considered as a covariate in the conditional likelihood function (4.1).

4.3.1 $1:m$ Matching

For the lth matched set with one case and m controls ($l = 1, \ldots, n$), let x_{1l} be the score for the case and x_{2lj} be the score for the jth control, $j = 1, \ldots, m$. The conditional likelihood function (4.1), $L(\beta|z)$, can be written as

$$L(\beta|z) = \prod_{l=1}^{n} \frac{\exp(\beta x_{1l})}{\exp(\beta x_{1l}) + \sum_{j=1}^{m} \exp(\beta x_{2lj})}.$$

The Score statistic for testing the null hypothesis of no association, $H_0 : \beta = 0$, can be written as (Problem 4.1)

$$Z_{\text{MTT}} = \frac{\sum_{l=1}^{n} \sum_{j=1}^{m} (x_{1l} - x_{2lj})}{[\sum_{l=1}^{n} \{\sum_{j=1}^{m} (x_{1l} - x_{2lj})^2 + \sum_{1 \le j_1 < j_2 \le m} (x_{2lj_1} - x_{2lj_2})^2\}]^{1/2}}. \tag{4.2}$$

Z_{MTT} is called the MTT, analogous to the trend test for unmatched case-control data (Sect. 3.3.1). Under H_0, $Z_{\text{MTT}} \sim N(0, 1)$ asymptotically for a given $x \in [0, 1]$. If the case and m controls in a matched set have the same genotype, then their scores are identical and

$$x_{1l} - x_{2lj} = x_{2lj_1} - x_{2lj_2} = 0.$$

Hence, this matched set does not contribute to the MTT.

$1:1$ Matching

When $m = 1$, (4.2) becomes

$$Z_{\text{MTT}} = \frac{\sum_{l=1}^{n} (x_{1l} - x_{2l})}{\sqrt{\sum_{l=1}^{n} (x_{1l} - x_{2l})^2}}, \tag{4.3}$$

where the subscript j is omitted in the score for the control $x_{2lj} = x_{2l}$. Using the data in Table 4.1, (4.3) can also be expressed as (Problem 4.3)

$$Z_{\text{MTT}} = \frac{\sum_{0 \le s < t \le 2} (m_{st} - m_{ts})(x_s - x_t)}{\sqrt{\sum_{0 \le s < t \le 2} (m_{st} + m_{ts})(x_s - x_t)^2}}, \tag{4.4}$$

where $(x_0, x_1, x_2) = (0, x, 1)$. From (4.4), it can be seen that the MTT is an extension of McNemar's test (4.5) for the matched design with three genotypes. The MTT depends on only the discordant matched sets, i.e. m_{st} for $s \ne t$.

Given the matched-pair data in Table 4.5 with two exposure levels, $+$ (the genetic susceptibility present) and $-$ (the genetic susceptibility not present), McNemar's test can be written as

$$T = \frac{(b - c)^2}{b + c} \sim \chi_1^2 \quad \text{under } H_0. \tag{4.5}$$

Table 4.5 Match pair data for McNemar's test

		Controls	
		+	−
Cases	+	a	b
	−	c	d

$1:2$ Matching

For $m = 2$, from Problem 4.4, the numerator of (4.2) using the data in Table 4.2 can be written as

$$\sum (x_{1l} - x_{2lj}) = x_{01}\{(m_{0,01} - 2m_{1,00}) + (2m_{0,11} - m_{1,01}) + (m_{0,12} - m_{1,02})\}$$
$$+ x_{02}\{(m_{0,02} - 2m_{2,00}) + (2m_{0,22} - m_{2,02}) + (m_{0,12} - m_{2,01})\}$$
$$+ x_{12}\{(m_{1,12} - 2m_{2,11}) + (2m_{1,22} - m_{2,12}) + (m_{1,02} - m_{2,01})\},$$

$$(4.6)$$

where $x_{st} = x_s - x_t$, and for the denominator of (4.2),

$$\sum (x_{1l} - x_{2lj})^2$$
$$= x_{01}^2\{(m_{0,01} + 2m_{1,00}) + (2m_{0,11} + m_{1,01}) + (m_{0,12} + m_{1,02})\}$$
$$+ x_{02}^2\{(m_{0,02} + 2m_{2,00}) + (2m_{0,22} + m_{2,02}) + (m_{0,12} + m_{2,01})\}$$
$$+ x_{12}^2\{(m_{1,12} + 2m_{2,11}) + (2m_{1,22} + m_{2,12}) + (m_{1,02} + m_{2,01})\}, \quad (4.7)$$

$$\text{and} \quad \sum (x_{2lj_1} - x_{2lj_2})^2 = x_{01}^2 s_{01} + x_{02}^2 s_{02} + x_{12}^2 s_{12}. \quad (4.8)$$

The ACCESS Example

Applying the MTT in (4.4) to Table 4.3 with a given x, the numerator of (4.4) is

$$(m_{01} - m_{10})(x_0 - x_1) + (m_{02} - m_{20})(x_0 - x_2) + (m_{12} - m_{21})(x_1 - x_2)$$
$$= (45 - 57)(0 - x) + (5 - 13)(0 - 1) + (9 - 13)(x - 1) = 8x + 12$$

and the denominator is

$$(m_{01} + m_{10})(x_0 - x_1)^2 + (m_{02} + m_{20})(x_0 - x_2)^2 + (m_{12} + m_{21})(x_1 - x_2)^2$$
$$= 102x^2 + 18 + 22(x - 1)^2 = 124x^2 - 44x + 40.$$

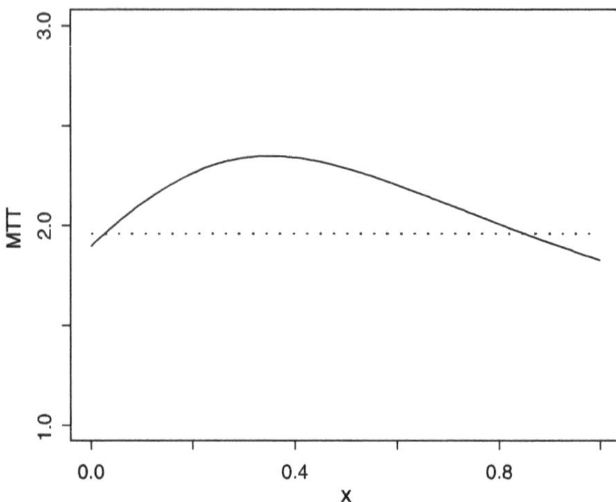

Fig. 4.1 Plot of the MTT given in (4.9) over the score $x \in [0, 1]$. The *dashed line* is the cut-off line for the 0.05 significance level

Hence, the MTT for a given x is

$$Z_{\mathrm{MTT}} = \frac{4x + 6}{\sqrt{31x^2 - 11x + 10}}. \tag{4.9}$$

Substituting $x = 0$, $1/2$ and 1, we obtain $Z_{\mathrm{MTT}} = 1.8974$, $Z_{\mathrm{MTT}} = 2.2857$, and $Z_{\mathrm{MTT}} = 1.8257$, respectively. If allele B of $KM(1, 3)$ is the risk allele, the corresponding p-values for the one-sided tests are 0.029, 0.011 and 0.034, all less than the significance level $\alpha = 0.05$. If the risk allele is unknown, then two-sided p-values are reported, which double the one-sided p-values. Therefore, only the test with the score $x = 1/2$ has a significant p-value. Although we consider $x = 0, 1/2, 1$ for various common genetic models, other values of $x \in [0, 1]$ can also be chosen.

Figure 4.1 plots the MTT over $x \in [0, 1]$ (the curve) with a dashed reference line corresponding to the significance level 0.05 (two-sided). For a given x, if the MTT is above the reference line, the test is significant at the 0.05 level (if multiple testing is ignored). Figure 4.1 shows that, except for the values near the endpoints of $x \in [0, 1]$, the MTT is significant at the 0.05 level. This example also shows that the result depends on the choice of score x. Robust tests studied in Chap. 6 are useful when the results depend on the choice of the score, i.e., the underlying genetic model.

4.3.2 A Variable Number of Controls and a Case Are Matched

Assume that, in some matched sets, a variable number of controls and a case are matched. For the lth matched set with one case and i controls, let x_{1il} be the score for the case and x_{2ilj} be the score for the jth control, $j = 1, \ldots, i$, $l = 1, \ldots, n_i$, and $i = 1, \ldots, m$. In this setting, we have n_i matched sets in which a case and i controls are matched. The total number of matched sets is $n = \sum_{i=1}^{m} n_i$. Under this setting, the conditional likelihood function (4.1), $L(\beta|z)$, can be written as

$$L(\beta|z) = \prod_{i=1}^{m} \prod_{l=1}^{n_i} \frac{\exp(\beta x_{1il})}{\exp(\beta x_{1il}) + \sum_{j=1}^{i} \exp(\beta x_{2ilj})}.$$

The Score test statistic for testing the null hypothesis of no association, $H_0 : \beta = 0$, can be written as

$$Z_{\mathrm{MTT}}$$

$$= \frac{\sum_{i=1}^{m} \frac{1}{1+i} \sum_{l=1}^{n_i} (i x_{1il} - \sum_{j=1}^{i} x_{2ilj})}{[\sum_{i=1}^{m} \frac{1}{(1+i)^2} \sum_{l=1}^{n_i} \{(1+i)(x_{1il}^2 + \sum_{j=1}^{i} x_{2ilj}^2) - (x_{1il} + \sum_{j=1}^{i} x_{2ilj})^2\}]^{1/2}}.$$

$$(4.10)$$

Under H_0, $Z_{\mathrm{MTT}} \sim N(0, 1)$ asymptotically for a given $x \in [0, 1]$. The MTT given in (4.2) is a special case of (4.10) given above.

For an alternative expression, let n_{il0} and n_{il1} be the numbers of AA and AB genotypes in the lth matched set with one case and i controls. Using the result in Problem 4.2, the MTT given in (4.10) can be written as

$$Z_{\mathrm{MTT}} = \frac{\sum_{i=1}^{m} \sum_{l=1}^{n_i} \{x_{1il} - \mathrm{E}_{H_0}(x_{1il}|n_{il0}, n_{il1})\}}{\sqrt{\sum_{i=1}^{m} \sum_{l=1}^{n_i} \mathrm{Var}_{H_0}(x_{1il}|n_{il0}, n_{il1})}}. \qquad (4.11)$$

Another expression for Z_{MTT} can also be obtained using the results in Problem 4.5.

4.4 Matching Disequilibrium Tests

For the matching disequilibrium test (MDT), the situation that a variable number of controls and a case are matched is not complicated. Hence, we first consider this case and obtain the $1 : m$ matching as a special case.

4.4.1 A Variable Number of Controls and a Case Are Matched

Using the notation of Sect. 4.3.2, consider a matched case-control design with n matched sets, where n_i matched sets contain one case and i matched controls, $i = 1, \ldots, m$ and $n = \sum_{i=1}^{m} n_i$. Let the following scores for genotypes be defined as in Sect. 4.3.2:

$$\{(x_{1il}, x_{2ilj}) : j = 1, \ldots, i; l = 1, \ldots, n_i; i = 1, \ldots, m\}.$$

For a matched set with one case and i controls, the average score for controls is $\sum_{j=1}^{i} x_{2ilj}/i$. Then, for this matched set, the difference of the mean scores between the case and controls is given by

$$d_{il} = x_{1il} - \frac{1}{i} \sum_{j=1}^{i} x_{2ilj}.$$

The average of d_{il} over all matched sets can be written as

$$D = \frac{1}{n} \sum_{i=1}^{m} \sum_{l=1}^{n_i} d_{il} = \frac{1}{n} \sum_{i=1}^{m} \sum_{l=1}^{n_i} \left(x_{1il} - \frac{1}{i} \sum_{j=1}^{i} x_{2ilj} \right).$$

The association can be tested based on D. Under the null hypothesis of no association H_0, $\mathrm{E}(D) = 0$. Thus, $\mathrm{Var}(D) = \mathrm{E}(D^2)$ where,

$$\mathrm{E}(D^2) = \frac{1}{n^2} \sum_{i=1}^{m} \sum_{l=1}^{n_i} \mathrm{E}_{H_0}(d_{il}^2) = \frac{1}{n} \mathrm{E}_{H_0}(d_{11}^2).$$

A consistent moment estimate of $\mathrm{Var}(D)$ under H_0 is given by

$$\widehat{\mathrm{Var}}(D) = \frac{1}{n^2} \sum_{i=1}^{m} \sum_{l=1}^{n_i} \left(x_{1il} - \frac{1}{i} \sum_{j=1}^{i} x_{2ilj} \right)^2.$$

The MDT can be written as

$$Z_{\mathrm{MDT}} = \frac{\sum_{i=1}^{m} \sum_{l=1}^{n_i} (x_{1il} - \sum_{j=1}^{i} x_{2ilj}/i)}{\sqrt{\sum_{i=1}^{m} \sum_{l=1}^{n_i} (x_{1il} - \sum_{j=1}^{i} x_{2ilj}/i)^2}}. \tag{4.12}$$

Under H_0, $Z_{\mathrm{MDT}} \sim N(0, 1)$ asymptotically for a given $x \in [0, 1]$.

4.4.2 1 : m Matching

For the special $1 : m$ matched design, denote the scores by (x_{1l}, x_{2lj}) for $l = 1, \ldots, n$ and $j = 1, \ldots, m$ as in Sect. 4.3.1. Then Z_{MDT} given in (4.12) can be simplified to

$$Z_{\mathrm{MDT}} = \frac{\sum_{l=1}^{n} (m x_{1l} - \sum_{j=1}^{m} x_{2lj})}{\sqrt{\sum_{l=1}^{n} (m x_{1l} - \sum_{j=1}^{m} x_{2lj})^2}}.$$

To calculate the above Z_{MDT}, we have

$$
Z_{\mathrm{MDT}}
$$

$$
= \frac{\sum_{l=1}^{n} \sum_{j=1}^{m} (x_{1l} - x_{2lj})}{\left[\sum_{l=1}^{n} \left\{ \sum_{j=1}^{m} (x_{1l} - x_{2lj})^2 + 2 \sum_{1 \le j_1 < j_2 \le m} (x_{1l} - x_{2lj_1})(x_{1l} - x_{2lj_2}) \right\}\right]^{1/2}},
$$

$$
(4.13)
$$

where $\sum (x_{1l} - x_{2lj})$ and $\sum (x_{1l} - x_{2lj})^2$ are given in (4.6) and (4.7), respectively, and $2 \sum (x_{1l} - x_{2lj_1})(x_{1l} - x_{2lj_2})$ can be written as

$$
2 \sum_{l=1}^{n} \sum_{1 \le j_1 < j_2 \le 2} (x_{1l} - x_{2lj_1})(x_{1l} - x_{2lj_2})
$$

$$
= 2x_{01}^2 (m_{0,11} + m_{1,00}) + 2x_{02}^2 (m_{0,22} + m_{2,00}) + 2x_{12}^2 (m_{1,22} + m_{2,11})
$$

$$
+ 2x_{01}x_{02}m_{0,12} + 2x_{02}x_{12}m_{2,01} - 2x_{01}x_{12}m_{1,02},
$$

where $x_{st} = x_s - x_t$.

Note that the original MDT only uses $x = 1/2$. Then the MDT in (4.12) is based on the difference of the average B allele counts between cases and controls. The MDT that we present in (4.12) generalizes the difference of the average allele counts to the difference of the average scores between cases and controls. The MTT and MDT are generally different in the variance calculations except for a matched pair design. Under the matched pair design, $Z_{\mathrm{MTT}} \equiv Z_{\mathrm{MDT}}$.

4.5 A Model-Free Test

For a given x, both Z_{MTT} and Z_{MDT} are one-degree-of-freedom tests but they depend on the underlying genetic model, or x. Like Pearson's test for an unmatched design, the two-degrees-of-freedom test for a matched design is often implemented in the commercial software, which uses two indicator variables to model the genetic effects. We first discuss matched case-control data in which matched sets have a variable number of controls matched to a case, as in Sect. 4.3.2 and Sect. 4.4. The $1 : m$ matching will be then obtained as a special case.

4.5.1 A Variable Number of Controls and a Case Are Matched

Analogous to the unmatched design with two indicator variables (Sect. 3.3.4), two indicator variables are used for cases and controls, respectively. For cases, define $(x_{1il1}, x_{1il2}) = (0, 0)$ for G_0, $(0, 1)$ for G_1, and $(1, 1)$ for G_2, and define (x_{2ilj1}, x_{2ilj2}) similarly for controls. Then the conditional likelihood function can be written as

$$
L(\beta_1, \beta_2 | z) = \prod_{i=1}^{m} \prod_{l=1}^{n_i} \frac{\exp(\beta_1 x_{1il1} + \beta_2 x_{1il2})}{\exp(\beta_1 x_{1il1} + \beta_2 x_{1il2}) + \sum_{j=1}^{i} \exp(\beta_1 x_{2ilj1} + \beta_2 x_{2ilj2})}.
$$

Denote the log-likelihood as $l = \log L(\beta_1, \beta_2|z)$. Then, the Score statistic for testing $H_0 : \beta_1 = \beta_2 = 0$ can be written as

$$T_{\chi_2^2,M} = \left[\frac{\partial l}{\partial \beta_1} \quad \frac{\partial l}{\partial \beta_2} \right] \left[\begin{array}{cc} -\frac{\partial^2 l}{\partial \beta_1^2} & -\frac{\partial^2 l}{\partial \beta_1 \beta_2} \\ -\frac{\partial^2 l}{\partial \beta_2 \beta_1} & -\frac{\partial^2 l}{\partial \beta_2^2} \end{array} \right]^{-1} \left[\begin{array}{c} \frac{\partial l}{\partial \beta_1} \\ \frac{\partial l}{\partial \beta_2} \end{array} \right] |_{H_0}, \qquad (4.14)$$

where expressions for the partial derivatives are given in Problem 4.7. Under H_0, $T_{\chi_2^2,M} \sim \chi_2^2$ asymptotically.

Denote

$$Z_i = (\partial l/\partial \beta_i)/\sqrt{-\partial^2 l/\partial \beta_i^2}|_{H_0}, \quad i = 1, 2.$$

Then, from Problem 4.7, Z_1 is the MTT with the score $x = 0$ and Z_2 is the MTT with the score $x = 1$. Denote

$$\rho = (-\partial^2 l/\partial \beta_1 \partial \beta_2)/\sqrt{(-\partial^2 l/\partial \beta_1^2)(-\partial^2 l/\partial \beta_2^2)}|_{H_0}.$$

From Problem 4.7,

$$T_{\chi_2^2,M} = \frac{1}{1-\rho^2}(Z_1^2 - 2\rho Z_1 Z_2 + Z_2^2). \qquad (4.15)$$

4.5.2 $1:m$ Matching

The two indicator variables for an individual take on the values $(0,0)$, $(0,1)$ and $(1,1)$ for the three genotypes G_0, G_1 and G_2, respectively. Because the indicators are either 0 or 1, we have $x_{1lk} = x_{1lk}^2$ and $\sum_{j=1}^m x_{2ljk}^2 = \sum_{j=1}^m x_{2ljk}$ for $k = 1, 2$. Moreover, $x_{1l1}x_{1l2} = x_{1l1}$ and $\sum_j x_{2lj1}x_{2lj2} = \sum_j x_{2lj1}$. Denote the average values for the first ($k = 1$) and second ($k = 2$) indicators in the lth stratum by

$$\bar{x}_{lk} = \frac{1}{m+1}\left(x_{1lk} + \sum_{j=1}^m x_{2ljk} \right), \quad k = 1, 2.$$

Then, using Problem 4.7, the second order partial derivatives given in (4.14) can be written as

$$-\frac{\partial^2 l}{\partial \beta_k^2}|_{H_0} = \sum_{l=1}^n \bar{x}_{lk}(1 - \bar{x}_{lk}), \qquad -\frac{\partial^2 l}{\partial \beta_1 \beta_2}|_{H_0} = \sum_{l=1}^n \bar{x}_{l1}(1 - \bar{x}_{l2}).$$

Hence, $T_{\chi^2,M}$ depends on (x_{1l1}, x_{1l2}) and $(\sum_{j=1}^m x_{2lj1}, \sum_{j=1}^m x_{2lj2})$.

Table 4.6 Values of d_{l1}^2 and d_{l2}^2 for a matched pair design

Matched pair genotype	d_{l1}^2	d_{l2}^2	Count
(AA, AA)	0	0	m_{00}
(AA, AB)	0	1	m_{01}
(AA, BB)	1	1	m_{02}
(AB, AA)	0	1	m_{10}
(AB, AB)	0	0	m_{11}
(AB, BB)	1	0	m_{12}
(BB, AA)	1	1	m_{20}
(BB, AB)	1	0	m_{21}
(BB, BB)	0	0	m_{22}

$1:1$ Matching

For a matched pair design with n matched sets, the scores for cases and controls
are denoted by x_{1lk} and x_{2lk} respectively, for the kth indicator variable and the lth
matched set, where $l = 1, \ldots, n$ and $k = 1, 2$. Let $d_{lk} = x_{1lk} - x_{2lk}$. Then, from
(4.3),

$$Z_k = \sum_{l=1}^{n} d_{lk} \Big/ \sqrt{\sum_{l=1}^{n} d_{lk}^2}.$$

In addition,

$$\bar{x}_{lk}(1 - \bar{x}_{lk}) = (x_{1lk} + x_{2lk})/2 - (x_{1lk} + x_{2lk})^2/4$$
$$= (x_{1lk} + x_{2lk})/2 - (x_{1lk} + x_{2lk})/4 - x_{1lk}x_{2lk}/2$$
$$= (x_{1lk} + x_{2lk})/4 - x_{1lk}x_{2lk}/2 = (x_{1lk}^2 + x_{2lk}^2)/4 - x_{1lk}x_{2lk}/2$$
$$= (x_{1lk} - x_{2lk})^2/4 = d_{lk}^2/4,$$
$$\bar{x}_{l1}(1 - \bar{x}_{l2}) = (x_{1l1} + x_{2l1})/2 - (x_{1l1} + x_{2l1})(x_{1l2} + x_{2l2})/4$$
$$= (x_{1l1} + x_{2l1} - x_{1l1}x_{2l2} - x_{2l1}x_{1l2})/4 = d_{l1}d_{l2}/4.$$

Thus,

$$\rho = \sum_{l=1}^{n}(d_{l1}d_{l2}) \Big/ \sqrt{\left(\sum_{l=1}^{n} d_{l1}^2\right)\left(\sum_{l=1}^{n} d_{l2}^2\right)}.$$

The values of $d_{l1}^2 = (x_{1l1} - x_{2l1})^2$ and $d_{l2}^2 = (x_{1l2} - x_{2l2})^2$ are given in Table 4.6,
from which we have $\sum_{l=1}^{n} d_{l1}^2 = m_{02} + m_{20} + m_{12} + m_{21}$, $\sum_{l=1}^{n} d_{l2}^2 = m_{01} + m_{10} + m_{02} + m_{20}$, and $\sum_{l=1}^{n} d_{l1}d_{l2} = m_{02} + m_{20}$.

Table 4.7 Computing ρ for $1:2$ matching

Count	$\bar{x}_{l1}$	$\bar{x}_{l2}$	$\bar{x}_{l1}(1-\bar{x}_{l1})$	$\bar{x}_{l2}(1-\bar{x}_{l2})$	$\bar{x}_{l1}(1-\bar{x}_{l2})$
$m_{0,00}$	0	0	0	0	0
$m_{0,01}$	0	1/3	0	2/9	0
$m_{0,02}$	1/3	1/3	2/9	2/9	2/9
$m_{0,11}$	0	2/3	0	2/9	0
$m_{0,12}$	1/3	2/3	2/9	2/9	1/9
$m_{0,22}$	2/3	2/3	2/9	2/9	2/9
$m_{1,00}$	0	1/3	0	2/9	0
$m_{1,01}$	0	2/3	0	2/9	0
$m_{1,02}$	1/3	2/3	2/9	2/9	1/9
$m_{1,11}$	0	1	0	0	0
$m_{1,12}$	1/3	1	2/9	0	0
$m_{1,22}$	2/3	1	2/9	0	0
$m_{2,00}$	1/3	1/3	2/9	2/9	2/9
$m_{2,01}$	1/3	2/3	2/9	2/9	1/9
$m_{2,02}$	2/3	2/3	2/9	2/9	2/9
$m_{2,11}$	1/3	1	2/9	0	0
$m_{2,12}$	2/3	1	2/9	0	0
$m_{2,22}$	1	1	0	0	0

$1:2$ Matching

To calculate ρ for $1:2$ matching, Table 4.7 can be used, where the first column contains the counts of the matched sets. Here is an example to illustrate how the entries in Table 4.7 are calculated. There are $m_{0,12}$ matched sets that each contains one case with genotype AA and two controls with genotypes AB and BB, respectively (see Table 4.2). Therefore, the case has the indicators $(x_{1l1}, x_{1l2}) = (0, 0)$ and controls have $(x_{2l11}, x_{2l12}) = (0, 1)$ and $(x_{2l21}, x_{2l22}) = (1, 1)$. Then, the mean values of the indicators for the first and second alleles are $\bar{x}_{l1} = (x_{1l1} + x_{2l11} + x_{2l21})/3 = 1/3$ and $\bar{x}_{l2} = (x_{1l2} + x_{2l12} + x_{2l22})/3 = 2/3$, respectively.

Using Table 4.7, $\sum_l \bar{x}_{lk}(1 - \bar{X}_{lk})$ and $\sum_l \bar{x}_{l1}(1 - \bar{X}_{l2})$ can be calculated as the sums of the corresponding columns weighted by the counts. For example,

$$\sum_{l=1}^{n} \bar{X}_{l1}(1 - \bar{X}_{l2}) = \frac{1}{9}(2m_{0,02} + 2m_{0,22} + 2m_{2,00} + 2m_{2,02} + m_{0,12} + m_{1,02} + m_{2,01}).$$

The ACCESS Example

Applying $T_{\chi_2^2,M}$ to the data given in Table 4.3 and using the results for the MTTs in Sect. 4.3, we have $Z_1 = 1.8974$ and $Z_2 = 1.8257$, and $\sum_{l=1}^{219} d_{l1}^2 = 5+9+13+13 = 40$, $\sum_{l=1}^{219} d_{l2}^2 = 45+5+57+13 = 140$, and $\sum_{l=1}^{219} d_{l1}d_{l2} = 5+13 = 18$. Therefore,

$$\rho = \sum_{l=1}^{219} d_{l1}d_{l2} \Big/ \sqrt{\sum_{l=1}^{219} d_{l1}^2 \sum_{l=1}^{219} d_{l2}^2} = 18/\sqrt{40 \times 120} = 0.2598.$$

Substituting these values into (4.15), we have $T_{\chi_2^2,M} = 5.5049$ with p-value $= 0.0638$.

4.6 Multiple Cases and Multiple Controls Are Matched

In Sects. 4.3–4.5, each matched set contains one case and at least one control. When a matched set has multiple cases and multiple controls, the previous test statistics need to be modified. We use the MTT and MDT as examples.

Assume the jth matched set contains m_{1j} cases and m_{2j} controls, $n_j = m_{1j} + m_{2j}$, $j = 1, \ldots, J$, and $n = \sum_j n_j$. The conditional likelihood function is

$$L(\beta|z) = \prod_{j=1}^{J} \frac{\exp(\beta \sum_{i=1}^{m_{1j}} x_{ij})}{\sum_{l=1}^{K_j} \exp(\beta \sum_{i(l)=1}^{m_{1j}} x_{i(l)j})},$$

where $K_j = \binom{n_j}{m_{1j}}$ is the total number of permutations of m_{1j} cases in a matched set with n_j subjects. For the lth permuted matched set ($l = 1, \ldots, K_j$), let $i(l) = 1, \ldots, m_{1j}$ indicate the permuted ranks of the cases. Then the MTT for testing $H_0: \beta = 0$ can be written as

$$Z_{\mathrm{MTT}} = \frac{\sum_{j=1}^{J}(K_j \sum_{i=1}^{m_{1j}} x_{ij} - \sum_{l=1}^{K_j} \sum_{i(l)=1}^{m_{1j}} x_{i(l)j})}{[\sum_{j=1}^{J}\{K_j \sum_{l=1}^{K_j}(\sum_{i(l)=1}^{m_{1j}} x_{i(l)j})^2 - (\sum_{l=1}^{K_j} \sum_{i(l)=1}^{m_{1j}} x_{i(l)j})^2\}]^{1/2}},$$

$$\tag{4.16}$$

which has an asymptotic $N(0, 1)$ distribution under H_0. Note that, if $n_j = 1 + m$ and $m_{1j} = 1$ for all j, then the MTT given in (4.16) is identical to the MTT for the $1:m$ matched design given in (4.2).

When the number of cases m_{1j} in each stratum or matched set is large, computing the MTT for all K_j permutations for $j = 1, \ldots, J$ may be intensive. The MDT studied in Sect. 4.4 is simple, because it replaces the score for the case in (4.12) by the averaged score for the cases in each stratum or matched set. The MDT can be written as

$$Z_{\text{MDT}} = \frac{\sum_{j=1}^{n}(\frac{1}{m_{1j}}\sum_{i=1}^{m_{1j}}x_{ij} - \frac{1}{m_{2j}}\sum_{i=m_{1j}+1}^{n_j}x_{ij})}{[\sum_{j=1}^{n}(\frac{1}{m_{1j}}\sum_{i=1}^{m_{1j}}x_{ij} - \frac{1}{m_{2j}}\sum_{i=m_{1j}+1}^{n_j}x_{ij})^2]^{1/2}}, \qquad (4.17)$$

which has an asymptotic $N(0, 1)$ distribution under H_0.

4.7 Simulating Matched Case-Control Data

We discuss simulation procedures for $1 : m$ matched designs. Examples are given for the $1 : 1$ and $1 : 2$ matched designs. The simulation studies discussed in Sect. 4.8 are based on these simulation methods.

Suppose the study population is divided into J strata based on the values of the confounding variable values $(z_1, \ldots, z_J)$. Denote $\pi_j = \Pr(z = z_j)$. Suppose n matched sets are sampled, each containing one case and m controls who have the same values of z. Let E_{ist} be the event that, given a matched set, the case has genotype G_i ($i = 0$, 1, or 2) and the m controls have genotype counts $(s, t, m - s - t)$ for (G_0, G_1, G_2). Denote $p_{ist} = \Pr(E_{ist})$ and the count for the event E_{ist} in n matched sets by y_{ist}. The following notation is also given in Sect. 4.1:

$$p_{ij} = \Pr(G_i | \text{case}, z_j) = g_{ij} f_{ij}/k_j; \qquad (4.18)$$

$$q_{ij} = \Pr(G_i | \text{control}, z_j) = g_{ij}(1 - f_{ij})/(1 - k_j). \qquad (4.19)$$

Then, by the independence of case and control genotypes given z,

$$p_{ist} = \binom{m}{s, t, m - r - s} \sum_{j=1}^{J} \pi_j p_{ij} q_{0j}^{s} q_{1j}^{t} q_{2j}^{m-s-t}, \quad i = 0, 1, \qquad (4.20)$$

and $\binom{m}{s, t, m-r-s} = m!/\{s!t!(m - s - t)!\}$.

To calculate the probabilities p_{ist}, the following parameters need to be specified: the number of strata J, π_j, k_j, MAFs p_j, and the GRRs $(\lambda_{1j}, \lambda_{2j})$ in the jth stratum. The following algorithm can be used to calculate p_{ist} for each combination of (i, s, t):

1. Specify J and the values of π_j, k_j, p_j, λ_{1j}, and λ_{2j} in the jth stratum for $j = 1, \ldots, J$.
2. Under HWE, calculate the genotype frequencies $g_{ij} = \Pr(G_{ij})$ in each stratum. Calculate $f_{0j} = k_j/(g_{0j} + \lambda_{1j}g_{1j} + \lambda_{2j}g_{2j})$, $f_{1j} = f_{0j}\lambda_{1j}$ and $f_{2j} = f_{0j}\lambda_{2j}$. Then $p_{ij} = g_{ij}f_{ij}/k_j$ and $q_{ij} = g_{ij}(1 - f_{ij})/(1 - k_{ij})$.
3. For each combination of (i, s, t) such that $i = 0, 1, 2$ and $s + t \le m$, calculate p_{ist} using (4.20).

Table 4.8 shows the probabilities p_{ist} for the matched pair design with $J = 5$ strata, where $\pi_j = 0.20$ for all j, $(k_1, k_2, k_3, k_4, k_5) = (0.01, 0.10, 0.15, 0.05, 0.20)$,

Table 4.8 Multinomial probabilities for simulating a matched pair design

Events E_{ist}	Genotypes		Count	Count[*]	p_{ist}
	Case	Control			
E_{010}	G_0	G_0	y_{010}	m_{00}	0.3212
E_{001}	G_0	G_1	y_{001}	m_{01}	0.1564
E_{000}	G_0	G_2	y_{000}	m_{02}	0.0225
E_{110}	G_1	G_0	y_{110}	m_{10}	0.2471
E_{101}	G_1	G_1	y_{101}	m_{11}	0.1422
E_{100}	G_1	G_2	y_{100}	m_{12}	0.0230
E_{210}	G_2	G_0	y_{210}	m_{20}	0.0498
E_{201}	G_2	G_1	y_{201}	m_{21}	0.0322
E_{200}	G_2	G_2	y_{200}	m_{22}	0.0056

[*]The counts are given in Table 4.1

Table 4.9 Simulated sample of 500 matched pairs

Cases	Controls			Total
	AA	AB	BB	
AA	163	63	12	238
AB	116	87	17	220
BB	20	18	4	42
Total	299	168	33	500

MAFs $(p_1, p_2, p_3, p_4, p_5) = (0.10, 0.30, 0.15, 0.25, 0.20)$, $\lambda_{1j} = 1.5$, and $\lambda_{2j} = 2$ for all j. Using the specified values and the above algorithm, p_{ist} can be calculated for each combination of (i, s, t) for $i = 0, 1, 2$ and $s + t \leq 1$. For reference, the symbols m_{st} for genotype counts given in Table 4.1 are also given in Table 4.8. To simulate matched pairs using Table 4.8, let

$$y = \{y_{010}, y_{001}, y_{000}, y_{110}, y_{101}, y_{100}, y_{210}, y_{201}, y_{200}\}$$

and

$$p = \{0.3212, 0.1564, 0.0225, 0.2471, 0.1422, 0.0230, 0.0498, 0.0322, 0.0056\}.$$

Then n matched pairs can be simulated from the multinomial distribution $y \sim Mul(n; p)$. Table 4.9 presents a simulated sample of 500 matched pairs using the probabilities given in Table 4.8.

In general, since $\sum_i \sum_{s+t \leq m} p_{ist} = 1$, the counts, $\{y_{ist} : i = 0, 1, 2; s + t \leq m\}$ for a $1 : m$ matched design can be generated from the multinomial distribution $Mul(n; \{p_{ist}, i = 0, 1, 2, s + t \leq m\})$. For $1 : 2$ matching, we use Table 4.10 when

Table 4.10 Multinomial probabilities for simulating $1:2$ matched design when the case genotype is G_i, $i = 0, 1, 2$

Events E_{ist}	Genotypes		Count	Count	p_{ist}
	Case	Control			
E_{i20}	G_i	(G_0, G_0)	y_{i20}	$m_{i,00}$	p_{i20}
E_{i11}	G_i	(G_0, G_1)	y_{i11}	$m_{i,01}$	p_{i11}
E_{i10}	G_i	(G_0, G_2)	y_{i10}	$m_{i,02}$	p_{i10}
E_{i02}	G_i	(G_1, G_1)	y_{i02}	$m_{i,11}$	p_{i02}
E_{i01}	G_i	(G_1, G_2)	y_{i01}	$m_{i,12}$	p_{i01}
E_{i00}	G_i	(G_2, G_2)	y_{i00}	$m_{i,22}$	p_{i00}

Table 4.11 $1:2$ matching: genotype counts of a single marker with alleles A and B

Cases	Controls						Total
	AA, AA	AA, AB	AA, BB	AB, AB	AB, BB	BB, BB	
AA	137	102	5	21	4	1	270
AB	91	77	10	20	5	0	203
BB	9	13	1	2	2	0	27
Total	237	192	16	43	11	1	500

the case genotype is G_i, $i = 0, 1, 2$. Therefore, a total of 18 probabilities have to be calculated for $m = 2$, and all the counts $\{y_{ist} : i = 0, 1, 2; s + t \leq 2\}$ for the 18 events $\{E_{ist} : i = 0, 1, 2; s + t \leq 2\}$ are simulated from the multinomial distribution. Table 4.11 presents a simulated $1:2$ matched dataset with the same parameter values as in Table 4.9.

4.8 Performance of the Three Test Statistics

We conduct simulations to compare the empirical power of the MTT (Z_{MTT}), the MDT (Z_{MDT}) and Pearson's test ($T_{\chi_2^2, M}$) under the null and alternative hypotheses for ADD, DOM and REC models. We only consider the matched pair and the $1:2$ matched designs. For the matched pair design, Z_{MTT} and $T_{\chi_2^2, M}$ are compared. For the $1:2$ matching, all three statistics are compared.

The values of the parameters for both designs are the same as those used in Tables 4.8 and 4.9 except that $\lambda_2 = 1.5$ in each stratum. The Type I error and empirical power are estimated using 10,000 replicates. The results for the matched pair and for the $1:2$ matching are presented in Figs. 4.2 and 4.3.

Note that, in Fig. 4.2, the empirical power of Z_{MTT} changes with the value of x, while the power of $T_{\chi_2^2, M}$ is independent of x. Z_{MTT} is expected to be most powerful when x approaches 0, 1/2 and 1 under the REC, ADD and DOM models,

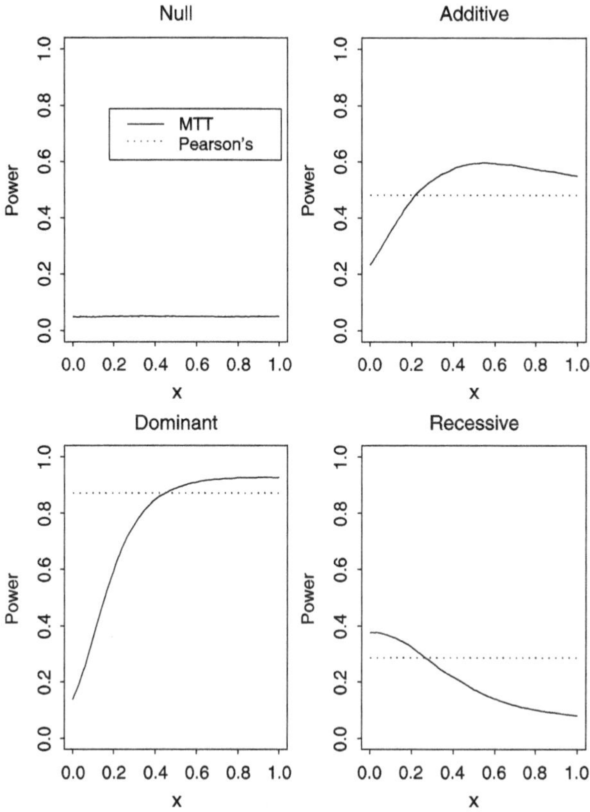

Fig. 4.2 Comparing the empirical power of the MTT and Pearson's test $(T_{\chi_2^2,M})$ for the matched pair design under the null and alternative hypotheses for ADD, DOM, and REC models. The power of the MTT changes with the value of x, where $x = 0, 1/2, 1$ correspond to the REC, ADD and DOM models, respectively

respectively. In addition, Z_{MTT} with the optimal x is more powerful than $T_{\chi_2^2,M}$. However, when x is not chosen appropriately, $T_{\chi_2^2,M}$ could be more powerful than Z_{MTT}. For example, under a REC model, $T_{\chi_2^2,M}$ is more powerful than Z_{MTT} when a larger x is chosen. Similar conclusions can be obtained for the $1:2$ matched design. However, Fig. 4.3 shows that the MTT is slightly more powerful than the MDT.

4.9 Estimates of Odds Ratios and Relative Risks

We discuss the estimates of ORs and RRs for a matched pair design. For RRs, we show that the estimates can be approximated by the estimates of ORs when the disease prevalence is small. The CIs for the estimates of ORs are also given.

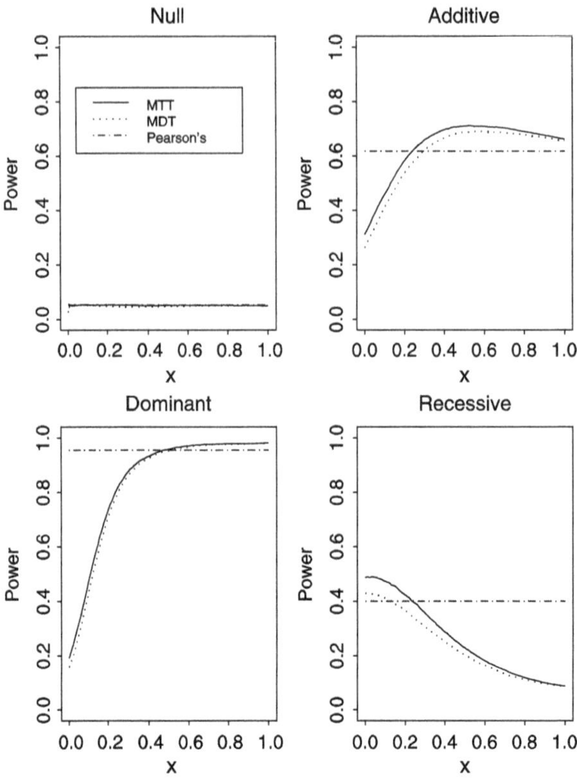

Fig. 4.3 Comparing the empirical power of the MTT, MDT and Pearson's test $(T_{\chi_2^2, M})$ for $1:2$ matching under the null and alternative hypotheses for ADD, DOM, and REC models. The power of the MTT and MDT changes with the value of x, where $x = 0, 1/2, 1$ correspond to the REC, ADD and DOM models, respectively

4.9.1 Conditional Odds Ratios

Suppose J strata are defined by the values $(z_1, \ldots, z_J)$ of confounding variables. Given z_j the conditional OR is defined as

$$
\begin{aligned}
\mathrm{OR}_{G_i:G_0|z_j} &= \frac{\Pr(G_i\,|\,\text{case},\, z_j)\,\Pr(G_0\,|\,\text{control},\, z_j)}{\Pr(G_0\,|\,\text{case},\, z_j)\,\Pr(G_i\,|\,\text{control},\, z_j)} \\[2mm]
&= \frac{\Pr(\text{case}\,|\,G_i,\, z_j)\,\Pr(\text{control}\,|\,G_0,\, z_j)}{\Pr(\text{case}\,|\,G_0,\, z_j)\,\Pr(\text{control}\,|\,G_i,\, z_j)}, \quad \text{for } i = 1, 2,
\end{aligned}
$$

i.e., the retrospective conditional OR equals the prospective conditional OR.

If $\mathrm{OR}_{G_i:G_0|z_{j_1}} = \mathrm{OR}_{G_i:G_0|z_{j_2}}$ for all $1 \le j_1 < j_2 \le J$ and $i = 1, 2$, there is a single pair of common ORs denoted as $\mathrm{OR}_{G_i:G_0}$ for $i = 1, 2$, and these can be consistently estimated. Using the data in Table 4.1, we have

$$\widehat{OR}_{G_1:G_0} = \frac{m_{10}}{m_{01}} \quad \text{and} \quad \widehat{OR}_{G_2:G_0} = \frac{m_{20}}{m_{02}}.$$

Asymptotic variances are better obtained for the logs of the above estimates, which can be obtained from

$$\widehat{Var}\{\log(\widehat{OR}_{G_i:G_0})\} = \frac{m_{i0} + m_{0i}}{m_{i0}m_{0i}}, \quad \text{for } i = 1, 2.$$

The CI for $OR_{G_i:G_0}$ can be obtained in a way similar to that under the unmatched design (Sect. 3.8). For $\log(OR_{G_i:G_0})$, the $100(1 - \alpha)\%$ CI is given by

$$\log(\widehat{OR}_{G_i:G_0}) \pm z_{1-\alpha/2}\sqrt{\widehat{Var}\{\log(\widehat{OR}_{G_i:G_0})\}},$$

from which the $100(1 - \alpha)\%$ CI for OR can be constructed.

The ACCESS Example

Using the data given in Table 4.3, $m_{10} = 57$, $m_{01} = 45$, $m_{20} = 13$, and $m_{02} = 5$. Thus, consistent estimates of the ORs are given by $\widehat{OR}_{G_1:G_0} = 57/45 \approx 1.27$ and $\widehat{OR}_{G_2:G_0} = 13/5 = 2.6$ with log ORs

$$\log(\widehat{OR}_{G_1:G_0}) = \log\left(\frac{57}{45}\right) \approx 0.2364,$$

$$\log(\widehat{OR}_{G_2:G_0}) = \log\left(\frac{13}{5}\right) \approx 0.9555.$$

Estimates of the variances of the above estimates can be calculated as

$$\widehat{Var}\{\log(\widehat{OR}_{G_1:G_0})\} = \frac{57 + 45}{57 \times 45} \approx 0.03977,$$

$$\widehat{Var}\{\log(\widehat{OR}_{G_2:G_0})\} = \frac{13 + 5}{13 \times 5} \approx 0.2769.$$

Thus, the 95% CI for $\log(OR_{G_1:G_0})$ is given by

$$0.2364 \pm 1.96\sqrt{0.03977} = (-0.1545, 0.6273),$$

which is converted to $(0.86, 1.87)$ for $OR_{G_1:G_0}$. The 95% CI for $\log(OR_{G_2:G_0})$ is given by

$$0.9555 \pm 1.96\sqrt{0.2769} = (-0.0759, 1.9869),$$

which is converted to $(0.93, 7.29)$ for $OR_{G_2:G_0}$.

If we display Table 4.1 in terms of alleles A and B, we obtain Table 4.12. A consistent estimate for the OR and the estimate of its asymptotic variance are given

Table 4.12 Allele-based table for the ACCESS data

Cases	Controls		Total
	A	B	
A	192	84	276
B	116	46	162
Total	308	130	438

by

$$\widehat{OR}_{B:A} = 116/84 \approx 1.381,$$

$$\widehat{Var}\{\log(\widehat{OR}_{B:A})\} \approx 0.0205.$$

Thus, the 95% CI for $\log(OR_{B:A})$ is $0.3228 \pm 1.96\sqrt{0.0205} = (0.0422, 0.6034)$, which is converted to $(1.04, 1.83)$ for the OR.

4.9.2 Relative Risks

It is known that, for an unmatched case-control design, the GRRs can be approximated by the ORs for rare diseases. This is also true for the matched case-control design. Consider the GRRs λ_{ij} conditional on z_j given by

$$\lambda_{ij} = \frac{f_{ij}}{f_{0j}} = \frac{\Pr(\text{case}\,|G_i, z_j)}{\Pr(\text{case}\,|G_0, z_j)} = \frac{\Pr(G_i|\,\text{case}, z_j)\,\Pr(G_0|z_j)}{\Pr(G_0|\,\text{case}, z_j)\,\Pr(G_i|z_j)},$$

where, for $i = 0, 1, 2$,

$$\Pr(G_i|z_j) = \Pr(\text{case}\,|z_j)\,\Pr(G_i|\,\text{case}, z_j) + \Pr(\text{control}\,|z_j)\,\Pr(G_i|\,\text{control}, z_j).$$

Thus the numerator of λ_{ij} can be written as

$$\Pr(G_i|\,\text{case}, z_j)\,\Pr(\text{case}\,|z_j)\,\Pr(G_0|\,\text{case}, z_j)$$

$$+ \{1 - \Pr(\text{case}\,|z_j)\}\,\Pr(G_i|\,\text{case}, z_j)\,\Pr(G_0|\,\text{control}, z_j),$$

which converges to $\Pr(G_i|\,\text{case}, z_j)\,\Pr(G_0|\,\text{control}, z_j)$ when $\Pr(\text{case}\,|z_j) \to 0$. Likewise, the denominator of λ_{ij} converges to $\Pr(G_0|\,\text{case}, z_j)\,\Pr(G_i|\,\text{control}, z_j)$ when $\Pr(\text{case}\,|z_j) \to 0$. Thus,

$$\lambda_{ij} \to \frac{\Pr(G_i|\,\text{case}, z_j)\,\Pr(G_0|\,\text{control}, z_j)}{\Pr(G_0|\,\text{case}, z_j)\,\Pr(G_i|\,\text{control}, z_j)} = OR_{G_i:G_0|z_j}.$$

4.10 Bibliographical Comments

The matched case-control design has been extensively studied in epidemiological studies [21, 39, 156, 270]. However, most results have dealt with binary exposures, equivalent to two alleles A and B in genetic studies. McNemar's test is often applied for the matched pair design with binary exposures [156]. These results have to be extended for three genotypes. Breslow and Day [21] and Lachin [156] discuss more general results for matched case-control designs, including $1 : m$ matching and the matching with a variable number of controls per case, estimation problems, etc. We used the matched prospective conditional likelihood to analyze matched retrospective case-control samples [156, 204]. Thus, our statistics can be applied to matched prospective case-control samples.

Breslow and Day [21] study general trend tests for matched case-control designs, which are derived as Score statistics in Lachin [156]. Zheng and Tian [346] study MTTs for testing genetic association for matched designs. The expression of the MTT, (4.11) in Sect. 4.3.2, can be found in Walter [296], who studied a general matched design where a matched set contains a variable number of controls per case. Lee [161] studied the MDT for an ADD model, which we generalized to any genetic model between the REC and DOM models by using $x \in [0, 1]$. See also Zang et al. [315].

In simulation studies, the multinomial distribution probabilities given in (4.20) were given in Ejigou and McHugh [70]. The ACCESS dataset given in Table 4.3 was from a matched pair case-control study for sarcoidosis [3]. Most of the estimation problems that are discussed here can be found in Lachin [156]. However, his results only considered binary exposures, which cannot be directly applied to analyses with three genotypes.

4.11 Problems

4.1 Derive the Score statistic MTT for the $1 : m$ matched design and show it can be written as (4.2).

4.2 Let n_{il0} and n_{il1} be the numbers of genotypes AA and AB in the lth matched set with one case and i controls. Then, for an integer v, show that, under H_0,

$$
E(x_{1il}^v | n_{il0}, n_{il1}) = E\left(x_{1il}^v \Big| x_{1il}^v + \sum_{j=1}^{i} x_{2ilj}^v \right) = \left(x_{1il}^v + \sum_{j=1}^{i} x_{2ilj}^v \right) \Big/ (1+i).
$$

4.3 For a matched pair design, using the data in Table 4.1, show that the MTT given in (4.2) can be written as

Table 4.13 Marginal genotype counts of a matched pair design based on Table 4.1

	Genotypes			Total
	AA	AB	BB	
Cases	$\sum_{j=0}^{2} m_{0j}$	$\sum_{j=0}^{2} m_{1j}$	$\sum_{j=0}^{2} m_{2j}$	$\sum_{i=1}^{2}\sum_{j=0}^{2} m_{ij}$
Controls	$\sum_{i=0}^{2} m_{i0}$	$\sum_{i=0}^{2} m_{i1}$	$\sum_{i=0}^{2} m_{i2}$	$\sum_{j=1}^{2}\sum_{i=0}^{2} m_{ij}$
Total	$\sum_{i=0}^{2}(m_{0i} + m_{i0})$	$\sum_{i=0}^{2}(m_{1i} + m_{i1})$	$\sum_{i=0}^{2}(m_{2i} + m_{i2})$	$2\sum_{i=1}^{2}\sum_{j=0}^{2} m_{ij}$

$$Z_{\text{MTT}} = \frac{\sum_{0 \le s < t \le 2}(m_{st} - m_{ts})(x_s - x_t)}{\sqrt{\sum_{0 \le s < t \le 2}(m_{st} + m_{ts})(x_s - x_t)^2}},$$

where $(x_0, x_1, x_2) = (0, x, 1)$.

4.4 Verify (4.6)–(4.8) for the MTT under the $1 : 2$ matching.

4.5 Let y_{vst} be defined as in Sect. 4.7 (see also Table 4.8). Denote $(x_0, x_1, x_1) = (0, x, 1)$. Prove that, for $k = 1, 2$,

$$\sum_{l=1}^{n_i} x_{1il}^{k} = \sum_{v=0}^{2} \sum_{s+t \le i} x_v^{k} y_{vst},$$

$$\sum_{l=1}^{n_i} \sum_{j=1}^{i} x_{2ilj}^{k} = \sum_{v=0}^{2} \sum_{s+t \le i} \{ix_2^k + s(x_0^k - x_2^k) + t(x_1^k - x_2^k)\} y_{vst},$$

$$\sum_{l=1}^{n_i} \left(x_{1il} + \sum_{j=1}^{i} x_{2ilj} \right)^2 = \sum_{v=0}^{2} \sum_{s+t \le i} \{x_v + rx_2 + s(x_0 - x_2) + t(x_1 - x_2)\}^2 y_{vst}.$$

Substituting the above formulas into (4.10), an alternative expression for the MTT can be obtained using all the observed y_{vst}.

4.6 The margins of the matched pair data in Table 4.1 form an unmatched case-control sample as presented in Table 4.13. Rewrite the trend test Z_{CATT} given in (3.8) for a given x using the data given in Table 4.13. Compare this Z_{CATT} to Z_{MTT} given in Problem 4.3 for a given x. Use the data in Table 4.3 as an example and plot the two test statistics as functions of x over $x \in [0, 1]$.

4.7 The two-degrees-of-freedom test.

(a) Show that the partial derivatives in (4.14) can be written as, for $k = 1, 2$,

$$\frac{\partial l}{\partial \beta_k}\Big|_{H_0} = \sum_{i=1}^{m} \sum_{l=1}^{n_i} \left\{ x_{1ilk} - \left(x_{1ilk} + \sum_{j=1}^{i} x_{2iljk} \right) \Big/ (1+i) \right\},$$

Table 4.14 Allele count for a matched pair design under the REC model

Cases	Controls	
	$AA + AB$	BB
$AA + AB$	a	b
BB	c	d

$a = m_{00} + m_{01} + m_{10} + m_{11}$

$b = m_{02} + m_{12}$

$c = m_{20} + m_{21}$

$d = m_{22}$

Table 4.15 Allele count for a matched pair design under the DOM model

Cases	Controls	
	$AA + AB$	BB
$AA + AB$	a	b
BB	c	d

$a = m_{00}$

$b = m_{01} + m_{02}$

$c = m_{10} + m_{20}$

$d = m_{11} + m_{12} + m_{21} + m_{22}$

$$-\frac{\partial^2 l}{\partial \beta_k^2}\Big|_{H_0} = \sum_{i=1}^{m}\sum_{l=1}^{n_i}\left\{\left(x_{1ilk}^2 + \sum_{j=1}^{i} x_{2iljk}^2\right)\Big/(1+i)\right.$$
$$\left. - \left(x_{1ilk} + \sum_{j=1}^{i} x_{2iljk}\right)^2\Big/(1+i)^2\right\},$$

$$-\frac{\partial^2 l}{\partial \beta_1 \beta_2}\Big|_{H_0} = \sum_{i=1}^{m}\sum_{l=1}^{n_i}\left\{\left(x_{1il1}x_{1il2} + \sum_{j=1}^{i} x_{2ilj1}x_{2ilj2}\right)\Big/(1+i)\right\}$$
$$- \sum_{i=1}^{m}\sum_{l=1}^{n_i}\left\{\left(x_{1il1} + \sum_{j=1}^{i} x_{2ilj1}\right)\left(x_{1il2} + \sum_{j=1}^{i} x_{2ilj2}\right)\Big/(1+i)^2\right\}.$$

(b) Prove (4.15) and show that, in (4.15), $Z_1 = Z_{MTT}$ with $x = 0$ and $Z_2 = Z_{MTT}$ with $x = 1$.

4.8 Consider a matched case-control design with J strata. The ith stratum contains n_i independent cases and each case is matched with m controls, a matched set ($i = 1, \ldots, J$). The total number of controls in the ith matched set is mn_i. Let $n = \sum_{i=1}^{J} n_i$ be the total number of cases. In the ith stratum, denote the scores for the lth case and the jth control matched to the lth case as x_{1il} and x_{2ilj}, respectively.

Then, using the conditional likelihood function

$$\prod_{i=1}^{J}\prod_{l=1}^{n_i} \frac{\exp(\beta x_{1il})}{\exp(\beta x_{1il}) + \sum_{j=1}^{m}\exp(\beta x_{2ilj})},$$

show that the Score statistic for testing $H_0 : \beta = 0$ can be written as

$$Z = \frac{\sum_{i=1}^{J}\sum_{l=1}^{n_i}(mx_{1l} - \sum_{j=1}^{m} x_{2lj})}{[\sum_{i=1}^{J}\sum_{l=1}^{n_i}\{(1+m)(x_{1l}^2 + \sum_{j=1}^{m} x_{2lj}^2) - (x_{1l} + \sum_{j=1}^{m} x_{2lj})^2\}]^{1/2}},$$

which is identical to the MTT, Z_{MTT}, given in (4.2). The MDT can be obtained similarly.

4.9 Show that, under REC ($x = 0$) and DOM models ($x = 1$), the MTTs given in (4.4) using the data in Table 4.1 are identical to McNemar's test (4.5) using the allele-based matched pair data in Tables 4.14 and 4.15.

Chapter 5
Bayes Factors for Case-Control Association Studies

Abstract Chapter 5 focuses on the Bayes factor with Laplace approximation and an approximate Bayes factor. The latter is the Bayes factor based on the maximum likelihood estimate of the odds ratio for the genetic effect. In this chapter, the underlying genetic model is assumed to be known (either a recessive, additive or dominant model). How to code the genetic effect in a Bayesian analysis is discussed. The result may depend on how the genetic effect is coded. Bayesian analysis based on a full saturated model is an alternative approach, which is also studied. Examples are given of using Bayes factors and approximate Bayes factors for the analysis of case-control association studies. Covariates can be adjusted out in the analysis. Results of simulation studies are presented.

In the previous two chapters, frequentist approaches for hypothesis testing have been discussed for case-control association studies, in which p-values of test statistics are calculated and used against a prespecified significance level to accept or reject the null hypothesis. The conventional significance level is 0.05 for testing a single hypothesis. In the analysis of GWAS, a small significance level, e.g. 5×10^{-7}, is used regardless of the power of the test statistic and the sample size of the study. Therefore, the null hypothesis can be rejected with a p-value less than 5×10^{-7} in a GWAS, even though the power to detect the association is low.

Unlike frequentist approaches, Bayesian approaches treat parameters (e.g., log OR) as random variables and use the observed data to update prior knowledge about the parameters. In Bayesian hypothesis testing, a Bayes factor is often calculated and used with the prior information to measure evidence in the data in favor of or against the null hypothesis. Bayes factors have been especially proposed for the analysis of GWAS because they incorporate both strong significance of associations (small p-values) and the power of associations. Calculating a Bayes factor can involve evaluating multiple integrations. In practice, approximations of Bayes factors are used, using asymptotic approximations (e.g., a Laplace approximation) or a Monte-Carlo Markov Chain technique. Approximate Bayes factors that model the distributions of test statistics are studied because they have closed forms and are computationally simple.

For the analysis of case-control data with a diallelic marker, the logistic regression model is used. When a genotype is the only covariate in the logistic regression

G. Zheng et al., *Analysis of Genetic Association Studies*,
Statistics for Biology and Health,
DOI 10.1007/978-1-4614-2245-7_5, © Springer Science+Business Media, LLC 2012

model, either the Laplace approximation or the approximate Bayes factor can be readily obtained. Bayesian hypothesis testing allows other covariates to be adjusted out, but the dimension of the parameter space then increases accordingly. In this case, intensive computation or the requirement of the Monte-Carlo Markov Chain technique may prevent us from using standard Bayesian techniques in GWAS, in which hundreds of thousands of markers are analyzed. The computation burden is greatly reduced if Bayes factors are only calculated for the top markers with the most significant p-values.

We focus on Bayes factors with Laplace approximation and a particular approximate Bayes factor. The latter is based on the MLEs of the parameters and their large sample properties. For this approximate Bayes factor, the data in the Bayes factor are replaced by a Wald statistic or the estimates of the parameters. Besides its simplicity and similar interpretation as a Bayes factor, another advantage of the approximate Bayes factor is that only the prior distributions for the parameters modeling the genetic effects have to be specified. The priors for the nuisance parameters (the intercept and the coefficients adjusting for other covariates in the logistic regression model) are not used.

In this chapter, we assume the underlying genetic model is known (either a REC, ADD or DOM model). Bayesian analysis based on a full saturated model is an alternative approach, which is also discussed. Examples using Bayes factors and approximate Bayes factors for the analysis of case-control association studies are given. Simulation studies are presented. Bibliographical comments and cited references are given at the end.

5.1 Introduction

Bayesian inference is based on the following Bayes theorem. For any two events A and B,

$$\Pr(A|B) = \Pr(B|A)\Pr(A)/\Pr(B). \tag{5.1}$$

Let $p(x|\theta)$ denote the likelihood for data x of the parameter θ, $p(\theta)$ denote the prior density, and $p(\theta|x)$ denote the posterior density. Then, using (5.1),

$$p(\theta|x) = p(x|\theta)p(\theta)/p(x) = p(x|\theta)p(\theta)/\int p(x|\theta)p(\theta)d\theta, \tag{5.2}$$

where $p(x) = \int p(x|\theta)p(\theta)d\theta$ is the marginal density of x. Equation (5.2) is often written as

$$p(\theta|x) \propto p(x|\theta)p(\theta).$$

Thus, the posterior is proportional to the likelihood multiplied by the prior. In this chapter, we use $\Pr(\cdot)$ to denote the probability of an event in general, and use $p(\cdot)$ for a likelihood or density. For discrete random variables, $\Pr(\cdot)$ and $p(\cdot)$ are also used.

5.2 Bayes Factor

5.2.1 Definition

Consider testing the null hypothesis H_0 against the alternative hypothesis H_1. The probabilities of observing data x under H_0 and H_1 are denoted by $\Pr(x|H_0)$ and $\Pr(x|H_1)$, respectively. The Bayes factor (BF) is defined as

$$\text{BF}_{01} = \frac{\Pr(x|H_0)}{\Pr(x|H_1)}. \tag{5.3}$$

In the literature, the BF may also be defined as

$$\text{BF}_{10} = \frac{\Pr(x|H_1)}{\Pr(x|H_0)}. \tag{5.4}$$

Define the prior odds and posterior odds of H_0 by

$$\text{prior odds}(H_0) = \Pr(H_0)/\Pr(H_1),$$

$$\text{posterior odds}(H_0) = \Pr(H_0|x)/\Pr(H_1|x).$$

From

$$\frac{\Pr(H_0|x)}{\Pr(H_1|x)} = \frac{\Pr(x|H_0)}{\Pr(x|H_1)}\frac{\Pr(H_0)}{\Pr(H_1)} = \text{BF}_{01} \times \frac{\Pr(H_0)}{\Pr(H_1)},$$

it follows that the BF is the ratio of the posterior odds to the prior odds. From (5.3), a smaller value of BF_{01} provides more evidence in the data in favor of H_1. If $\text{BF}_{01} = 1$, it implies that the data are equally likely under H_0 or H_1. Further interpretation of the BF is discussed later.

Assume the data are drawn from the probability model $p(x|\theta)$, where $\theta = \theta_i$ under H_i, $i = 0, 1$. Then

$$\text{BF}_{01} = \frac{\Pr(x|H_0)}{\Pr(x|H_1)} = \frac{\int_{\Theta_0} p(x|\theta_0, H_0)p(\theta_0|H_0)d\theta_0}{\int_{\Theta_1} p(x|\theta_1, H_1)p(\theta_1|H_1)d\theta_1}, \tag{5.5}$$

where $p(\theta_i|H_i)$ is a prior density and Θ_i is the parameter space under the hypothesis H_i for $i = 0, 1$. From (5.5), the parameter θ is averaged out in the integrations over the parameter space rather than maximized.

5.2.2 Interpreting Bayes Factors

The BF is often used as a measure of evidence in the data in favor of the null or alternative hypotheses. It has to be interpreted together with the prior odds. If one has negligible prior evidence for or against H_0, then the prior odds is 1 (i.e., the prior probability of H_0 is $1/2$), and the posterior odds equals the BF. If $\text{BF}_{01} < 0.05$, then the posterior odds in favor of H_0 is less than 5% of the prior odds, and this is evidence against H_0.

Without the prior information, $\text{BF}_{01} = 0.05$ itself does not provide evidence against H_0. If the prior odds is large, then $\text{BF}_{01} = 0.05$ could still be in favor of H_0. In fact, an important distinction between Bayesian and frequentist approaches is that the BF depends on the prior information to provide evidence in the data, while a p-value alone does not measure strength of association. However, when comparing strength of association of two genetic markers (within a study or across studies), their BFs can be compared if they have the same priors for H_0.

Given the prior probability of H_0 as $\pi_0 = \Pr(H_0)$, the posterior probability of H_0, $\pi_1 = \Pr(H_0|x)$, can be obtained using the BF as follows:

$$\pi_1 = \frac{\text{BF}_{01} \times \text{prior odds}(H_0)}{1 + \text{BF}_{01} \times \text{prior odds}(H_0)}. \tag{5.6}$$

Hence, when the prior odds of H_0 is 1 and the BF is less than 0.05, the posterior probability of H_0 is less than 0.0476, which is in favor of H_1. Some practical guidelines are provided to interpret the BF as evidence against H_0. Using the logarithm to base 10 of BF_{01}, the evidence against H_0 is positive if $-2\log_{10}(\text{BF}_{01})$ is between 2 and 6, strong if it is between 6 and 10, and very strong if it is greater than 10. Hence, $\text{BF}_{01} < 0.05$ corresponds to strong evidence in the data against H_0. This interpretation, however, is for testing a single hypothesis. The posterior probability of H_0, $\pi_1 = \Pr(H_0|x)$, is also referred to as a Bayesian false discovery probability (BFDP).

Alternatively, one specifies $1 - \pi_0 = \Pr(H_1)$, the prior probability of H_1, and reports $1 - \pi_1 = \Pr(H_1|x)$ as the posterior probability of association (PPA). Then

$$\text{PPA} = \frac{1}{1 + \text{BF}_{01} \times \text{prior odds}(H_0)} = \frac{\text{BF}_{10} \times \text{prior odds}(H_1)}{1 + \text{BF}_{10} \times \text{prior odds}(H_1)}, \tag{5.7}$$

where the prior $\text{odds}(H_1) = \Pr(H_1)/\Pr(H_0)$. In testing association with a single marker, a negligible prior $\pi_0 = 0.50$ may be used. In GWAS, however, $\pi_0 = 0.999$ to 0.9999 has been suggested. That is, $\Pr(H_1) = 1 - \pi_0$ is about 10^{-4} to 10^{-5}.

Given a threshold, H_1 is claimed as noteworthy if the PPA exceeds the threshold. The probability that H_1 is claimed as noteworthy under H_1 is called Bayesian power. Given a threshold t, Bayesian power is $\Pr(\text{PPA} > t) = \Pr(\pi_1 < 1 - t) = \Pr(\text{BFDP} < 1 - t)$.

5.2.3 Approximations of Bayes Factors

To evaluate the BF, the following integrals need to be evaluated:

$$\Pr(x|H_i) = \int p(x|\theta_i, H_i)p(\theta_i|H_i)d\theta_i, \quad i = 0, 1. \tag{5.8}$$

For case-control genetic association studies, a logistic regression model is often used, and evaluating the above integral may not be trivial, particularly with a large number of covariates. Various approximations of the BF have been commonly used. Some of them are considered below. More details of the first two approaches will be given for case-control genetic association studies.

Laplace Approximation

Let $\widetilde{\theta}_i$ maximize $p(x|\theta_i, H_i)p(\theta_i|H_i) = p(x, \theta_i|H_i)$, which is referred to as the maximum a posteriori (MAP) estimate of θ_i. Note that $p(x, \theta_i|H_i) = p(x|H_i)p(\theta_i|x, H_i)$ and that $p(x|H_i)$ does not contain the parameter. Thus, the MAP estimate is also the posterior mode, which maximizes $p(\theta_i|x, H_i)$.

Expand $h(\theta_i) = \log\{p(x, \theta_i|H_i)\}$ as a quadratic function about the MAP estimate $\widetilde{\theta}_i$:

$$h(\theta_i) \approx h(\widetilde{\theta}_i) - \frac{1}{2}(\theta_i - \widetilde{\theta}_i)^T \left(-\frac{\partial^2 h}{\partial\theta_i \partial\theta_i^T} \right)(\theta_i - \widetilde{\theta}_i).$$

Denote

$$\widetilde{\Sigma}_i = -\left(\frac{\partial^2 h}{\partial\theta_i \partial\theta_i^T} \right)^{-1} \Big|_{\theta_i = \widetilde{\theta}_i}.$$

Then

$$p(x|\theta_i, H_i)p(\theta_i|H_i) \approx p(x|\widetilde{\theta}_i, H_i)p(\widetilde{\theta}_i|H_i) \exp\left\{ -\frac{1}{2}(\theta_i - \widetilde{\theta}_i)^T \widetilde{\Sigma}_i^{-1}(\theta_i - \widetilde{\theta}_i) \right\}.$$

Integrating both sides and using the multivariate normal distribution, we have

$$\int p(x|\theta_i, H_i)p(\theta_i|H_i)d\theta_i \approx p(x|\widetilde{\theta}_i, H_i)p(\widetilde{\theta}_i|H_i)$$

$$\times \int \exp\left\{ -\frac{1}{2}(\theta_i - \widetilde{\theta}_i)^T \widetilde{\Sigma}_i^{-1}(\theta_i - \widetilde{\theta}_i) \right\}d\theta_i$$

$$= p(x|\widetilde{\theta}_i, H_i)p(\widetilde{\theta}_i|H_i)(2\pi)^{d_i/2}|\widetilde{\Sigma}_i|^{1/2},$$

where d_i is the dimension of θ_i. This yields the following Laplace approximation of $\Pr(x|H_i)$:

$$\log\{\Pr(x|H_i)\} \approx \frac{d_i}{2}\log(2\pi) + \frac{1}{2}\log|\widetilde{\Sigma}_i| + \log\{p(x|\widetilde{\theta}_i, H_i)p(\widetilde{\theta}_i|H_i)\}. \quad (5.9)$$

The MAP estimate $\widetilde{\theta}_i$ can be obtained using the Newton-Raphson optimization algorithm or by a grid search over the parameter space.

Approximate Bayes Factors

The BF given in (5.3) models the data with the distributions (likelihoods) of the data under H_0 and H_1, where the parameters in the distributions are averaged out with respect to the prior distributions under H_0 and H_1. A simple modification of the BF in (5.3) is to model a test statistic T with its asymptotic distributions under H_0 and H_1, where the parameters are also averaged out with respective to the prior distributions. This modified BF, referred to as approximate BF (ABF), can be written as

$$\mathrm{ABF}_{01} = \frac{\mathrm{Pr}(T \mid H_0)}{\mathrm{Pr}(T \mid H_1)} = \frac{\int_{\Theta_0} p(T; \theta_0, H_0) p(\theta_0 \mid H_0) d\theta_0}{\int_{\Theta_1} p(T; \theta_1, H_1) p(\theta_1 \mid H_1) d\theta_1}, \tag{5.10}$$

where $p(T; \theta_i, H_i)$ is the asymptotic distribution of T under H_i and $p(\theta \mid H_i)$ is the prior density of θ under H_i. Note that the parameter in (5.3) and the parameter in (5.10) can be different. So the priors $p(\theta \mid H_i)$, $i = 0, 1$, can also be different. The above ABF has an interpretation similar to that of BF in (5.3). For example, given the prior odds, a similar posterior probability of H_1 and PPA can be obtained as follows:

$$\mathrm{Pr}(H_0 \mid T) = \frac{\mathrm{ABF}_{10} \times \text{prior odds}(H_0)}{1 + \mathrm{ABF}_{10} \times \text{prior odds}(H_0)},$$

and PPA $= \mathrm{Pr}(H_1 \mid T) = 1 - \mathrm{Pr}(H_0 \mid T)$. The ABF can be regarded as a measure of evidence in T for or against H_0.

The ABF can be useful if we replace T by the MLE of the parameter of interest θ. In this case, the large sample distributions of the MLE under H_0 and H_1 can be applied in computing the ABF. Hence, from (5.10),

$$\mathrm{ABF}_{01} = \frac{\mathrm{Pr}(\widehat{\theta} \mid H_0)}{\mathrm{Pr}(\widehat{\theta} \mid H_1)},$$

in which $\widehat{\theta}$ is the MLE of θ. As $n \to \infty$, ignoring negligible terms,

$$\sqrt{n}(\widehat{\theta} - \theta) \to N_d(0, I_1^{-1}(\theta)) \tag{5.11}$$

in distribution, where d is the dimension of θ and $I_1(\theta)$ is the Fisher information matrix contained in a single sample. For applications, the observed Fisher information matrix $i_1(\widehat{\theta})$ is used to replace $I_1(\theta)$, where the parameter θ is replaced by its MLE. Thus, without negligible terms,

$$\widehat{\theta} \sim N_{d_i}(\theta_i, i_1^{-1}(\widehat{\theta})/n) \quad \text{under } H_i \text{ for } i = 0, 1.$$

Then

$$\mathrm{ABF}_{01} = \frac{\mathrm{Pr}(\widehat{\theta} \mid H_0)}{\mathrm{Pr}(\widehat{\theta} \mid H_1)} = \frac{\int p(\widehat{\theta} \mid \theta_0, H_0) p(\theta_0 \mid H_0) d\theta_0}{\int p(\widehat{\theta} \mid \theta_1, H_1) p(\theta_1 \mid H_1) d\theta_1}, \tag{5.12}$$

where the multivariate normal density in (5.11) can be used for $p(\widehat{\theta} \mid \theta_i, H_i)$ rather than using the logistic regression model $p(x \mid \theta_i, H_i)$ as in the BF.

Monte Carlo and Importance Sampling

One approach to approximate the integral (5.8) is to use a random sample of size M drawn from the prior density $p(\theta_i|H_i)$. Denote the random sample by

$$\theta_i^{(1)}, \ldots, \theta_i^{(M)} \sim p(\theta_i|H_i).$$

Then, when M is large, one has

$$\widehat{\Pr}(x|H_i) \approx \frac{1}{M} \sum_{m=1}^{M} \Pr(x|\theta_i^{(m)}, H_i). \tag{5.13}$$

The approximation in (5.13) may not be efficient when the random samples $\theta_i^{(m)}$, $m = 1, \ldots, M$ have small likelihood values so that the convergence of (5.13) to a Gaussian distribution can be slow. One approach to improve this is to draw random samples from the so-called importance sampling function $p^*(\theta_i|H_i)$. Then define $w_m = p(\theta_i^{(m)}|H_i)/p^*(\theta_i^{(m)}|H_i)$, and estimate the integral (5.8) as

$$\widehat{\Pr}(x|H_i) \approx \frac{\sum_{m=1}^{M} w_m \Pr(x|\theta_i^{(m)}, H_i)}{\sum_{m=1}^{M} w_m}. \tag{5.14}$$

One choice for $p^*(\theta_i|H_i)$ is the posterior density

$$p^*(\theta_i|H_i) = p(\theta_i|x, H_i) = p(x|\theta_i, H_i)p(\theta_i|H_i)/p(x|H_i).$$

Then, using the above equation, $w_m = p(x|H_i)/p(x|\theta_i^{(m)}, H_i)$, and (5.14) becomes the harmonic mean of the likelihood values:

$$\widehat{\Pr}(x|H_i) \approx \left[\frac{1}{M} \sum_{m=1}^{M} \{\Pr(x|\theta_i^{(m)}, H_i)\}^{-1} \right]^{-1}.$$

Drawing a random sample from the posterior density is usually not feasible. Other techniques, such as Markov Chain Monte Carlo, in particular the Metropolis-Hastings algorithm or Gibbs sampler, are used to draw a dependent sample $\theta_i^{(m)}$, $m = 1, \ldots, M$, which form a Markov chain.

5.3 Bayes Factor for Genetic Association Studies

Let $d = 1$ indicate a case and $d = 0$ indicate a control. Denote the three genotypes for a diallelic marker with alleles A and B by $(G_0, G_1, G_2) = (AA, AB, BB)$. Let $P_i = \Pr(d = 1|\theta, G_i)$, which is given by

$$P_i = \frac{\exp\{\alpha + \beta I(G_i)\}}{1 + \exp\{\alpha + \beta I(G_i)\}}, \tag{5.15}$$

where $\theta = (\alpha, \beta)^T$ and $I(G_i)$ is a known function of genotype G_i for $i = 0, 1, 2$. For example, $I(G_i) = i$ for the ADD model, $I(G_0) = I(G_1) = 1$ and $I(G_2) = 1$ for the REC model, and $I(G_0) = 0$ and $I(G_1) = I(G_2) = 1$ for the DOM model. Because a single parameter β is used for the genetic effect, we assume the genetic model is known, i.e., the function $I(G)$ is well defined given one of the three genetic models. In general, we can write

$$
\begin{aligned}
I(G) = 0, \quad &\text{if } G = AA, \\
= t_1, \quad &\text{if } G = AB, \\
= t_2, \quad &\text{if } G = AB.
\end{aligned}
\tag{5.16}
$$

Assume B is the risk allele under H_1. Then $(t_1, t_2) = (0, 1)$ for the REC model, $(t_1, t_2) = (1, 1)$ for the DOM model, and $(t_1, t_2) = (1, 2)$ for the ADD model. Under the null hypothesis of no association H_0, $\beta = 0$ and α is a nuisance parameter. In the above logistic regression model, we have only an intercept α and a covariate β for the genetic effect. Therefore, the dimension of θ here is $d_0 = 1$ under H_0 and $d_1 = 2$ under H_1. Later we will describe models to adjust out other covariates.

5.3.1 Laplace Approximation

Suppose that r cases and s controls are drawn from the population with genotype counts (r_0, r_1, r_2) and (s_0, s_1, s_2) for (G_0, G_1, G_2). The following prospective likelihood function can be used for case-control data:

$$
\Pr(\text{data}|\theta) = \prod_{j=1}^{n} P_j^{d_j}(1 - P_j)^{1-d_j} = \frac{\exp\{\alpha r + \beta \sum_{i=0}^{2} r_i I(G_i)\}}{\prod_{i=0}^{2}[1 + \exp\{\alpha + \beta I(G_i)\}]^{n_i}}, \tag{5.17}
$$

where $n_i = r_i + s_i$ is the total genotype count for G_i and $n = r + s$ is the total sample size. Under the alternative hypothesis H_1, $\theta_1 = (\alpha, \beta)^T$ and the likelihood function is given in (5.17), which is rewritten as

$$
\Pr(\text{data}|\theta_1, H_1) = \frac{\exp\{\alpha r + \beta \sum_{i=0}^{2} r_i I(G_i)\}}{\prod_{i=0}^{2}[1 + \exp\{\alpha + \beta I(G_i)\}]^{n_i}}.
$$

Under H_0, $\theta_0 = \alpha$ and the likelihood function is given by

$$
\Pr(\text{data}|\theta_0, H_0) = \frac{e^{\alpha r}}{(1 + e^{\alpha})^n}.
$$

The prior distributions for α and β can be specified as

$$
\alpha \sim N(\mu_1, \sigma_1^2),
$$

$$
\beta \sim N(\mu_2, \sigma_2^2),
$$

where (μ_1, σ_1) and (μ_2, σ_2) are prespecified. Choosing $\mu_1 = \mu_2 = 0$, their densities are given by

$$p(\theta_0|H_0) \propto \frac{1}{\sigma_1} \exp\left(-\frac{\alpha^2}{2\sigma_1^2}\right),$$

$$p(\theta_1|H_1) \propto \frac{1}{\sigma_1} \exp\left(-\frac{\alpha^2}{2\sigma_1^2}\right) \frac{1}{\sigma_2} \exp\left(-\frac{\beta^2}{2\sigma_2^2}\right).$$

The denominator of the BF involves double integration with respect to $\theta_1 = (\alpha, \beta)^T$,

$$\int \Pr(\text{data}|\theta_1, H_1) p(\theta_1|H_1) d\theta_1.$$

We use the Laplace approximation to evaluate the above integral. Under H_1, with $\mu_1 = \mu_2 = 0$, the MAP estimate $\widetilde{\theta}_1 = (\widetilde{\alpha}, \widetilde{\beta})^T$ satisfies (Problem 5.2)

$$r - \frac{\widetilde{\alpha}}{\sigma_1^2} - \sum_{i=0}^{2} \frac{n_i \exp\{\widetilde{\alpha} + \widetilde{\beta} I(G_i)\}}{1 + \exp\{\widetilde{\alpha} + \widetilde{\beta} I(G_i)\}} = 0, \qquad (5.18)$$

$$\sum_{i=0}^{2} r_i I(G_i) - \frac{\widetilde{\beta}}{\sigma_2^2} - \sum_{i=0}^{2} \frac{n_i I(G_i) \exp\{\widetilde{\alpha} + \widetilde{\beta} I(G_i)\}}{1 + \exp\{\widetilde{\alpha} + \widetilde{\beta} I(G_i)\}} = 0, \qquad (5.19)$$

and $|\widetilde{\Sigma}_1^{-1}| = 1/|\widetilde{\Sigma}_1|$ is given by

$$|\widetilde{\Sigma}_1^{-1}| = \begin{vmatrix} \frac{1}{\sigma_1^2} + \sum_{i=0}^{2} n_i \Delta_i(\widetilde{\alpha}, \widetilde{\beta}) & \sum_{i=0}^{2} n_i I(G_i) \Delta_i(\widetilde{\alpha}, \widetilde{\beta}) \\ \sum_{i=0}^{2} n_i I(G_i) \Delta_i(\widetilde{\alpha}, \widetilde{\beta}) & \frac{1}{\sigma_2^2} + \sum_{i=0}^{2} n_i I^2(G_i) \Delta_i(\widetilde{\alpha}, \widetilde{\beta}) \end{vmatrix}, \qquad (5.20)$$

where $\Delta_i(\alpha, \beta) = \exp\{\alpha + \beta I(G_i)\}/[1 + \exp\{\alpha + \beta I(G_i)\}]^2$.

The numerator of the BF is equal to

$$E_{\theta_0|H_0}\left[\frac{\exp(\alpha r)}{\{1 + \exp(\alpha)\}^n}\right] = \frac{1}{\sqrt{2\pi}\sigma_1} \int \frac{\exp(\alpha r)}{\{1 + \exp(\alpha)\}^n} \exp\left(-\frac{\alpha^2}{2\sigma_1^2}\right) d\alpha,$$

which contains a single integral. However, the integrand is usually too small to integrate in the range $\alpha \in (-\infty, \infty)$. For example, if $r = 100$ and $n = 200$ with $\sigma_1 = 1$, the integrand is 2.4826×10^{-61} when $\alpha = 0$, 5.5558×10^{-72} when $\alpha = 1$, and 3.87×10^{-457} when $\alpha = 10$. To approximate the numerator of the BF, we can also use the Laplace approximation with $\beta = 0$. Under H_0, the MAP estimate for α, $\widetilde{\alpha}_0$, satisfies

$$\frac{\widetilde{\alpha}_0}{\sigma_1^2} + \frac{n e^{\widetilde{\alpha}_0}}{1 + e^{\widetilde{\alpha}_0}} = r$$

and

$$\Sigma_0^{-1} = 1/\sigma_1^2 + ne^{\tilde{\alpha}_0}/(1 + e^{\tilde{\alpha}_0})^2. \tag{5.21}$$

Then BF_{01} can be computed with Laplace approximations using the above approximations, (5.3) and (5.9).

5.3.2 An Example

For illustration, we compute a BF using the Laplace approximation for the SNP rs10510126 which has shown association with breast cancer in a GWAS (see Table 3.10). The genotype counts for the SNP are $(r_0, r_1, r_2) = (10, 180, 955)$ and $(s_0, s_1, s_2) = (14, 272, 854)$. Thus, $r = 1145$, $s = 1140$, and $n = 2285$, where $(n_0, n_1, n_2) = (24, 452, 1809)$. For the function $I(G)$ defined in (5.16), in addition to choosing $(t_1, t_2) = (0, 1)$, $(1, 1)$, and $(1, 2)$, we also chose $(t_1, t_2) = (1/2, 1)$ for comparison with $(t_1, t_2) = (1, 2)$.

Given σ_1^2, σ_2^2 and (t_1, t_2), and $\mu_1 = \mu_2 = 0$, Eqs. (5.18) and (5.19) become

$$\frac{\alpha}{\sigma_1^2} + \frac{24e^{\alpha}}{1 + e^{\alpha}} + \frac{452e^{\alpha+\beta t_1}}{1 + e^{\alpha+\beta t_1}} + \frac{1809e^{\alpha+\beta t_2}}{1 + e^{\alpha+\beta t_2}} = 1145,$$

$$\frac{\beta}{\sigma_2^2} + \frac{452t_1 e^{\alpha+\beta t_1}}{1 + e^{\alpha+\beta t_1}} + \frac{1809t_2 e^{\alpha+\beta t_2}}{1 + e^{\alpha+\beta t_2}} = 180t_1 + 955t_2.$$

We solve these two equations for $\theta = (\alpha, \beta)^T$ to obtain the MAP estimates under H_1. Under $H_0 : \beta = 0$, only Eq. (5.18) is available. Thus, the MAP estimate for α satisfies

$$\frac{\alpha}{\sigma_1^2} + \frac{2285e^{\alpha}}{1 + e^{\alpha}} = 1145.$$

The numerical values of MAP estimates $\tilde{\theta}_1 = (\tilde{\alpha}_1, \tilde{\beta}_1)^T$ under H_1 and $\tilde{\theta}_0 = \tilde{\alpha}_0$ under H_0 depend on σ_1^2, σ_2^2 and (t_1, t_2). Table 5.1 reports the values of the MAP estimates.

To use Laplace approximations, $|\tilde{\Sigma}_i|$ and $L(\tilde{\theta}_i) = p(\text{data}|\tilde{\theta}_i, H_i)p(\tilde{\theta}_i|H_i)$, $i = 0, 1$ are calculated. $|\tilde{\Sigma}_i|$ is calculated using (5.20) and (5.21). $L(\tilde{\theta}_i)$ is given by

$$L(\tilde{\theta}_0) = \frac{e^{1145\tilde{\alpha} - \tilde{\alpha}^2/(2\sigma_1^2)}}{\sqrt{2\pi}\,\sigma_1(1 + e^{\tilde{\alpha}})^{2285}},$$

$$L(\tilde{\theta}_1) = \frac{e^{1145\tilde{\alpha} + (180t_1 + 955t_2)\tilde{\beta} - \tilde{\alpha}^2/(2\sigma_1^2) - \tilde{\beta}^2/(2\sigma_2^2)}}{2\pi\,\sigma_1\sigma_2(1 + e^{\tilde{\alpha}})^{24}(1 + e^{\tilde{\alpha}+\tilde{\beta}t_1})^{452}(1 + e^{\tilde{\alpha}+\tilde{\beta}t_2})^{1809}}.$$

The BFs in Table 5.1 are obtained from $BF_{01} = \Pr(\text{data}|H_0)/\Pr(\text{data}|H_1)$ with the Laplace approximation (5.9).

Table 5.1 MAP estimate, BF and posterior probability of H_0, $\Pr(H_0|\text{data})$, when $\Pr(H_0) = 0.5$, using Laplace approximations given $\sigma_1 = 1.0$ (a negligible prior for α), σ_2 and (t_1, t_2). PPA can be obtained from $1 - \Pr(H_0|\text{data})$

σ_2	(t_1, t_2)	$\widetilde{\alpha}_0$	$\widetilde{\alpha}_1$	$\widetilde{\beta}_1$	BF_{01}	$\Pr(H_0|\text{data})$
0.10	$(0, 1)$	0.0043	-0.1928	0.2493	0.0033	0.0033
	$(1, 2)$		-0.4191	0.2381	0.0036	0.0036
	$(1, 1)$		-0.0144	0.0190	1.0142	0.5035
	$(\frac{1}{2}, 1)$		-0.1710	0.1972	0.0936	0.0856
0.20	$(0, 1)$	0.0043	-0.3178	0.4070	0.0001	0.0001
	$(1, 2)$		-0.6537	0.3698	0.0002	0.0002
	$(1, 1)$		-0.0585	0.0636	1.0591	0.5143
	$(\frac{1}{2}, 1)$		-0.4190	0.4761	0.0036	0.0036
0.40	$(0, 1)$	0.0043	-0.3792	0.4843	$3\mathrm{e}{-5}$	$3\mathrm{e}{-5}$
	$(1, 2)$		-0.7611	0.4300	$9\mathrm{e}{-5}$	$9\mathrm{e}{-5}$
	$(1, 1)$		-0.1473	0.1553	1.2404	0.5537
	$(\frac{1}{2}, 1)$		-0.6537	0.7396	0.0002	0.0002

A smaller BF_{01} indicates more evidence in the data in favor of H_1. Table 5.1 shows that the BFs in this example are fairly robust across various choices of the prior parameter σ_2^2 but they are strongly dependent on the underlying genetic model, i.e., the values of (t_1, t_2). Here we assume the genetic model is known. In practice, when the genetic model is unknown, we need to be cautious about which values of (t_1, t_2) are used in calculating BFs. The BFs are different when $(t_1, t_2) = (1, 2)$ and $(t_1, t_2) = (1/2, 1)$ are used. This indicates that, when the same priors are used, the BF is not invariant under a scaled transformation of (t_1, t_2). The reason for this will be discussed in the next section. On the other hand, the trend tests in Chap. 3 are invariant under any scaled transformation of the scores (t_1, t_2).

In Table 5.1, a negligible prior for $\alpha | H_0 \sim N(0, 1)$ is used (i.e., $\sigma_1 = 1$). For $\beta | H_1 \sim N(0, \sigma_2^2)$, the choice of σ_2 is related to the genetic effect. In Sect. 5.5, we see that $\sigma_2 = 0.174$ and $\sigma_2 = 0.557$ correspond to small and large genetic effects, respectively, determined by the upper bounds of the small and large genetic effects. Thus when σ_2 increases, the upper bound for the genetic effect increases accordingly.

Some parameter values are not reported in Table 5.1, e.g., $L(\widetilde{\theta}_i)$. These values are extremely small in the calculations. Corresponding to the first entry of the table (row 1), $L(\widetilde{\theta}_1) = 9.4712 \times 10^{-686}$ and $L(\widetilde{\theta}_0) = 5.620 \times 10^{-689}$. In Table 5.1, we chose $\sigma_2 = 0.1, 0.2$ and 0.4. For comparison, we calculate the trend tests (3.8) for the same SNP, and obtain $Z_{\mathrm{CATT}}(0) = 4.999$ (REC model), $Z_{\mathrm{CATT}}(1/2) = 4.827$ (ADD model), and $Z_{\mathrm{CATT}}(1) = 0.832$ (DOM model). The results from using BFs and trend tests are consistent.

Assuming the prior odds of H_0 is 1 (a negligible prior with $\pi_0 = 0.50$), the posterior probability of H_0 is $\Pr(H_0|\text{data}) = \mathrm{BF}_{01}/(1 + \mathrm{BF}_{01})$, which is also presented in Table 5.1 (the last column). There is very strong evidence for association of this

SNP with breast cancer under the REC model, and strong evidence under the ADD model. However, the result is not in favor of H_1 under the DOM model.

5.3.3 Coding the Genetic Effect

In Table 5.1, the BFs with genotype codes $(t_1, t_2) = (1, 2)$ and $(t_1, t_2) = (1/2, 1)$ are different when the same priors are used. The first code is used to count the number of B alleles in the genotypes, while the second one uses the proportion of B alleles in the genotypes.

Consider one genotype code

$$(I^{(1)}(G_0), I^{(1)}(G_1), I^{(1)}(G_2)) = (0, t_1, t_2), \tag{5.22}$$

where $t_2 \geq t_1 \geq 0$ and $t_2 > 0$, and another genotype code

$$(I^{(2)}(G_0), I^{(2)}(G_1), I^{(2)}(G_2)) = (0, t, 1), \tag{5.23}$$

where $t \in [0, 1]$. Let $t = t_1/t_2$ and (α_i, β_i) denote the parameters for the ith genotype code. Suppose one chooses the same priors for α, $\alpha_i | H_0 \sim N(0, \sigma_1^2)$ and $\alpha_i | H_1 \sim N(0, \sigma_1^2)$ for $i = 1, 2$, but different priors for β, $\beta_1 | H_1 \sim N(0, \sigma_2^2)$ and $\beta_2 | H_1 \sim N(0, \tilde{\sigma}_2^2)$. Denote the BF with parameters σ_1^2 and σ_2^2 and the genotype code (t_1, t_2) by $\mathrm{BF}_{01}(\sigma_1, \sigma_2; t_1, t_2)$. Then (Problem 5.7)

$$\mathrm{BF}_{01}(\sigma_1, \sigma_2; t_1, t_2) = \mathrm{BF}_{01}(\sigma_1, t_2\sigma_2; t_1/t_2, 1). \tag{5.24}$$

The above result shows that the BF with the code (t_1, t_2) equals the BF with the code $(t, 1) = (t_1/t_2, 1)$ if the priors $\beta_1 | H_1 \sim N(0, \sigma_2^2)$ and $\beta_2 | H_1 \sim N(0, t_2^2\sigma_2^2)$ are used, respectively. To prove (5.24), one can use the two transformations $\alpha_1 = \alpha_2$ and $\beta_1 = \beta_2/t_2$. The second one implies that $\tilde{\sigma}_2^2 = \mathrm{Var}(\beta_2) = t_2^2 \mathrm{Var}(\beta_1) = t_2^2\sigma_2^2$. Therefore, using $\beta_1 | H_1 \sim N(0, \sigma_2^2)$ and $\beta_2 | H_1 \sim N(0, t_2^2\sigma_2^2)$ ensures that comparable priors are used for both codes under which the BFs are identical.

As an example, in Table 5.1, the BF with $(t_1, t_2) = (1/2, 1)$ and $\sigma_2 = 0.20$ (or 0.40) is identical to the BF with $(t_1, t_2) = (1, 2)$ and $\sigma_2 = 0.10$ (or 0.20).

5.4 Approximate Bayes Factor for Genetic Association Studies I

In this section we consider the ABF when a single parameter is used to model the genetic effect of the marker. We start with the model that has only an intercept and a single parameter for the genetic model. Then the simple model is extended to have other covariates. In the next section, a saturated model with two parameters is considered.

5.4.1 No Covariates

Denote the log-likelihood as $l = \log \Pr(\text{data}|\theta)$, where $\Pr(\text{data}|\theta)$ is given in (5.17). The function $I(G)$ defined in (5.16) is used.

The MLE of θ, denoted by $\widehat{\theta} = (\widehat{\alpha}, \widehat{\beta})^T$, satisfies $\partial l/\partial\theta = 0$. The expressions for $\partial l/\partial\theta = 0$ are given in Problem 5.3 (a). The elements of the observed Fisher information matrix evaluated at $\widehat{\theta}$ can be written as $i_n(\widehat{\theta}) = -\partial l^2/\partial\theta\partial\theta^T|_{\theta=\widehat{\theta}}$, which is also given in Problem 5.3 (a). When the underlying genetic model is REC with $(t_1, t_2) = (0, 1)$ or DOM with $(t_1, t_2) = (1, 1)$, simple closed forms for $\widehat{\theta}$ can be obtained (see Problem 5.3 (b)). For the ADD model with $(t_1, t_2) = (1, 2)$, $\widehat{\theta}$ can be found numerically. When HWE proportions hold in the population, one may consider a 2×2 table for the ADD model comparing the two alleles between cases and controls. In this case, the closed form $\widehat{\theta}$ is available.

By the large sample property of the MLE $\widehat{\theta}$, we have, as $n = r + s \to \infty$ (and $r/n \to \varepsilon \in (0, 1)$), without negligible terms,

$$\widehat{\theta} = \begin{bmatrix} \widehat{\alpha} \\ \widehat{\beta} \end{bmatrix} \sim N_2(\theta, i_n^{-1}(\widehat{\theta})) = N_2\left(\begin{bmatrix} \alpha \\ \beta \end{bmatrix}, \begin{bmatrix} i_{00}(\widehat{\theta}) & i_{01}(\widehat{\theta}) \\ i_{10}(\widehat{\theta}) & i_{11}(\widehat{\theta}) \end{bmatrix}^{-1} \right),$$

where $i_n(\widehat{\theta})$ is based on n case-control samples. For comparison, $i_1(\theta)$ in (5.11) is based on a single sample. Using the transformation $\alpha^* = \alpha + (i_{01}(\widehat{\theta})/i_{00}(\widehat{\theta}))\beta$, which is estimated by $\widehat{\alpha}^* = \widehat{\alpha} + (i_{01}(\widehat{\theta})/i_{00}(\widehat{\theta}))\widehat{\beta}$, we have

$$\begin{bmatrix} \widehat{\alpha}^* \\ \widehat{\beta} \end{bmatrix} \sim N_2\left(\begin{bmatrix} \alpha^* \\ \beta \end{bmatrix}, \begin{bmatrix} i_{00}^{-1}(\widehat{\theta}) & 0 \\ 0 & (i_{11}(\widehat{\theta}) - i_{01}^2(\widehat{\theta})/i_{00})^{-1}(\widehat{\theta}) \end{bmatrix} \right).$$

Then the ABF is given by

$$\text{ABF} = \frac{\int p(\widehat{\alpha}^*, \widehat{\beta}|\alpha^*, H_0)p(\alpha^*|H_0)d\alpha^*}{\int \int p(\widehat{\alpha}^*, \widehat{\beta}|\alpha^*, \beta, H_1)p(\alpha^*, \beta|H_1)d\alpha^* d\beta},$$

where the numerator of the ABF can be written as

$$p(\widehat{\beta}|H_0) \int p(\widehat{\alpha}^*|\alpha^*, H_0)p(\alpha^*|H_0)d\alpha^*$$

and the denominator of the ABF can be written as

$$\int p(\widehat{\beta}|\beta, H_1)p(\beta|H_1)d\beta \times \int p(\widehat{\alpha}^*|\alpha^*, H_1)p(\alpha^*|H_1)d\alpha^*.$$

The same prior density can be used for α^* under either model H_i, i.e. $p(\alpha^*|H_0) = p(\alpha^*|H_1)$. Then the ABF can be simplified to

$$\text{ABF} = \frac{p(\widehat{\beta}|H_0)}{\int p(\widehat{\beta}|\beta, H_1)p(\beta|H_1)d\beta},$$

where $p(\widehat{\beta}|H_0)$ is the density $N(0, V)$, $p(\widehat{\beta}|\beta, H_1)$ is the density $N(\beta, V)$, where

$$V = (i_{11}(\widehat{\theta}) - i_{01}^2(\widehat{\theta})/i_{00}(\widehat{\theta}))^{-1},$$

and $p(\beta|H_1)$ is the prior density $N(0, \sigma_2^2)$, where σ_2^2 is prespecified. Then (Problem 5.3)

$$\text{ABF} = \sqrt{\frac{V + \sigma_2^2}{V}} \exp\left(-\frac{1}{2}\frac{\widehat{\beta}^2}{V}\frac{\sigma_2^2}{\sigma_2^2 + V}\right), \tag{5.25}$$

where $\widehat{\beta}^2/V$ is the Wald statistic for testing $H_0 : \beta = 0$. The ABF in (5.25) depends on the underlying genetic model, specified by (t_1, t_2).

5.4.2 With Covariates

Let z be a vector of m covariates, including an intercept, to adjust for in the logistic regression model. It takes the value $z_{ij} = (z_{ij1}, \ldots, z_{ijm})^T$ with $z_{ij1} = 1$ for the jth individual with genotype G_{ij}, $j = 1, \ldots, n_i$ and $i = 0, 1, 2$. Without loss of generality, assume the first r individuals are cases. Thus, the covariates for the cases with genotypes G_{ij} are z_{ij}, $j = 1, \ldots, r$, and for the controls with genotypes G_{ij} they are z_{ij}, $j = r + 1, \ldots, n$. Then the likelihood function (5.17) becomes

$$\text{Pr}(\text{data}|\theta, z, H_1) = \frac{\exp\{\sum_{i=0}^{2}\sum_{j=1}^{r_i}\alpha^T z_{ij} + \beta\sum_{i=0}^{2} r_i I(G_i)\}}{\prod_{i=0}^{2}\prod_{j=1}^{n_i}[1 + \exp\{\alpha^T z_{ij} + \beta I(G_{ij})\}]}, \tag{5.26}$$

where $\alpha = (\alpha_1, \ldots, \alpha_m)^T$ and $(G_0, G_1, G_2) = (G_{0j}, G_{1j}, G_{2j})$. Under $H_0 : \beta = 0$,

$$\text{Pr}(\text{data}|\theta, z, H_0) = \frac{\exp(\sum_{i=0}^{2}\sum_{j=1}^{r_i}\alpha^T z_{ij})}{\prod_{i=0}^{2}\prod_{j=1}^{n_i}\{1 + \exp(\alpha^T z_{ij})\}}. \tag{5.27}$$

The equations for the MLEs of $\theta = (\alpha, \beta)^T$ and observed Fisher information matrix are given in Problem 5.3 (c). It can be shown that the ABF with covariates has the same form as (5.25) (Problem 5.5) given by

$$\text{ABF} = \sqrt{\frac{V^* + \sigma_2^2}{V^*}} \exp\left(-\frac{1}{2}\frac{\widehat{\beta}^{*2}}{V^*}\frac{\sigma_2^2}{\sigma_2^2 + V^*}\right), \tag{5.28}$$

where $\widehat{\beta}^*$ is the MLE of β satisfying

$$\frac{\partial}{\partial\theta}\log\text{Pr}(\text{data}|\theta, z) = 0,$$

σ_2^2 is specified in the prior $\beta|H_1 \sim N(0, \sigma_2^2)$ and is also given in (5.25), and V^* is given in Problem 5.5 with the covariates.

5.4.3 An Alternative Derivation

In deriving the ABF in Sect. 5.4.1, the parameter θ in the ABF contains $(\alpha, \beta)^T$, where α is the nuisance parameter and β (the log OR) is the parameter of interest. Note that the linear transformation $\alpha^* = \alpha + (i_{01}(\widehat{\theta})/i_{00}(\widehat{\theta}))\beta$ was used in the derivation to eliminate α in the ABF. Thus, the ABF given by (5.25) can also be obtained by replacing the statistic T in the ABF with $\widehat{\beta}$, i.e.,

$$\text{ABF} = \frac{\Pr(\widehat{\beta}|H_0)}{\Pr(\widehat{\beta}|H_1)} = \sqrt{\frac{V + \sigma_2^2}{V}} \exp\left(-\frac{1}{2}\frac{\widehat{\beta}^2}{V}\frac{\sigma_2^2}{\sigma_2^2 + V}\right).$$

A similar result holds when covariates are adjusted out in the ABF.

5.4.4 Coding the Genetic Effect

Suppose the genotype codes (5.22) and (5.23) are used. We show that a result similar to (5.24) can be obtained:

$$\text{ABF}(\sigma_1, \sigma_2; t_1, t_2) = \text{ABF}(\sigma_1, t_2\sigma_2; t_1/t_2, 1). \tag{5.29}$$

In (5.29), covariates are assumed to be present. Let $(\widehat{\alpha}_1^*, \widehat{\beta}_1^*)$ and $(\widehat{\alpha}_2^*, \widehat{\beta}_2^*)$ be the MLEs using (5.22) and (5.23), respectively, with covariates. Then using Problem 5.3 (c), it can be shown that $\widehat{\alpha}_1^* = \widehat{\alpha}_2^*$ and $\widehat{\beta}_1^* = \widehat{\beta}_2^*/t_2$. Denote the observed Fisher information matrix corresponding to $(\widehat{\alpha}_j^*, \widehat{\beta}_j^*)$ by $i_{00}^{(j)}$, $i_{01}^{(j)}$ and $i_{11}^{(j)}$, $j = 1, 2$. Then, using Problem 5.3 (c), it can be shown that $i_{00}^{(1)} = i_{00}^{(2)}$, $i_{01}^{(1)} = t_2 i_{01}^{(2)}$, and $i_{11}^{(1)} = t_2^2 i_{11}^{(2)}$. Hence,

$$V^{*(1)} = \left(i_{11}^{(1)} - i_{10}^{(1)}\left(i_{00}^{(1)}\right)^{-1}i_{01}^{(1)}\right)^{-1} = \frac{1}{t_2^2}\left(i_{11}^{(2)} - i_{10}^{(2)}\left(i_{00}^{(2)}\right)^{-1}i_{01}^{(2)}\right)^{-1} = V^{*(2)}/t_2^2.$$

Thus,

$$\text{ABF}(\sigma_1, \sigma_2; t_1, t_2) = \sqrt{\frac{V^{*(1)} + \sigma_2^2}{V^{*(1)}}} \exp\left(-\frac{1}{2}\frac{(\widehat{\beta}_1^*)^2}{V^{*(1)}}\frac{\sigma_2^2}{\sigma_2^2 + V^{*(1)}}\right)$$

$$= \sqrt{\frac{V^{*(2)}/t_2^2 + t_2^2\sigma_2^2/t_2^2}{V^{*(2)}/t_2^2}} \exp\left(-\frac{1}{2}\frac{(\widehat{\beta}_2^*)^2/t_2^2}{V^{*(2)}/t_2^2}\frac{t_2^2\sigma_2^2/t_2^2}{t_2^2\sigma_2^2/t_2^2 + V^{*(2)}/t_2^2}\right)$$

$$= \sqrt{\frac{V^{*(2)} + t_2^2\sigma_2^2}{V^{*(2)}}} \exp\left(-\frac{1}{2}\frac{(\widehat{\beta}_2^*)^2}{V^{*(2)}}\frac{t_2^2\sigma_2^2}{t_2^2\sigma_2^2 + V^{*(2)}}\right)$$

$$= \text{ABF}(\sigma_1, t_2\sigma_2; t_1/t_2, 1).$$

5.4.5 An Example

The example studied in Sect. 5.3.2 is revisited using the ABFs with REC, ADD and DOM models. Based on the results of the previous section, we only consider the genotype codes $(t_1, t_2) = (0, 1)$ for the REC model, $(1, 2)$ for the ADD model and $(1, 1)$ for the DOM model. Across the three genetic models, the same σ_2^2 is used in the prior distribution of β.

We apply the ABF (5.28) to the SNP for a given genetic model. The MLEs $\widehat{\alpha}$ and $\widehat{\beta}$ can be solved from the following equations (see Problem 5.3 (a) and (b))

$$\frac{24e^{\widehat{\alpha}}}{1 + e^{\widehat{\alpha}}} + \frac{452e^{\widehat{\alpha}+t_1\widehat{\beta}}}{1 + e^{\widehat{\alpha}+t_1\widehat{\beta}}} + \frac{1809e^{\widehat{\alpha}+t_2\widehat{\beta}}}{1 + e^{\widehat{\alpha}+t_2\widehat{\beta}}} = 1145,$$

$$\frac{452t_1 e^{\widehat{\alpha}+t_1\widehat{\beta}}}{1 + e^{\widehat{\alpha}+t_1\widehat{\beta}}} + \frac{1809t_2 e^{\widehat{\alpha}+t_2\widehat{\beta}}}{1 + e^{\widehat{\alpha}+t_2\widehat{\beta}}} = 180t_1 + 955t_2.$$

Under the REC or DOM models, closed forms for $\widehat{\alpha}$ and $\widehat{\beta}$ are available. Under the ADD model, we apply the Newton-Raphson procedure to find $\widehat{\alpha}$ and $\widehat{\beta}$.

For illustration, consider the REC model. Numerical results show that $\widehat{\alpha} = -0.4090$ and $\widehat{\beta} = 0.5207$. Given $\widehat{\alpha}$ and $\widehat{\beta}$, $\widehat{\Delta}_0 = \exp(\widehat{\alpha})/\{1 + \exp(\widehat{\alpha})\}^2 = 0.2398$, $\widehat{\Delta}_1 = \exp(\widehat{\alpha} + t_1\widehat{\beta})/\{1 + \exp(\widehat{\alpha} + t_1\widehat{\beta})\}^2 = 0.2398$ and $\widehat{\Delta}_2 = \exp(\widehat{\alpha} + t_2\widehat{\beta})/\{1 + \exp(\widehat{\alpha} + t_2\widehat{\beta})\}^2 = 0.2492$, where $t_1 = 0$ and $t_2 = 1$. The observed Fisher information can be evaluated using

$$i_{00}(\widehat{\theta}) = 24\widehat{\Delta}_0 + 452\widehat{\Delta}_1 + 1809\widehat{\Delta}_2 = 564.9476,$$

$$i_{01}(\widehat{\theta}) = 452t_1\widehat{\Delta}_1 + 1809t_2\widehat{\Delta}_2 = 450.8028,$$

$$i_{11}(\widehat{\theta}) = 452t_1^2\widehat{\Delta}_1 + 1809t_2^2\widehat{\Delta}_2 = 450.8028.$$

Hence, the asymptotic variance for $\widehat{\beta}$ is $V = 1/(i_{11}(\widehat{\theta}) - i_{01}^2(\widehat{\theta})/i_{00}(\widehat{\theta})) = 0.01098$. Finally, the ABF given by (5.28) is computed. The results are reported in Table 5.2. Comparing the results in Table 5.2 with those in Table 5.1, we notice that the ABFs are similar to the BFs. The ABFs are again fairly robust to the choices of σ_2 but they are very sensitive to the underlying genetic model through the values of (t_1, t_2).

5.5 Approximate Bayes Factor for Genetic Association Studies II

In this section, we consider a saturated model with two parameters to model the genetic effect of a single marker. In this case, the underlying genetic model is not required. We start with the case where there are covariates to adjust out. Then we consider the special case with only an intercept and two coefficients for the genetic effect.

Table 5.2 MLEs and ABFs given σ_2 and a genetic model

σ_2	(t_1, t_2)	$\widehat{\alpha}$	$\widehat{\beta}$	V	ABF_{01}
0.10	$(0, 1)$	-0.4090	0.5207	0.0110	0.0038
	$(1, 2)$	-0.8315	0.4686	0.0096	0.0041
	$(1, 1)$	-0.3365	0.3444	0.1732	1.0094
0.20	$(0, 1)$	-0.4090	0.5207	0.0110	0.0001
	$(1, 2)$	-0.8315	0.4686	0.0096	0.0002
	$(1, 1)$	-0.3365	0.3444	0.1732	1.0404
0.40	$(0, 1)$	-0.4090	0.5207	0.0110	$3\mathrm{e}{-5}$
	$(1, 2)$	-0.8315	0.4686	0.0096	$8\mathrm{e}{-5}$
	$(1, 1)$	-0.3365	0.3444	0.1732	1.1767

5.5.1 With Covariates

In Sect. 5.3, Sect. 5.4.1, and Sect. 5.4.2, an indicator function $I(G)$ is used for genotype G with $I(AA) = 0$, $I(AB) = t_1$, and $I(BB) = t_2$, where the values of (t_1, t_2) depend on the underlying genetic model. A single coefficient β is used for the genetic effect. That setting requires the underlying genetic model. When the genetic model is unknown, one can use two indicator functions with two coefficients, as in Sect. 3.3.4.

Define $I_1(G) = 0, 0, 1$ for $G = AA, AB, BB$, and $I_2(G) = 0, 1, 1$ for $G = AA, AB, BB$. Let z_{ij}, $j = 1, \ldots, n$, be covariates as defined before. The likelihood function (5.17) with covariates becomes

$$\Pr(\text{data}|\theta, z, H_1) = \frac{\exp\{\sum_{i=0}^{2} \sum_{j=1}^{r_i} \alpha^T z_{ij} + \sum_{i=1}^{2} \sum_{h=1}^{2} r_i \beta_h I_h(G_i)\}}{\prod_{i=0}^{2} \prod_{j=1}^{n_i} [1 + \exp\{\alpha^T z_{ij} + \sum_{h=1}^{2} \beta_h I_h(G_{ij})\}]},$$

where $(G_0, G_1, G_2) = (G_{0j}, G_{1j}, G_{2j}) = (AA, AB, BB)$. Under $H_0 : \beta_1 = \beta_2 = 0$,

$$\Pr(\text{data}|\theta, z, H_0) = \frac{\exp(\sum_{i=0}^{2} \sum_{j=1}^{r_i} \alpha^T z_{ij})}{\prod_{i=0}^{2} \prod_{j=1}^{n_i} \{1 + \exp(\alpha^T z_{ij})\}}.$$

Denote

$$E_{ij}(\theta) = \exp\left\{\alpha^T z_{ij} + \sum_{h=1}^{2} \beta_h I_h(G_{ij})\right\}, \quad j = 1, \ldots, n_i, \; i = 0, 1, 2.$$

Let $l(\theta)$ denote the log-likelihood function. The MLEs of $\theta = (\alpha, \beta_1, \beta_2)^T$, denoted by $\widehat{\theta} = (\widehat{\alpha}, \widehat{\beta}_1, \widehat{\beta}_2)$, can be solved from $\partial l(\theta)/\partial \alpha = 0$ and $\partial l(\theta)/\partial \beta_h = 0$, $h = 1, 2$, which are given by

$$\sum_{i=0}^{2}\sum_{j=1}^{r_i} z_{ij} = \sum_{i=0}^{2}\sum_{j=1}^{n_i} \frac{z_{ij} E_{ij}(\theta)}{1 + E_{ij}(\theta)}, \tag{5.30}$$

$$\sum_{i=1}^{2} r_i I_h(G_i) = \sum_{i=0}^{2}\sum_{j=1}^{n_i} \frac{I_h(G_{ij}) E_{ij}(\theta)}{1 + E_{ij}(\theta)}, \quad h = 1, 2. \tag{5.31}$$

Denote $\delta_{ij} = E_{ij}(\theta)/\{1 + E_{ij}(\theta)\}^2$. Then the observed Fisher information matrix for $\widehat{\theta} = (\widehat{\alpha}, \widehat{\beta}_1, \widehat{\beta}_2)^T$ can be written as

$$i_n(\widehat{\theta}) = \begin{bmatrix} i_{00} & i_{01} & i_{02} \\ i_{10} & i_{11} & i_{12} \\ i_{20} & i_{21} & i_{22} \end{bmatrix}_{\theta=\widehat{\theta}}$$

$$= \begin{bmatrix} \sum\sum z_{ij} z_{ij}^T \delta_{ij} & \sum\sum z_{ij} I_1 \delta_{ij} & \sum\sum z_{ij} I_2 \delta_{ij} \\ \sum\sum z_{ij} I_1 \delta_{ij} & \sum\sum I_1 \delta_{ij} & \sum\sum I_1 I_2 \delta_{ij} \\ \sum\sum z_{ij} I_2 \delta_{ij} & \sum\sum I_1 I_2 \delta_{ij} & \sum\sum I_2 \delta_{ij} \end{bmatrix}_{\theta=\widehat{\theta}} \tag{5.32}$$

where $I_h = I_1(G_{ij})$ for $h = 1, 2$, and θ is replaced by $\widehat{\theta}$. Then, asymptotically,

$$\widehat{\theta} \sim N_{m+2}(\theta, i_n^{-1}(\widehat{\theta})),$$

where m is the number of covariates, including the intercept.

Partition the matrix $i(\widehat{\theta})$ as $i(\widehat{\theta}) = (B_{ij})_{2\times 2}$, where $B_{11} = i_{00}$, $B_{12} = (i_{01}, i_{02})$, $B_{21} = B_{12}^T$, and

$$B_{22} = \begin{bmatrix} i_{11} & i_{12} \\ i_{12} & i_{22} \end{bmatrix}.$$

Consider the transformation $\alpha^* = \alpha + B_{11}^{-1} B_{12}\beta$, where $\beta = (\beta_1, \beta_2)^T$. Let $\widehat{\alpha}^* = \widehat{\alpha} + B_{11}^{-1} B_{12}\widehat{\beta}$. Then, asymptotically,

$$\begin{bmatrix} \widehat{\alpha}^* \\ \widehat{\beta} \end{bmatrix} \sim N_{m+2}\left(\begin{bmatrix} \alpha^* \\ \beta \end{bmatrix}, \begin{bmatrix} \mathrm{Var}(\widehat{\alpha}^*) & 0 \\ 0 & (B_{22} - B_{21} B_{11}^{-1} B_{12})^{-1} \end{bmatrix} \right). \tag{5.33}$$

Using a similar argument as for the ABF in Sect. 5.4.1, we have

$$\mathrm{ABF} = \frac{\int p(\widehat{\alpha}^*, \widehat{\beta} | \alpha^*, H_0) p(\alpha^* | H_0) d\alpha^*}{\int\int p(\widehat{\alpha}^*, \widehat{\beta} | \alpha^*, \beta, H_1) p(\alpha^*, \beta | H_1) d\alpha^* d\beta}$$

$$= \frac{p(\widehat{\beta} | H_0)}{\int p(\widehat{\beta} | \beta, H_1) p(\beta | H_1) d\beta}.$$

Denote

$$V = (B_{22} - B_{21} B_{11}^{-1} B_{12})^{-1}.$$

Then $\widehat{\beta}|H_0 \sim N_2(0, V)$ and $\widehat{\beta}|\beta, H_1 \sim N_2(\beta, V)$. Let $\beta|H_1 \sim N_2(0, W)$. Then

$$p(\widehat{\beta}|H_0) = \frac{1}{2\pi |V|^{1/2}} \exp\left(-\frac{1}{2}\widehat{\beta}^T V^{-1}\widehat{\beta}\right),$$

and, using the results of Problem 5.6,

$$\int p(\widehat{\beta}|\beta, H_1) p(\beta|H_1) d\beta$$

$$= \frac{1}{(2\pi)^2 |VW|^{1/2}} \int \exp\left[-\frac{1}{2}\{(\beta - \widehat{\beta})^T V^{-1}(\beta - \widehat{\beta}) + \beta^T W^{-1}\beta\}\right] d\beta$$

$$= \frac{1}{2\pi |V + W|^{1/2}} \exp\left\{-\frac{1}{2}\widehat{\beta}^T (V + W)^{-1}\widehat{\beta}\right\}.$$

Thus, the ABF can be written as

$$\text{ABF} = \frac{|V + W|^{1/2}}{|V|^{1/2}} \exp\left[-\frac{1}{2}\widehat{\beta}^T \{V^{-1} - (V + W)^{-1}\}\widehat{\beta}\right]. \tag{5.34}$$

5.5.2 No Covariates

When the logistic regression model only contains an intercept α and two parameters (β_1, β_2) for the genetic effect, the likelihood function (5.17) becomes

$$\text{Pr}(\text{data}|\theta, H_1) = \frac{\exp\{\alpha r + \sum_{i=1}^{2} \sum_{h=1}^{2} r_i \beta_h I_h(G_i)\}}{\prod_{i=0}^{2} \prod_{j=1}^{n_i} [1 + \exp\{\alpha + \sum_{h=1}^{2} \beta_h I_h(G_{ij})\}]}.$$

Under $H_0 : \beta_1 = \beta_2 = 0$,

$$\text{Pr}(\text{data}|\theta, H_0) = \frac{\exp(\alpha r)}{\{1 + \exp(\alpha)\}^n}.$$

The MLEs $\widehat{\theta}$ can be written as

$$\widehat{\alpha} = \log\left(\frac{r_0}{s_0}\right), \qquad \widehat{\beta}_1 = \log\left(\frac{r_2 s_1}{r_1 s_2}\right), \qquad \widehat{\beta}_2 = \log\left(\frac{r_1 s_0}{r_0 s_1}\right). \tag{5.35}$$

Note that $\widehat{\beta}_1$ and $\widehat{\beta}_2$ are log ORs of genotype $G_2 = BB$ relative to $G_1 = AB$ and genotype $G_1 = AB$ relative to $G_0 = AA$. Using the Delta method, we can obtain the asymptotic covariance matrix of $\widehat{\beta}_1$ and $\widehat{\beta}_2$ directly. Following the derivation used before with the linear transformation, the observed Fisher information matrix $i(\widehat{\theta})$ in (5.32) can be obtained and used to find $V = (B_{22} - B_{21}B_{11}^{-1}B_{12})^{-1}$ given in (5.33). Let $a_i = r_i s_i / n_i$ for $i = 0, 1, 2$. Then (5.32) can be written as

$$i_n(\widehat{\theta}) = \begin{bmatrix} \sum_{i=0}^{2} a_i & a_2 & \sum_{i=1}^{2} a_i \\ a_2 & a_2 & a_2 \\ \sum_{i=1}^{2} a_i & a_2 & \sum_{i=1}^{2} a_i \end{bmatrix} \quad \text{and}$$

$$i_n^{-1}(\widehat{\theta}) = \begin{bmatrix} \frac{1}{a_0} & 0 & -\frac{1}{a_0} \\ 0 & \frac{1}{a_1} + \frac{1}{a_2} & -\frac{1}{a_1} \\ -\frac{1}{a_0} & -\frac{1}{a_1} & \frac{1}{a_0} + \frac{1}{a_1} \end{bmatrix}$$

with the determinant $|i_n(\widehat{\theta})| = a_0 a_1 a_2$. Thus, V is given by

$$V = (B_{22} - B_{21}B_{11}^{-1}B_{12})^{-1}$$

$$= \begin{bmatrix} \frac{1}{r_1} + \frac{1}{s_1} + \frac{1}{r_2} + \frac{1}{s_2} & -\frac{1}{r_1} - \frac{1}{s_1} \\ -\frac{1}{r_1} - \frac{1}{s_1} & \frac{1}{r_0} + \frac{1}{s_0} + \frac{1}{r_1} + \frac{1}{s_1} \end{bmatrix}. \tag{5.36}$$

A direct approach to derive V is to find the asymptotic covariance matrix of $\widehat{\beta} = (\widehat{\beta}_1, \widehat{\beta}_2)^T$ using multinomial distributions for case genotype counts and control genotype counts and the fact that cases and controls are independent. Using the prior $\beta | H_1 \sim N(0, W)$, the ABF in (5.34) can be computed.

5.5.3 An Example

We revisit the SNP rs10510126 studied before with genotype counts $(r_0, r_1, r_2) = (10, 180, 955)$ and $(s_0, s_1, s_2) = (14, 272, 854)$. The estimate $\widehat{\alpha}$ is not used in the ABF. Thus, we only calculate the estimates for β_1 and β_2, which are given by $\widehat{\beta}_1 = 0.5246$ and $\widehat{\beta}_2 = -0.07637$. The matrix V in (5.36) is given by

$$V = \begin{bmatrix} 0.01145 & -0.009232 \\ -0.009232 & 0.1807 \end{bmatrix}.$$

For the prior we choose $(\beta_1, \beta_2)^T \sim N_2(0, W)$ with

$$W = \begin{bmatrix} \sigma_2^2/1.5^2 & -\sigma_2^2/1.5 \\ -\sigma_2^2/1.5 & \sigma_2^2 \end{bmatrix}. \tag{5.37}$$

The choice of the above covariance matrix is for illustration. How to choose prior distributions is discussed in the next section. The ABFs are 0.0051, 0.0002, and 5e−5 for $\sigma_2 = 0.1$, 0.2, and 0.4, respectively.

5.6 Prior Specification

5.6.1 Prior for Using a Single Parameter

Priors need to be specified in Bayesian hypothesis testing. The BF given in Sect. 5.3 and the ABF given in Sect. 5.4 depend on the prior distributions. The results change when different priors are used. Hence, as shown in Tables 5.1 and 5.2, a sensitivity analysis with different priors is essential to draw meaningful conclusions using a BF or an ABF.

In Sect. 5.3, the priors for α and β are specified for the BF, while in Sect. 5.4, only the prior for β is specified for the ABF. In the logistic regression model (5.15), α is the log odds of baseline genotype $G_0 = AA$, which contains 0 risk alleles,

$$\alpha = \log\left(\frac{\text{Pr(case}\,|G_0)}{1 - \text{Pr(case}\,|G_0)}\right).$$

Therefore, a normal prior is reasonable for α. In practice, to have a negligible prior for α,

$$\alpha \sim N(0, \sigma_1^2) = N(0, 1)$$

can be used. Both the BF and ABF require a prior for β, which is the log OR of genotype G_i relative to the baseline genotype G_0. More specifically,

$$\log\left\{\frac{\text{Pr(case}\,|G_i)}{1 - \text{Pr(case}\,|G_i)} \middle/ \frac{\text{Pr(case}\,|G_0)}{1 - \text{Pr(case}\,|G_0)}\right\} = \beta I(G_i), \quad \text{for } i = 1, 2.$$

For the ADD model, $I(G_1) = 1$ and β is the log OR of genotype $G_1 = AB$ relative to $G_0 = AA$, given by

$$\beta = \log\left\{\frac{\text{Pr(case}\,|G_1)}{1 - \text{Pr(case}\,|G_1)} \middle/ \frac{\text{Pr(case}\,|G_0)}{1 - \text{Pr(case}\,|G_0)}\right\}.$$

Hence, a normal prior can be used for β. In practice, one may choose

$$\beta \sim N(0, \sigma_2^2).$$

There are many ways to determine the value for σ_2^2. One approach is based on the OR of the genotype G_1 relative to G_0. For many common diseases, the OR is in the range of 1.1 to 2 with more weight on the range of 1.1 to 1.5. If we assume that the probability of an OR greater than 2 is 0.05, then from

$$\text{Pr}(\exp(\beta) \leq 2) = \text{Pr}(\beta \leq \log 2) = \text{Pr}(\beta/\sigma_2 \leq \log 2/\sigma_2) = 0.95,$$

and $\beta/\sigma_2 \sim N(0, 1)$, we have

$$\sigma_2 = \log(2)/\Phi^{-1}(0.95) \approx 0.421. \tag{5.38}$$

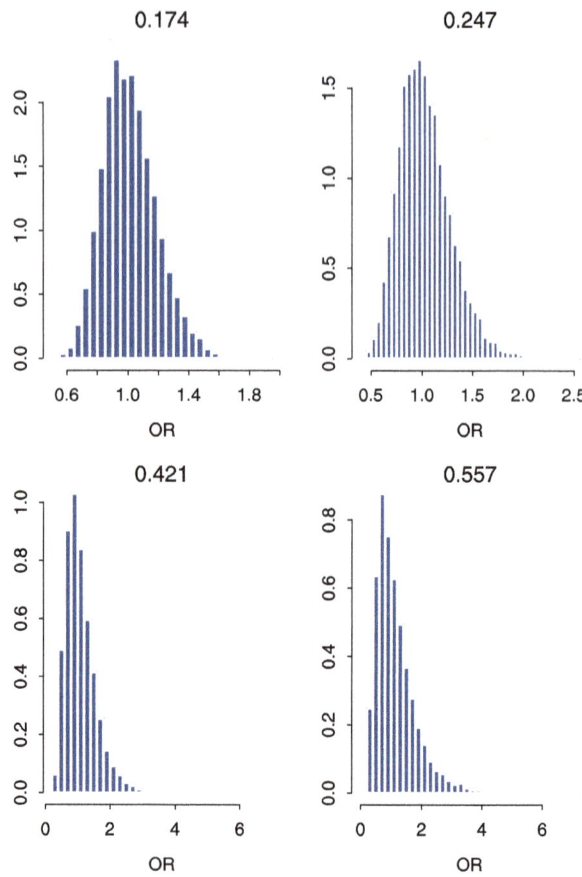

Fig. 5.1 Histogram plots of the ORs OR $= e^{\beta}$ with $\sigma_2 = 0.174, 0.247, 0.421,$ and 0.557. Each plot is based on 10,000 random variates $\beta \sim N(0, \sigma_2^2)$

If a two-sided OR is considered, then

$$\sigma_2 = \log(2)/\Phi^{-1}(0.975) \approx 0.354.$$

In general, we can give an upper bound U_β for β with a small probability p_β such that $\Pr(\exp(\beta) \le U_\beta) = 1 - p_\beta$, from which σ_2 can be obtained in a similar manner to (5.38). Table 5.3 presents σ_2 for some choices of U_β and p_β. The choices of σ_2 range from 0.174 for a small genetic effect to 0.557 for a large genetic effect. Figure 5.1 plots histograms of the OR e^{β} simulated from $\beta \sim N(0, \sigma_2^2)$ with different choices of σ_2. Because the BF and ABF would change with different σ_2, it is important to conduct sensitivity analysis and calculate the BF and ABF with different σ_2^2 or even with different priors.

Table 5.3 Choosing priors for the log OR β with a risk allele given the upper bound of the OR U_β and the probability p_β that the OR is greater than the upper bound

U_β	p_β	σ_2
1.5	0.01	0.174
	0.05	0.247
2.0	0.01	0.298
	0.05	0.421
2.5	0.01	0.394
	0.05	0.557

Table 5.4 Median (standard deviation) of the posterior probability of H_0 under H_0, given the prior probability of H_0 0.99 with allele frequency $p = \Pr(B)$ and σ_2^2. We used $t = 0$, 1/2, and 1 for the BFs calculated under the REC, ADD, and DOM models, respectively

p	σ_2	$t = 0$	$t = 1/2$	$t = 1$
0.1	0.1	0.9901	0.9911	0.9909
		(0.0001)	(0.0032)	(0.0028)
	0.2	0.9902	0.9931	0.9928
		(0.0004)	(0.0142)	(0.0123)
	0.4	0.9907	0.9957	0.9954
		(0.0013)	(0.0202)	(0.0199)
0.3	0.1	0.9905	0.9921	0.9914
		(0.0013)	(0.0086)	(0.0054)
	0.2	0.9918	0.9947	0.9936
		(0.0049)	(0.0149)	(0.0121)
	0.4	0.9942	0.9970	0.9962
		(0.0138)	(0.0170)	(0.0205)
0.5	0.1	0.9911	0.9924	0.9911
		(0.0031)	(0.0077)	(0.0032)
	0.2	0.9931	0.9951	0.9931
		(0.0106)	(0.0166)	(0.0121)
	0.4	0.9958	0.9973	0.9958
		(0.0199)	(0.0226)	(0.0198)

5.7   Simulation Studies Using Approximate Bayes Factors

We present simulation results to compare the posterior probabilities of H_0 when H_0 is true. The prior probability of H_0 is fixed at 0.99 in the simulation. Under H_1, we consider the PPA. In all the simulations, we use $r = s = 500$ with disease prevalence 0.1 and the different MAFs $p = 0.1$, 0.3 or 0.5. The standard deviations ($\sigma_2 = 0.1$, 0.2 and 0.4) in the normal prior distribution for the genetic effect are used. In the simulations, HWE proportions in the population are assumed. The results are based on 10,000 case-control datasets.

Table 5.5 Medians of PPA under H_1, given the prior probability of H_1 0.01 with the allele frequency $p = \text{Pr}(B)$, σ_2^2 and GRR λ_2 with a genetic model. We used $t = 0$, $1/2$, and 1 for the REC, ADD, and DOM models, respectively

Model	p	Measures	$\sigma_2 = 0.2$			$\sigma_2 = 0.4$		
			λ_2			λ_2		
			1.2	1.5	2.0	1.2	1.5	2.0
REC	0.3	$t = 0$	0.009	0.023	0.252	0.007	0.031	0.685
		$t = 1/2$	0.006	0.012	0.169	0.003	0.008	0.161
		$t = 1$	0.006	0.007	0.011	0.004	0.004	0.007
	0.5	$t = 0$	0.011	0.160	0.996	0.008	0.255	0.999
		$t = 1/2$	0.008	0.092	0.992	0.004	0.079	0.997
		$t = 1$	0.007	0.009	0.024	0.004	0.006	0.024
ADD	0.3	$t = 0$	0.009	0.013	0.041	0.006	0.013	0.075
		$t = 1/2$	0.007	0.044	0.871	0.004	0.037	0.923
		$t = 1$	0.008	0.030	0.609	0.005	0.028	0.813
	0.5	$t = 0$	0.008	0.021	0.158	0.005	0.019	0.252
		$t = 1/2$	0.007	0.049	0.830	0.004	0.042	0.879
		$t = 1$	0.008	0.024	0.238	0.005	0.024	0.466
DOM	0.3	$t = 0$	0.008	0.010	0.014	0.006	0.007	0.014
		$t = 1/2$	0.010	0.172	0.994	0.006	0.180	0.998
		$t = 1$	0.013	0.295	0.999	0.010	0.441	0.999
	0.5	$t = 0$	0.007	0.008	0.011	0.004	0.005	0.008
		$t = 1/2$	0.007	0.035	0.429	0.004	0.023	0.462
		$t = 1$	0.011	0.079	0.795	0.008	0.123	0.973

The medians and the standard deviations of the posterior probability of H_0 from 10,000 replicates simulated under H_0 are reported in Table 5.4. The results show that the medians and the standard deviations are comparable among the three ABFs.

The simulation results under H_1 are reported in Table 5.5 for the three ABFs. We only considered $p = 0.3$ and 0.4 with $\sigma_2 = 0.2$ and 0.4. Under H_1, given the prior probability of H_1 to be 0.01, a greater PPA indicates stronger association. The results show that the PPA with correctly chosen t is largest under that model, and the PPA with $t = 1/2$ is fairly robust across the three genetic models.

Results presented in Table 5.5 are based on median PPAs. In Table 5.6, we report Bayesian power, the proportion of PPA for a given method being greater than 0.20, which is a threshold of PPA that we chose to claim association given the prior of H_1 is 0.01. Only $\sigma_2 = 0.2$ was considered. The conclusions are similar to those obtained from Table 5.5. The results also show that using $t = 1/2$ is fairly robust across the three genetic models.

Table 5.6 Proportion of PPA greater than 0.20 (Bayesian power) under H_1, given the prior probability of H_1 0.01

Model	p	Measures	λ_2		
			1.2	1.5	2.0
REC	0.3	$t = 0$	0.001	0.034	0.575
		$t = 1/2$	0.006	0.066	0.468
		$t = 1$	0.002	0.006	0.036
	0.5	$t = 0$	0.025	0.451	0.991
		$t = 1/2$	0.026	0.349	0.963
		$t = 1$	0.002	0.011	0.086
ADD	0.3	$t = 0$	0.000	0.054	0.102
		$t = 1/2$	0.019	0.231	0.870
		$t = 1$	0.010	0.153	0.766
	0.5	$t = 0$	0.006	0.077	0.441
		$t = 1/2$	0.021	0.251	0.847
		$t = 1$	0.006	0.086	0.543
DOM	0.3	$t = 0$	0.002	0.001	0.009
		$t = 1/2$	0.039	0.473	0.980
		$t = 1$	0.045	0.588	0.996
	0.5	$t = 0$	0.014	0.007	0.246
		$t = 1/2$	0.017	0.180	0.665
		$t = 1$	0.017	0.275	0.885

5.8 Bibliographical Comments

Many classical textbooks on Bayesian analysis contain BFs [25, 99]. We present BFs and related results for the analysis of case-control genetic association studies. Therefore the review paper of BFs by Kass and Raftery [140] serves as our primary reference. The BF in the context of case-control genetic association studies was discussed by the WTCCC [301] and Stephens and Balding [259]. The ABFs of Wakefield [284, 285] are simple for analyzing case-control data. Because of using the estimate of the parameter instead of using the observed data, the ABFs may be less powerful than the BF. The ABF is a special case of the BF based on a test statistic proposed by Johnson [133, 134], who considered modeling the distributions of a test statistic under H_0 and H_1 instead of the distributions of the observed data in the original BF. Bayesian analysis for categorical data by Congdon [42] is also a useful reference. Sawcer [226] provided a good review of using BFs in complex genetics and showed that the BF integrates the p-value (significance) and the observed power of association. Simulations in Sawcer [226] show that case-control studies with different sample sizes and GRRs can have the same p-values but different BFs.

In other words, the simulations demonstrate that BFs are more comparable across studies than p-values.

The Laplace approximation of integrals and its properties were described in Tierney and Kadane [273]. It is a reasonable approach when the posterior density is unimodal or has a dominant single mode. The advantage of the ABF is that it has a closed form, so its computation is usually simpler.

Both the WTCCC [301] and Wakefield [285] discussed the choice of priors. The prior model for β described in (5.38) was proposed in Wakefield [285], who also proposed several other models for the prior, e.g., a prior depending on the MAF or related to the p-value. Stephens and Balding [259] also discussed using a normal mixture prior, $0.9N(0, 0.2^2) + 0.05N(0, 0.4^2) + 0.05N(0, 0.8^2)$, for β, with a small probability and a large variance 0.64. When the variance σ_2^2 in the normal prior $N(0, \sigma_2^2)$ for β is unknown, a hyper-prior can be used, for example the inverse of σ_2^2 following a gamma distribution Gamma(u, v) with two additional parameters u and v (see Sect. 1.1.3), which can be determined *a prior*. See the discussion in Fridley et al. [92]. Sensitivity analysis with different priors is important in Bayesian analysis. Kass and Raftery [140] cover more on how to conduct sensitivity analysis.

In this chapter, we assumed that the underlying genetic model is known (REC, ADD (or MUL), or DOM models). Hence, a single parameter β is used for the genetic effect in either the BF or ABF. When the genetic model is unknown, we have shown in numerical examples and simulations that BFs and ABFs are sensitive to the underlying genetic model. Some standard treatments of model uncertainty in Bayesian analysis can be found in Kass and Raftery [140]. Bayesian model averaging was discussed in Stephens and Balding [259]. For the situation that the true genetic model is unknown, the WTCCC [301] and Wakefield [284] discussed the BF and ABF, respectively, based on the two parameters β_1 and β_2, which model the genetic effects of both $G_1 = AB$ and $G_2 = BB$, where B is the risk allele. This approach is model-free but the computation is more complex than using a single parameter β. In addition, the two-parameter model in the WTCCC [301] is different from the one we discussed here owing to using different parameterizations.

Other approaches to deal with genetic model uncertainty have also been discussed in the literature (e.g., Hoeting et al. [121]; Kass and Raftery [140]). For example, in the context of the three possible genetic models (the REC, ADD and DOM models), the posterior of each model is calculated and the following set is defined as the one containing the models for consideration

$$\left\{ H_l : \frac{\max_{i=1,2,3} \Pr(H_i|\text{data})}{\Pr(H_l|\text{data})} \leq C; \ l = 1, 2, 3 \right\},$$

where C is a given number, e.g., $C = 20$. That is, if a genetic model is not included in the above set, it will be excluded. For the genetic models included in the above set, a sensitivity analysis can be conducted to examine how the BFs and ABFs depend on the genetic models.

In the analysis of GWAS, although p-values are still the main tool used to report association of a genetic marker with a disease, BFs or ABFs have been increasingly reported to support the results obtained based on p-values alone. When a small p-value is found, either the conditional power of the test statistic is calculated for that marker and reported, or a BF or ABF for that marker is reported to support the observed p-value. Therefore, a BF or ABF is only calculated for the top markers in GWAS.

5.9 Problems

5.1 Show that

$$\Pr(H_0|x) = \frac{\mathrm{BF}_{01} \times \text{prior odds}}{1 + \mathrm{BF}_{01} \times \text{prior odds}}.$$

5.2 Verify that the MAP estimates satisfy (5.18) and (5.20).

5.3 MLEs and information matrices.

(a) No covariates. Denote $\Delta_i = \exp(\alpha + \beta I(G_i))/[1 + \exp\{\alpha + \beta I(G_i)\}]^2$. Show that the MLE of $\theta = (\alpha, \beta)^T$ in Sect. 5.4 satisfies

$$r = \sum_{i=0}^{2} n_i \frac{\exp\{\alpha + \beta I(G_i)\}}{1 + \exp\{\alpha + \beta I(G_i)\}},$$

$$\sum_{i=0}^{2} r_i I(G_i) = \sum_{i=0}^{2} n_i I(G_i) \frac{\exp\{\alpha + \beta I(G_i)\}}{1 + \exp\{\alpha + \beta I(G_i)\}},$$

and the observed Fisher information matrix $i_n(\theta)$ can be obtained from

$$i_{00} = -\frac{\partial^2 l}{\partial \alpha^2} = \sum_{i=0}^{2} n_i \Delta_i,$$

$$i_{01} = i_{10} = -\frac{\partial^2 l}{\partial \alpha \partial \beta} = \sum_{i=0}^{2} n_i I(G_i) \Delta_i,$$

$$i_{11} = -\frac{\partial^2 l}{\partial \beta^2} = \sum_{i=0}^{2} n_i I^2(G_i) \Delta_i,$$

where θ is to be replaced by its MLE.
(b) No covariates (continued). Under the REC model, show that the MLEs are given by $\widehat{\alpha} = \log\{(r_0 + r_1)/(s_0 + s_1)\}$ and $\widehat{\beta} = \log[\{r_2(s_0 + s_1)\}/\{s_2(r_0 + r_1)\}]$. Under the DOM model, show that $\widehat{\alpha} = \log(r_0/s_0)$ and $\widehat{\beta} = \log[\{s_0(r_1 + r_2)\}/\{r_0(s_1 + s_2)\}]$.

(c) With covariates. Show that the MLEs satisfy

$$\sum_{i=0}^{2}\sum_{j=1}^{r_i} z_{ij} = \sum_{i=0}^{2}\sum_{j=1}^{n_i} \frac{z_{ij}\exp\{\alpha^T z_{ij} + \beta I(G_{ij})\}}{1+\exp\{\alpha^T z_{ij} + \beta I(G_{ij})\}},$$

$$\sum_{i=1}^{2} r_i I(G_i) = \sum_{i=0}^{2}\sum_{j=1}^{n_i} \frac{I(G_{ij})\exp\{\alpha^T z_{ij} + \beta I(G_{ij})\}}{1+\exp\{\alpha^T z_{ij} + \beta I(G_{ij})\}}.$$

Denote $\Delta_{ij} = \exp(\alpha^T z_{ij} + \beta I(G_{ij}))/[1+\exp\{\alpha^T z_{ij} + \beta I(G_{ij})\}]^2$. Show

$$i_{00} = -\frac{\partial^2 l}{\partial \alpha^2} = \sum_{i=0}^{2}\sum_{j=1}^{n_i} z_{ij} z_{ij}^T \Delta_{ij},$$

$$i_{01} = -\frac{\partial^2 l}{\partial \alpha \partial \beta} = \sum_{i=0}^{2}\sum_{j=1}^{n_i} z_{ij} I(G_{ij}) \Delta_{ij},$$

$$i_{11} = -\frac{\partial^2 l}{\partial \beta^2} = \sum_{i=0}^{2}\sum_{j=1}^{n_i} z_{ij} I^2(G_{ij}) \Delta_{ij}.$$

5.4 Derive the ABF given in (5.25).

5.5 From Sect. 5.4 with covariates, let

$$i(\theta) = \begin{bmatrix} i_{00} & i_{01} \\ i_{10} & i_{11} \end{bmatrix},$$

where $i_{10}^T = i_{01}$. Denote $\Delta = i_{11} - i_{10} i_{00}^{-1} i_{01}$. Show that the inverse of i can be written as

$$i^{-1}(\theta) = \begin{bmatrix} i_{00}^{-1} + i_{00}^{-1}\Delta^{-1} i_{10} i_{00}^{-1} & -i_{00}^{-1} i_{01}\Delta^{-1} \\ -\Delta^{-1} i_{10} i_{00}^{-1} & \Delta^{-1} \end{bmatrix}.$$

Show that, using the transformation $\alpha^* = \alpha + i_{00}^{-1} i_{01}\beta$, the ABF when covariates are adjusted for in the logistic regression model can be written as (5.28), where $V^* = \Delta^{-1}$.

5.6 ABF with two indicator functions.

(a) Prove that $V^{-1} - V^{-1}(V^{-1} + W^{-1})^{-1} V^{-1} = (V + W)^{-1}$ by multiplying both sides by V from the left, followed by multiplying by $V^{-1} + W^{-1}$ from the left. Finally, multiply both sides by $V + W$ from the right.

(b) Show that

$$(\beta - \widehat{\beta})^T V^{-1} (\beta - \widehat{\beta}) + \beta^T W^{-1} \beta$$
$$= \widehat{\beta}^T (V + W)^{-1} \widehat{\beta}$$
$$+ [\beta - (V^{-1} + W^{-1})^{-1} V^{-1} \widehat{\beta}]^T (V^{-1} + W^{-1})$$
$$\times [\beta - (V^{-1} + W^{-1})^{-1} V^{-1} \widehat{\beta}].$$

(c) Let $(r_0, r_1, r_2) \sim Mul(r; p_0, p_1, p_2)$ and $(s_0, s_1, s_2) \sim Mul(s; q_0, q_1, q_2)$. Suppose genotype counts (r_0, r_1, r_2) in cases are independent of those in controls (s_0, s_1, s_2). Let $(\widehat{\beta}_1, \widehat{\beta}_2)$ be given as in (5.35). Show that, omitting higher order terms,

$$\mathrm{Var}(\widehat{\beta}_1) = \frac{1}{rp_1} + \frac{1}{rp_2} + \frac{1}{sq_1} + \frac{1}{sq_2},$$

$$\mathrm{Var}(\widehat{\beta}_2) = \frac{1}{rp_0} + \frac{1}{rp_1} + \frac{1}{sq_0} + \frac{1}{sq_1}.$$

In addition, show that $\mathrm{Cov}(\widehat{\beta}_1, \widehat{\beta}_2) = -1/(rp_1) - 1/(sq_1)$.

5.7 Let $\alpha_i | H_0 \sim N(0, \sigma_1^2)$ and $\alpha_i | H_1 \sim N(0, \sigma_1^2)$ for $i = 1, 2$. Let $\beta_1 | H_1 \sim N(0, \sigma_2^2)$ and $\beta_2 | H_1 \sim N(0, t_2^2 \sigma_2^2)$. The codes for genotypes are (t_1, t_2) and $(t_1/t_2, 1)$ respectively. Show that $p(x | H_i) = \int p(x | \theta_i, H_i) p(\theta_i | H_i) d\theta_i$ using the first code with the above priors for $(\alpha_1, \beta_1)^T$ equals $p(x | H_i)$ using the second code with the above priors for $(\alpha_2, \beta_2)^T$.

5.8 The allele counts for (A, B) are $(2r_0 + r_1, 2r_2 + r_1)$ in cases and $(2s_0 + s_1, 2s_2 + s_1)$ in controls. Then the logistic regression model based on the allele counts is given by

$$\mathrm{logit}\{\Pr(\text{case} \,|\text{allele})\} = \alpha + \beta I (\text{allele})$$

where $I(A) = 0$ and $I(B) = 1$. The likelihood function is given by

$$\frac{\exp(2r\alpha) + (2r_2 + r_1)\beta}{(1 + \exp(\alpha))^{2n_0 + n_1} (1 + \exp(\alpha + \beta))^{2n_2 + n_1}}.$$

This leads to

$$\widehat{\alpha} = \log\left(\frac{2r_0 + r_1}{2s_0 + s_1}\right), \qquad \widehat{\beta} = \log\left\{\frac{(2r_2 + r_1)(2s_0 + s_1)}{(2s_2 + s_1)(2r_0 + r_1)}\right\},$$

and the elements of the observed Fisher information matrix are

$$i_{00} = (2r_0 + r_1)(2s_0 + s_1)/(2n_0 + n_1) + (2r_2 + r_1)(2s_2 + s_1)/(2n_2 + n_1),$$
$$i_{01} = i_{10} = i_{11} = (2r_2 + r_1)(2s_2 + s_1)/(2n_2 + n_1),$$

where $\theta = (\alpha, \beta)^T$ is replaced by its estimate $\widehat{\theta} = (\widehat{\alpha}, \widehat{\beta})^T$. Derive the ABF based on the allele counts, which is an allele-based ABF. Compare the allele-based ABF with the genotype-based ABF under the ADD model, given in (5.25), in simulations with and without HWE in the population.

5.9 Find the ABF for the SNP (rs10510126) given in Sect. 5.5.3 with the prior $(\beta_1, \beta_2)^T \sim N_2(0, W)$, where

$$W = \sigma_2^2 \begin{bmatrix} 1 & 0 \\ 0 & 1 \end{bmatrix}$$

with $\sigma^2 = 0.1, 0.2$ and 0.4, respectively.

5.10 Let $Z_{\mathrm{CATT}}(x)$ be the trend test given in (3.8) for a given genetic model x, where $x = 0, 1/2$ and 1 for the REC, ADD and DOM model, respectively. Define an approximate BF as

$$\mathrm{ABF} = \frac{\Pr(Z_{\mathrm{CATT}}(x)|H_0)}{\Pr(Z_{\mathrm{CATT}}(x)|H_1)}.$$

Derive expressions for the above ABF with and without covariates and compare then with the ABFs given in (5.25) and (5.28) for the same genetic model.

Chapter 6
Robust Procedures

Abstract Robust procedures for the analysis of case-control association are presented in Chap. 6, starting with an introduction to robust hypothesis testing. The definition of the maximin efficiency is given. This chapter discusses how to find the maximum efficiency robust test (MERT). Several maximum tests based on the maximum of trend tests are studied, including MAX2, MAX3 and a more general MAX. Connections among MAX, Pearson's test and the trend test are given. Other robust tests are also studied, including MIN2, the constrained likelihood ratio test, and tests based on genetic model selection or exclusion. Simulation studies are conducted to compare the different robust tests. All results in this chapter are presented for unmatched case-control data except for MAX3, which is also applied to a matched case-control design.

For testing association between a diallelic marker and a disease in case-control studies, the null hypothesis of no association is equivalent to the three penetrances being equal to the disease prevalence in the population (see Sect. 3.1). Therefore, under the alternative hypothesis of association, at least one of the three penetrances is not equal to the disease prevalence. In this case, a genetic model refers to the mode of inheritance, which defines some relationship among the risks of having the disease given different genotypes (penetrances). The common genetic models include, but are not limited to, REC, ADD, MUL and DOM models. Under the alternative hypothesis, if the three penetrances increase with the numbers of risk alleles in the genotype, the penetrances are ordered. In this case, one can restrict the alternative hypotheses to the collection of models formed by the above four genetic models, which includes any genetic model between the REC and DOM models. Though less common, genetic models outside the above collection may also occur, for example, the over-dominant and under-dominant models (Sect. 3.1). Because the MUL model can be approximated by the ADD model, some results may not be presented for the MUL model.

In Chap. 3, the trend test and Pearson's test were discussed, which are the most common statistics for the analysis of case-control association studies. To apply the trend test, increasing scores are specified *a priori* for the three genotypes. If the underlying genetic model is known, the asymptotically optimal trend test can be used. Otherwise, a single trend test is not robust when the scores are misspecified. On the

G. Zheng et al., *Analysis of Genetic Association Studies*,
Statistics for Biology and Health,
DOI 10.1007/978-1-4614-2245-7_6, © Springer Science+Business Media, LLC 2012

other hand, Pearson's test does not require specifying the genetic model. Hence, it is more robust than a single trend test. More insight regarding the robustness of Pearson's test will be discussed later in this chapter. Pearson's test, however, ignores that the penetrances are often ordered under the alternative hypothesis. Thus, it is less powerful compared to the trend test when the genetic model can be approximately specified. The trade-off of power and robustness between the trend test and Pearson's test will be studied in this chapter. Robust tests are useful when the underlying genetic model is unknown. Several robust tests will be studied in this chapter.

We first present a general discussion of robust hypothesis testing and maximin efficiency robustness. A class of simple, linear maximin efficiency robust tests (MERTs) is first introduced. Several maximal statistics (e.g., MAX3 and MAX) based on the trend tests will be studied next. Distributions and approximations of the tails of the maximal statistics will be discussed. Relationships and insight among the trend tests, Pearson's test and MAX will be provided. A constrained likelihood ratio test statistic will also be discussed, which has power performance similar to MAX. Next, a genome-wide scan statistic proposed by the Wellcome Trust Case-Control Consortium is reviewed. Its asymptotic null distribution and p-value are provided. Other approaches that are considered in this chapter include genetic model selection and genetic model exclusion. Simulation results and applications to real data will be used to illustrate how to apply the above methods in real data analysis.

6.1 Robust Hypothesis Testing

6.1.1 Discrete Numbers of Alternative Hypotheses

Consider testing a null hypothesis H_0 against a family of alternative hypotheses $\{H_{1i} : i = 1, \ldots, M\}$. Each of the M alternative hypotheses corresponds to a scientifically plausible model under which the data are generated. Given model i ($i = 1, \ldots, M$), an asymptotically normally distributed test Z_i is obtained and used to test H_0. We assume Z_i is asymptotically optimal (most efficient) when i is the true model under the alternative hypothesis. The efficiency of a test is defined using the asymptotic relative efficiency (ARE) (Sect. 1.7). In testing case-control genetic association, H_{11}, H_{12}, and H_{13} correspond to REC, ADD, and DOM models, respectively. The trend tests $Z_{\text{CATT}}(0)$, $Z_{\text{CATT}}(1/2)$ and $Z_{\text{CATT}}(1)$ are respectively used to test H_0 against H_{11}, H_{12}, and H_{13}. It is shown that $Z_{\text{CATT}}(0)$ and $Z_{\text{CATT}}(1)$ are asymptotically optimal under the REC and DOM models. For the ADD model, $Z_{\text{CATT}}(1/2)$ is asymptotically optimal when the proportion of cases in the data is close to the disease prevalence. Otherwise, $Z_{\text{CATT}}(1/2)$ is approximately optimal under the ADD model.

Denote the ARE of Z_j to Z_i by $\text{ARE}(Z_j, Z_i)$ for $i, j = 1, \ldots, M$. If the true model is i^* and $1 \le i^* \le M$, then Z_{i^*} is used to test H_0. On the other hand, when the true model is unknown, any test in the family of normally distributed statistics $T = \{Z_i : i = 1, \ldots, M\}$ could be optimal. In the analysis of case-control genetic associations, T contains all three trend tests $Z_{\text{CATT}}(x)$ with scores $x = 0$, $1/2$, and 1. If the true model is i^* but this is unknown, and we choose the test statistic Z_i, sub-optimal results may be obtained and Z_i may not be efficient when $i^* \neq i$. The loss of efficiency is measured by

$$e(i, i^*) = \text{ARE}(Z_i, Z_i^*).$$

For studying robust tests, we assume that any two tests out of $\{Z_i, i = 1, \ldots, M\}$ follow asymptotically bivariate normal distributions under H_0 and H_1 with the asymptotic null correlations given by $\rho_{ij} = \text{Corr}_{H_0}(Z_i, Z_j)$ for any $i, j = 1, \ldots, M$ with $\rho_{ii} = 1$ and $\rho_{ij} > 0$ for $i \neq j$.

6.1.2 Alternative Hypothesis Indexed by an Interval

The model described in the previous section assumes that H_1 contains a finite number of possible models. In many applications, H_1 is also indexed by an interval $x \in [a, b]$, where the endpoints of the interval are known. For example, in the analysis of case-control association using the trend test $Z_{\text{CATT}}(x)$, the parameter x belongs to $[0, 1]$, where $x = 0$, $x = 1/2$, and $x = 1$ correspond to the REC, ADD, and DOM models, respectively (Sect. 3.3.1). In this case, the family of normally distributed test statistics is given by $T = \{Z_x : x \in [a, b]\}$. When H_{1x} is the true model for $x \in [0, 1]$, Z_x is asymptotically optimal when the proportion of cases in the data is close to the disease prevalence or approximately optimal otherwise. For any $x, y \in [a, b]$, we assume (Z_x, Z_y) follow bivariate normal distributions under H_0 and H_1. Denote the asymptotic null correlation by $\rho_{xy} = \text{Corr}_{H_0}(Z_x, Z_y) > 0$. When x^* is the true model and Z_x is used but $x \neq x^*$, the ARE of Z_x to Z_{x^*} is given by

$$e(x, x^*) = \text{ARE}(Z_x, Z_{x^*}).$$

6.1.3 Maximin Efficiency

For each alternative hypothesis H_{1i}, $i = 1, \ldots, M$, Z_i is asymptotically (approximately) optimal, and $Z_i \sim N(0, 1)$ under H_0. In this case, there is no uniformly optimal test for a family of alternative hypotheses, because each test would be optimal when the true model is specified. A similar argument can be made for alternative hypotheses indexed by an interval: H_{1x}, $x \in [a, b]$. In the following, without loss of generality, we only consider $[a, b] = [0, 1]$. Thus, tests cannot be compared with respect to their highest efficiency or power. *Maximin efficiency* can be used to compare the tests: finding a test with most efficiency in its worst performance when the model is misspecified.

Let $i = i^* \in \{1, \ldots, M\}$ be the index for the true model. We focus on the case with a finite number of alternative hypotheses. The results can be readily extended to the case when the alternative hypothesis is indexed by $x \in [0, 1]$. Thus, Z_{i*} is asymptotically optimal, but the optimal model i^* is unknown. Suppose Z_i is chosen to test H_0. Then the ARE of Z_i to Z_{i*} is $e(i, i^*) = \rho_{ii*}^2$, for $i = 1, \ldots, M$. Because i^* is unknown, the *worst* ARE when using Z_i is given by

$$\min_{1 \leq i^* \leq M} e(i, i^*). \tag{6.1}$$

For each $i = 1, \ldots, M$, the worst ARE in (6.1) can be evaluated. Among the M worst AREs, the *best* is given by

$$\max_{1 \leq i \leq M} \min_{1 \leq i^* \leq M} e(i, i^*),$$

which is referred to as the maximin efficiency. If Z_j has the best worst ARE, i.e.,

$$\min_{1 \leq i^* \leq M} e(j, i^*) = \max_{1 \leq i \leq M} \min_{1 \leq i^* \leq M} e(i, i^*), \tag{6.2}$$

then Z_j is the maximin efficiency robust test (MERT) among $T = \{Z_i : i = 1, \ldots, M\}$. However, we often do not find the MERT restricted to the tests in $T = \{Z_i : i = 1, \ldots, M\}$ (Problem 6.14). Instead, we are interested in finding the MERT in a larger set $T^* = \{w_i Z_i + w_j Z_j : w_i, w_j \geq 0, Z_i, Z_j \in T\}$. See Sect. 6.2.1 for the definition of the MERT based on T^*.

Note that if test Z_1 is more efficient than test Z_2, Z_1 is usually more powerful than Z_2 under local alternatives. A relationship between power and efficiency is given in Sect. 1.7. Thus, the maximin efficiency of tests can be demonstrated by the empirical power of the tests. For case-control genetic association studies, when the trend test is used, $T = \{Z_{\text{CATT}}(x) : x \in [0, 1]\}$ is given in (3.8) with $(x_0, x_1, x_2) = (0, x, 1)$ and $x \in [0, 1]$, which is also given by

$$Z_{\text{CATT}}(x) = \frac{\sqrt{\frac{rs}{n}}\{(xr_1/r + r_2/r) - (xs_1/s + s_2/s)\}}{\sqrt{(x^2 n_1/n + n_2/n) - (xn_1/n + n_2/n)^2}}, \tag{6.3}$$

where (r_0, r_1, r_2) and (s_0, s_1, s_2) are genotype counts of (AA, AB, BB) in r cases and s controls, $n_i = r_i + s_i$ and $n = r + s$.

In Table 6.1, the empirical power of the three trend tests, $Z_{\text{CATT}}(x)$ with $x = 0, 1/2, 1$, is obtained under the REC, ADD and DOM models with 250 cases and 250 controls and disease prevalence 0.1. Assuming HWE proportions in the population, under H_1 with a given genetic model, the GRRs are chosen so that the asymptotically optimal trend test has about 80% power. Then empirical power is estimated for each of the three trend tests using the data simulated using the same GRRs. The results reported in Table 6.1 are grouped by the MAF for the risk allele. For each MAF, the empirical power of each trend test is estimated from the simulation for each genetic model. The minimum power (min power) of each trend test across the three genetic models is also presented. Finally, the largest power among the minimum powers is reported, which is the maximin power across the genetic models given the MAF and other parameters. From Table 6.1, it is seen that the three trend tests cannot be compared by their maximum power, because each test is optimal under one genetic model. However, among the three trend tests, $Z_{\text{CATT}}(1/2)$ has

Table 6.1 Empirical power of three trend tests $Z_{\text{CATT}}(x)$ for a given MAF of the risk allele under three genetic models: the REC, ADD, and DOM models

MAF	True model	$Z_{\text{CATT}}(x)$		
		$x = 0$	$x = \frac{1}{2}$	$x = 1$
0.1	REC	0.813	0.364	0.138
	ADD	0.223	0.813	0.802
	DOM	0.108	0.796	0.813
	min power	0.108	0.364	0.138
	maximin power		0.364	
0.3	REC	0.793	0.537	0.177
	ADD	0.433	0.812	0.684
	DOM	0.133	0.717	0.787
	min power	0.133	0.537	0.177
	maximin power		0.537	
0.5	REC	0.810	0.662	0.177
	ADD	0.575	0.802	0.684
	DOM	0.131	0.574	0.787
	min power	0.131	0.574	0.177
	maximin power		0.574	

the maximin power across the three genetic models. Hence, it is more robust than $Z_{\text{CATT}}(0)$ and $Z_{\text{CATT}}(1)$.

For H_1 indexed by $x \in [0, 1]$ using a family of test statistics $T = \{Z_x : x \in [0, 1]\}$, the maximin efficiency, restricted to T, is given by

$$\sup_{x \in [0,1]} \inf_{x^* \in [0,1]} e(x, x^*),$$

where $e(x, y) = \text{ARE}(Z_x, Z_y)$ and x^* is the true unknown model and x is the selected model. A test Z_y is the MERT among T if it reaches the maximin efficiency, i.e.

$$\inf_{x^* \in [0,1]} e(y, x^*) = \sup_{x \in [0,1]} \inf_{x^* \in [0,1]} e(x, x^*).$$

Finding the MERT from $T = \{Z_x : x \in [0, 1]\}$ is much more complicated than the case with a finite number of tests, $T = \{Z_i : i = 1, \ldots, M\}$.

6.2 Maximin Efficiency Robust Test

6.2.1 The MERT as a Robust Test

The MERT of a Family of Test Statistics

In Sect. 6.1.2, the maximin efficiency and the MERT are introduced. But the discussions are focused on the MERT among the families of statistics

$$T = \{Z_i : i = 1, \ldots, M\} \quad \text{and}$$
$$T = \{Z_x : x \in [0, 1]\}.$$

However, we are interested in finding the MERT of all convex linear combinations of test statistics among T (Problem 6.14), denoted by

$$T^* = \left\{ \sum_{j=1}^{M} c_j Z_j : c_j \geq 0 \right\} \quad \text{and} \tag{6.4}$$

$$T^* = \left\{ \sum_{j=1}^{m} c_j Z_{x_j} : c_j \geq 0, \ x_j \in [0, 1], \ m \geq 1 \right\}. \tag{6.5}$$

Hence $T \subset T^*$. Then the maximin efficiency is modified to

$$\sup_{Z_i \in T^*} \inf_{Z_j \in T} \text{ARE}(Z_i, Z_j) \quad \text{or} \quad \sup_{Z_x \in T^*} \inf_{Z_y \in T} \text{ARE}(Z_x, Z_y).$$

In this case, the MERT may not belong to the family of test statistics T. Note that the test statistics contained in T^* are consistent and asymptotically normally distributed. T^* can be further expanded to T^{**}, which contains all consistent tests. When T is fixed, the maximin efficiency is increased if the family of test statistics is expanded.

Extreme Pair

Two test statistics Z_i and Z_j are called the extreme pair of the family of test statistics T if their correlation is the minimum among any pair of two test statistics in T. Denote the minimum correlation by $\rho_0 > 0$. Then, for any test Z_i and the optimal test Z_{i*} for the alternative hypothesis H_{1i*} with asymptotic null correlation $\rho_{i,i*}$, $\text{ARE}(Z_i, Z_{i*}) = \rho_{i,i*}^2 \geq \rho_0^2$. Thus, the minimum correlation of the extreme pair of test statistics provides a lower bound for the ARE when the underlying model is misspecified. Therefore, a larger ρ_0^2 implies a "smaller" family of test statistics, in the sense that using a test statistic in the family with larger ρ_0 may lose less efficiency compared to using a test in a "larger" family of test statistics with smaller ρ_0. Applications and empirical studies have shown that the minimum correlation is high if $\rho_0 \geq 0.75$ and low if $\rho_0 \leq 0.50$.

Let $x, y \in [0, 1]$ and $\rho_{x,y}$ be the asymptotic null correlation of $Z_{\text{CATT}}(x)$ and $Z_{\text{CATT}}(y)$. Then (Problem 6.1)

$$\rho_{x,y} = \frac{(xyp_1 + p_2) - (xp_1 + p_2)(yp_1 + p_2)}{\sqrt{(x^2 p_1 + p_2) - (xp_1 + p_2)^2}\sqrt{(y^2 p_1 + p_2) - (yp_1 + p_2)^2}}, \qquad (6.6)$$

where (p_0, p_1, p_2) are the probabilities of genotypes $(G_0, G_1, G_2) = (AA, AB, BB)$ in the population, which can be written as functions of the MAF under HWE proportions. An estimate of $\rho_{x,y}$ can be obtained by replacing (p_0, p_1, p_2) with their consistent estimates under H_0, e.g., $\widehat{p}_i = n_i/n$ for $i = 0, 1, 2$, where n_i is the count of genotype G_i and $n = n_0 + n_1 + n_2$. Note that $\rho_{x,y} = \rho_{y,x}$ for any $x, y \in [0, 1]$.

For the three trend tests with $x = 0, 1/2, 1$, we have

$$\rho_{0,1/2} = \frac{p_2(p_1 + 2p_0)}{\sqrt{p_2(1 - p_2)}\sqrt{(p_1 + 2p_2)p_0 + (p_1 + 2p_0)p_2}}, \qquad (6.7)$$

$$\rho_{1/2,1} = \frac{p_0(p_1 + 2p_2)}{\sqrt{p_0(1 - p_0)}\sqrt{(p_1 + 2p_2)p_0 + (p_1 + 2p_0)p_2}}, \qquad (6.8)$$

$$\rho_{0,1} = \sqrt{\frac{p_0 p_2}{(1 - p_0)(1 - p_2)}}. \qquad (6.9)$$

Expressions for the above correlations under HWE proportions are given in Problem 6.11. Consistent estimates of $\rho_{0,1/2}$, $\rho_{0,1}$ and $\rho_{1/2,1}$ under H_0 are given by

$$\widehat{\rho}_{0,1/2} = \frac{n_2(n_1 + 2n_0)}{\sqrt{n_2(n - n_2)}\sqrt{(n_1 + 2n_2)n_0 + (n_1 + 2n_0)n_2}},$$

$$\widehat{\rho}_{1/2,1} = \frac{n_0(n_1 + 2n_2)}{\sqrt{n_0(n - n_0)}\sqrt{(n_1 + 2n_2)n_0 + (n_1 + 2n_0)n_2}},$$

$$\widehat{\rho}_{0,1} = \sqrt{\frac{n_0 n_2}{(n - n_0)(n - n_2)}}.$$

Using (6.7) to (6.9), it can be shown that (Problem 6.2)

$$1 + 2\rho_{0,1/2}\rho_{0,1}\rho_{1/2,1} = \rho_{0,1/2}^2 + \rho_{0,1}^2 + \rho_{1/2,1}^2. \qquad (6.10)$$

Define the following matrix

$$\Sigma = \begin{bmatrix} 1 & \rho_{0,1/2} & \rho_{0,1} \\ \rho_{0,1/2} & 1 & \rho_{1/2,1} \\ \rho_{0,1} & \rho_{1/2,1} & 1 \end{bmatrix}.$$

Then (6.10) shows that the determinant of Σ is 0, i.e. $|\Sigma| = 0$.

Table 6.2 reports the values of $\rho_{x,y}$ for the three trend tests under HWE. The results show that, among the three trend tests, $Z_{CATT}(0)$ and $Z_{CATT}(1)$ are the extreme pair with minimum correlation in the range 0.20 to 0.35, while $Z_{CATT}(1/2)$ and $Z_{CATT}(1)$ have the largest correlation, greater than 0.80 across various MAFs. Note that if we switch the labels for the two alleles, i.e., switching alleles A and B, then (r_0, r_1, r_2) and (s_0, s_1, s_2) are genotype counts for (BB, AB, AA) in cases and controls. Accordingly, $\rho_{0,1/2}$ and $\rho_{1/2,1}$ are switched, but $\rho_{0,1}$ does not change. Figure 6.1 plots three correlation curves for various values of MAFs. The top, middle and bottom plots correspond to $\rho_{1/2,1}$, $\rho_{0,1/2}$ and $\rho_{0,1}$, respectively.

Table 6.2 The asymptotic null pair-wise correlations among the three trend tests $\rho_{x,y} = \mathrm{Corr}(Z_{\mathrm{CATT}}(x), Z_{\mathrm{CATT}}(y))$ under HWE proportions. The correlations are functions of the MAF

MAF	$\rho_{x,y}$		
	$\rho_{0,\frac{1}{2}}$	$\rho_{\frac{1}{2},1}$	$\rho_{0,1}$
0.10	0.4264	0.9733	0.2075
0.20	0.5774	0.9428	0.2722
0.25	0.6325	0.9258	0.2928
0.30	0.6794	0.9075	0.3083
0.40	0.7559	0.8660	0.3273
0.50	0.8165	0.8165	0.3333

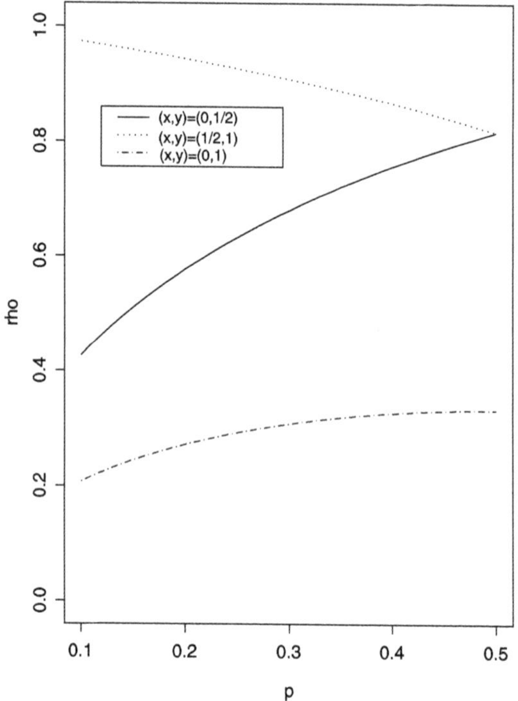

Fig. 6.1 Plots of the three pair-wise correlations $\rho_{x,y}$ of the three trend tests against the MAF p for the REC, ADD and DOM models. The *top*, *middle* and *bottom* plots across p correspond to $\rho_{1/2,1}$, $\rho_{0,1/2}$ and $\rho_{0,1}$, respectively, when B is the risk allele

Finding the MERT

Let $T = \{Z_i : i = 1, \ldots, M\}$ or $T = \{Z_x : x \in [0,1]\}$ be a family of consistent test statistics that we discussed before. The pair-wise correlation is defined by ρ_{ij} of Z_i and Z_j or ρ_{xy} of Z_x and Z_y. Let T^* be defined as in (6.4) or (6.5). Denote the minimum correlation by ρ_0. If $\rho_0 > \delta > 0$, where δ is some positive number (independent of the sample size), then the MERT in T^* exists and is unique. It can be written as a linear combination of test statistics in T.

A simple algorithm to find the MERT of T^* is to find the MERT for the extreme pair. Let Z_{i_0} and Z_{i_1} be the extreme pair ($1 \le i_0 < i_1 \le M$ or $i_0, i_1 \in [0, 1]$). Then the MERT of the extreme pair is given by (Problem 6.14)

$$Z_{\mathrm{MERT}} = \frac{Z_{i_0} + Z_{i_1}}{\sqrt{2(1 + \rho_0)}}. \tag{6.11}$$

A necessary and sufficient condition for the MERT of the extreme pair in (6.11), Z_{MERT}, to be the MERT of T^* is one of the following inequalities:

$$\rho_{i_0,i} + \rho_{i,i_1} \ge 1 + \rho_{i_0,i_1}, \quad \text{for any } i = 1, \ldots, M, \tag{6.12}$$

$$\rho_{i_0,x} + \rho_{x,i_1} \ge 1 + \rho_{i_0,i_1}, \quad \text{for any } x \in [0, 1]. \tag{6.13}$$

In general, (6.12) and (6.13) are not easy to verify. Note that if (6.13) holds, (6.12) also holds. If condition (6.13) holds, the ARE of Z_{MERT} to the optimal test in T^* is at least $(1 + \rho_0)/2$. Thus, if $\rho_0 \ge 0.75$, the MERT has high ARE, at least 0.875. On the other hand, if $\rho_0 < 0.50$, then the ARE of Z_{MERT} is at most 0.75. Even when (6.13) cannot be confirmed, Z_{MERT} may also be used as a robust test. Based on the minimum correlations in Table 6.2, when the MERT Z_{MERT} is used for testing case-control association, the ARE of the MERT to the optimal test would be in the range of $(1 + 0.208)/2 = 0.604$ to $(1 + 0.333)/2 = 0.667$ for MAFs of 0.1 to 0.5.

6.2.2 The MERT Versus a Single Trend Test for Genetic Association

In Table 6.2 and Fig. 6.1, it is shown numerically that ρ_{01} is the minimum correlation. Using the result in Problem 6.3, condition (6.13) holds. Thus, $Z_{\mathrm{CATT}}(0)$ and $Z_{\mathrm{CATT}}(1)$ are the extreme pair for case-control association studies with $x \in [0, 1]$. In addition, the MERT for case-control genetic association studies can be written as

$$Z_{\mathrm{MERT}} = \frac{Z_{\mathrm{CATT}}(0) + Z_{\mathrm{CATT}}(1)}{\sqrt{2(1 + \rho_{0,1})}}, \tag{6.14}$$

which has an asymptotic normal distribution $N(0, 1)$ under H_0. The ARE of the MERT to the optimal test for genetic association is between 0.60 and 0.67.

Table 6.3 reports simulated power of the three trend tests with $x = 0, 1/2, 1$ and the MERT under the four genetic models: REC, ADD/MUL, and DOM models. Under each model, the GRR, $\lambda_2 = \Pr(\text{case}\,|G_2)/\Pr(\text{case}\,|G_0)$, is chosen so that the optimal trend test has about 80% power. The sample sizes for the simulation studies are $r = 1{,}000$ (cases) and $s = 1{,}000$ (controls) with disease prevalence 0.1. HWE in the population is assumed. The results in Table 6.3 show that the MERT is more efficiency robust than any single trend test. It can be seen that the MERT has higher efficiency than the trend test $Z_{\mathrm{CATT}}(1/2)$ because the REC model is included in the family of models. The trend test $Z_{\mathrm{CATT}}(1/2)$ is more powerful than the MERT under the ADD/MUL and DOM models. When the MAF is 0.5, the MERT and $Z_{\mathrm{CATT}}(1/2)$ have similar power performance. Later in Sect. 6.3.2 we will express

Table 6.3 Empirical power of $Z_{\mathrm{CATT}}(x)$ and the MERT for a given GRR and MAF with 1,000 cases and 1,000 controls under four genetic models: the REC, ADD/MUL, and DOM models

MAF	True model	$Z_{\mathrm{CATT}}(x)$			Z_{MERT}	GRR
		$x = 0$	$x = \frac{1}{2}$	$x = 1$		
0.1	REC	0.811	0.299	0.115	0.597	2.43
	ADD	0.210	0.813	0.799	0.721	1.60
	MUL	0.242	0.798	0.775	0.720	1.65
	DOM	0.093	0.788	0.806	0.601	1.32
min power		0.093	0.299	0.115	0.597	
maximin power					0.597	
0.3	REC	0.808	0.504	0.154	0.625	1.44
	ADD	0.465	0.808	0.746	0.789	1.40
	MUL	0.500	0.802	0.714	0.788	1.41
	DOM	0.132	0.722	0.814	0.622	1.26
min power		0.132	0.504	0.154	0.622	
maximin power					0.622	
0.5	REC	0.818	0.659	0.170	0.650	1.29
	ADD	0.606	0.800	0.647	0.801	1.38
	MUL	0.652	0.803	0.618	0.803	1.38
	DOM	0.144	0.609	0.791	0.618	1.31
min power		0.144	0.609	0.170	0.618	
maximin power					0.618	

$Z_{\mathrm{CATT}}(1/2)$ as a weighted sum of the extreme pair, $Z_{\mathrm{CATT}}(0)$ and $Z_{\mathrm{CATT}}(1)$, with more weight on $Z_{\mathrm{CATT}}(1)$. This could explain why $Z_{\mathrm{CATT}}(1/2)$ is more powerful for the ADD to DOM models. Table 6.3 also shows that the MERT has maximin power from 0.597 to 0.622, which is consistent with our previous statement that the ARE of the MERT is in the range of 0.60 to 0.67 owing to low null correlations of the extreme pair.

Figures 6.2, 6.3, 6.4 plot the empirical power of the MERT and $Z_{\mathrm{CATT}}(1/2)$ under various genetic models with different MAFs. These plots also show that the MERT is often more powerful than the trend test under the REC model, while the trend test is more powerful under the ADD and DOM models. The loss of power of the MERT under the ADD and DOM models is less than that of the trend test under the REC model. In practice, if the REC model is more of interest, then the MERT seems to be more robust than the trend test $Z_{\mathrm{CATT}}(1/2)$. On the other hand, if the ADD or DOM models are of interest, then $Z_{\mathrm{CATT}}(1/2)$ is preferable. In general, we prefer using $Z_{\mathrm{CATT}}(1/2)$ because, under an imperfect LD model, a REC model at the functional locus is usually not presented at the marker locus as the same REC model, but is in fact *closer* to the ADD model at the marker (see Sect. 2.2.1 and Table 2.2).

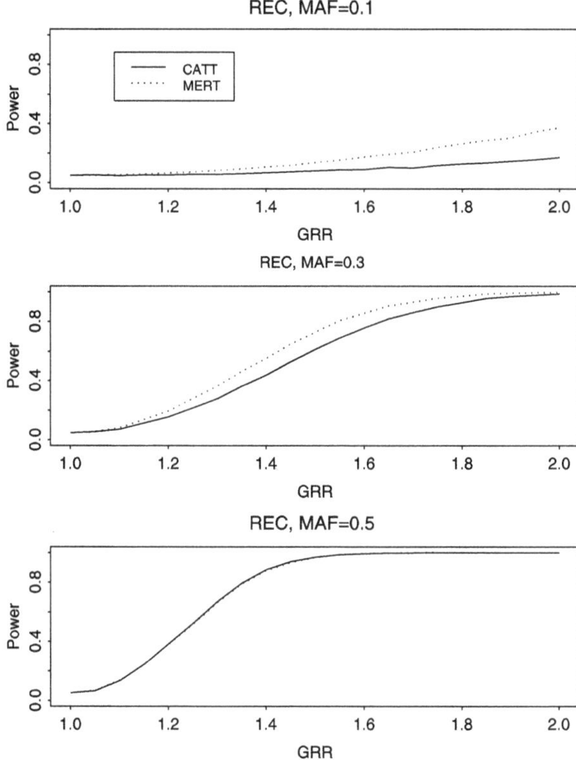

Fig. 6.2 Empirical power of the MERT and $Z_{CATT}(1/2)$ under the REC model with various MAFs

The above discussions are based on normally distributed test statistics (the trend tests and MERT). In the next section, we discuss more robust tests that are based on maximum statistics. These maximum-type statistics are computationally more intensive than the trend tests and MERT. We also compare the trend tests and the maximum-type statistics with Pearson's chi-squared test.

6.3 Max Statistics

The minimum correlation among the trend tests presented in Table 6.2 is in the range of 0.20 to 0.35. The maximin efficiency robust theory shows that the MERT of this family of trend tests would have asymptotic efficiency relative to the optimal trend test below 0.70. One advantage of the MERT given in (6.14) is that it asymptotically follows $N(0, 1)$ under H_0. Therefore, it is easy to use. More robust tests have been studied that are computationally more intensive than any single trend test and the MERT. Maximum-type statistics are among them. We first introduce MAX3 followed by a general MAX, which may also be used in the literature for MAX3. Other robust tests will be discussed in later sections of this chapter.

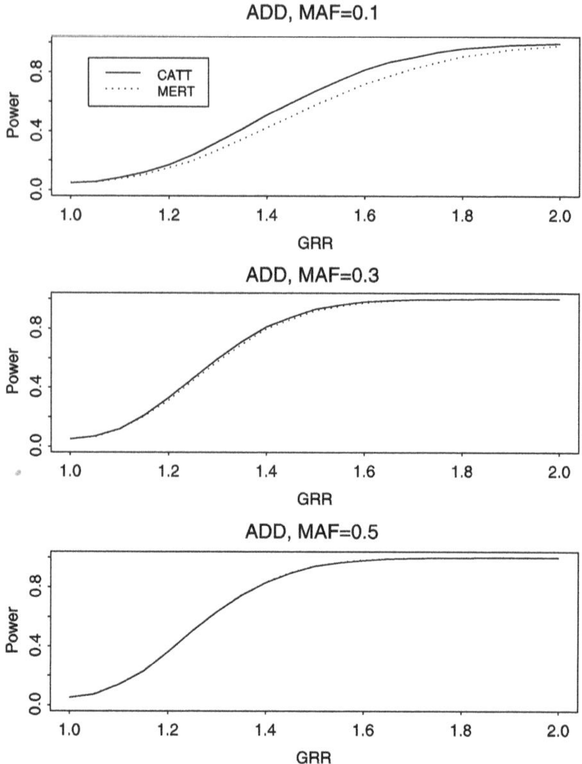

Fig. 6.3 Empirical power of the MERT and $Z_{\text{CATT}}(1/2)$ under the ADD model with various MAFs

6.3.1 MAX3

Denote the family of trend statistics for testing H_0 by $\{Z_x : x \in [0, 1]\}$. For a given $x \in [0, 1]$, $Z_x \sim N(0, 1)$ under H_0. When the risk allele is unknown, MAX3 is defined by

$$\text{MAX3} = \max\{|Z_{\text{CATT}}(0)|, |Z_{\text{CATT}}(1/2)|, |Z_{\text{CATT}}(1)|\}. \tag{6.15}$$

MAX3 can also be defined by

$$\text{MAX3} = \max\{Z^2_{\text{CATT}}(0), Z^2_{\text{CATT}}(1/2), Z^2_{\text{CATT}}(1)\}. \tag{6.16}$$

Both definitions result in the same p-value. Thus, we use the definition given in (6.15). If the risk allele is known, from Problem 6.4, the trend tests are one-sided for any scores under H_1. Thus, when allele B is the risk allele, MAX3 is given by

$$\text{MAX3} = \max\{Z_{\text{CATT}}(0), Z_{\text{CATT}}(1/2), Z_{\text{CATT}}(1)\}. \tag{6.17}$$

From (6.15), when one of the REC, ADD/MUL or DOM models is the true data-generating model, the corresponding Score statistic is asymptotically optimal under that model. MAX3 will be likely to take the value of that trend test statistic. Thus, using a single trend test may lose efficiency by misspecifying the underlying genetic

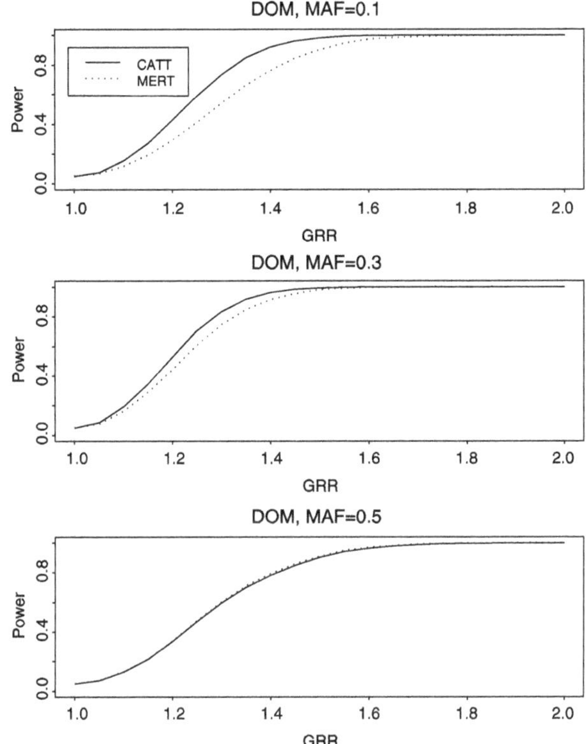

Fig. 6.4 Empirical power of the MERT and $Z_{\mathrm{CATT}}(1/2)$ under the DOM model with various MAFs

model. But MAX3 covers a wider range of genetic models and is more robust than a single trend test.

Under H_1, a large value of MAX3 is in favor of H_1. Although each trend test has an asymptotic $N(0, 1)$ under H_0, MAX3 does not follow the same distribution as the trend test. Figure 6.5 plots empirical densities of the three trend tests $|Z_{\mathrm{CATT}}(x)|$ and MAX3 with sample sizes $r = s = 500$, and MAF of 0.3 assuming HWE in the population. The plots, based on 1,000 replicates, show the distribution of MAX3 is different from those of the trend tests. The medians of the four distributions are 1.02, 0.66, 0.64 and 0.70 for MAX3, $|Z_{\mathrm{CATT}}(0)|$, $|Z_{\mathrm{CATT}}(1/2)|$ and $|Z_{\mathrm{CATT}}(1)|$, respectively.

Moreover, due to the multiple testing issue (testing association in each of the three models, see the discussion in Sect. 1.2.5), the significance level $\alpha = 0.05$ for a single trend test is no longer a correct size for MAX3. Applying the Bonferroni correction and testing MAX3 at the level $\alpha/3$ using $N(0, 1)$ is too conservative because of the positive correlations among the three trend tests.

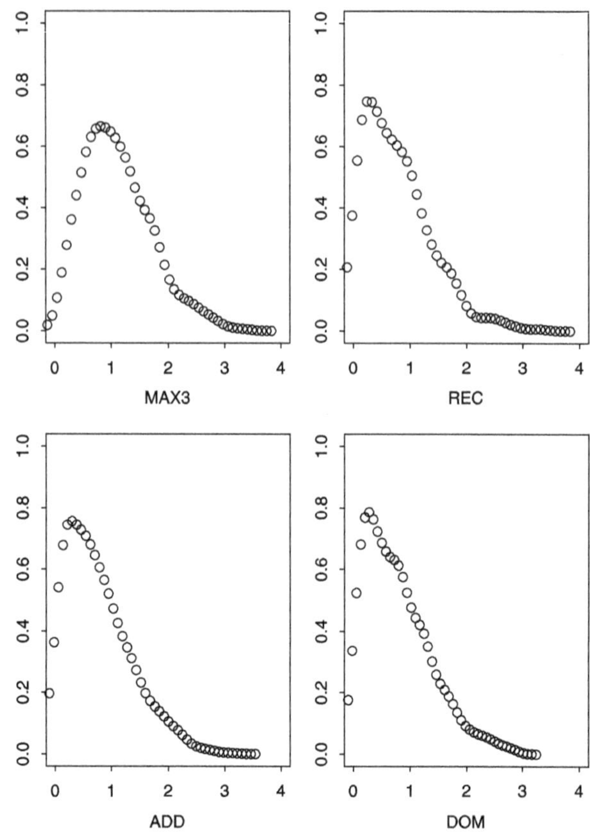

Fig. 6.5 Densities of the absolute value of $Z_{\mathrm{CATT}}(x)$ for $x = 0, 1/2, 1$ and MAX3 under H_0; MAF is 0.3, with 500 cases and 500 controls

6.3.2 Monte-Carlo Approaches for MAX3

Monte-Carlo approaches can be used to simulate the empirical null distribution of MAX3 and approximate its empirical power. Two approaches are discussed in this section. One is the parametric bootstrap (Sect. 3.5.3 and Sect. 3.9) and the other is based on the asymptotic joint distribution of trend test statistics.

Parametric Bootstrap Approach

The parametric bootstrap approach that we discussed in Sect. 3.5.3 can be applied to simulate the distribution of MAX3. Suppose the genotype counts of $(G_0, G_1, G_2) = (AA, AB, BB)$ in cases and controls are denoted by (r_0, r_1, r_2) and (s_0, s_1, s_2), respectively. The total number of genotype counts are (n_0, n_1, n_2), where $n_i = r_i + s_i$. Let $n = n_0 + n_1 + n_2$, $r = r_0 + r_1 + r_2$ and $s = s_0 + s_1 + s_2$. Note that under H_0 $(r_0, r_1, r_2) \sim Mul(r; p_0, p_1, p_2)$ and $(s_0, s_1, s_2) \sim Mul(s; p_0, p_1, p_2)$, where the probabilities p_i are estimated under H_0 by $\widehat{p}_i = n_i/n$ for $i = 0, 1, 2$.

In the bootstrap procedure, case-control datasets of the same size (r, s) are simulated from $(r_0, r_1, r_2) \sim Mul(r; \widehat{p}_0, \widehat{p}_1, \widehat{p}_2)$ and $(s_0, s_1, s_2) \sim Mul(s; \widehat{p}_0, \widehat{p}_1, \widehat{p}_2)$, respectively. The MAX3 statistic is calculated using each simulated dataset. After this procedure has been done m times, the m MAX3 values form an empirical null distribution for MAX3, which can be used to determine a critical value for MAX3 or an approximate p-value.

The above method is used to find the critical value or p-value for MAX3 after the case-control data are observed. The critical value and p-value found by this approach may vary from SNP to SNP. In simulation studies, because replicates of case-control data are simulated with the same parameter values, the same critical value can be used for all replicates. In this case, $p_i = \Pr(G_i)$ under H_0 for both cases and controls, which can be calculated under HWE or using Wright's inbreeding coefficient when HWE does not hold. In addition, the parametric bootstrap method described here can be used to approximate the null distribution for any test statistics, e.g., the constrained likelihood ratio test that we describe later.

The parametric bootstrap approach can also be used to approximate empirical power in simulation studies, in which (p_0, p_1, p_2) and (q_0, q_1, q_2) are calculated by

$$p_i = \frac{\Pr(G_i) f_i}{k} \quad \text{and} \quad q_i = \frac{\Pr(G_i)(1 - f_i)}{1 - k},$$

for $i = 0, 1, 2$ (see Eq. (3.2) in Sect. 3.1). The empirical power is estimated using case-control data simulated from $(r_0, r_1, r_2) \sim Mul(r; p_0, p_1, p_2)$ and $(s_0, s_1, s_2) \sim Mul(s; q_0, q_1, q_2)$. For other simulations of case-control data, see Sect. 3.9.

Simulating Trend Tests from the Bivariate Normal Distribution

From (6.10) of Sect. 6.2.1, under H_0 $Z_{\mathrm{CATT}}(0)$, $Z_{\mathrm{CATT}}(1/2)$ and $Z_{\mathrm{CATT}}(1)$ do not asymptotically follow a joint multivariate normal distribution because the covariance matrix Σ is not positive definite. The covariance matrix is given by

$$\Sigma = \begin{bmatrix} 1 & \rho_{0,1/2} & \rho_{0,1} \\ \rho_{0,1/2} & 1 & \rho_{1/2,1} \\ \rho_{0,1} & \rho_{1/2,1} & 1 \end{bmatrix},$$

where the correlations are given in (6.6). That is, there exists a non-zero vector $\mathbf{a}$ such that $\mathbf{a}^T \Sigma \mathbf{a} = 0$. In other words, $\mathbf{a}^T \mathbf{Z} = 0$, where

$$\mathbf{Z} = (Z_{\mathrm{CATT}}(0), Z_{\mathrm{CATT}}(1/2), Z_{\mathrm{CATT}}(1))^T.$$

Let $\mathbf{a} = (a_1, a_2, a_3)^T \neq 0$. Then $a_1 Z_{\mathrm{CATT}}(0) + a_2 Z_{\mathrm{CATT}}(1/2) + a_3 Z_{\mathrm{CATT}}(1) = 0$. It can be shown that $a_2 \neq 0$; otherwise a_1 and a_3 must be 0 too (Problem 6.5). Without loss of generality, we write

$$Z_{\mathrm{CATT}}(1/2) = w_0 Z_{\mathrm{CATT}}(0) + w_1 Z_{\mathrm{CATT}}(1).$$

Then

$$\rho_{0,1/2} = w_0 + w_1\rho_{0,1},$$

$$\rho_{1/2,1} = w_0\rho_{0,1} + w_1.$$

Solving the above equations, we obtain

$$w_0^* = \frac{\rho_{0,1/2} - \rho_{0,1}\rho_{1/2,1}}{1 - \rho_{0,1}^2}, \tag{6.18}$$

$$w_1^* = \frac{\rho_{1/2,1} - \rho_{0,1}\rho_{0,1/2}}{1 - \rho_{0,1}^2}. \tag{6.19}$$

See Problem 6.11 for w_0^* and w_1^* under HWE. Therefore,

$$Z_{\text{CATT}}(1/2) = w_0^* Z_{\text{CATT}}(0) + w_1^* Z_{\text{CATT}}(1). \tag{6.20}$$

From Problems 6.3 and 6.5, $w_0^* > 0$, $w_1^* > 0$ and $w_0^* + w_1^* \geq 1$. Hence, $Z_{\text{CATT}}(1/2)$ can be written as a weighted sum of the extreme pair $Z_{\text{CATT}}(0)$ and $Z_{\text{CATT}}(1)$. When B (or A) is the risk allele $w_1^* > $ (or $<$) w_0^*. Thus, more weight is on $Z_{\text{CATT}}(1)$ (or $Z_{\text{CATT}}(0)$) when B (or A) is the risk allele. For comparison, the MERT gives equal weights to the extreme pair.

An algorithm to generate the three trend tests and MAX3 is given as follows.

i) Generate $(Z_{\text{CATT}}(0), Z_{\text{CATT}}(1))^T$ from the bivariate normal distribution,

$$\begin{bmatrix} Z_{\text{CATT}}(0) \\ Z_{\text{CATT}}(1) \end{bmatrix} \sim N\left(\begin{bmatrix} 0 \\ 0 \end{bmatrix}, \begin{bmatrix} 1 & \rho_{0,1} \\ \rho_{0,1} & 1 \end{bmatrix} \right). \tag{6.21}$$

ii) Calculate $Z_{\text{CATT}}(1/2)$ from (6.20). All correlations are estimated by replacing p_i with n_i/n for $i = 0, 1, 2$.

iii) Find MAX3 once the three trend tests are obtained.

Unlike simulating case-control samples in the parametric bootstrap procedure, the above method can be used to simulate the trend test statistics without simulating case-control data. Hence, it is more efficient computationally. Like the parametric bootstrap method, in simulation studies, the genotype frequencies in the correlations in (6.21) and (w_0^*, w_1^*) can be calculated using the MAF under HWE, or together with Wright's inbreeding coefficient without assuming HWE. Table 6.4 reports critical values for MAX3 using the two simulation-based approaches under HWE. The critical values calculated using both approaches match very well except for MAF 0.1. Otherwise, the critical values are not sensitive to change in the MAF. In these simulations, a sample size of 500 cases and 500 controls was used in the parametric bootstrap method, while the sample size was not used in the bivariate normal approach.

6.3.3 Asymptotic Distribution of MAX3

The asymptotic null distribution of MAX3 can be derived using (6.21). Denote the joint density of $(Z_{\text{CATT}}(0), Z_{\text{CATT}}(1))^T$ by $f(z_0, z_1; \Sigma_0)$, where $\Sigma_0 = \begin{bmatrix} 1 & \rho_{0,1} \\ \rho_{0,1} & 1 \end{bmatrix}$ is the covariance matrix of $(Z_{\text{CATT}}(0), Z_{\text{CATT}}(1))^T$ given in (6.21). Then

Table 6.4 Critical values for MAX3 with various MAFs using the parametric bootstrap (boot) and bivariate normal distribution (BVN) under HWE. The nominal level is α. Each critical value is based on 1,000,000 replicates

MAF	α	Critical values		MAF	α	Critical values	
		boot	BVN			boot	BVN
0.10	0.05	2.23	2.26	0.30	0.05	2.28	2.28
	0.01	2.73	2.84		0.01	2.86	2.85
0.20	0.05	2.26	2.27	0.40	0.05	2.28	2.27
	0.01	2.84	2.85		0.01	2.86	2.86
0.25	0.05	2.28	2.27	0.50	0.05	2.28	2.27
	0.01	2.85	2.85		0.01	2.86	2.87

$$\Pr(\text{MAX3} > t) = 1 - \Pr(|Z_0| < t, |Z_{1/2}| < t, |Z_1| < t)$$

$$= 1 - \Pr(|Z_0| < t, |w_0^* Z_0 + w_1^* Z_1| < t, |Z_1| < t)$$

$$= 1 - \int\!\!\int_{\Omega} f(z_0, z_1; \Sigma_0) dz_0 dz_1, \tag{6.22}$$

where $\Omega = \{(z_0, z_1) : |Z_0| < t, |w_0^* Z_0 + w_1^* Z_1| < t, |Z_1| < t\}$. The integration region Ω is the shaded area shown in Fig. 6.6, where the coordinates for the points u and v on the Z_0-axis are $-t(1 - w_1^*)/w_0^*$ and $t(1 - w_1^*)/w_0^*$, respectively. The probability in (6.22) requires double integration. Based on the symmetry of the bivariate normal distribution, the above integrals are only calculated for the right half-space of Ω. Thus,

$$\int\!\!\int_{\Omega} f(z_0, z_1; \Sigma_0) dz_0 dz_1 = 2 \int_0^{\frac{t(1-w_1^*)}{w_0^*}} dz_0 \int_{-t}^{t} f(z_0, z_1; \Sigma_0) dz_1$$

$$+ 2 \int_{\frac{t(1-w_1^*)}{w_0^*}}^{t} dz_0 \int_{-t}^{\frac{t - w_0^* z_0}{w_1^*}} f(z_0, z_1; \Sigma_0) dz_1.$$

Note that

$$f(z_0, z_1; \Sigma_0) = f(z_0) f(z_1 | z_0; \rho_{0,1}),$$

where $f(z_0) = \phi(z_0)$ is the density $N(0, 1)$ and $f(z_1 | z_0; \rho_{0,1})$ is the density of the conditional normal distribution $N(\rho_{0,1} z_0, 1 - \rho_{0,1}^2)$ (Sect. 1.1.3). That is,

$$f(z_1 | z_0; \rho_{0,1}) = \frac{1}{\sqrt{1 - \rho_{0,1}^2}} \phi\left(\frac{z_1 - \rho_{0,1} z_0}{\sqrt{1 - \rho_{0,1}^2}}\right).$$

Applying the above densities, we have

$$2 \int_0^{\frac{t(1-w_1^*)}{w_0^*}} dz_0 \int_{-t}^{t} f(z_0, z_1; \Sigma_0) dz_1$$

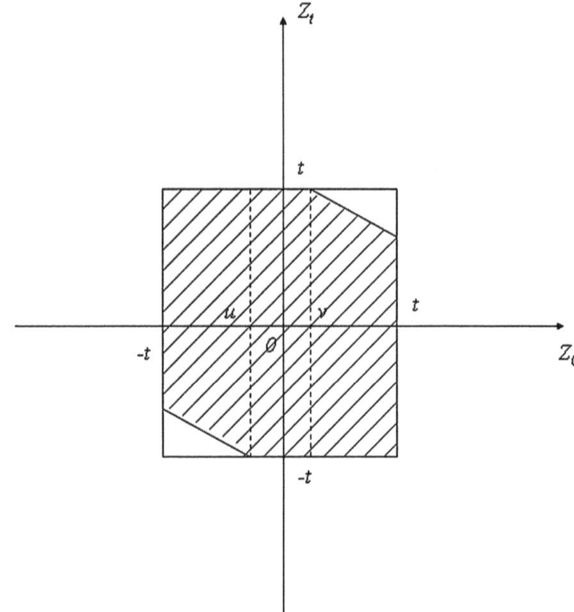

Fig. 6.6 The integration region Ω bounded by $|Z_0| < t$, $|w_0^* Z_0 + w_1^* Z_1| < t$, and $|Z_1| < t$, where $w_0^* + w_1^* \geq 1$

$$= 2 \int_0^{\frac{t(1-w_1^*)}{w_0^*}} \left\{ \Phi\left(\frac{t - \rho_{0,1} z_0}{\sqrt{1 - \rho_{0,1}^2}} \right) - \Phi\left(\frac{-t - \rho_{0,1} z_0}{\sqrt{1 - \rho_{0,1}^2}} \right) \right\} \phi(z_0) dz_0$$

and

$$2 \int_{\frac{t(1-w_1^*)}{w_0^*}}^{t} dz_0 \int_{-t}^{\frac{t - w_0^* z_0}{w_1^*}} f(z_0, z_1; \Sigma_0) dz_1$$

$$= 2 \int_{\frac{t(1-w_1^*)}{w_0^*}}^{t} \left\{ \Phi\left(\frac{(t - w_0^* z_0)/w_1^* - \rho_{0,1} z_0}{\sqrt{1 - \rho_{0,1}^2}} \right) - \Phi\left(\frac{-t - \rho_{0,1} z_0}{\sqrt{1 - \rho_{0,1}^2}} \right) \right\} \phi(z_0) dz_0.$$

Finally,

$$\int \int_\Omega f(z_0, z_1; \Sigma_0) dz_0 dz_1 = 2 \int_0^{\frac{t(1-w_1^*)}{w_0^*}} \Phi\left(\frac{t - \rho_{0,1} z_0}{\sqrt{1 - \rho_{0,1}^2}} \right) \phi(z_0) dz_0$$

$$+ 2 \int_{\frac{t(1-w_1^*)}{w_0^*}}^{t} \Phi\left(\frac{(t - w_0^* z_0)/w_1^* - \rho_{0,1} z_0}{\sqrt{1 - \rho_{0,1}^2}} \right) \phi(z_0) dz_0$$

$$- 2 \int_0^{t} \Phi\left(\frac{-t - \rho_{0,1} z_0}{\sqrt{1 - \rho_{0,1}^2}} \right) \phi(z_0) dz_0. \tag{6.23}$$

The asymptotic null distribution of MAX3 is a function of genotype frequencies through the correlation $\rho_{0,1}$, where the genotype frequencies can be estimated by

$\widehat{p}_i = n_i/n$ under H_0. Hence it may vary from SNP to SNP with different MAFs. If $t^* = \text{MAX3}$ is observed, then the p-value of MAX3 is given by $\Pr(\text{MAX3} > t^*)$.

6.3.4 Approximation of the Tail of the Distribution of MAX3: The Rhombus Formula

Monte-Carlo approaches, in particular the parametric bootstrap method that generates complete case-control data, have limitations when the significance level is small. In GWAS, the significance levels would be $\alpha = 1 \times 10^{-5}$ for moderate associations and $\alpha = 5 \times 10^{-7}$ for strong associations. P-values much smaller than 5×10^{-7} are often observed. To find a p-value about $\alpha = 5 \times 10^{-7}$, at least 10 million replicates per SNP are required in the simulation. When testing 500,000 to more than a million SNPs in GWAS, Monte-Carlo approaches could be computationally prohibitive given the current computer capacity. Finding p-values using the asymptotic distribution of MAX3 requires computing multiple integrations for each marker. This may also be computationally intensive in GWAS. Simpler approaches have been proposed. We introduce one here.

The approach we introduce here approximates the p-value of MAX3 by an upper bound of the tail probability of MAX3. Consider three normally distributed test statistics T_1, T_2 and T_3, $T_i \sim N(0, 1)$, with correlations $\rho_{ij} = \text{Corr}(T_i, T_j)$. Let $L_{i,j} = \arccos(\rho_{ij})$ and $i \neq j$. Denote $\text{MAX3} = \max_{1 \leq i \leq 3}(|T_i|)$. Define

$$I_{i,i+1} = 2\Phi\left(\frac{tL_{i,i+1}}{2}\right) + e^{-\frac{t^2 L_{i,i+1}^2}{8}}\left\{\Phi\left(\frac{t(\pi - L_{i,i+1})}{2}\right) - \Phi\left(\frac{tL_{i,i+1}}{2}\right)\right\};$$

$$I_{i,i+1}^c = 2\Phi\left(\frac{t(\pi - L_{i,i+1})}{2}\right) + e^{-\frac{t^2(\pi - L_{i,i+1})^2}{8}}\left\{\Phi\left(\frac{tL_{i,i+1}}{2}\right)\right.$$
$$\left. - \Phi\left(\frac{t(\pi - L_{i,i+1})}{2}\right)\right\}.$$

Then,

$$\Pr(\text{MAX3} > t)$$
$$\leq \frac{4\phi(t)}{t}\sum_{i=1}^{2}\{L_{i,i+1}I_{(L_{i,i+1}\in[0,\pi/2])} + L_{i,i+1}^c I_{(L_{i,i+1}\in[\pi/2,\pi])} - 1\} - 2\Phi(-t),$$

where ϕ and Φ are the PDF and CDF of $N(0, 1)$, respectively and $I_{(.)}$ is an indicator. The above bound, referred to as the Rhombus formula, can be used to find the approximate p-value for MAX3 when the three normally distributed tests are replaced by the three trend test statistics and t is replaced by the observed MAX3.

Note that the order of three tests T_1, T_2 and T_3 is not specified in the above approximation. Therefore, for the three trend tests, 6 upper bounds could be obtained using the above formula. The smallest upper bound, which gives the best approximation, is reported.

6.3.5 MAX

MAX3 takes the maximum of the trend tests over three genetic models: REC, ADD and DOM models. A more general statistic is to take the maximum over all genetic models in the constrained genetic model space Λ:

$$\Lambda = \{(\lambda_1, \lambda_2) : \lambda_2 \geq \lambda_1 \geq 1, \text{ and } \lambda_2 > 1\}, \tag{6.24}$$

where $\lambda_i = f_i/f_0$ is the GRR and $f_i = \Pr(\text{case}\,|\,G_i)$ is the penetrance for $i = 0, 1, 2$. For the discussion of a family of genetic models, see Sect. 3.2. We assume B is the risk allele. The constrained genetic model space Λ contains four common genetic models: the REC ($\lambda_1 = 1$), ADD ($\lambda_1 = (1 + \lambda_2)/2$), MUL ($\lambda_1 = \lambda_2^{1/2}$), and DOM ($\lambda_1 = \lambda_2$) models (see Fig. 3.1). The REC, ADD and DOM models can also be expressed using a linear function of λ_1 and λ_2 by $\lambda_1 = 1 - \theta + \theta\lambda_2$ for $\theta \in [0, 1]$, which is also given in (3.4). Then the REC, ADD and DOM models correspond to $\theta = 0, 1/2, 1$, respectively. Using this parameterization, the REC and DOM models correspond to the boundaries of $\theta \in [0, 1]$ and the ADD model is in the middle. The score $x = \theta$ is used in the trend test $Z_{\mathrm{CATT}}(x)$. When $(\lambda_1, \lambda_2) \approx (1, 1)$, the MUL model is approximately close to the ADD model in the middle of $[0, 1]$.

The MAX for $\{Z_x : x \in [0, 1]\}$ can be written as

$$\mathrm{MAX} = \max_{x \in [0, 1]} |Z_x|.$$

For the trend tests, we have

$$\mathrm{MAX} = \max_{x \in [0, 1]} |Z_{\mathrm{CATT}}(x)|.$$

A simple closed expression for MAX is given in Sect. 6.3.7, where we relate MAX to the trend test and Pearson's test. The asymptotic null distribution of MAX is more complicated than MAX3. The parametric bootstrap procedure (Sect. 6.3.2) can be used to find the asymptotic null distribution or p-value for MAX.

6.3.6 Comparing MAX2, MAX3 and MAX

To compare the empirical power of MAX3 and MAX, we add a simpler maximum test $\mathrm{MAX2} = \max(Z_{\mathrm{CATT}}(0), Z_{\mathrm{CATT}}(1))$. The data are simulated similarly to those under H_0 but with GRRs $(\lambda_1, \lambda_2) \neq (1, 1)$ for a given genetic model under H_1. We choose $\lambda_2 = 1.25$ and 1.5 with MAFs 0.1, 0.3, or 0.5. Prevalence is 0.1 and 500 cases and 500 controls are used. The empirical power is estimated using 10,000 replicates. Results are reported in Table 6.5.

The results are consistent with how the maximum tests are constructed. MAX2 only considers the REC and DOM models. Thus, it is slightly more powerful under these two models. MAX3 and MAX are often more powerful under the ADD model. Moreover, MAX is slightly more powerful than MAX3. Overall, the three maximum tests perform similarly. The difference in power is usually less than 2% under the REC or DOM models and less than 5% under the ADD model.

Table 6.5 Empirical power of MAX2, MAX3 and MAX given MAF and a genetic model (REC, ADD or DOM); 500 cases and 500 controls with prevalence 0.1

MAF	Model	$\lambda_2 = 1.25$			$\lambda_2 = 1.5$		
		MAX2	MAX3	MAX	MAX2	MAX3	MAX
0.1	REC	0.063	0.062	0.062	0.097	0.092	0.099
	ADD	0.121	0.122	0.120	0.342	0.346	0.340
	DOM	0.290	0.288	0.281	0.795	0.789	0.780
0.3	REC	0.173	0.172	0.175	0.524	0.516	0.523
	ADD	0.235	0.240	0.244	0.611	0.633	0.640
	DOM	0.429	0.427	0.426	0.914	0.912	0.912
0.5	REC	0.350	0.352	0.354	0.854	0.857	0.855
	ADD	0.242	0.259	0.263	0.617	0.656	0.663
	DOM	0.312	0.314	0.315	0.768	0.766	0.770

6.3.7 Relationship Among MAX, Trend Test and Pearson's Test

In Chap. 3, e.g., Tables 3.8 and 3.9, we compared the trend test, which is optimal for the ADD model, and Pearson's test $T_{\chi_2^2}$. We showed that the trend test $Z_{\mathrm{CATT}}(1/2)$ is more powerful under the ADD and DOM models while $T_{\chi_2^2}$ is more powerful under the REC model. Simulation results presented in Table 6.6 show that MAX3 has greater efficiency robustness than $Z_{\mathrm{CATT}}(1/2)$ and $T_{\chi_2^2}$. In fact, among the five tests considered in Table 6.6, MAX3 is the test that has the maximin efficiency, and it outperforms Pearson's test for each of the four genetic models. From Table 6.5, MAX3 and MAX have similar power performance. Thus, we study MAX here and discuss the relationship among the trend test, MAX and Pearson's test. The results can be used to explain why MAX3 (or MAX, as expected) is always more powerful than Pearson's test over the four common genetic models, and the trade-off between the trend test and Pearson's test.

Let the scores used in the trend test be (x_0, x_1, x_2). We used scores $(0, x, 1)$ with $x \in [0, 1]$ because the trend test is invariant after a linear transformation of the scores. That is, provided that $x_2 > x_0$, the trend test is identical if the two scores (x_0, x_1, x_2) and $(0, (x_1 - x_0)/(x_2 - x_0), 1)$ are used (Problem 6.6). Scores in the trend tests are prespecified. For the REC, ADD/MUL and DOM models, $x = 0, 1/2, 1$, respectively.

When case-control data (r_0, r_1, r_2) and (s_0, s_1, s_2) are observed, we define a set of new scores as

$$(x_0^*, x_1^*, x_2^*) = (r_0/n_0, r_1/n_1, r_2/n_2).$$

These scores are not prespecified but random. Let $x^* = (x_1^* - x_0^*)/(x_2^* - x_0^*)$, which is not necessarily in $[0,1]$. We are interested in what the trend test is if the score $(0, x^*, 1)$ is used. The following result (Problem 6.7) shows that the trend test with this random score is identical to Pearson's test, i.e.,

Table 6.6 Power of the trend tests $Z_{CATT}(x)$ with $x = 0, 1/2, 1$, Pearson's test $T_{\chi_2^2}$ and MAX3 with prevalence 0.1, MAF 0.3, 500 cases and 500 controls, and 10,000 replicates: GRRs are chosen so that the optimal trend test has about 80% power

Model	$Z_{CATT}(x)$			$T_{\chi_2^2}$	MAX3
	$x = 0$	$x = 1/2$	$x = 1$		
REC	0.797	0.516	0.162	0.711	0.733
ADD	0.389	0.818	0.805	0.742	0.786
MUL	0.508	0.799	0.718	0.711	0.748
DOM	0.131	0.712	0.797	0.690	0.735
min	0.131	0.516	0.162	0.690	0.733
maximin					0.733

$$T_{\chi_2^2} \equiv Z_{CATT}^2(x^*). \tag{6.25}$$

Hence Pearson's test is also a trend test, with the random score $(0, x^*, 1)$ and, owing to the randomness, the degrees of freedom of its asymptotic null distribution increase from 1 to 2. The random score r_i/n_i is the proportion of cases among sampled individuals with genotype G_i. In a prospective case-control (cohort) study, r_i/n_i is the MLE of the penetrance $f_i = \Pr(\text{case} \,|\, G_i)$. When we consider retrospective case-control data, i.e., cases and controls are sampled from case and control populations, r_i/n_i is a biased estimate of f_i. Because it is data-driven, the trend test with this score (Pearson's test) is more robust than the trend test with a prespecified fixed score. On the other hand, its robustness that is due to randomness leads to a higher degree of freedom test and loses power compared to $Z_{CATT}(1/2)$ when the model with $x = 1/2$ is correctly specified.

Let

$$\text{MAX} = \max_{x \in [0,1]} Z_{CATT}^2(x),$$

which is slightly different from the one defined before as

$$\text{MAX} = \max_{x \in [0,1]} |Z_{CATT}(x)|.$$

The random score x^* used in Pearson's test can be any real number, $x^* \in (-\infty, \infty)$. However, if $x^* \in [0, 1]$, then the following holds (Problem 6.7):

$$\text{MAX} \equiv T_{\chi_2^2} = Z_{CATT}^2(x^*), \quad \text{if } x^* \in [0, 1]. \tag{6.26}$$

Hence, MAX itself is a constrained trend test, or Pearson's test when the random score is constrained. When case-control data are generated under the four genetic models in a constrained genetic model space Λ, MAX would be more powerful using this constraint than Pearson's test without any constraint. However, if the true genetic model is outside of Λ, Pearson's test would be more powerful.

Note that, when $x^* \notin [0, 1]$, $\text{MAX} = \max(Z_{CATT}^2(0), Z_{CATT}^2(1))$ on taking the maximum on the boundary, or the extreme pair.

Table 6.7 SNPs reported from GWAS of prostate cancer and breast cancer (see Table 3.10)

Cancer	SNP IDs	Cases			Controls			$\widehat{p}_0$	$\widehat{p}_1$
		r_0	r_1	r_2	s_0	s_1	s_2		
Prostate	rs1447295	25	283	864	10	218	929	0.0150	0.2151
	rs6983267	223	598	351	301	579	277	0.2250	0.5044
	rs7837688	27	283	861	11	206	939	0.0163	0.2101
Breast	rs10510126	10	180	955	14	272	854	0.0105	0.1978
	rs12505080	50	477	608	99	408	628	0.0656	0.3899
	rs17157903	18	316	777	26	220	862	0.0198	0.2416
	rs1219648	250	543	352	170	538	433	0.1837	0.4729
	rs7696175	187	605	353	249	496	396	0.1907	0.4816
	rs2420946	242	546	357	165	537	440	0.1780	0.4736

6.3.8 Examples

In this section, we illustrate the use of MAX3 to test association when the true
genetic model is unknown. The SNPs that were reported with associations in GWAS
of prostate cancer and breast cancer are used (see Table 3.10). Table 6.7 presents the
genotype counts for these SNPs along with their SNP ID numbers and the estimates
of genotype frequencies in case-control samples given by

$$\widehat{p}_i = \frac{n_i}{n_0 + n_1 + n_2}, \quad \text{for } i = 0, 1,$$

where $n_j = r_j + s_j$, $j = 0, 1, 2$ and $\widehat{p}_2 = 1 - \widehat{p}_0 - \widehat{p}_1$. For the SNPs in Table 6.7,
neither the underlying genetic models nor the risk alleles are known *a priori*.

The trend tests for a given score $(x_0, x_1, x_2) = (0, x, 1)$ are given in (3.8) or
(6.3). Using the data in Table 6.7, three trend statistics are calculated under the REC
($x = 0$), ADD ($x = 1/2$), and DOM ($x = 1$) models. The results are reported in Ta-
ble 6.8 along with MAX3 $= \max_{x=0,1/2,1} |Z_{\text{CATT}}(x)|$. Using the estimated genotype
frequencies in Table 6.7 and the formulas (6.7) to (6.9), we arrive at the estimated
pair-wise correlations also given in Table 6.8. Because the risk allele is unknown,
$\rho_{0,1/2} > \rho_{1/2,1}$ when A is the risk allele. The results in Table 6.8 indicate that A is
the risk allele under H_1.

To determine the p-values for MAX3, we consider four approaches: (i) the parametric bootstrap, (ii) simulation using the bivariate normal, (iii) asymptotic distribution of MAX3, and (iv) the approximation using the Rhombus formula. For the
first two methods, 1 million and 10 million replicates are used, respectively. We use
the first SNP in Tables 6.7 and 6.8 for illustration.

i) Fix the total numbers of cases and controls at $r = 25 + 283 + 864 = 1172$
and $s = 10 + 218 + 929 = 1157$. To apply the parametric bootstrap, we simulate
genotype counts (r_{0l}, r_{1l}, r_{2l}) in cases and genotype counts in controls (s_{0l}, s_{1l}, s_{2l})
from

Table 6.8 Trend tests $Z_{\text{CATT}}(x)$ for $x = 0, 1/2, 1$, their estimated pair-wise correlations $\rho_{x,y}$, and MAX3 for the SNPs in Table 6.7

SNP IDs	$|Z_{\text{CATT}}(x)|$			$\rho_{x,y}$			MAX3
	$x = 0$	$x = \frac{1}{2}$	$x = 1$	$\rho_{0,\frac{1}{2}}$	$\rho_{0,1}$	$\rho_{\frac{1}{2},1}$	
rs1447295	3.768	4.080	2.516	0.9668	0.2259	0.4673	4.080
rs6983267	3.267	4.468	4.038	0.8270	0.3274	0.8019	4.468
rs7837688	4.438	4.694	2.577	0.9644	0.2381	0.4866	4.694
rs10510126	4.999	4.827	0.832	0.9737	0.2009	0.4189	4.999
rs12505080	0.843	0.986	4.153	0.9233	0.2898	0.6352	4.153
rs17157903	4.214	3.417	1.227	0.9614	0.2391	0.4972	4.214
rs1219648	3.628	4.773	4.281	0.8580	0.3431	0.7768	4.773
rs7696175	1.975	0.546	3.341	0.8524	0.3389	0.7809	3.341
rs2420946	3.688	4.759	4.180	0.8602	0.3403	0.7723	4.759

$$(r_{0l}, r_{1l}, r_{2l}) \sim Mul(1172; 0.015, 0.2151, 0.7699),$$

$$(s_{0l}, s_{1l}, s_{2l}) \sim Mul(1157; 0.015, 0.2151, 0.7699), \quad \text{for } l = 1, \ldots, m.$$

For each replicate ($l = 1, \ldots, m$), we calculate the three trend tests and MAX3. Then the p-value of MAX3 is estimated by the proportion of simulated MAX3 values greater than or equal to the observed one in Table 6.8. We choose $m = 1,000,000$ for the bootstrap method.

ii) Apply (6.21) to generate three test statistics directly from the bivariate normal distribution:

$$\begin{bmatrix} Z_{0,l} \\ Z_{1,l} \end{bmatrix} \sim N\left(\begin{bmatrix} 0 \\ 0 \end{bmatrix}, \begin{bmatrix} 1 & 0.2259 \\ 0.2259 & 1 \end{bmatrix} \right), \quad \text{for } l = 1, \ldots, m.$$

The weights in (6.18) and (6.19) are given by $w_0^* = 0.9075$ and $w_1^* = 0.2623$. Then, using (6.20), we have $Z_{1/2,l} = w_0^* Z_{0,l} + w_1^* Z_{1,l}$ for $l = 1, \ldots, m$. Finally, for each l, we calculate MAX3 $= \max(|Z_{0,l}|, |Z_{1/2,l}|, |Z_{1,l}|)$, from which the empirical distribution of MAX3 is obtained. The p-value of MAX3 can also be obtained. We choose $m = 10,000,000$ for the bivariate normal approach. We choose a larger m because generating test statistics is less simulation-intensive than simulating case-control data in the parametric bootstrap approach.

iii) To apply the asymptotic null distribution of MAX3 to find p-values, let t be an observed MAX3. Formula (6.23) is used to calculate the p-value $\Pr(\text{MAX3} > t)$ for each SNP. Using SNP rs1447295 for illustration, given $t = 4.080$, $w_0^* = 0.9075$, $w_1^* = 0.2623$, and the estimated $\widehat{\rho}_{0,1} = 0.2259$, the three double integrals in (6.23) with 10 decimal places are obtained as

$$I_1 = 2 \int_0^{\frac{t(1-w_1^*)}{w_0^*}} \Phi\left(\frac{t - \widehat{\rho}_{0,1} z_0}{\sqrt{1 - \widehat{\rho}_{0,1}^2}} \right) \phi(z_0) dz_0 = 0.9990509524,$$

$$I_2 = 2 \int_{\frac{t(1-w_1^*)}{w_0^*}}^{t} \Phi\left(\frac{(t - w_0^* z_0)/w_1^* - \widehat{\rho}_{0,1} z_0}{\sqrt{1 - \widehat{\rho}_{0,1}^2}}\right) \phi(z_0) dz_0 = 0.000847540775,$$

$$I_3 = 2 \int_0^t \Phi\left(\frac{-t - \widehat{\rho}_{0,1} z_0}{\sqrt{1 - \widehat{\rho}_{0,1}^2}}\right) \phi(z_0) dz_0 = 7.184633976 \times 10^{-6}.$$

Then the p-value is $1 - I_1 - I_2 + I_3 = 1.0869 \times 10^{-4}$, which is reported as $1.1e{-}4$ in Table 6.9.

iv) The last method is to apply the Rhombus formula (Sect. 6.3.3). We first set $T_1 = Z_{CATT}(0)$, $T_2 = Z_{CATT}(1/2)$ and $T_3 = Z_{CATT}(1)$. Using $\pi \approx 3.14159$,

$$L_{1,2} = \arccos(\rho_{0,1/2}) = \arccos(0.9668) = 0.2584 \in [0, \pi/2],$$

$$L_{2,3} = \arccos(\rho_{1/2,1}) = \arccos(0.4673) = 1.0846 \in [0, \pi/2].$$

Based on the formulas in Sect. 6.3.4, when $L_{i,i+1} \in [0, \pi/2]$ for $i = 1, 2$, we only need to calculate $I_{1,2}$ and $I_{2,3}$, not $I_{1,2}^c$ and $I_{2,3}^c$ which will only be used when $L_{i,i+1} \in [\pi/2, \pi]$ for $i = 1, 2$. Thus, using $t = 4.080$ and $L_{1,2} = 0.2584$,

$$I_{1,2} = 2\Phi\left(\frac{tL_{1,2}}{2}\right) + \exp\left(-\frac{t^2 L_{1,2}^2}{8}\right)\left\{\Phi\left(\frac{t(\pi - L_{1,2})}{2}\right) - \Phi\left(\frac{tL_{1,2}}{2}\right)\right\}$$

$$= 1.6622.$$

$I_{2,3} = 1.9742$ can be obtained using $L_{2,3} = 1.0846$ to replace $L_{1,2}$ in the above formula. Finally, the p-value is approximately given by

$$\Pr(\text{MAX3} > t) \approx \frac{4\phi(t)}{t}(I_{1,2} - 1 + I_{2,3} - 1) - 2\Phi(-t) \approx 0.0001104.$$

The p-value calculated by the Rhombus formula depends on the order of the three tests. All six permutations are used and the minimum p-value of the six permutations is reported as the approximate p-value of MAX3. For the first SNP in Table 6.8, the other five approximate p-values are 0.0001419, 0.0001122, 0.000112, 0.0001104, and 0.0001122. The minimum p-value reported in Table 6.9 is $1.1e{-}4$.

In Table 6.9, the p-values of all four methods are presented. Note that p-values using the asymptotic distribution and the Rhombus formulas match particularly well. P-values of both approaches also match that of using the bivariate normal simulation (using 10 million replicates). The parametric bootstrap method using 1 million replicates does not match well with the other three methods in some cases. It is also the most computationally intensive among the four methods. Applying the asymptotic distribution of MAX3 requires integrations while using the Rhombus formula only requires calculations of normal distribution functions. The parametric bootstrap method can be easily used in candidate-gene association studies, but the asymptotic distribution of MAX3 or the Rhombus formula are preferred for large-scale association studies such as GWAS. The last two methods are also useful in simulation studies at genome-wide scales.

Table 6.9 P-values of MAX3 from four approaches: bootstrap (boot), bivariate normal distribution (BVN), asymptotic distribution (ASYM) and the approximation using Rhombus formula (Rhombus). For the simulation-based p-values, the numbers of replicates are 1 million for the bootstrap method (boot) and 10 million for using the bivariate normal method (BVN)

SNP IDs	P-values of MAX3			
	boot	BVN	ASYM	Rhombus
rs1447295	8.2e−5	1.1e−4	1.1e−4	1.1e−4
rs6983267	2.2e−5	2.0e−5	2.2e−5	2.1e−5
rs7837688	4.0e−6	7.0e−6	6.7e−6	6.7e−5
rs10510126	1.0e−6	1.4e−6	1.4e−6	1.4e−6
rs12505080	8.7e−5	8.2e−5	8.5e−5	8.3e−5
rs17157903	4.6e−5	6.2e−5	6.2e−5	6.2e−5
rs1219648	6.0e−6	6.5e−6	5.0e−6	4.8e−6
rs7696175	2.1e−3	2.1e−3	2.1e−3	2.0e−3
rs2420946	8.0e−6	6.8e−6	5.3e−6	5.2e−6

6.4 MIN2

6.4.1 Joint Distribution and P-Value

An alternative robust test, which borrows strengths from Pearson's test under the REC model and the trend test under the ADD or DOM models, is the minimum of the p-values of Pearson's test and the trend test that is optimal for the ADD model. This robust test is referred to as MIN2, given by

$$\text{MIN2} = \min(p_{\chi_2^2}, p_{\text{CATT}}), \tag{6.27}$$

where $p_{\chi_2^2}$ is the p-value of Pearson's test $T_{\chi_2^2}$ and p_{CATT} is the p-value of $Z_{\text{CATT}}^2(1/2)$.

Both p-values are calculated based on the same case-control data. Hence they are correlated. To find the asymptotic distribution and p-value of MIN2 under the null hypothesis H_0 of no association, the correlation is usually required. However, using a property of Pearson's test and trend test (Problem 6.8), $Z_{\text{CATT}}^2(1/2)/T_{\chi_2^2}$ and $T_{\chi_2^2}$ are asymptotically independent under H_0. Hence, the joint distribution of $T_{\chi_2^2}$ and $Z_{\text{CATT}}^2(1/2)$ under H_0 can be obtained (Problem 6.8) as

$$\Pr\left(Z_{\text{CATT}}^2\left(\frac{1}{2}\right) < t_1, T_{\chi_2^2} < t_2\right) = 1 - \frac{1}{2}e^{-\frac{t_1}{2}} - \frac{1}{2}e^{-\frac{t_2}{2}}$$
$$+ \frac{1}{2\pi}\int_{t_1}^{t_2} e^{-\frac{v}{2}} \arcsin\left(\frac{2t_1}{v} - 1\right) dv \tag{6.28}$$

when $t_1 < t_2$, and $\Pr(Z_{\text{CATT}}^2(1/2) < t_1, T_{\chi_2^2} < t_2) = 1 - \exp(-t_2/2)$ when $t_1 > t_2$. Let F_i denote the distribution function of χ_i^2 with $i = 1, 2$ degrees of freedom. Then

$$p_{\text{CATT}} = 1 - F_1(Z^2_{\text{CATT}}(1/2)),$$

$$p_{\chi^2_2} = 1 - F_2(T_{\chi^2_2}).$$

Hence,

$$\Pr(\text{MIN2} > t) = \Pr\left(Z^2_{\text{CATT}}\left(\frac{1}{2}\right) < F_1^{-1}(1-t), T_{\chi^2_2} < F_2^{-1}(1-t) \right).$$

Thus, (6.28) can be used to find the distribution of MIN2 under H_0 and its p-value, denoted by $p_{\text{MIN2}} = \Pr(\text{MIN2} < t_{\min2})$, where $t_{\min2}$ is the observed value of MIN2. Then the p-value of MIN2 can be written as

$$p_{\text{MIN2}} = \frac{1}{2}e^{-F_1^{-1}(1-t_{\min2})/2} + \frac{1}{2}t_{\min2}$$
$$- \frac{1}{2\pi}\int_{F_1^{-1}(1-t_{\min2})}^{-2\log(t_{\min2})} e^{-\frac{v}{2}} \arcsin\left(\frac{2F_1^{-1}(1-t_{\min2})}{v} - 1\right) dv. \quad (6.29)$$

Note that, from (6.29), the p-value of MIN2 only depends on the value of MIN2 and is independent of the MAF of the genetic marker. Computation of the p-value of MIN2 only involves the evaluation of a single integral.

6.4.2 MIN2 Versus the P-Value of MIN2

In Problem 6.8, it is shown that Pearson's test $T_{\chi^2_2}$ and the trend test $Z^2_{\text{CATT}}(1/2)$ are positively correlated, and that MIN2 is always greater than its p-value p_{MIN2}. That is, MIN2 itself is not a valid p-value. Using MIN2 as a p-value would inflate Type I error in testing association. For example, if the significance level is $\alpha = 0.05$ and MIN2 $= 0.05$ is observed, then the p-value of MIN2 using (6.29) is 0.0751. In order to have the p-value $p_{\text{MIN2}} < 0.05$, the significance level has to be no more than $\alpha = 0.0328$, which is smaller than the typical 0.05 level but greater than 0.025, the level obtained on applying the Bonferroni correction.

Table 6.10 reports thresholds for MIN2 to be significant given the significance levels (or p-values of MIN2). For example, to have an association to be significant at the level 5×10^{-5}, i.e., $p_{\text{MIN2}} < 5 \times 10^{-5}$, the observed MIN2 has to be no more than 2.97×10^{-5}.

6.4.3 Examples

For illustration, we apply MIN2 to the SNPs reported in Table 6.9 from two GWAS of cancer. For comparison, the p-values of MAX3 reported in Table 6.9 using the asymptotic null distribution are also presented. The p-value of MIN2 is calculated from (6.29) for each SNP. Results are presented in Table 6.11.

Table 6.10 The thresholds for MIN2 to be significant given the significance levels (p-values of MIN2)

Threshold	p_{MIN2}
3.28×10^{-2}	5.00×10^{-2}
3.12×10^{-3}	5.00×10^{-3}
3.03×10^{-4}	5.00×10^{-4}
2.97×10^{-5}	5.00×10^{-5}
2.93×10^{-6}	5.00×10^{-6}
2.90×10^{-7}	5.00×10^{-7}
9.62×10^{-8}	1.67×10^{-7}
5.76×10^{-8}	1.00×10^{-7}

Table 6.11 P-values of MAX3 and MIN2 for the SNPs reported in Table 6.9. The p-values of MAX3, which are also reported in Table 6.9, are based on the asymptotic null distribution (ASYM)

SNP IDs	P-values			
	$Z_{\text{CATT}}(\frac{1}{2})$	$T_{\chi_2^2}$	MAX3	MIN2
rs1447295	4.5e−5	1.9e−4	1.1e−4	7.6e−5
rs6983267	7.9e−6	3.5e−5	2.2e−5	1.3e−5
rs7837688	2.7e−6	1.6e−5	6.7e−6	4.6e−5
rs10510126	1.4e−6	3.7e−6	1.4e−6	2.4e−6
rs12505080	0.3240	1.8e−5	8.5e−5	3.1e−5
rs17157903	6.3e−4	9.9e−6	6.2e−5	1.7e−5
rs1219648	1.8e−6	7.5e−6	5.0e−6	3.1e−6
rs7696175	0.5851	1.6e−5	2.1e−3	2.7e−3
rs2420946	1.9e−6	8.8e−6	5.3e−6	3.3e−6

Table 6.11 shows that the trend test is not robust. The two SNPs, rs12505080 and rs7696175, have p-values 0.3240 and 0.5851, respectively. The trend test and Pearson's test also have p-values that disagree: when a p-value of the trend test is smallest in Table 6.11, the p-value of Pearson's test is largest, and vice versa. MIN2 borrows strength from both the trend test and Pearson's test and is more robust in the sense that its p-values are always between those of the trend test and Pearson's test. The results also show that MIN2 could have smaller p-values than MAX3, but not always. More comparison between MAX3 and MIN2 will be presented later in this chapter, along with other robust tests.

6.5 The Constrained Likelihood Ratio Test

The idea of the constrained likelihood ratio test (CLRT) is similar to MAX. It constrains the GRRs (λ_1, λ_2) to the genetic model space Λ given in (6.24). Note that $(\lambda_1, \lambda_2) \in \Lambda$ indicates that $f_0 \leq f_1 \leq f_2$ when B is the risk allele. When A is the risk allele, the constrained genetic model space would correspond to $f_0 \geq f_1 \geq f_2$. In other words, the constrained genetic model corresponds to ordered penetrances.

6.5.1 Restricted Maximum Likelihood Estimates of Penetrances

Note that the frequencies of G_i genotype in cases and controls are $p_i = g_i f_i / k$ and $q_i = g_i(1 - f_i)/(1 - k)$, respectively, for $i = 0, 1, 2$, where g_i is the population frequency of G_i, f_i is a penetrance, and k is the prevalence. The likelihood for the case-control data (r_i, s_i), $i = 0, 1, 2$ is proportional to $\prod_{i=0}^{2} p_i^{r_i} q_i^{s_i}$. Thus, the log-likelihood function is proportional to

$$l_2(f_0, f_1, f_2) = \sum_{i=0}^{2} \{r_i \log f_i + s_i \log(1 - f_i)\}.$$

Under H_0, the log-likelihood function has a maximum

$$l_0 = r \log(\widehat{f_0}) + s \log(1 - \widehat{f_0}),$$

where $\widehat{f_0} = r/n$. Therefore, the CLRT is given by

$$T_{\text{CLRT}} = 2\left(\max_{\substack{(f_0, f_1, f_2) \\ \text{are ordered}}} l_2(f_0, f_1, f_2) - l_0 \right).$$

An algorithm to obtain T_{CLRT} is as follows:

(i) Denote $\widehat{f_i} = r_i/n_i$ for $i = 0, 1, 2$. If $\widehat{f_i}$, $i = 0, 1, 2$ are ordered (increasing or decreasing), T_{CLRT} can be directly calculated using the estimates as

$$T_{\text{CLRT}} = 2(l_2(\widehat{f_0}, \widehat{f_1}, \widehat{f_2}) - l_0).$$

(ii) Otherwise, estimate $\widehat{f_0} = \widehat{f_1} = (r_0 + r_1)/(n_0 + n_1)$ and $\widehat{f_2} = r_2/n_2$ under the REC model and calculate $T_{\text{CLRTR}} = 2(l_2(\widehat{f_0}, \widehat{f_0}, \widehat{f_2}) - l_0)$. Next, estimate them by $\widehat{f_0} = r_0/n_0$ and $\widehat{f_1} = \widehat{f_2} = (r_1 + r_2)/(n_1 + n_2)$ under the DOM model, and calculate $T_{\text{CLRTD}} = 2(l_2(\widehat{f_0}, \widehat{f_2}, \widehat{f_2}) - l_0)$. Finally, $T_{\text{CLRT}} = \max(T_{\text{CLRTR}}, T_{\text{CLRTD}})$.

Under H_0, the asymptotic distribution of T_{CLRT} is a mixture of chi-squared distributions with degrees of freedom 0, 1 and 2. The bootstrap procedure used for MAX and MAX3 can be also used to find the asymptotic null distribution for T_{CLRT}.

Note that, under case (i), the estimates $\widehat{f_i} = r_i/n_i$, $i = 0, 1, 2$ are the random scores (x_0^*, x_1^*, x_2^*) used in Pearson's test, for which the random scores do not need to be ordered. However, when the random scores are ordered as in case (i), the trend test becomes MAX. When the random scores are not ordered, T_{CLRT} takes on the maximum value of the trend tests for the REC model (case (ii)) or DOM model (case (iii)). Hence, the CLRT and MAX are expected to have similar power performance.

6.5.2 Examples

For illustration, we use the first SNP in Table 6.7 with $(r_0, r_1, r_2) = (25, 283, 864)$ in $r = 1172$ cases, $(s_0, s_1, s_2) = (10, 218, 929)$ in $s = 1157$ controls, $(n_0, n_1, n_2) = (35, 501, 1793)$, and $n = 2329$. First, we calculate l_0 by

Table 6.12 P-values of MAX3 and the CLRT for the SNPs reported in Table 6.9

SNP IDs	P-values	
	MAX3	CLRT
rs1447295	1.1e−4	1.1e−4
rs6983267	2.2e−5	1.9e−5
rs7837688	6.7e−6	8.4e−5
rs10510126	1.4e−6	2.4e−6
rs12505080	8.5e−5	8.7e−5
rs17157903	6.2e−5	8.4e−5
rs1219648	5.0e−6	4.5e−6
rs7696175	2.1e−3	2.3e−3
rs2420946	5.3e−6	3.9e−6

$$l_0 = 1172 \log\left(\frac{1172}{2329}\right) + 1157 \log\left(\frac{1157}{2329}\right) = -1614.29.$$

Next, we calculate the random scores $\widehat{f}_i$ for $i = 0, 1, 2$ and obtain $\widehat{f}_0 = 25/35 = 0.7143$, $\widehat{f}_1 = 283/501 = 0.5649$, and $\widehat{f}_2 = 864/1793 = 0.4819$, which are decreasing. Thus, case (i) applies and l_2 is obtained

$$l_2 = 25 \log(0.7143) + 283 \log(0.5649) + 864 \log(0.4819)$$
$$+ 10 \log(1 - 0.7143) + 218 \log(1 - 0.5649) + 929 \log(1 - 0.4819)$$
$$= -1605.61.$$

Then, $T_{\mathrm{CLRT}} = 2(l_2 - l_0) = 17.36$. The parametric bootstrap can be applied to find the p-value for $T_{\mathrm{CLRT}} = 17.36$. In Table 6.12, p-values of the CLRT are reported for all the SNPs in Table 6.7. The p-values of the CLRT are similar to those of MAX3.

6.6 Genetic Model Selection

The genetic model selection (GMS) approach is an adaptive procedure that has two steps. In step 1, an underlying genetic model is selected based on the difference in HWD between cases and controls. The selected genetic model is either REC, DOM or ADD (MUL). Then the score, 0, 1/2, or 1 for the trend test is determined based on the selected genetic model. In step 2, the trend test with the score corresponding to the selected model is used to test for association. The correlation between the two steps is taken into account to control the overall Type I error.

The HWD coefficient and the HWDTT for association have been discussed in Sect. 3.6. Here we discuss the relationship between HWD and genetic models. Then we present how to use the HWDTT to select a genetic model and test for association.

6.6.1 Hardy-Weinberg Disequilibrium and Genetic Models

Using the notation in Sect. 3.6, $p_i = \Pr(G_i|\text{case})$ and $q_i = \Pr(G_i|\text{control})$ for genotypes $(G_0, G_1, G_2) = (AA, AB, BB)$. The HWD coefficients in cases (Δ_p), controls (Δ_q), and the population (Δ) are given by $\Delta_p = p_2 - (p_2 + p_1/2)^2$, $\Delta_q = q_2 - (q_2 + q_1/2)^2$, and $\Delta = \Pr(BB) - \{\Pr(BB) + \Pr(AB)/2\}^2$. We are interested in the relationship between (Δ_p, Δ_q) and genetic models when HWE holds in the population $(\Delta = 0)$.

Under HWE, $g_i = \Pr(G_i)$ can be calculated by

$$(g_0, g_1, g_2) = ((1 - p)^2, 2p(1 - p), p^2),$$

where $p = \Pr(B)$. Substituting $p_i = g_i f_i/k$ and $q_i = g_i(1 - f_i)/(1 - k)$, where $k = \Pr(\text{case})$, into Δ_p and Δ_q, we have

$$\Delta_p = \frac{f_0^2 p^2 (1 - p)^2}{k^2}(\lambda_2 - \lambda_1^2), \tag{6.30}$$

$$\Delta_q = \frac{f_0^2 p^2 (1 - p)^2}{(1 - k)^2}(2\lambda_1 - 1 - \lambda_2 - f_0\lambda_1^2 + f_0\lambda_2). \tag{6.31}$$

Under a REC model $\lambda_1 = 1$,

$$\lambda_2 - \lambda_1^2 = \lambda_2 - 1 > 0,$$
$$2\lambda_1 - 1 - \lambda_2 - f_0\lambda_1^2 + f_0\lambda_2 = -(\lambda_2 - 1)(1 - f_0) < 0.$$

Thus, from (6.30) and (6.31), $\Delta_p > 0$ and $\Delta_q < 0$. On the other hand, under a DOM model $\lambda_1 = \lambda_2$,

$$\lambda_2 - \lambda_1^2 = -\lambda_2(\lambda_2 - 1) < 0,$$
$$2\lambda_1 - 1 - \lambda_2 - f_0\lambda_1^2 + f_0\lambda_2 = (\lambda_2 - 1)(1 - f_0\lambda_2) = (\lambda_2 - 1)(1 - f_2) > 0.$$

Thus $\Delta_p < 0$ and $\Delta_q > 0$.

Note that, when B is the risk allele, the signs of Δ_p and Δ_q are the opposite of those under the REC model $(\Delta_p, \Delta_q) = (+, -)$ and DOM model $(\Delta_p, \Delta_q) = (-, +)$. However, the signs of Δ_p and Δ_q are independent of which allele is the risk allele. If A is the risk allele, using the same definitions of G_i and f_i, $i = 0, 1, 2$, then $\lambda_2 \le \lambda_1 \le 1$ and $\lambda_2 < 1$. In addition Δ_p and Δ_q have the same expressions as in (6.30) and (6.31). Under the REC model $(\lambda_1 = \lambda_2)$, $\lambda_1 = \lambda_2$, and under the DOM model, $\lambda_1 = 1$. Hence, under the REC model, $\lambda_2 - \lambda_1^2 = \lambda_2(1 - \lambda_2) > 0$ and $2\lambda_1 - 1 - \lambda_2 - f_0\lambda_1^2 + f_0\lambda_2 = -(1 - \lambda_2)(1 - f_2) < 0$. Under the DOM model $(\lambda_1 = 1)$, $\lambda_2 - \lambda_1^2 < 0$ and $2\lambda_1 - 1 - \lambda_2 - f_0\lambda_1^2 + f_0\lambda_2 > 0$.

Although the signs of Δ_p and Δ_q can be used to determine the genetic model, a simple approach is to consider the difference $\Delta_p - \Delta_q$, which can be normalized to the HWDTT, Z_{HWDTT}, given in (3.20) and is also given below:

$$Z_{\text{HWDTT}} = \frac{\sqrt{rs/n}(\widehat{\Delta}_p - \widehat{\Delta}_q)}{\{1 - n_2/n - n_1/(2n)\}\{n_2/n + n_1/(2n)\}}. \tag{6.32}$$

Table 6.13 Performance of the GMS under HWE given MAF. True genetic models include REC, ADD, MUL, and DOM models. The ADD or MUL models are grouped as A/M when neither REC or DOM is selected. The sample sizes are $r = s = 250$ with $\lambda_2 = 2$

True model	MAF	Selected model		
		REC	A/M	DOM
REC	0.1	20.28%	79.21%	0.51%
	0.3	66.86%	33.13%	0.01%
	0.5	66.28%	33.71%	0.01%
ADD	0.1	2.02%	90.24%	7.74%
	0.3	2.27%	87.94%	9.79%
	0.5	2.36%	89.22%	8.42%
MUL	0.1	2.95%	92.14%	4.91%
	0.3	5.00%	90.27%	4.73%
	0.5	5.64%	90.20%	4.16%
DOM	0.1	0.03%	61.48%	38.49%
	0.3	0.00%	31.73%	68.27%
	0.5	0.03%	34.91%	65.06%

Under H_0, $Z_{\mathrm{HWDTT}} \sim N(0, 1)$. We assume the underlying genetic model is ADD or MUL unless there is strong evidence that it is REC when $Z_{\mathrm{HWDTT}} > c^*$ or DOM when $Z_{\mathrm{HWDTT}} < -c^*$, where the threshold $c^* = 1.645$, corresponding to the upper 95% percentile of $N(0, 1)$, can be used.

6.6.2 Performance of the Genetic Model Selection

To examine the performance of the GMS under H_1, we conduct a simulation study. The parameters in the simulation study are given below. We first examine the performance under HWE. The sample sizes are $r = s = 250$ when GRR $\lambda_2 = 2.0$ or $r = s = 1000$ when $\lambda_2 = 1.5$. The GRR λ_1 is determined by the underlying genetic model and the value of λ_2. Next, we examine it without HWE by choosing Wright's coefficient of inbreeding $F = 0.10$. In all simulations, the prevalence is $k = 0.10$. The frequencies of selecting genetic models are reported in Table 6.13 and Table 6.14 for sample sizes 500 and 2,000, respectively.

The GMS mostly performs well for moderate to common allele frequencies. The frequencies of correctly selecting the REC or DOM models range from 65% to 80% in the simulations. They are higher for the ADD or MUL models, because the GMS procedure assumes the genetic model is ADD or MUL unless there is strong evidence indicating a REC or DOM model.

The signs of the HWD coefficients in cases and controls presented in Sect. 6.6.1 require HWE in the population. We also conduct simulations with Wright's coefficient of inbreeding in the population $F = 0.10$. Results corresponding to Table 6.13

Table 6.14 Performance of the GMS under HWE given MAF. True genetic models include REC, ADD, MUL, and DOM models. The ADD or MUL models are grouped as A/M when neither REC or DOM is selected. The sample sizes are $r = s = 1000$ with $\lambda_2 = 1.5$

True model	MAF	Selected model		
		REC	A/M	DOM
REC	0.1	25.26%	74.36%	0.38%
	0.3	75.08%	24.92%	0.00%
	0.5	79.90%	20.10%	0.00%
ADD	0.1	3.37%	90.41%	6.22%
	0.3	3.06%	88.92%	8.02%
	0.5	3.13%	89.27%	7.60%
MUL	0.1	4.47%	90.62%	4.91%
	0.3	5.25%	89.71%	5.04%
	0.5	5.59%	89.88%	4.53%
DOM	0.1	0.13%	64.15%	35.72%
	0.3	0.00%	23.22%	76.78%
	0.5	0.00%	21.65%	78.15%

Table 6.15 Performance of the GMS without HWE. Wright's coefficient of inbreeding is $F = 0.10$. Other parameter values are the same as those in Table 6.13

True model	MAF	Selected model		
		REC	A/E	DOM
REC	0.1	35.18%	64.74%	0.08%
	0.3	74.91%	25.09%	0.00%
	0.5	61.56%	38.44%	0.00%
ADD	0.1	8.91%	89.12%	1.97%
	0.3	4.16%	90.62%	5.22%
	0.5	2.08%	88.40%	9.52%
MUL	0.1	12.12%	86.51%	1.32%
	0.3	8.74%	88.81%	2.45%
	0.5	4.55%	89.91%	5.54%
DOM	0.1	1.17%	86.10%	12.73%
	0.3	0.02%	43.31%	56.67%
	0.5	0.00%	33.14%	66.86%

are reported in Table 6.15. They show that there is no strong influence of HWD on the performance of genetic model selection.

6.6.3 Testing Association After the Genetic Model Selection

The idea of the GMS is to enhance the power to detect true association after the model selection. If the selected model is REC, ADD/MUL or DOM, the trend test optimal for the selected model can be used to test the null hypothesis. Because the same case-control data are used for both model selection and testing association, the two steps are statistically correlated. Therefore, we need to first derive the correlation between the model selection and a trend test. Then an association test can be applied with an adjusted level, or a critical value, to control the overall significance level.

Correlation Between the Model Selection and a Trend Test

The GMS is based on the HWDTT, Z_{HWDTT}, given by (6.32). The trend test $Z_{\mathrm{CATT}}(x)$ is given by (6.3). The model index x in the trend test is determined by Z_{HWDTT}. In order to control the Type I error, the correlation between Z_{HWDTT} and $Z_{\mathrm{CATT}}(x)$ is helpful for deriving analytical results.

We describe how the asymptotic null correlation of Z_{HWDTT} and $Z_{\mathrm{CATT}}(x)$ can be derived. Denote, under H_0,

$$\rho_x = \mathrm{Corr}(Z_{\mathrm{HWDTT}}, Z_{\mathrm{CATT}}(x)).$$

Assume the proportion of cases has a limit: $r/n \to \eta \in (0, 1)$ as $n \to \infty$. Then, under H_0,

$$\frac{n_i}{n} = \frac{r}{n}\frac{r_i}{r} + \frac{s}{n}\frac{s_i}{s} \to \eta p_i + (1 - \eta)q_i = p_i.$$

Therefore, the denominator of Z_{HWDTT} converges in probability:

$$\{1 - n_2/n - n_1/(2n)\}\{n_2/n + n_1/(2n)\} \to (1 - p_2 - p_1/2)(p_2 + p_1/2).$$

Likewise, the denominator of $Z_{\mathrm{CATT}}(x)$ converges in probability:

$$\sqrt{(x^2 n_1/n + n_2/n) - (x n_1/n + n_2/n)^2} \to \sqrt{(x^2 p_1 + p_2) - (x p_1 + p_2)^2}.$$

Under H_0, the expections of the numerators of the trend test and the HWDTT are 0. Hence we focus on the asymptotic null correlation between the numerator of the trend test (denoted by U_x) and that of the HWDTT (denoted by D) (see Problem 1.1), which are given by

$$U_x = \sqrt{rs/n^2}\sqrt{n}\{(x r_1/r + r_2/r) - (x s_1/s + s_2/s)\},$$

$$D = \sqrt{rs/n^2}\sqrt{n}\{r_2/r - (r_2/r + r_1/r)^2 - s_2/s + (s_2/s + s_2/s)^2\}.$$

Note that $\sqrt{rs/n^2} \to \sqrt{\eta(1 - \eta)}$. The null correlation of U_x and D can be obtained by applying the multinomial distributions for (r_0, r_1, r_2) and (s_0, s_1, s_2) and the independence of genotype counts between cases and controls.

With HWE in the population and $p = \Pr(B)$, it can be shown that (see Problem 3.11)

$$\rho_0 = \sqrt{\frac{1-p}{1+p}} + O(n^{-1}),\tag{6.33}$$

$$\rho_{\frac{1}{2}} = O(n^{-1}),\tag{6.34}$$

$$\rho_1 = -\sqrt{\frac{p}{2-p}} + O(n^{-1}).\tag{6.35}$$

The higher order terms are omitted in the above expressions. Note that $\rho_{1/2}$ is asymptotically 0, which was given in (3.21) of Sect. 3.7 and was used to combine Z_{HWDTT} and $Z_{\text{CATT}}(1/2)$.

The Genetic Model Selection Test

Let B be the risk allele. The genetic model index $x = 0$ if $Z_{\text{HWDTT}} > c^*$, $x = 1$ if $Z_{\text{HWDTT}} < -c^*$, and $x = 1/2$ otherwise, where $c^* = 1.645$. Denote the index for the selected model by x^*. Then the trend test $Z_{\text{CATT}}(x^*)$ is used to test association. The genetic model selection (GMS) test, denoted by Z_{GMS}, is given by

$$\begin{aligned}
Z_{\text{GMS}} &= Z_{\text{CATT}}(0), &&\text{if } Z_{\text{HWDTT}} > c^*;\\
&= Z_{\text{CATT}}(1), &&\text{if } Z_{\text{HWDTT}} < -c^*;\\
&= Z_{\text{CATT}}(1/2), &&\text{if } |Z_{\text{HWDTT}}| < c^*.
\end{aligned}$$

Because we assume B is the risk allele, we test association for a one-sided alternative with significance level $\alpha/2$. In this case, each allele can be tested as the risk allele at the $\alpha/2$ level, by the Bonferroni correction.

Asymptotic Distribution

The null hypothesis H_0 is rejected when $Z_{\text{GMS}} = Z_{\text{CATT}}(x^*) > c$. Note that $Z_{\text{CATT}}(x^*)$ does not follow $N(0, 1)$ asymptotically under H_0. We need to determine c under H_0 from

$$\Pr(Z_{\text{GMS}} > c) = \Pr(Z_{\text{CATT}}(x^*) > c) = \alpha/2,\tag{6.36}$$

where

$$\begin{aligned}
\Pr(Z_{\text{CATT}}(x^*) > c) = {}&\Pr(Z_{\text{HWDTT}} > c^*, Z_{\text{CATT}}(0) > c)\\
&+ \Pr(Z_{\text{HWDTT}} < -c^*, Z_{\text{CATT}}(1) > c)\\
&+ \Pr(-c^* < Z_{\text{HWDTT}} < c^*, Z_{\text{CATT}}(1/2) > c).
\end{aligned}\tag{6.37}$$

All the above probabilities are evaluated under H_0, under which the asymptotic distribution of $(Z_{\text{CATT}}(x), Z_{\text{HWDTT}})^T$ is the bivariate normal

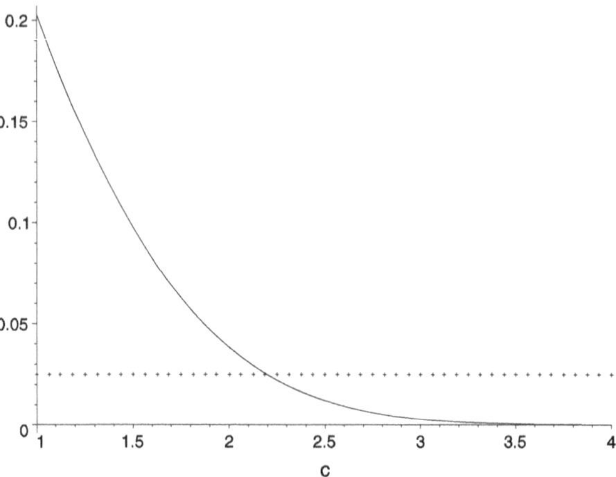

Fig. 6.7 Type I error (*solid*) of the GMS test $\Pr(Z_{\text{GMS}} > c)$ over $c \in [1, 4]$ under H_0 when HWE holds in the population. The reference line (*point*) is the for the nominal level $\alpha/2 = 0.025$

$$
\begin{bmatrix} Z_{\text{CATT}}(x) \\ Z_{\text{HWDTT}} \end{bmatrix} \sim N\left(\begin{bmatrix} 0 \\ 0 \end{bmatrix}, \begin{bmatrix} 1 & \rho_x \\ \rho_x & 1 \end{bmatrix} \right),
$$

where ρ_x is given in (6.33)–(6.35). Let the density of $(Z_{\text{CATT}}(x), Z_{\text{HWDTT}})^T$ be $f(u, v; x)$ given by

$$
f(u, v; x) = \frac{1}{2\pi\sqrt{1 - \rho_x^2}} \exp\left\{ -\frac{1}{2(1 - \rho_x^2)}(u^2 - 2\rho_x uv + v^2) \right\}
$$

$$
= \frac{1}{\sqrt{2\pi(1 - \rho_x^2)}} \exp\left\{ -\frac{1}{2}\left(\frac{v - \rho_x u}{\sqrt{1 - \rho_x^2}} \right)^2 \right\} \frac{1}{\sqrt{2\pi}} \exp(-u^2/2).
$$

Then the equation in (6.36) can be written as:

$$
2\Phi(c^*)\{1 - \Phi(c)\} + \int_c^{\infty} \left\{ \Phi\left(\frac{-c^* - \rho_1 u}{\sqrt{1 - \rho_1^2}} \right) - \Phi\left(\frac{c^* - \rho_0 u}{\sqrt{1 - \rho_0^2}} \right) \right\} d\Phi(u) = \frac{\alpha}{2},
$$

$$
(6.38)
$$

where $\Phi(c^*) = 0.95$ when $c^* = 1.645$, and c is unknown. Both c and c^* appear in (6.37).

Let the left hand side of (6.38) be a function of the critical value c. Then it can be shown that the derivative of that function with respect to c is strictly negative (Problem 6.9). Note that, under H_0, $\Pr(Z_{\text{CATT}}(x^*) > -\infty) = 1 > \alpha/2$ and $\Pr(Z_{\text{CATT}}(x^*) > \infty) = 0 < \alpha/2$. Thus, there exists a unique c satisfying (6.38).

To obtain the p-value of Z_{GMS}, calculate the left hand side of (6.38) separately with A and B being the risk allele by substituting the observed Z_{GMS} for c, which must be greater than 0 (otherwise the p-value is greater than 0.5), and replacing ρ_0 and ρ_1 with their estimates respectively. Take the minimum of the two p-values. Then the p-value of Z_{GMS} is twice the minimum. Figure 6.7 plots $\Pr(Z_{\text{GMS}} > c)$ over $c \in [1, 4]$ under H_0 with the reference line for $\alpha/2 = 0.025$. Numerical values of the critical values c are reported in Table 6.16. In general, the critical values

Table 6.16 Critical values c for the GMS test Z_{GMS} when HWE holds in the population

MAF	α	c	MAF	α	c
0.05	0.05	2.2396	0.30	0.05	2.1974
	0.01	2.8107		0.01	2.8186
0.10	0.05	2.2333	0.35	0.05	2.1916
	0.01	2.8171		0.01	2.8168
0.15	0.05	2.2235	0.40	0.05	2.1875
	0.01	2.8205		0.01	2.8152
0.20	0.05	2.2136	0.45	0.05	2.1851
	0.01	2.8212		0.01	2.8141
0.25	0.05	2.2047	0.50	0.05	2.1843
	0.01	2.8203		0.01	2.8138

change with the frequency of allele B. Table 6.16 only presents critical values for $p \leq 0.50$. For $p > 0.50$, the critical value is identical to the one for $1 - p$ (Problem 6.10).

6.6.4 Examples

For illustration, we apply Z_{GMS} to the SNPs in Table 6.7. We also use the first SNP as an example to show detailed calculations. Given the genotype counts for (AA, AB, BB) as $(r_0, r_1, r_2) = (25, 283, 864)$ in cases and $(s_0, s_1, s_2) = (10, 218, 929)$ in controls, we calculate Z_{HWDTT} using (6.32) and obtain $Z_{HWDTT} = 0.6919$, which satisfies $|Z_{HWDTT}| < c^* = 1.645$. Thus, there is no strong evidence for a REC model or a DOM model underlying the data. We choose $x^* = 0.5$ for the trend test and obtain $Z_{GMS} = Z_{CATT}(0.5) = -4.080 < 0$. This implies that A is the risk allele under H_1. If we switch alleles A and B, the sign of the trend test $Z_{CATT}(0.5)$ will change to positive. (Note, however, for $x^* = 0$ and $x^* = 1$, $Z_{CATT}(0)$ and $Z_{CATT}(1)$ are also switched.) If we set $(r_2, r_1, r_0) = (25, 283, 864)$ and $(s_2, s_1, s_0) = (10, 218, 929)$, Z_{HWDTT} does not change but $Z_{CATT}(0.5) = 4.080$.

Next, we estimate $\widehat{p} = (n_1 + 2n_2)/(2n) = 0.1226$ as the allele frequency and

$$\widehat{\rho}_0 = \sqrt{\frac{1 - \widehat{p}}{1 + \widehat{p}}} = 0.8841,$$

$$\widehat{\rho}_1 = -\sqrt{\frac{\widehat{p}}{2 - \widehat{p}}} = 0.2555.$$

Evaluate the left hand side of (6.38) with $c = 4.080$ and ρ_0 and ρ_1 being replaced by 0.8841 and 0.2555, respectively. The p-value is twice the left hand side of (6.38), which is 0.0000984 and reported in Table 6.17 as 9.8e−5.

Table 6.17 P-value of Z_{GMS} for SNPs reported in Table 6.7. The p-values of MAX3 are also reported for comparison

SNP IDs	Z_{HWDTT}	x^*	Z_{GMS}	P-values	
				MAX3	GMS
rs1447295	0.692	0.5	4.080	1.1e−4	9.8e−5
rs6983267	−0.752	0.5	4.468	2.2e−5	2.1e−5
rs7837688	0.579	0.5	4.694	6.7e−6	6.0e−6
rs10510126	1.506	0.5	4.827	1.4e−6	3.1e−6
rs12505080	−4.515	1.0	4.153	8.5e−5	7.9e−5
rs17157903	−3.371	1.0	4.214	6.2e−5	5.6e−5
rs1219648	0.975	0.5	4.773	5.0e−6	5.0e−6
rs7696175	−4.672	1.0	3.341	2.1e−3	1.9e−3
rs2420946	0.853	0.5	4.759	5.3e−6	5.3e−6

To illustrate how $Z_{CATT}(0)$ and $Z_{CATT}(1)$ are switched with opposite signs when the alleles A and B are switched, we use SNP rs17157903 (Table 6.17). With genotype counts $(r_0, r_1, r_2) = (18, 316, 777)$ and $(s_0, s_1, s_2) = (26, 220, 862)$, we obtain $Z_{HWDTT} = -3.371 < -1.645$. Thus, the DOM model is selected with $x^* = 1.0$. However, which trend test, $Z_{CATT}(0)$ or $Z_{CATT}(1)$, is for the DOM model is relative to the risk allele. $Z_{CATT}(1)$ is optimal when B is the risk allele while $Z_{CATT}(0)$ is optimal when A is the risk allele. Numerical results show that $Z_{CATT}(0) = -4.214$ and $Z_{CATT}(1) = 1.227$. Using $Z_{GMS} = 1.227$, its p-value is 0.1529. If we switch the alleles with $(r_2, r_1, r_0) = (18, 316, 777)$ and $(s_2, s_1, s_0) = (26, 220, 862)$, Z_{HWDTT} does not change, but $Z_{CATT}(0) = -1.227$ and $Z_{CATT}(1) = 4.214$. Using $Z_{GMS} = 4.214$, the p-value is 0.00002799. The final reported p-value is $2 \times 0.00002799 = 0.00005597$ or 5.6e-5 as in Table 6.17.

Results in Table 6.17 show that the p-values of Z_{GMS} are slightly smaller than or equal to those of MAX3 except for SNP rs10510126. For that SNP, $x^* = 0.5$ is selected but $Z_{CATT}(0) = 4.999 > Z_{CATT}(1/2) = 4.827$. Thus, $Z_{GMS} = 4.827$ and MAX3 $= 4.999$, which leads to a smaller p-value for MAX3.

6.6.5 Choice of Thresholds for the Genetic Model Selection

The GMS procedure depends on the threshold c^* for model selection. So far we have used the threshold $c^* = 1.645$ for model selection with Z_{HWDTT}, which corresponds to the upper 95th percentile of $N(0, 1)$. We consider some other values here. In particular, we choose $c^* = 1.285$ and 1.96, which correspond to the upper 90th and 97.5th percentiles of $N(0, 1)$, respectively. Intuitively, a larger value of c^* would select stronger REC or DOM effects than a smaller c^*. Therefore, there is a trade-off between selecting ADD/MUL models and REC or DOM models, in particular when Z_{HWDTT} is close to the threshold c^*.

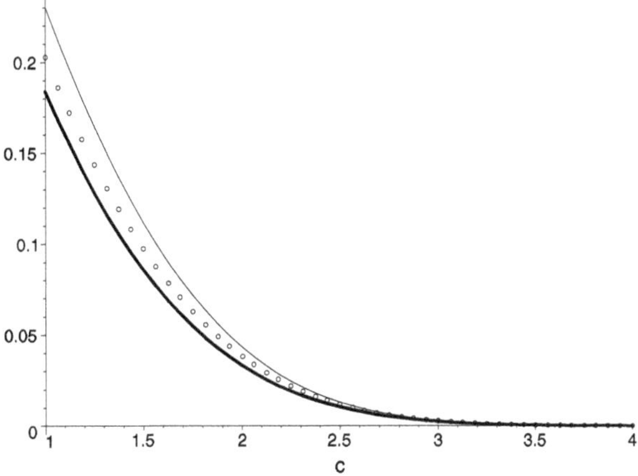

Fig. 6.8 Type I error rates of the GMS test $\Pr_{H_0}(Z_{\mathrm{GMS}} > c)$ over $c \in [1, 4]$ with different choices of threshold c^*. The *light solid*, *point* and *dark solid curves* correspond to $c^* = 1.285$, 1.645, and 1.96, respectively

Table 6.18 P-values of Z_{GMS} for SNPs reported in Table 6.7 with three different choices of threshold c^*

SNP IDs	c^*		
	1.285	1.645	1.96
rs1447295	1.0e−4	9.8e−5	9.6e−5
rs6983267	2.1e−5	2.1e−5	2.0e−5
rs7837688	6.1e−6	6.0e−6	5.8e−6
rs10510126	1.3e−6	3.1e−6	3.1e−6
rs12505080	8.1e−5	7.9e−5	7.6e−5
rs17157903	5.7e−5	5.6e−5	5.5e−5
rs1219648	4.9e−6	5.0e−6	4.8e−6
rs7696175	2.0e−3	1.9e−3	1.7e−3
rs2420946	5.3e−6	5.3e−6	5.1e−6

Figure 6.8 plots Type I error rates, the left hand side of (6.38), for the three different values of c^*. The light solid, point and dark solid curves correspond to $c^* = 1.285$, 1.645 and 1.96, respectively. The plots show that, given α, the critical value becomes smaller when the threshold c^* increases. P-values with these three thresholds are reported in Table 6.18. Overall, p-values are not that sensitive to the thresholds. P-values with $c^* = 1.96$ are smaller than those with smaller c^* except for SNP rs10510126, in which the REC model is selected with $c^* = 1.285$, but not with the other two thresholds. In practice, it would be helpful to conduct a sensitivity analysis with different values of c^* as in Table 6.18.

6.6.6 Simulating the Null Distribution

In Sect. 6.6.3, we derived the asymptotic null distribution for the GMS test Z_{GMS}. To obtain p-values and critical values, we need to evaluate single integrals or double integrals (with the CDF of $N(0, 1)$).

The parametric bootstrap procedure discussed in Sect. 6.3.2 can still be applied. As shown for MAX3 (Sect. 6.3.2), directly simulating test statistics under H_0 with their correlations is simpler. Throughout this section, we assume HWE holds in the population. First, we show that $Z_{\text{CATT}}(0)$, $Z_{\text{CATT}}(1)$ and Z_{HWDTT} are linearly dependent. From $\rho_0 = \sqrt{(1-p)/(1+p)}$, $\rho_1 = -\sqrt{(1-q)/(1+q)}$, and $\rho_{0,1} = \sqrt{pq/\{(1+p)(1+q)\}}$ (Problem 6.11), we have

$$\rho_0^2 + \rho_1^2 + \rho_{0,1}^2 - 2\rho_0\rho_1\rho_{0,1} = 1.$$

Thus,

$$\begin{vmatrix} 1 & \rho_{0,1} & \rho_0 \\ \rho_{0,1} & 1 & \rho_1 \\ \rho_0 & \rho_1 & 1 \end{vmatrix} = 0.$$

Writing $Z_{\text{HWDTT}} = u^* Z_{\text{CATT}}(0) + v^* Z_{\text{CATT}}(1)$ leads to

$$u^* = \frac{\rho_0 - \rho_1\rho_{0,1}}{1 - \rho_{0,1}^2}, \tag{6.39}$$

$$v^* = \frac{\rho_1 - \rho_0\rho_{0,1}}{1 - \rho_{0,1}^2}. \tag{6.40}$$

To estimate u^* and v^*, we use $\widehat{p} = (n_1 + 2n_2)/(2n)$.

The following algorithm can be used to simulate Z_{GMS} given the observed case-control data.

i) Estimate p, ρ_0, ρ_1, and $\rho_{0,1}$. Calculate (w_0^*, w_1^*) given in (6.18) and (6.19) and (u^*, v^*);

ii) Simulate $(Z_{\text{CATT}}(0), Z_{\text{CATT}}(1))^T$ from the bivariate normal distribution

$$\begin{bmatrix} Z_0 \\ Z_1 \end{bmatrix} \sim N\left(\begin{bmatrix} 0 \\ 0 \end{bmatrix}, \begin{bmatrix} 1 & \rho_{0,1} \\ \rho_{0,1} & 1 \end{bmatrix}\right);$$

iii) Calculate

$$Z_{\text{CATT}}(1/2) = w_0^* Z_0 + w_1^* Z_1,$$

$$Z_{\text{HWDTT}} = u^* Z_0 + v^* Z_1.$$

iv) Find the one-sided test, Z_{GMS}, as follows: $Z_{\text{GMS}} = Z_0$ if $Z_{\text{HWDTT}} > 1.645$; $Z_{\text{GMS}} = Z_1$ if $Z_{\text{HWDTT}} < -1.645$; and $Z_{\text{GMS}} = Z_{\text{CATT}}(1/2)$ if $|Z_{\text{HWDTT}}| < 1.645$.

Table 6.19 Simulated p-values of Z_{GMS} for the SNPs reported in Table 6.7 with $c^* = 1.645$. p is the frequency of the risk allele B. P-values in Table 6.18 are also included for comparison. The number of replicates is 10 million for each SNP

SNP IDs	p	u^*	v^*	w_0^*	w_1^*	Analytical	Simulated
rs1447295	0.123	0.992	−0.480	0.262	0.908	9.8e−5	9.6e−5
rs6983267	0.522	0.853	−0.879	0.631	0.594	2.1e−5	2.3e−5
rs7837688	0.121	0.993	−0.478	0.261	0.908	6.0e−6	5.6e−6
rs10510126	0.891	0.455	−0.994	0.918	0.246	3.1e−6	3.0e−6
rs12505080	0.739	0.673	−0.965	0.802	0.405	7.9e−5	7.4e−5
rs17157903	0.141	0.990	−0.511	0.283	0.894	5.6e−5	5.5e−5
rs1219648	0.420	0.907	−0.815	0.546	0.677	5.0e−6	5.4e−6
rs7696175	0.568	0.823	−0.902	0.668	0.556	1.9e−3	1.9e−3
rs2420946	0.415	0.910	−0.811	0.542	0.681	5.3e−6	5.8e−6

Repeat the above steps to generate empirical distribution of Z_{GMS} under H_0 and HWE, from which the proportion of simulated Z_{GMS} greater than the observed Z_{GMS} can be calculated. The p-value is twice that proportion.

The above simulation procedure is applied to the SNPs reported in Table 6.18. To obtain small p-values, 10 million replicates are used for each SNP. Results are presented in Table 6.19. The analytical p-values and the simulated p-values match very well.

6.7 Genetic Model Exclusion

Unlike the GMS procedure which selects a genetic model using the HWDTT Z_{HWDTT}, based on which the appropriate trend test is applied for testing association, the genetic model exclusion (GME) procedure is to exclude unlikely model(s) based on Z_{HWDTT}, and then test association with a smaller range of possible models.

6.7.1 Reducing the Genetic Model Space

From Tables 6.13 to 6.15, the frequencies of correctly selecting the REC or DOM models are in the range of 65–80% with GRRs from 1.5 to 2.0. The frequencies could be even lower when the GRRs are smaller. Although it may not be possible to correctly select the true genetic model with high frequency, it is relatively easy to exclude the most unlikely genetic model(s). Consider the following algorithm for GME:

i) Assume B is the risk allele. Let $c^* = 1.645$. If $Z_{\text{HWDTT}} > c^*$, the DOM model is excluded. The possible models are REC or ADD/MUL;

Table 6.20 Frequencies of correctly excluding unlikely genetic model(s) under HWE in the population given MAF. True genetic models include REC, ADD, MUL, and DOM models. R/D denotes REC or DOM models and A/M denotes ADD or MUL models. The sample sizes are $r = s = 250$ with $\lambda_2 = 2$

True model	MAF	GMS selects			Frequencies of correct exclusion	
		REC	A/M	DOM		
REC	0.1	20.28%	79.21%	0.51%	DOM	99.49%
	0.3	66.86%	33.13%	0.01%		99.99%
	0.5	66.28%	33.71%	0.01%		99.99%
ADD	0.1	2.02%	90.24%	7.74%	R/D	90.24%
	0.3	2.27%	87.94%	9.79%		87.94%
	0.5	2.36%	89.22%	8.42%		89.22%
MUL	0.1	2.95%	92.14%	4.91%	R/D	92.14%
	0.3	5.00%	90.27%	4.73%		90.27%
	0.5	5.64%	90.20%	4.16%		90.20%
DOM	0.1	0.03%	61.48%	38.49%	REC	99.97%
	0.3	0.00%	31.73%	68.27%		100%
	0.5	0.03%	34.91%	65.06%		99.97%

ii) If $Z_{\mathrm{HWDTT}} < -c^*$, the REC model is excluded. The possible models are DOM or ADD/MUL models;

iii) Otherwise ($|Z_{\mathrm{HWDTT}}| < c^*$), the REC and DOM models are both excluded. The possible models are ADD or MUL.

Re-organizing Table 6.13 to show the above GME, we have Table 6.20, in which the last column is the frequency of correctly excluding unlikely genetic model(s). The frequencies of correctly excluding REC or DOM models are much higher than correctly selecting them.

6.7.2 The MERT-Based Genetic Model Exclusion Test

Testing After Model Exclusion

After some genetic models are excluded, we test association based on a set of reduced genetic models. We apply the MERT to a smaller set of genetic models. The MERT-based GME trend test, denoted by Z_{GME1}, is defined as follows. Assume B is the risk allele.

$$Z_{\mathrm{GME1}} = \frac{Z_{\mathrm{CATT}}(0) + Z_{\mathrm{CATT}}(1/2)}{\sqrt{2(1 + \widehat{\rho}_{0,1/2})}}, \quad \text{if } Z_{\mathrm{HWDTT}} > c^*; \tag{6.41}$$

$$= \frac{Z_{\mathrm{CATT}}(1/2) + Z_{\mathrm{CATT}}(1)}{\sqrt{2(1 + \widehat{\rho}_{1/2,1})}}, \quad \text{if } Z_{\mathrm{HWDTT}} < -c^*; \tag{6.42}$$

$$= Z_{\text{CATT}}(1/2), \quad \text{if } |Z_{\text{HWDTT}}| < c^*. \tag{6.43}$$

In (6.41) and (6.42), the MERT (Sect. 6.2) is applied to the REC and ADD models and to the DOM and ADD models, respectively.

Asymptotic Null Distribution

The null hypothesis H_0 is rejected for a large value of Z_{GME1}. Because Z_{GME1} does not follow $N(0,1)$ asymptotically under H_0, we need to determined c under H_0 such that

$$\Pr(Z_{\text{GME1}} > c) = \alpha/2.$$

Z_{GME1} only depends on the three trend tests $Z_{\text{CATT}}(x)$ with $x = 0, 1/2, 1$ and Z_{HWDTT}. The trend test $Z_{\text{CATT}}(1/2)$ and Z_{HWDTT} are linear combinations of the extreme pair $Z_{\text{CATT}}(0)$ and $Z_{\text{CATT}}(1)$. Denote

$$Z_{\text{CATT}}(1/2) = w_0^* Z_{\text{CATT}}(0) + w_1^* Z_{\text{CATT}}(1),$$

$$Z_{\text{HWDTT}} = u^* Z_{\text{CATT}}(0) + v^* Z_{\text{CATT}}(1),$$

where w_0^* and w_1^* are given in (6.18) and (6.19), and u^* and v^* are given in (6.39) and (6.40). After omitting the terms converging to 0 arising from replacing $\widehat{\rho}_{0,1/2}$ by $\rho_{0,1/2}$ and $\widehat{\rho}_{1,1/2}$ by $\rho_{1,1/2}$, we have

$$\Pr(Z_{\text{GME1}} > c)$$

$$= \Pr\left(\frac{Z_{\text{CATT}}(0) + Z_{\text{CATT}}(\tfrac{1}{2})}{\sqrt{2(1 + \rho_{0,\frac{1}{2}})}} > c, \; Z_{\text{HWDTT}} > c^* \right) \tag{6.44}$$

$$+ \Pr\left(\frac{Z_{\text{CATT}}(1) + Z_{\text{CATT}}(\tfrac{1}{2})}{\sqrt{2(1 + \rho_{1,\frac{1}{2}})}} > c, \; Z_{\text{HWDTT}} < -c^* \right) \tag{6.45}$$

$$+ \Pr(Z_{\text{CATT}}(1/2) > c, \; |Z_{\text{HWDTT}}| < c^*). \tag{6.46}$$

The last term in (6.46) can be easily obtained as $\{1 - \Phi(c)\}\{2\Phi(c^*) - 1\}$ by the asymptotic independence of $Z_{\text{CATT}}(1/2)$ and Z_{HWDTT}. The other two probabilities in (6.44)–(6.45) can be written as double integrals using the joint density of the extreme pair. However, the integration regions are not simple. We take a simpler approach to compute these two probabilities.

Let $T_x = \{Z_{\text{CATT}}(x) + Z_{\text{CATT}}(1/2)\}/\sqrt{2(1 + \rho_{x,1/2})}$ for $x = 0, 1$. Under H_0, $T_x \sim N(0,1)$ for a given x. Assume that, for a given x, T_x and Z_{HWDTT} follow jointly a bivariate normal distribution. Then, under H_0,

$$\text{Corr}\left(\frac{Z_{\text{CATT}}(x) + Z_{\text{CATT}}(\tfrac{1}{2})}{\sqrt{2(1 + \rho_{x,\frac{1}{2}})}}, \; Z_{\text{HWDTT}} \right) = \frac{\rho_x}{\sqrt{2(1 + \rho_{x,\frac{1}{2}})}}.$$

Denote the above correlation by $\widetilde{\rho}_x$ for $x = 0, 1$. The joint density of $(T_x, Z_{\text{HWDTT}})^T$ can then be written as

Table 6.21 Critical values c of the GME test Z_{GME1} when HWE holds in the population

MAF	α	c	MAF	α	c
0.05	0.05	2.0933	0.30	0.05	2.0566
	0.01	2.7226		0.01	2.6820
0.10	0.05	2.0802	0.35	0.05	2.0540
	0.01	2.7088		0.01	2.6789
0.15	0.05	2.0714	0.40	0.05	2.0522
	0.01	2.6991		0.01	2.6767
0.20	0.05	2.0650	0.45	0.05	2.0511
	0.01	2.6919		0.01	2.6755
0.25	0.05	2.0602	0.50	0.05	2.0508
	0.01	2.6863		0.01	2.6751

$$f(u, v; \widetilde{\rho}_x) = \frac{1}{2\pi\sqrt{1 - \widetilde{\rho}_x^2}} \exp\left\{ -\frac{1}{2(1 - \widetilde{\rho}_x^2)}(u^2 - 2\widetilde{\rho}_x uv + v^2) \right\}.$$

Hence, (6.44) can be written as

$$\Pr(T_0 > c,\ Z_{\text{HWDTT}} > c^*) = \int_c^\infty \left\{ \int_{c^*}^\infty f(u, v; \widetilde{\rho}_0) dv \right\} du$$

$$= 1 - \Phi(c) - \int_c^\infty \Phi\left(\frac{c^* - \widetilde{\rho}_0 u}{\sqrt{1 - \widetilde{\rho}_0^2}} \right) d\Phi(u).$$

Similarly, (6.45) can be written as

$$\Pr(T_1 > c,\ Z_{\text{HWDTT}} < -c^*) = \int_c^\infty \Phi\left(\frac{-c^* - \widetilde{\rho}_1 u}{\sqrt{1 - \widetilde{\rho}_1^2}} \right) d\Phi(u).$$

Combining the above probabilities, we obtain

$$\Pr(Z_{\text{GME1}} > c)$$
$$= 2\Phi(c^*)\{1 - \Phi(c)\} + \int_c^\infty \left\{ \Phi\left(\frac{-c^* - \widetilde{\rho}_1 u}{\sqrt{1 - \widetilde{\rho}_1^2}} \right) - \Phi\left(\frac{c^* - \widetilde{\rho}_0 u}{\sqrt{1 - \widetilde{\rho}_0^2}} \right) \right\} d\Phi(u).$$

$$(6.47)$$

Note that this probability has the same form as that of the GMS test $\Pr(Z_{\text{GMS}} > c)$, given as the left hand side of (6.38), except for the correlations. In (6.38), ρ_x for $x = 0, 1$ are used, but in (6.47) $\widetilde{\rho}_x$ are used. Thus, the previous computation program to find c for using Z_{GMS} can also be used to find c for Z_{GME1} such that $\Pr(Z_{\text{GME1}} > c) = \alpha/2$ by substituting the new correlations.

Table 6.21 reports critical values c for various MAFs. Note that the critical values for Z_{GME1} are smaller than the corresponding critical values for Z_{GMS}. This is not surprising, because selecting a single genetic model in Z_{GMS} is more likely to

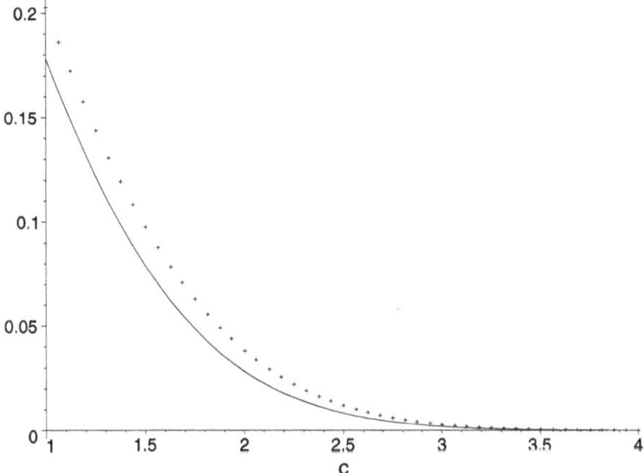

Fig. 6.9 Type I error rate of the GMS test $\Pr(Z_{GMS} > c)$ (*point curve*) and the GME test $\Pr(Z_{GME1} > c)$ (*solid curve*) over $c \in [1, 4]$

increase Type I error than selecting two genetic models (or excluding one model) in Z_{GME1}. Figure 6.9 plots $\Pr(Z_{GMS} > c)$ (point curve) and $\Pr(Z_{GME1} > c)$ (solid curve) over $c \in [1, 4]$ for a MAF $p = 0.3$. It also shows that the critical value of Z_{GME1} is smaller than that of Z_{GMS}.

From the expressions of Z_{GMS} and Z_{GME1}, we see that the only difference between them occurs when $|Z_{HWDTT}| > c^*$. When $|Z_{HWDTT}| < c^*$, both tests use $Z_{HWDTT}(1/2)$. But the smaller critical value of Z_{GME1} indicates that its p-value could be smaller than that of Z_{GMS}. However, when $|Z_{HWDTT}| > c^*$, MERT is used by Z_{GME1}. Because Z_{HWDTT} has low power under the ADD model, $Z_{CATT}(1/2)$ may be much smaller than $Z_{CATT}(0)$ or $Z_{CATT}(1)$, which may yield a larger p-value for Z_{GME1} than Z_{GMS} when $|Z_{HWDTT}| > c^*$. For illustration, consider SNPs rs12505080 and rs7696175. From Table 6.8, both SNPs have $|Z_{CATT}(1/2)| < 1$ but their $Z_{HWDTT} = -4.515$ and -4.672, respectively (Table 6.17). Thus, Z_{GME1} for these two SNPs would be much smaller than Z_{GMS}, with larger p-values, even though the critical values of Z_{GME1} are smaller.

6.7.3 Examples

We apply Z_{GME1} to the SNPs in Table 6.9. For comparison, we also show the GMS test Z_{GMS} with three choices of $c^* = 1.285$, 1.645, and 1.96 that were reported in Table 6.18, but we only report Z_{GME1} with $c^* = 1.645$. The results are presented in Table 6.22. As expected, Z_{GME1} always has smaller p-values than Z_{GMS} (with $c^* = 1.645$) when the ADD/MUL models are selected. Three p-values (indicated with *) for Z_{GME1} become much larger than those for Z_{GMS} when the DOM model is selected and $Z_{CATT}(1/2)$ is relatively small. In Table 6.22, Z_{GME2} is the MAX-based GME test described in the next section. For all the three SNPs, $|Z_{HWDTT}|$ is much larger than 1.645. We will examine the performance of Z_{GME1} in simulations later for relatively smaller $|Z_{HWDTT}|$ and $|Z_{HWDTT}| > 1.645$.

Table 6.22 P-values of Z_{GMS}, Z_{GME1} (the MERT-based), and Z_{GME2} (the MAX-based) for the SNPs reported in Table 6.9. For Z_{GMS}, $c^* = 1.285$, 1.645, and 1.96 are used but only $c^* = 1.645$ is used for Z_{GME1} and Z_{GME2}

SNP IDs	Z_{GMS}			Z_{GME1}	Z_{GME2}
	1.285	1.645	1.96	1.645	1.645
rs1447295	1.0e−4	9.8e−5	9.6e−5	8.0e−5	1.1e−4
rs6983267	2.1e−5	2.1e−5	2.0e−5	1.4e−5	2.0e−5
rs7837688	6.1e−6	6.0e−6	5.8e−6	5.1e−6	4.6e−6
rs10510126	1.3e−6	3.1e−6	3.1e−6	2.7e−6	4.2e−6
rs12505080	8.1e−5	7.9e−5	7.6e−5	0.0120*	8.3e−5
rs17157903	5.7e−5	5.6e−5	5.5e−5	2.0e−4*	5.7e−5
rs1219648	4.9e−6	5.0e−6	4.8e−6	3.2e−6	5.0e−6
rs7696175	2.0e−3	1.9e−3	1.7e−3	0.0537*	1.9e−3
rs2420946	5.3e−6	5.3e−6	5.1e−6	3.5e−6	5.8e−6

*Power of $Z_{CATT}(1/2)$ is low with large values of Z_{HWDTT}, which affects Z_{GME1}

6.7.4 The MAX-Based Genetic Model Exclusion Test

Instead of using the MERT in Z_{GME1}, we now take the maximum of the trend tests over the remaining two models after one model is excluded. We denote this test by Z_{GME2}. Assume B is the risk allele. Z_{GME2} can be written as

$$Z_{GME2} = \max(Z_{CATT}(0), Z_{CATT}(1/2)), \quad \text{if } Z_{HWDTT} > c^*;$$
$$= \max(Z_{CATT}(1), Z_{CATT}(1/2)), \quad \text{if } Z_{HWDTT} < -c^*;$$
$$= Z_{CATT}(1/2), \quad \text{if } |Z_{HWDTT}| < c^*.$$

The null hypothesis is rejected when $Z_{GME2} > c$, where c satisfies

$$\Pr(Z_{GME2} > c) = \alpha/2.$$

The derivation of $\Pr(Z_{GME2} > c)$ is more tedious than that of $\Pr(Z_{GME1} > c)$. A simulation procedure similar to that for Z_{GMS} can be used. The p-values for Z_{GME2} reported in Table 6.22 (last column) are obtained using simulation with 10 million replicates. These p-values are comparable to those of Z_{GME1}.

6.8 Simulation Studies with Robust Tests

6.8.1 Critical Values and Type I Errors

We conduct simulation studies to compare several robust tests. The true genetic model in the simulations is unknown. It is indexed by $x = \theta$ satisfying (Sect. 6.3.5)

Table 6.23 Critical values used in the simulations given a MAF

Statistics	MAF		
	0.1	0.3	0.5
MAX3	2.2661	2.2740	2.2753
MIN2	0.0328	0.0328	0.0328
CLRT*	4.1982	5.3735	5.3297
Z_{GMS}	2.2333	2.1974	2.1843
Z_{GME1}	2.0802	2.0566	2.0508
Z_{GME2}*	1.9235	2.1964	2.1837

*Based on 1 million replicates

Table 6.24 Simulated Type I error rate given MAF based on 10,000 replicates

Statistics	MAF		
	0.1	0.3	0.5
$T_{\chi_2^2}$	0.0215	0.0470	0.0500
MAX3	0.0222	0.0486	0.0492
MIN2	0.0272	0.0470	0.0503
CLRT	0.0486	0.0486	0.0493
Z_{GMS}	0.0200	0.0497	0.0506
Z_{GME1}	0.0300	0.0470	0.0501
Z_{GME2}	0.0491	0.0497	0.0508

$$\lambda_1 = 1 - x + x\lambda_2,$$

where λ_1 and λ_2 are GRRs. We focus on $x \in [0, 1]$. The REC, ADD and DOM models correspond to $x = 0, 1/2, 1$, respectively. We fix $\lambda_2 = 1.5$ or 2.0 with sample size $r = s = 250$. λ_1 is calculated using the above equation given x and λ_2. The disease prevalence is $k = 0.1$. Three MAFs $p = 0.1, 0.3$, and 0.5 are used. The risk allele is also assumed to have the MAF. The significance level in the simulations is $\alpha = 0.05$.

The critical values used in the simulations for Pearson's test, MAX3, MIN2, Z_{GMS}, and Z_{GME1} are obtained from the asymptotic distributions of the test statistics. The critical values for the CLRT and Z_{GME2} are obtained from simulations with 1 million replicates. Table 6.23 reports the critical values used in the simulations. Except for MIN2, the critical values depend on minor allele frequencies. Table 6.24 reports the estimated Type I error rate for each test statistic using these critical values with 10,000 replicates. Type I error rates are close to the nominal level 0.05 for the MAFs $p = 0.3$ and 0.5. For small allele frequencies, the Type I error rates based on the asymptotic distributions are smaller than 0.05 except for the CLRT and Z_{GME2}, whose Type I error rates are based on the simulated critical values. Based on Table 6.24, we suggest using simulated critical values or simulated p-values for very small MAFs.

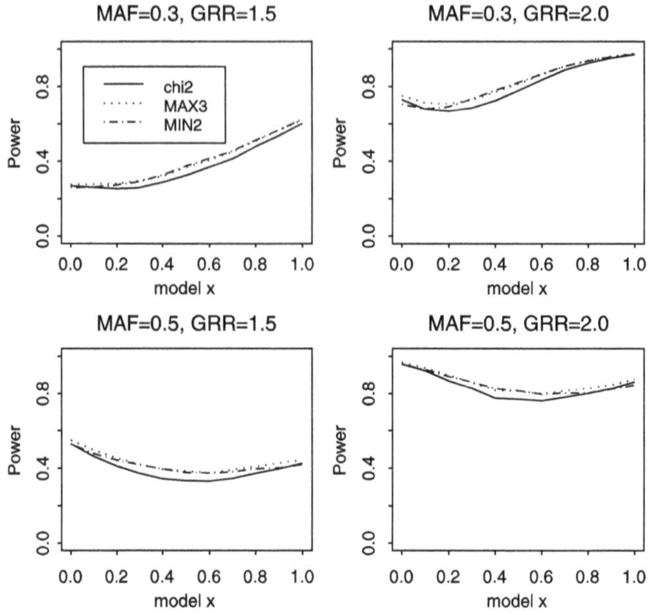

Fig. 6.10 Power of Person's test $T_{\chi_2^2}$ (chi2), MAX3, and MIN2

6.8.2 Empirical Power

The empirical power comparisons are grouped by test statistics. For a test statistic in each group, 10,000 replicates are run to estimate the empirical power as the proportion of simulations exceeding the critical value. Only MAFs 0.3 and 0.5 are considered.

MAX3, Pearson's Test, MIN2, and the CLRT

We first compare MAX3, Pearson's test and MIN2 over $x \in [0, 1]$. The empirical power is plotted in Fig. 6.10. The plots show that Pearson's test is least powerful among the three tests when the genetic models are restricted to lie between the REC and DOM models, and that MAX3 and MIN2 have comparable power except when x is close to 0 (the REC model) or 1 (the DOM model), under which MAX3 is slightly more powerful. Figure 6.11 plots the empirical power of MAX3 and the CLRT. As expected, they have nearly identical power across all values of x.

MAX3, the GMS test and GMEs

The power of MAX3 and Z_{GMS} is presented in Fig. 6.12, and that of Z_{GMS} and GMEs (Z_{GME1} and Z_{GME2}) is given in Fig. 6.13. The figures show that MAX3 and

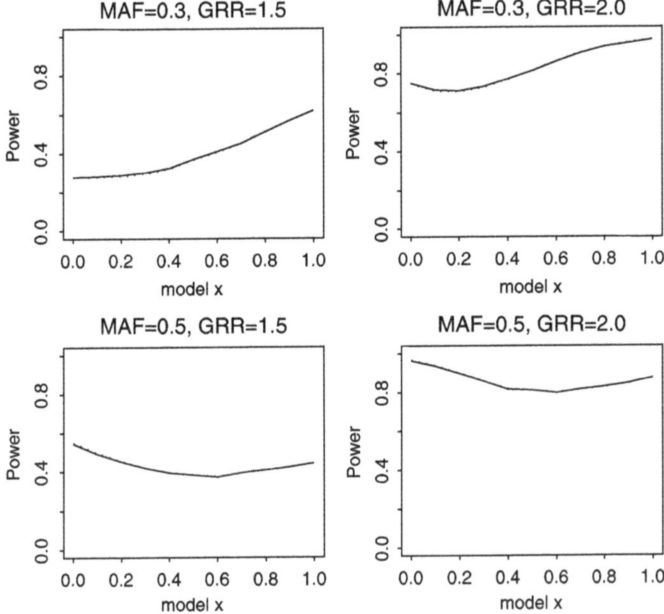

Fig. 6.11 Power of MAX3 (*dashed*) and the CLRT (*solid*). MAX3 and the CLRT have nearly identical power

Z_{GMS} have very comparable power for most genetic models, and that Z_{GME1} seems to outperform Z_{GMS}, which has very comparable power with Z_{GME2}. This finding is slightly different from the p-values reported in Table 6.22, in which for some SNPs the p-value for Z_{GME1} is much larger owing to a smaller value of the trend test for the ADD model $Z_{CATT}(1/2)$, with larger Z_{HWDTT}.

6.8.3 Discussion

From the simulation studies, we have shown that MAX3, MIN2, the CLRT, Z_{GMS} and Z_{GME2} have similar performance, which outperform Pearson's test when the genetic models are restricted to the range that includes the REC, ADD/MUL, and DOM models. Z_{GME1} seems to outperform the other tests. However, real applications demonstrate that Z_{GME1} could lead to larger p-values for SNPs under REC or DOM models, with larger Z_{HWDTT} and small $Z_{CATT}(1/2)$.

Our simulation studies are done under a candidate-gene setting with significance level 0.05. For GWAS, the significance level is much smaller. Moreover, the SNPs with association need to be detected among a large number of null SNPs. The performance of these robust tests would be different under this setting.

In practice, we recommend MAX3, MIN2, Z_{GMS} and Z_{GME1}. One could apply any one of them or several of them. However, the multiple testing issue for a single

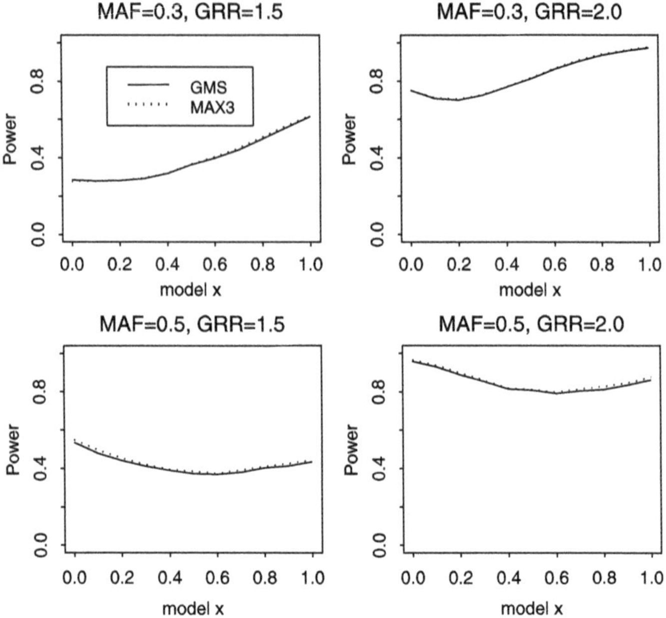

Fig. 6.12 Power of MAX3 and Z_{GMS}. They have very comparable power

SNP is a concern when more than one test is applied to each SNP. Other evidence (e.g., through haplotype analysis and meta-analysis) and independent replication studies are very important in this situation.

6.9 MAX3 for Matched Pair Designs

From Sect. 6.2 to Sect. 6.7, we have discussed robust test statistics for unmatched case-control designs. Robust procedures for matched case-control designs (Chap. 4) have not been well studied. We only discuss the use of MAX3 for a matched case-control design. The MTTs (Sect. 4.3) will be used in MAX3. The correlations among the three MTTs will be given. The simulation procedure for matched case-control data was presented in Sect. 4.7. The simulation results for MAX3, however, will now be presented for matched designs.

Pair-matching is the most common of matched case-control designs. Thus, we focus on MAX3 for the matched pair design. Using the matched pair data given in Table 6.25 (see Table 4.1), the MTT can be written as

$$Z_{\mathrm{MTT}}(x) = \frac{\sum_{0 \le s < t \le 2}(m_{st} - m_{ts})(x_s - x_t)}{\sqrt{\sum_{0 \le s < t \le 2}(m_{st} + m_{ts})(x_s - x_t)^2}}$$

where $x_0 = 0$, $x_1 = x \in [0, 1]$, and $x_2 = 1$. The above test is also given in (4.4).

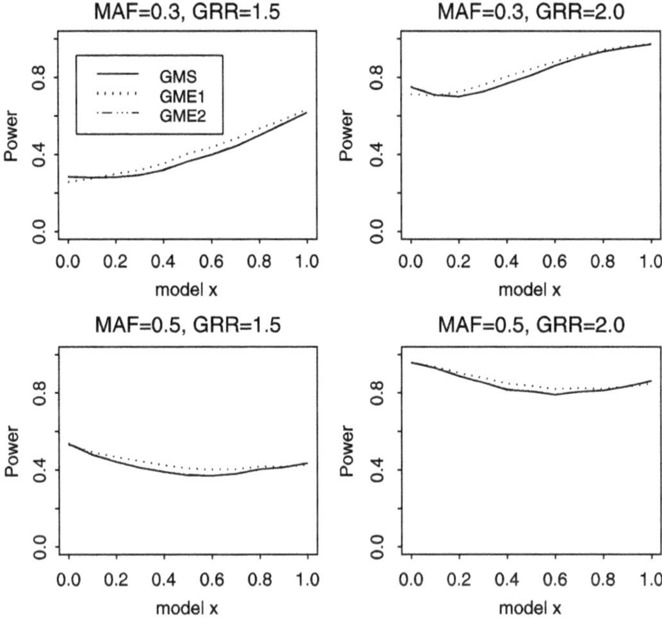

Fig. 6.13 Power of the GMS test and GMEs. Z_{GMS} and Z_{GME2} have nearly identical power

Table 6.25 Genotype counts for a single marker with alleles A and B in a matched pair design with n matched sets

Cases	Controls			Total
	AA	AB	BB	
AA	m_{00}	m_{01}	m_{02}	r_0
AB	m_{10}	m_{11}	m_{12}	r_1
BB	m_{20}	m_{21}	m_{22}	r_2
Total	s_0	s_1	s_2	n

Let $x \in [0, 1]$ and $y \in [0, 1]$, and $x \neq y$. The asymptotic null correlation between $Z_{\mathrm{MTT}}(x)$ and $Z_{\mathrm{MTT}}(y)$ can be written as (omitting higher order terms)

$$\rho_{x,y}^{M} = \frac{\sum_{s<t}(x_s - x_t)(y_s - y_t)(m_{st} + m_{ts})}{\sqrt{\sum_{s<t}(x_s - x_t)^2(m_{st} + m_{ts})}\sqrt{\sum_{s<t}(y_s - y_t)^2(m_{st} + m_{ts})}}, \quad (6.48)$$

where $(x_0, x_1, x_2) = (0, x, 1)$ and $(y_0, y_1, y_2) = (0, y, 1)$.

Applying the correlation in (6.48) to the MTT under the REC, ADD and DOM models, we have

$$\rho_{0,1}^{M} = \frac{M_{20}}{\sqrt{(M_{20} + M_{21})(M_{20} + M_{10})}},$$

$$\rho_{0,\frac{1}{2}}^{M} = \frac{M_{20} + M_{21}/2}{\sqrt{(M_{20} + M_{21}/4 + M_{10}/4)(M_{20} + M_{21})}},$$

$$\rho^{M}_{\frac{1}{2},1} = \frac{M_{20} + M_{10}/2}{\sqrt{(M_{20} + M_{21}/4 + M_{10}/4)(M_{20} + M_{10})}},$$

where $M_{st} = m_{st} + m_{ts}$.

MAX3 for the matched pair design can be written as

$$\text{MAX3} = \max(|Z_{\text{MTT}}(0)|, |Z_{\text{MTT}}(1/2)|, |Z_{\text{MTT}}(1)|).$$

Like unmatched designs, the three MTTs, $Z_{\text{MTT}}(0)$, $Z_{\text{MTT}}(1/2)$ and $Z_{\text{MTT}}(1)$, are linearly dependent (Problem 6.13). Thus, $Z_{\text{MTT}}(1/2)$ can be expressed as the linear sum of $Z_{\text{MTT}}(0)$ and $Z_{\text{MTT}}(1)$. Using this result (Problem 6.13), the asymptotic null distribution of MAX3 can be simulated without simulating the raw matched data.

6.10 Bibliographical Comments

We have discussed many robust procedures for testing single marker case-control association studies. When the underlying genetic model is known, the CATT with an appropriately chosen set of scores is asymptotically optimal and can be employed [223, 248]. The trend test, however, uses prespecified scores and is not robust to genetic model misspecification when the model is unknown [91, 334]. A general discussion of the sensitivity of using scores in ordered categorical data can be found in Graubard and Korn [106]. Pearson's chi-squared test is robust because it does not specify any genetic model and uses data-driven scores [338]. However, this ignores that the alternative hypothesis of association could be ordered in terms of penetrances. Hence, it is usually less powerful, especially under the ADD model.

Efficient robust testing is useful in the situation that the alternative hypothesis contains several scientifically plausible models. The MERT was proposed by Gastwirth [95]. The algorithm to find the MERT was studied by Gastwirth [95, 96] and Birnbaum et al. [18]. The general conditions for the MERT of the extreme pair to be the MERT of a larger family of models was given in Gastwirth [95, 96]. The Bayesian version of the MERT was studied in [19]. In addition to applications of the MERT in genetics, it has applications in other areas, including survival analysis [90, 116, 356].

Owing to their higher efficiency robustness, MAX3 or a general maximum test (MAX) are more commonly used as robust tests. Davies [55, 56] studied MAX with a parameter over a closed interval. His results were proposed for general hypothesis testing when a nuisance parameter is present only under the alternative. For example, if the nuisance parameter refers to the genetic model, it is only defined under the alternative hypothesis. MAX3 is a simple version of MAX. MAX3 and MAX have been applied to many genetic studies, including the family-based trio design [51, 243, 331, 333], linkage studies [97, 243, 244], and case-control association studies [91, 334]. Zheng and Chen [330] compared MAX3 and MAX for several genetic studies and found they have comparable power performance. MAX3 has been applied to GWAS as a scan in initial analysis [170, 247]. The computations of MAX3 using the asymptotic null distribution and simulated null distribution are derived by

Zang et al. [316], and the Rhombus formula was obtained by Li et al. [168]. Conneely and Boehnke [43] also proposed a simple approach to correct p-values after multiple correlated tests have been applied. A comparison between the MERT and MAX3 and suggestions for choosing between the MERT and MAX3 were provided by Freidlin et al. [90]. The relationships among the trend test, MAX and Pearson's test are given by Zheng et al. [338]. In particular, they show that all three are trend tests, depending on whether they use fixed scores or random scores and whether or not the scores are constrained. Yamada and Okada [309] obtain similar results. We focused on MAX3 based on the trend tests. Gonzalez et al. [102] considered MAX3 based on the LRTs under REC, ADD and DOM models.

The CLRT is another common robust test. It was first studied by Chernoff [35] and Chernoff and Lander [36]. Much statistical theory of constrained inference has been developed since then, e.g., Self and Liang [238]. Wang and Sheffield [288] applied the method of Prentice and Pyke [204] to the retrospective case-control data and obtained the CLRT. The performance of the CLRT is similar to that of MAX or MAX3, because both approaches (CLRT and MAX3 or MAX) use the restricted data-driven scores as the estimates of penetrances.

MIN2, taking the minimum p-values of the trend test and Pearson's test, was first proposed by the Wellcome Trust Case-Control Consortium (WTCCC) [301]. MIN2 was later further developed by Joo et al. [135], who also derived the asymptotic null distribution. Song and Elston [251] studied using the HWDTT and the trend test for association studies. Asymptotic results of estimates of the HWD coefficient using cases and controls can be found in Weir [299]. The results of Song and Elston [251] were later used to develop a GMS procedure [344] and GMEs [137]. Although both the GMS test and the GME procedures require the risk allele to be known, this assumption can be relaxed in replication studies if the same risk allele is replicated as in the original study. Moreover, in the GMS test and GMEs, the HWDTT uses the difference of HWD between cases and controls. It is expected that it might be more efficient to construct a HWDTT based on the deviation from HWE in only cases because controls mimic the general population when the disease prevalence is small (e.g. for a rare disease) so that the HWD in controls is approximate 0 when HWE holds in the general population (see Problem 3.13).

Other robust tests have also been studied in the literature. Zheng et al. [345] studied an adaptive procedure, in which they used two independent test statistics (the HWDTT and the trend test that is optimal for the ADD model) in two stages. In stage 1, they determined the significance level for the conditional power of the HWDTT to be at least 80%. The significance level to be used in stage 2 is then determined by the independence of the two statistics and the level used in stage 1. This adaptive test is more robust than a single trend test. Similar adaptive two-stage (two-phase) analysis was also considered by Zheng et al. [343]. Donegani [61] also considered some powerful adaptive randomization tests, which can be modified to test case-control genetic association.

We also briefly discussed MAX3 for the matched pair design. For more results of robust tests for the matched designs, derivations, simulation studies, and asymptotic power, refer to Zheng and Tian [346] and Zang et al. [315]. The real data used for illustrations were taken from GWAS for breast cancer [127] and prostate cancer [313].

6.11 Problems

6.1 Let $Z_{\text{CATT}}(x)$ be the trend test given by (6.3) with $x \in [0, 1]$. Denote the denominator of $Z_{\text{CATT}}(x)$ by $v^{1/2}(x, n_1/n, n_2/n)$ and the numerator by $u(x, r_i, s_i, r, s, n)$. Note that, as $n \to \infty$,

$$v^{1/2}(x, n_1/n, n_2/n) \to v^{1/2}(x, p_1, p_2)$$

in probability, where $p_i = \Pr(\text{case}\,|\,G_i)$ for genotype G_i, $i = 1, 2$. Assume $r/n \to \phi \in (0, 1)$ as $n \to \infty$. Derive the asymptotic null correlation (6.6) of $Z_{\text{CATT}}(x)$ and $Z_{\text{CATT}}(y)$ for $x, y \in [0, 1]$ and $x \neq y$ by applying Problem 1.11.

6.2 Properties of asymptotic null correlations $\rho_{x,y}$.

1) Using (6.7) to (6.9), prove $|\Sigma| = 0$.
2) Show that $\rho_{0,1/2} > \rho_{0,1}\rho_{1/2,1}$ and $\rho_{1/2,1} > \rho_{0,1}\rho_{0,1/2}$.
3) Show that $\rho_{1/2,1} > \rho_{0,1/2}$ if and only if $p_0 > p_2$. Under HWE, this implies that B is the allele with allele frequency less than 1/2.
4) Let w_0^* and w_1^* be given as in (6.18) and (6.19). Then show that $w_0^* < w_1^*$ if and only if $p_2 < p_0$.

6.3 For case-control studies, show that for $x \in [0, 1]$

$$\rho_{0,x} + \rho_{x,1} \geq 1 + \rho_{0,1},$$

where $\rho_{x,y}$ is given in (6.6).

6.4 If B is the risk allele under H_1, i.e., $f_2 \geq f_1 \geq f_0$ and $f_2 > f_0$, show that $E(Z_{\text{CATT}}(x)) > 0$ for any $x \in [0, 1]$ under H_1.

6.5 Assume $|\Sigma| = 0$. Then there exists $\mathbf{a} \neq 0$ such that $a_1 Z_{\text{CATT}}(0) + a_2 Z_{\text{CATT}}(\frac{1}{2}) + a_3 Z_{\text{CATT}}(1) = 0$. Show that, if $a_2 = 0$, then $\rho_{01} = 1$. This implies that $a_2 \neq 0$.

6.6 Let $Z_{\text{CATT}}(x_0, x_1, x_2)$ be the trend test defined in (3.8). Show that the trend test is invariant under a linear transformation of the scores. That is $Z_{\text{CATT}}(x_0, x_1, x_2) = Z_{\text{CATT}}(0, x, 1)$, where $x = (x_1 - x_0)/(x_2 - x_1)$, provided that $x_2 \neq x_0$.

6.7 Prove (6.25) and (6.26).

6.8 Properties of the trend test, Pearson's test and MIN2.

1) Prove that $Z_{\text{CATT}}^2(1/2)/T_{\chi_2^2}$ and $T_{\chi_2^2}$ are asymptotically independent under H_0 (Zheng et al. [343]) and derive (6.28).

2) Show that

$$\Pr\left(Z_{\mathrm{CATT}}^2(1/2) > t_1, T_{\chi_2^2} > t_2\right) > \Pr\left(Z_{\mathrm{CATT}}^2(1/2) > t_1\right)\Pr(T_{\chi_2^2} > t_2).$$

Use this result to show that $Z_{\mathrm{CATT}}^2(1/2)$ and $T_{\chi_2^2}$ are positively correlated.

3) Use the result in Problem 1.9 and the above result to show MIN2 > p_{MIN2}, where p_{MIN2} is the p-value of MIN2.

6.9 Let $\Pr(Z_{\mathrm{CATT}}(x^*) > c) = p(c)$ be the left hand side of (6.38). Then

$$\frac{\partial p(c)}{\partial c} = -2\Phi(c^*)\phi(c) - \Phi\left(\frac{-c^* - \rho_1 c}{\sqrt{1 - \rho_1^2}}\right)\phi(c) + \Phi\left(\frac{c^* - \rho_0 c}{\sqrt{1 - \rho_0^2}}\right)\phi(c).$$

Show that $\partial p(c)/\partial c < \{1 - 2\Phi(c^*)\}\phi(c) < 0$ for $c^* = 1.645$.

6.10 Show that the critical value c solved from (6.38) does not change with p replaced by $1 - p$.

6.11 Correlations under HWE in the population.

1) Show that, under HWE, the correlations given in (6.7)–(6.9) can be written as

$$\rho_{0,1/2} = \sqrt{\frac{2p}{1+p}}, \qquad \rho_{1/2,1} = \sqrt{\frac{2q}{1+q}},$$

$$\rho_{0,1} = \sqrt{\frac{pq}{(1+p)(1+q)}},$$

where $p = \Pr(B)$ and $q = 1 - p$.

2) Show that the weights w_0^* and w_1^* given in (6.18) and (6.19) can be written as

$$w_0^* = \sqrt{\frac{p(1+p)}{2}}, \qquad w_1^* = \sqrt{\frac{q(1+q)}{2}}.$$

3) Using $Z_{\mathrm{CATT}}(1/2) = w_0^* Z_{\mathrm{CATT}}(0) + w_1^* Z_{\mathrm{CATT}}(1)$, and ρ_0 and ρ_1 as given in (6.33) and (6.35), show that, under H_0,

$$\rho_{\frac{1}{2}} = \mathrm{Corr}(Z_{\mathrm{CATT}}(1/2), Z_{\mathrm{HWDTT}}) = w_0^* \rho_0 + w_1^* \rho_1 = 0.$$

4) Show that

$$1 + 2\rho_0\rho_1\rho_{0,1} = \rho_0^2 + \rho_1^2 + \rho_{0,1}^2.$$

6.12 How can you simulate critical values and p-values for the genetic model exclusion trend test without simulating case-control data?

6.13 Matched trend tests.

1) Show that $Z_{\mathrm{MTT}}(0)$, $Z_{\mathrm{MTT}}(1/2)$, and $Z_{\mathrm{MTT}}(1)$ are linearly dependent.

2) Write $Z_{\mathrm{MTT}}(1/2) = \alpha^* Z_{\mathrm{MTT}}(0) + \beta^* Z_{\mathrm{MTT}}(1)$. Determine the weights α^* and β^* in terms of the correlations among the MTTs under H_0.

3) Derive the asymptotic null distribution for MAX3 and design a simulation procedure for MAX3.

6.14 The MERT.

Let both Z_1 and Z_2 have a $N(0, 1)$ distribution and the correlation $\rho > 0$ under H_0. Under H_1, one of them corresponds to the true model (more powerful). The ARE of Z_1 (or Z_2) relative to Z_2 (or Z_1) when Z_2 (or Z_1) is based on the true model is ρ^2. Show that

1) $(Z_1 + Z_2)/\sqrt{2(1 + \rho)}$ has ARE $(1 + \rho)/2 > \rho^2$.

2) The MERT for all linear combinations of Z_1 and Z_2, $(w_1 Z_1 + w_2 Z_2)\sqrt{w_1^2 + 2w_1 w_2 \rho + w_2^2}$, with $w_1, w_2 \geq 0$ is $(Z_1 + Z_2)/\sqrt{2(1 + \rho)}$.

Part III
Multi-marker Analyses for Case-Control Data

Chapter 7
Haplotype Analysis for Case-Control Data

Abstract Chapter 7 covers haplotype analysis. It starts with haplotype inference, including an introduction to phase and phase ambiguity and estimation of haplotype frequencies. Haplotype disequilibrium, testing for linkage disequilibrium (LD), haplotype blocks and tagging SNPs are discussed. Two types of tests are considered. The first is haplotype-based association analysis, including the likelihood ratio test, regression method, and haplotype similarity. The second comprise LD contrast tests, including composite LD measures and contrasting LD measures.

Association analysis attempts to identify genetic variants that predispose to complex diseases. The identified genetic variants either could be the causal variants or are in LD with the casual variants. Alleles at different loci or sites on the same chromosome (i.e., in *cis* position) within a gene may create a "super allele" that has a larger effect than any of the single alleles. The "super allele" composed of a sequence of alleles at different loci or sites on the same chromosome is known as a haplotype. As noted in Sect. 2.1, SNPs occur at sites rather than at loci. In this chapter, we will use the word locus to denote either a locus or a site. The LD information of the alleles on the same haplotype can be thought of as representing allelic *cis* interaction that captures the genetic variations of human traits. Therefore, haplotype analysis is valuable in characterizing human genetic variations.

Alleles on the same chromosome are said to be in phase. But phase information is not observable with most of the current genotyping platforms and only unphased genotypes can be observed. Although molecular haplotyping methods can be used to derive phase information, they are very costly and not applicable to large scale studies. Therefore, recovering phase information from unphased multi-locus genotypes is a crucial step in haplotype analysis. Many algorithms have been proposed for this, among which the EM algorithm for solving the MLEs of haplotype frequencies is one of the popular haplotype inference methods. Other methods include a combinatorial method, a Bayesian method and other evolution-based methods. We focus on the combinatorial algorithm and the EM algorithm.

Association analysis using haplotypes is expected to provide useful information of allelic interaction across different loci and, by using a regression model, can detect haplotype effects on disease susceptibility. Three major difficulties occur with haplotype-based association analysis using unphased genotypes. First, phase

G. Zheng et al., *Analysis of Genetic Association Studies*,
Statistics for Biology and Health,
DOI 10.1007/978-1-4614-2245-7_7, © Springer Science+Business Media, LLC 2012

ambiguity of genotype data makes haplotype analysis complicated; second, the over-sampling of cases in a case-control design needs to be allowed for in the analysis; third, high-dimensionality of the haplotype space may cause standard statistical analysis methods to be problematic. In this chapter, we will introduce a retrospective likelihood approach, in which the retrospective sampling nature of genotype data is accounted for by a retrospective likelihood method; the high-dimensionality problem is solved by introducing haplotype-specific covariates for one or a group of haplotypes; and a conditional EM method is used to maximize the retrospective likelihood function of the unphased genotypes. We will also introduce association analysis methods that are based on contrasting haplotype similarity measures or LD patterns between cases and controls.

This chapter is organized as follows. We first introduce methods for estimating haplotype frequencies in the population followed by definitions of LD measures. Then we discuss haplotype-based case-control association analysis using a retrospective likelihood approach. Finally, we consider an association analysis method based on contrasting the LD patterns between cases and controls.

7.1 Haplotype Inference

Haplotypes provide a useful tool in dissecting the genetic basis of complex diseases. A haplotype is a sequence of alleles at different loci on the same chromosome that are transmitted together as a block. If phase information is observable by molecular methods or other haplotyping methods, haplotype-based analysis can be directly implemented using observed haplotypes. However, phase information cannot be observed in most studies. Therefore, reconstructing haplotypes for each individual or estimating haplotype frequencies from genotype observations in the studied population is an inevitable step in any haplotype-based studies.

7.1.1 Phase and Phase Ambiguity

When phase is known, the haplotype pairs of each individual can be directly observed. Based on such data, the population haplotype frequencies can be estimated by the counting method. Let h_{i1} and h_{i2} be the two haplotypes of individual i, and denote the (unordered) haplotype pair by $H_i = \{h_{i1}, h_{i2}\}$, $i = 1, \ldots, n$, where n is the number of individuals. Then the frequency of haplotype h can be estimated by the gene counting method

$$\widehat{p}_h = \frac{1}{2n} \sum_{i=1}^{n} \delta_h(H_i),$$

where $\delta_h(H_i)$ denotes the number of haplotypes h in H_i, and the variances and covariances are given by

Table 7.1 Two-locus genotypes and haplotypes

	BB	Bb	bb
AA	AB/AB	AB/Ab	Ab/Ab
Aa	AB/aB	AB/ab or Ab/aB	Ab/ab
aa	aB/aB	aB/ab	ab/ab

$$\mathrm{Var}(\widehat{p}_h) = p_h(1 - p_h)/2n,$$
$$\mathrm{Cov}(\widehat{p}_h, \widehat{p}_{h'}) = -p_h p_{h'}/2n, \quad h \neq h'.$$

Molecular methods are costly and only applicable for obtaining phase information of haplotypes with short lengths. Therefore, in most population-based association analyses, the phase information is usually unknown to the researchers and only genotypes are available. Many methods for haplotype inference and haplotype association analysis have been developed. See the discussion in the Bibliographical comments.

Table 7.1 illustrates the issue of phase ambiguity in estimating two-locus haplotypes from genotype data. The alleles at the two loci are denoted as A, a and B, b, respectively. The genotypes at the first and second loci are one of AA, Aa, aa and one of BB, Bb, bb, respectively. Therefore, there are in total 9 genotype combinations. Except for the double-heterozygous cell in the middle of the table, the remaining 8 genotype combinations are heterozygous at no more than one locus and their haplotype pairs can be uniquely determined. For the genotype combination (Aa, Bb), there are two possible haplotype pairs, $\{AB, ab\}$ or $\{Ab, aB\}$, as shown in the table.

7.1.2 Haplotype Reconstruction

Clark's parsimony method attempts to find the smallest (and hence the most parsimonious) set of haplotypes that are consistent with the observed genotypes. It was the first method for reconstructing haplotypes from genotype data and still remains an efficient approach for resolving haplotypes, especially when the number of loci is large. If we code the two alleles at each locus by 0 and 1, then a haplotype is a binary vector and the genotypes at all loci is a vector with each element being 0, 1 or 2. Given genotypes at multiple loci, the parsimony approach, as well as other combinatorial algorithms, essentially solves a set of linear equations. For example, given genotypes $G = (2, 1, 1, 2, 0)$, one solves haplotype pairs $\{h, h'\}$ such that $h + h' = G$. The two possible solutions for this G are $h = (1, 0, 1, 1, 0)$, $h' = (1, 1, 0, 1, 0)$, and $h = (1, 0, 0, 1, 0)$, $h' = (1, 1, 1, 1, 0)$. We say that a haplotype h can resolve, or is compatible with, genotype G if $h' = G - h$ is also a haplotype; that is, all elements of h and h' are either 0 or 1.

Given the observed ambiguous genotypes G_i, $i = 1, \ldots, n$, the combinatorial methods solve the linear equations $h_{i1} + h_{i2} = G_i$, $i = 1, \ldots, n$, under some constraints on the solutions. The parsimony approach repeats the following three steps:

(a) Resolve into haplotypes all the genotypes of individuals who are homozygotes or single-locus heterozygotes, and store these haplotypes in R, as the initial set of resolved haplotypes;
(b) Determine in turn whether each of the haplotypes in R can resolve any unresolved genotypes. If it can, then another haplotype, either in R or not, can be identified (Clark's Inference Rule);
(c) If the haplotype identified in step (b) is not in R, add it to R and remove the resolved genotype from the ambiguous genotypes.

The above procedure is repeated until either all the genotypes are resolved or no further genotype can be resolved. Remaining unresolved genotypes are called "orphans". This method has the drawback that multiple solutions can occur if different orders of resolving genotypes are applied. Clark showed that the solution with the fewest orphans is the most accurate one and suggested that the solution with the maximum parsimony, which solves the maximum number of ambiguous genotypes, is unique and has high accuracy. The rationale behind this approach is that unambiguous genotypes and their corresponding haplotypes are probably common and a phase-ambiguous genotype is likely to have one or two such common haplotypes in it.

The parsimony algorithm can be reformulated into a maximum resolution (MR) problem, which can be reduced to an integer linear programming problem. The parsimony algorithm is quite simple and easy to implement. However, in many situations, not all genotypes can be unambiguously resolved by the algorithm. In addition, the algorithm implicitly requires the random mating assumption and is quite sensitive to deviation from HWE. Furthermore, Clark's algorithm cannot properly handle missing data.

Since, in most situations, it is impossible to resolve the haplotypes perfectly by any of the combinatorial methods, the MLE method, which does not aim to resolve all the haplotype pairs, but rather attempts to estimate the probabilities of the haplotype pairs, is often used in practice. We introduce the MLE method in the next section.

7.1.3 Estimating Haplotype Frequencies

The EM algorithm is a classical method for estimating haplotype frequencies from the observed genotype data. The EM algorithm breaks up into two steps, namely, the E-step and the M-step (Sect. 1.5). In the E-step, the unobserved haplotype pair or phase information is estimated by using its conditional expectation given an initial guess of haplotype frequencies. Then, with the phase information imputed, in the M-step one can apply the gene counting method to obtain the sample proportions of haplotypes and update the initial guess of the haplotype frequencies. These two steps are repeated until the haplotype frequencies converge to some stable values, which are usually the MLEs. In what follows, we first show the EM algorithm in a two-locus case, and then introduce the EM method for multiple loci.

Table 7.2 Two-locus genotype counts

	BB	Bb	bb	Total
AA	n_{11}	n_{12}	n_{13}	n_{1+}
Aa	n_{21}	n_{22}	n_{23}	n_{2+}
aa	n_{31}	n_{32}	n_{33}	n_{3+}
Total	n_{+1}	n_{+2}	n_{+3}	n

EM Algorithm for Two-Locus Haplotype Estimation

We first illustrate the EM method with the two-locus case. Denote the alleles at the first locus by A, a and those at the second locus by B, b. There are 4 possible haplotypes, AB, Ab, aB, ab, and their frequencies are denoted as p_{AB}, p_{Ab}, p_{aB}, p_{ab}. Table 7.2 presents genotype counts for the 9 genotype combinations. Only the genotype combination (Aa, Bb) is ambiguous in reconstructing the haplotype pair, which leads to the possible haplotype pair $\{AB, ab\}$ or $\{Ab, aB\}$.

The probability of each of the two possible pairs depends on the haplotype frequencies in the population, which may be inferred from the other, unambiguous, genotypes. Let x be the (unobserved) count for haplotype pair $\{AB, ab\}$ and y for the pair $\{Ab, aB\}$. Note that $x + y = n_{22}$. If the haplotype frequencies are known, then under the assumption of HWE, x and y are expected to be proportional to $p_{AB}p_{ab}$ and $p_{Ab}p_{aB}$, respectively. They can be estimated as

$$x = n_{22}\frac{p_{AB}p_{ab}}{p_{AB}p_{ab} + p_{Ab}p_{aB}}, \qquad y = n_{22} - x, \tag{7.1}$$

which is the E-step in the EM algorithm. On the other hand, if x and y are known, then the haplotype frequencies can be obtained by the gene counting method as follows

$$
\begin{aligned}
p_{AB} &= \frac{2n_{11} + n_{12} + n_{21} + x}{2n}, \\[4pt]
p_{Ab} &= \frac{n_{12} + 2n_{13} + y + n_{23}}{2n}, \\[4pt]
p_{aB} &= \frac{n_{21} + y + 2n_{31} + n_{32}}{2n}, \\[4pt]
p_{ab} &= \frac{x + n_{23} + n_{32} + 2n_{33}}{2n},
\end{aligned}
\tag{7.2}
$$

which is the M-step in the EM algorithm. The MLEs of the haplotype frequencies can be solved by iterating the above two steps (7.1) and (7.2) starting from some arbitrary initial frequencies. The iterating procedure converges in a few steps, and the final values of $(p_{AB}, p_{Ab}, p_{aB}, p_{ab})$ are the MLEs of the haplotype frequencies. An application of this procedure to real data is given in Sect. 7.5.

General EM Algorithm

To understand the EM algorithm for m loci, suppose that each locus has two alleles denoted by 0 and 1. A haplotype is a vector of 0's and 1's and there are totally 2^m haplotypes. We denote all the haplotypes at the m loci by $h_1 = (0, 0, 0, \ldots, 0)$, $h_2 = (1, 0, 0, \ldots, 0), \ldots, h_{2^m} = (1, 1, 1, \ldots, 1)$, corresponding to the binary expansions of $0, 1, 2, \ldots, 2^m - 1$, respectively. For example, for $m = 3$ loci, the 8 haplotypes are given below

Locus	h_1	h_2	h_3	h_4	h_5	h_6	h_7	h_8
1	0	1	0	1	0	1	0	1
2	0	0	1	1	0	0	1	1
3	0	0	0	0	1	1	1	1

Let $p_h = \Pr(h)$ be the relative frequency of a haplotype h and

$$\mathbf{p} = (p_{h_1}, p_{h_2}, \ldots, p_{h_{2^m}}).$$

Suppose there are n individuals. Let genotype $G_{ij} \in \{0, 1, 2\}$ be the number of copies of allele 1 in the genotype at locus j for individual i ($1 \le i \le n$). The observed genotypes at all m loci for individual i are denoted by a vector $G_i = (G_{i1}, G_{i2}, \ldots, G_{im})$. We denote the set of compatible haplotype pairs for a genotype G by

$$S(G) = \{\{h, h'\} | h + h' = G\}. \tag{7.3}$$

To simplify notation, let $S_i = S(G_i)$ be the set of haplotype pairs that are compatible with G_i.

Under HWE, the probability of haplotype pair $H = \{h, h'\}$ is $\pi_H = 2 p_h p_{h'}$ if $h \ne h'$ and $\pi_H = p_h^2$ if $h = h'$. The likelihood function for the observed genotypes is given by

$$L(\mathbf{p}) = \prod_{i=1}^{n} \left(\sum_{H \in S_i} \pi_H \right). \tag{7.4}$$

Instead of maximizing the above likelihood function directly, the EM algorithm maximizes the expected complete-data likelihood as described below.

Let $X_H^{(i)}$ be the (unobservable) indicator function that individual i has the haplotype pair H. Then the likelihood function for the complete data is given by

$$L_c(\mathbf{p}) = \prod_{i=1}^{n} \prod_{H \in S_i} \pi_H^{X_H^{(i)}}. \tag{7.5}$$

Assuming $\mathbf{p}$ is known, the E-step of the EM algorithm predicts the unobserved random variable $X_H^{(i)}$ by using its conditional expectation given $\mathbf{p}$ and the genotype data:

$$\widehat{X_H^{(i)}} = \mathrm{E}(X_H^{(i)} | G, \mathbf{p}) = \Pr(X_H^{(i)} = 1 | G_i, \mathbf{p}) = \frac{\pi_H}{\sum_{\tilde{H} \in S_i} \pi_{\tilde{H}}} 1_{(H \in S_i)}, \tag{7.6}$$

which is the posterior probability of individual i having haplotype pair H, given the genotype G_i, where $1_{(H \in S_i)}$ is the indicator function of $H \in S_i = S(G_i)$. With the predicted value $\widehat{X_H^{(i)}}$, the M-step maximizes the conditional expectation of the log of the complete-data likelihood (7.5), given the observed genotype data and the current value of the haplotype frequencies. The maximizer of (7.5) is given by

$$p_h^{\text{new}} = \frac{\sum_{i=1}^{n} \sum_{H \in S_i} \delta_h(H) \widehat{X_H^{(i)}}}{2n}, \tag{7.7}$$

which updates the haplotype frequencies, where $\delta_h(H)$ is the number of h haplotypes in H. Starting from an initial value of $\mathbf{p}$, the EM algorithm iterates between the E-step (7.6) and the M-step (7.7) until convergence is achieved.

It is well known that the EM algorithm is stable and always converges in the sense that the likelihood function (7.4) always increases in the iterating procedure, but the convergence is usually very slow when the number of loci is large. In addition, the EM algorithm may converge to a local maximum and a typical solution for this problem of local maximization is to try different initial values of haplotype frequencies and find the solution with the overall maximal likelihood.

The EM algorithm allows random missing genotypes. For example, it can handle completely missing data (no genotype observed at some loci) and partially missing data (only one allele A or a present but not the other). When there are missing data, the above EM algorithm can be applied in the same way except that the compatible haplotype set (7.3) for genotypes G_i containing missing elements is enlarged.

7.2 Linkage Disequilibrium

LD refers to the non-independence of alleles at different loci. When a particular allele at one locus is found together more often than expected with a specific allele on the same chromosome at a second locus, the two loci are in disequilibrium. LD is a special case of gametic phase disequilibrium (Sect. 2.1).

7.2.1 Linkage Disequilibrium Coefficients

For two loci with alleles A and a at the first locus and B and b at the second locus, let the allele frequencies be p_A, p_a, p_B, p_b. The two-locus haplotype frequencies are denoted by p_{AB}, p_{Ab}, p_{aB} and p_{ab}. The (gametic) LD coefficient is defined as

$$D_{AB} = p_{AB} - p_A p_B = p_{AB} p_{ab} - p_{Ab} p_{aB}. \tag{7.8}$$

The LD coefficient can also be defined using other haplotypes, denoted as D_{Ab}, D_{aB} and D_{ab}. It is easy to see that $D_{AB} = -D_{Ab} = -D_{aB} = D_{ab}$. The measure D_{AB} is not standardized, which makes it difficult to use to compare LD patterns. There are many standardized measures of LD proposed in the literature, among which the LD coefficient proposed by Lewontin and the correlation coefficient are widely used.

Since $0 \leq p_{AB} \leq \min\{p_A, p_B\}$, we have

$$\max(-p_A p_B, -p_a p_b) = D_{\min} \leq D_{AB} \leq D_{\max} = \min(p_A p_b, p_a p_B),$$

which is used to standardize D_{AB} to yield Lewontin's LD coefficient (see also (2.1) in Sect. 2.1)

$$D'_{AB} = \begin{cases} D_{AB}/D_{\max} & \text{if } D_{AB} \geq 0 \\ D_{AB}/|D_{\min}| & \text{if } D_{AB} < 0. \end{cases}$$

This measure lies between -1 and 1. If $|D'_{AB}| = 1$, then the loci are in complete LD and at least one haplotype has 0 frequency. If $D'_{AB} = 0$ or $D_{AB} = 0$, the two loci are in linkage equilibrium and the haplotype frequencies are the products of allele frequencies.

By applying the Cauchy-Schwartz inequality, one can bound LD by

$$|D_{AB}| = |p_{AB} - p_A p_B| \leq \sqrt{p_A p_a p_B p_b},$$

which leads to another commonly used standardized LD coefficient

$$r_{AB} = \frac{D_{AB}}{\sqrt{p_A p_a p_B p_b}},$$

which is known as Pearson's correlation coefficient. This measure also lies between -1 and 1, and $r = 0$ corresponds to linkage equilibrium and $r_{AB} = \pm 1$ corresponds to perfect correlation, for which at most two haplotypes are possibly present.

The "fundamental formula for LD mapping" asserts that the allelic test statistic at a marker locus is related to the allelic test at the disease locus by the LD coefficient (squared correlation coefficient) between the two loci. Therefore, significance of a test at a marker may imply that the marker is in strong LD with a disease locus.

7.2.2 Testing for Linkage Equilibrium

Non-LD can be tested based on the estimated LD coefficients. Let $\widehat{p}_{AB}$ be the sample frequency of haplotype AB and $\widehat{p}_A, \widehat{p}_B, \widehat{p}_a = 1 - \widehat{p}_A, \widehat{p}_b = 1 - \widehat{p}_B$ be the sample allele frequencies estimated from n individuals. Then the sample LD coefficient is defined as $\widehat{D}_{AB} = \widehat{p}_{AB} - \widehat{p}_A \widehat{p}_B$. Its mean is $E(\widehat{D}_{AB}) = (2n - 1)D_{AB}/2n$, and its variance is (see Weir [299])

$$\text{Var}(\widehat{D}_{AB}) = \{p_A p_B p_a p_b + (1 - 2p_A)(1 - 2p_B)D_{AB} - D_{AB}^2\}/2n.$$

Under the null hypothesis of linkage equilibrium $H_0 : D_{AB} = 0$, $\text{Var}(\widehat{D}_{AB}) = (p_A p_B p_a p_b)/2n$. The chi-squared test statistic for H_0 can be written as

$$\chi^2 = \frac{\widehat{D}_{AB}^2}{\widehat{\text{Var}}(\widehat{D}_{AB})} = \frac{2n(\widehat{p}_{AB} - \widehat{p}_A \widehat{p}_B)^2}{\widehat{p}_A \widehat{p}_B \widehat{p}_a \widehat{p}_b} = 2n(\widehat{r}_{AB})^2,$$

which asymptotically follows χ_1^2 under H_0.

7.2.3 *Haplotype Block and Haplotype-Tagging SNPs*

Empirical studies have shown that the human genome is structured as haplotype blocks. Each block represents a region with high LD and a small number of haplotypes. The haplotype blocks are separated by short regions known as recombination hotspots, in which recombinations occur frequently and therefore LD between two contiguous blocks is relatively low. The block structure of the human genome can explain a large proportion of the haplotype diversity.

Within a haplotype block, the SNPs are in tight LD and there are only a few haplotypes present. Within a block or a small region with low haplotype diversity, it is anticipated that most SNPs may be redundant and only a few representative SNPs are necessary to capture the LD information in this region. These representative SNPs are called haplotype-tagging SNPs (htSNPs). In order to select a set of htSNPs, we need to quantitatively measure how informative the selected subset of SNPs is about the haplotypes formed by all the SNPs. A haplotype certainty measure was introduced for this purpose, denoted as R_h^2, which measures the haplotype information retained in the subset. The following materials are based on Stram et al. [263].

Haplotype Certainty Measure

For a specific haplotype h, let δ_h be the number of copies of h in the haplotype pair of an individual, which is a random variable and takes on the value 0, 1 or 2. Under HWE, it is apparent that δ_h has a binomial distribution $B(2; p_h)$ with mean $2p_h$ and variance $2p_h(1 - p_h)$, where p_h is the probability of h. Let $\delta_h(H)$ be the number of copies of h in a specific haplotype pair H, then the predicted number of copies of haplotype h conditional on genotype G is given by

$$\widehat{\delta}_h = \mathrm{E}(\delta_h | G) = \sum_{H \in S(G)} \delta_h(H) \Pr(H|G) = \sum_{H \in S(G)} \left\{ \delta_h(H) \pi_H \Big/ \sum_{H \in S(G)} \pi_H \right\},$$

where, for $H = \{h_1, h_2\}$, $\pi_H = 2 p_{h_1} p_{h_2}$ if $h_1 \neq h_2$ and $\pi_H = p_{h_1}^2$ if $h_1 = h_2$, and $\Pr(G) = \sum_{H \in S(G)} \pi_H$, $\Pr(H|G) = \pi_H 1_{(H \in S(G))} / \sum_{H \in S(G)} \pi_H$ as given in (7.6). Variability of the prediction is measured by its variance

$$\mathrm{Var}(\widehat{\delta}_h) = \sum_G \{\mathrm{E}(\delta_h | G)\}^2 \Pr(G) - (2 p_h)^2 = \sum_G \widehat{\delta}_h^2 \Pr(G) - 4 p_h^2 \qquad (7.9)$$

where the outer summation is over all genotypes G that are compatible with haplotype h.

Define the certainty measure $R_h^2 = \mathrm{Corr}(\widehat{\delta}_h, \delta_h)^2$ to be the squared correlation of $\widehat{\delta}_h$ and δ_h. It measures how well the compatible genotypes can predict the specific haplotype h. Since $\mathrm{E}(\widehat{\delta}_h) = \mathrm{E}(\delta_h) = 2 p_h$, and $\mathrm{Cov}(\widehat{\delta}_h, \delta_h) = \mathrm{Var}(\widehat{\delta}_h)$ (Problem 7.5),

$$R_h^2 = \frac{\mathrm{Var}(\widehat{\delta}_h)}{\mathrm{Var}(\delta_h)} = \frac{\mathrm{Var}(\widehat{\delta}_h)}{2 p_h (1 - p_h)}, \qquad 0 < p_h < 1 \qquad (7.10)$$

Table 7.3 Details of the calculation of $\mathrm{Var}(\widehat{\delta}_h)$ and R_h^2 for two SNPs (reproduced from Stram et al. [263])

G	$(0,0)$	$(0,1)$	$(0,2)$	$(1,0)$	$(1,1)$	$(1,2)$	$(2,0)$	$(2,1)$	$(2,2)$
$S(G)$	$\{h_1,h_1\}$	$\{h_1,h_3\}$	$\{h_3,h_3\}$	$\{h_1,h_2\}$	$\{h_2,h_3\}$ $\{h_1,h_4\}$	$\{h_3,h_4\}$	$\{h_2,h_2\}$	$\{h_2,h_4\}$	$\{h_4,h_4\}$
$P(G)$	$p_{h_1}^2$	$2p_{h_1}p_{h_3}$	$p_{h_3}^2$	$2p_{h_1}p_{h_2}$	$2(p_{h_1}p_{h_4}+p_{h_2}p_{h_3})$	$2p_{h_3}p_{h_4}$	$p_{h_2}^2$	$2p_{h_2}p_{h_4}$	$p_{h_4}^2$
$\widehat{\delta}_{h_1}$	2	1	0	1	$\dfrac{p_{h_1}p_{h_4}}{p_{h_1}p_{h_4}+p_{h_2}p_{h_3}}$	0	0	0	0
$\widehat{\delta}_{h_2}$	0	0	0	1	$\dfrac{p_{h_2}p_{h_3}}{p_{h_1}p_{h_4}+p_{h_2}p_{h_3}}$	0	2	1	0
$\widehat{\delta}_{h_3}$	0	1	2	0	$\dfrac{p_{h_2}p_{h_3}}{p_{h_1}p_{h_4}+p_{h_2}p_{h_3}}$	1	0	0	0
$\widehat{\delta}_{h_4}$	0	0	0	0	$\dfrac{p_{h_1}p_{h_4}}{p_{h_1}p_{h_4}+p_{h_2}p_{h_3}}$	1	0	1	2

and, for $p_h = 0$ or $p_h = 1$, R_h^2 is defined to be 1. Because $\mathrm{Var}(\delta_h) = \mathrm{Var}(\widehat{\delta}_h) + \mathrm{E}\{\mathrm{Var}(\delta_h|G)\}$, it follows that $0 \le R_h^2 \le 1$ and, in view of (7.10), R_h^2 is the proportion of the total haplotype variability explained by the observed genotypes. Obviously, $1 - R_h^2$ can be regarded as a haplotype uncertainty measure. Empirical studies show that, typically, R_h^2 decreases as the number of loci increases or as the LD coefficient decreases.

Table 7.3 illustrates calculation of the conditional variances and the certainty measure for two SNPs. For brevity, we use the binary notation for alleles and use $\{h, h'\}$ to represent an unordered haplotype pair. The four haplotypes are $h_1 = (0, 0)$, $h_2 = (1, 0)$, $h_3 = (0, 1)$, and $h_4 = (1, 1)$. Calculation of the predictions is straightforward, for example, for $G = (1, 1)$, $S(G) = \{H_a = \{h_1, h_4\}, H_b = \{h_2, h_3\}\}$,

$$\widehat{\delta}_{h_1} = \mathrm{E}(\delta_{h_1}|G = (1, 1)) = \frac{1 \times \pi_{H_a} + 0 \times \pi_{H_b}}{\pi_{H_a} + \pi_{H_b}} = \frac{p_{h_1}p_{h_4}}{p_{h_1}p_{h_4} + p_{h_2}p_{h_3}},$$

and by (7.9)

$$\mathrm{Var}(\widehat{\delta}_{h_1}) = 4p_{h_1}^2 + 2p_{h_1}p_{h_3} + 2p_{h_1}p_{h_2} + \frac{2p_{h_1}^2 p_{h_4}^2}{p_{h_1}p_{h_4} + p_{h_2}p_{h_3}} - 4p_{h_1}^2$$

$$= 2p_{h_1}(1 - p_{h_1}) - \frac{2p_{h_1}p_{h_2}p_{h_3}p_{h_4}}{p_{h_1}p_{h_4} + p_{h_2}p_{h_3}},$$

then the certainty measure of h_1 is

$$R_{h_1}^2 = 1 - \frac{p_{h_2}p_{h_3}p_{h_4}}{(1 - p_{h_1})(p_{h_1}p_{h_4} + p_{h_2}p_{h_3})}, \qquad 0 < p_{h_1} < 1.$$

Generally,

$$R_{h_k}^2 = 1 - \frac{p_{h_1}p_{h_2}p_{h_3}p_{h_4}}{p_{h_k}(1 - p_{h_k})(p_{h_1}p_{h_4} + p_{h_2}p_{h_3})}, \qquad 0 < p_{h_k} < 1, \; k = 1, 2, 3, 4$$

and $R_{h_k} = 1$ for $p_{h_k} = 0$ or 1. From the above formulas, we can see that the certainty measures are all 1 if and only if at least one of $p_{h_1}, p_{h_2}, p_{h_3}, p_{h_4}$ is 0, or equivalently $D' = 1$.

Table 7.4 Details of the calculation of $\mathrm{Var}(\widehat{\delta_h})$ and R_h^2 for two SNPs when only the first SNP is used for prediction

G	$(0,-)$	$(1,-)$	$(2,-)$
$S(G)$	$(\{h_1,h_1\},\{h_1,h_3\},\{h_3,h_3\})$	$(\{h_1,h_2\},\{h_2,h_3\},$ $\{h_1,h_4\},\{h_3,h_4\})$	$(\{h_2,h_2\},\{h_2,h_4\},\{h_4,h_4\})$
$P(G)$	$(p_{h_1}+p_{h_3})^2$	$2(p_{h_1}+p_{h_3})(p_{h_2}+p_{h_4})$	$(p_{h_2}+p_{h_4})^2$
$\widehat{\delta}_{h1}$	$\dfrac{2p_{h_1}}{p_{h_1}+p_{h_3}}$	$\dfrac{p_{h_1}}{p_{h_1}+p_{h_3}}$	0
$\widehat{\delta}_{h2}$	0	$\dfrac{p_{h_2}}{p_{h_2}+p_{h_4}}$	$\dfrac{2p_{h_2}}{p_{h_2}+p_{h_4}}$
$\widehat{\delta}_{h3}$	$\dfrac{2p_{h_3}}{p_{h_1}+p_{h_3}}$	$\dfrac{p_{h_3}}{p_{h_1}+p_{h_3}}$	0
$\widehat{\delta}_{h4}$	0	$\dfrac{p_{h_4}}{p_{h_2}+p_{h_4}}$	$\dfrac{2p_{h_4}}{p_{h_2}+p_{h_4}}$

Tagging Haplotypes

When a subset of SNPs is used, called htSNPs, information is lost and the certainty measure decreases in magnitude. Proper candidates for htSNPs should not reduce the original certainty measure of the whole set of SNPs to a large extent. For each subset, S, of all available SNPs and each haplotype h, one can compute the certainty measure $R_h^2(S)$ similar to the above calculations. The only difference is that, for a reduced subset of SNPs, there are more haplotype pairs that are compatible with the genotypes in the reduced set. The set of htSNPs should keep the certainty measure as much as possible. One approach is to select m htSNPs out of all the available SNPs by maximizing $\min_h R_h^2(S)$ over all possible subsets S with size m.

We illustrate this procedure using two SNPs, where we want to keep just one of the two SNPS. Table 7.4 shows details of the calculation of the predictions $\widehat{\delta}_h$ using information from the first SNP. For example, for $G = (0, -)$, $S(G) = \{\{h_1, h_1\}, \{h_1, h_3\}, \{h_3, h_3\}\}$,

$$\widehat{\delta}_{h_1} = \frac{2 \times p_{h_1}^2 + 1 \times 2p_{h_2}p_{h_3} + 0 \times p_{h_3}^2}{p_{h_1}^2 + 2p_{h_2}p_{h_3} + p_{h_3}^2} = \frac{2p_{h_1}}{p_{h_1} + p_{h_3}},$$

then

$$\mathrm{Var}(\widehat{\delta}_{h_1}) = \frac{2p_{h_1}^2(p_{h_2} + p_{h_4})}{p_{h_1} + p_{h_3}}$$

and

$$R_{h_1}^2(1) = \frac{p_{h_1}(p_{h_2} + p_{h_4})}{(1 - p_{h_1})(p_{h_1} + p_{h_3})} = \frac{p_{h_1}/(1 - p_{h_1})}{(p_{h_1} + p_{h_3})/(1 - p_{h_1} - p_{h_3})}.$$

Note that $p_{h_1} + p_{h_3}$ is the frequency of allele 0 at the first locus. To be more transparent, we write the probabilities of alleles 0 and 1 at the locus as p_{0-} and p_{1-}, respectively, and the allele probabilities at the second locus as p_{-0} and p_{-1}, and use the notation $p_{00} = p_{h_1}$, $p_{10} = p_{h_2}$, $p_{10} = p_{h_3}$ and $p_{11} = p_{h_4}$. Then the above formula is expressed as an OR (two-locus versus first locus only):

$$R^2_{h_1}(1) = \frac{p_{00}/(1 - p_{00})}{p_{0-}/(1 - p_{0-})}.$$

Generally, for haplotype $h = (i, j)$, $i, j = 0, 1$, the certainty measure when the first locus is chosen as the htSNP is

$$R^2_{ij}(1) = \frac{p_{ij}/(1 - p_{ij})}{p_{i-}/(1 - p_{i-})}$$

and for the second locus

$$R^2_{ij}(2) = \frac{p_{ij}/(1 - p_{ij})}{p_{-j}/(1 - p_{-j})}.$$

This tagging method first finds the minimal value among all the 4 certainty measures for each of the two SNPs. Let $R^2(1) = \min_h R^2_h(1)$ for the first locus and $R^2(2) = \min_h R^2_h(2)$ for the second, where the minimizations are over all the 4 haplotypes. Then the first SNP is chosen as htSNP if $R^2(1) > R^2(2)$ and otherwise the second SNP is chosen to be the htSNP.

7.3 Haplotype-Based Population Association Analysis

In single-marker analysis, one tests association based on the genotype by comparing the genotype frequencies between cases and controls. On the other hand, the allelic test that compares allele frequencies between cases and controls can be more powerful but requires that HWE holds in the population. Similarly, for a multi-locus study, association analysis can be based on comparing frequencies of either joint genotypes or haplotypes, which play the role of "super-alleles".

7.3.1 Likelihood Ratio Test

The LRT for testing association between haplotypes and disease can be constructed from the maximum likelihood functions for cases, controls and the pooled data of cases and controls. The null hypothesis is that the haplotype frequencies in cases and controls have no difference. Let the maximum likelihood for cases, controls and the pooled data be L_{case}, L_{control}, L_{total}, respectively. Then the LRT is

$$\text{LRT} = 2\{\log(L_{\text{case}}) + \log(L_{\text{control}}) - \log(L_{\text{total}})\}.$$

The LRT statistic has an asymptotic chi-squared distribution with degrees of freedom one less than the number of haplotypes present in the data.

The LRT works well for a small number of loci but, when the number of loci is relatively large, the approximation of the null distribution using a chi-squared distribution may not be accurate owing to the existence of rare haplotypes for loci with high LD coefficients. Another limitation of the LRT is that HWE is assumed when estimating haplotype frequencies from the data, which may bias the estimates. Furthermore, since the LRT is a global test, it does not provide inference on the effects of haplotypes. Therefore a variety of regression methods have been proposed to model the haplotype effects. The retrospective likelihood method of Epstein and Satten [78] will be discussed next.

7.3.2 Regression Method

The Retrospective Likelihood

Let H be the (unordered) haplotype pair for an individual. Define $\pi_H = \Pr(H|D = 0)$, $\rho_H = \Pr(H|D = 1)$ as the probabilities of observing H in controls and cases, respectively. For individual i, denote the observed genotype by G_i and the disease status by D_i $(i = 1, \ldots, n)$. Then the retrospective likelihood function is given by

$$L = \prod_{i=1}^{n} \Pr(G_i|D_i = 1)^{D_i} \Pr(G_i|D_i = 0)^{1-D_i}$$

$$= \prod_{i=1}^{n} \left(\sum_{H \in S_i} \rho_H \right)^{D_i} \left(\sum_{H \in S_i} \pi_H \right)^{1-D_i}.$$

Let the odds of disease for haplotype pair H be

$$\theta_H = \frac{\Pr(D = 1|H)}{\Pr(D = 0|H)}.$$

Then we have $\Pr(H, D = 1) = \Pr(D = 1|H)\Pr(H) = \theta_H \Pr(D = 0|H)\Pr(H) = \theta_H \pi_H \Pr(D = 0)$. Hence ρ_H can be expressed as a function of π's and θ's as

$$\rho_H = \frac{\Pr(H, D = 1)}{\Pr(D = 1)} = \frac{\Pr(H, D = 1)}{\sum_{H'} \Pr(H', D = 1)} = \frac{\theta_H \pi_H}{\sum_{H'} \theta_{H'} \pi_{H'}}. \tag{7.11}$$

Thus, the retrospective likelihood function can be written as

$$L = \prod_{i=1}^{n} \left(\sum_{H \in S_i} \frac{\pi_H \theta_H}{\sum_{H'} \pi_{H'} \theta_{H'}} \right)^{D_i} \left(\sum_{H \in S_i} \pi_H \right)^{1-D_i}. \tag{7.12}$$

In order to assess haplotype-specific effects, we assume the following logistic model

$$\theta_H = \alpha + x_H^T \beta, \tag{7.13}$$

where x_H is the design vector for haplotype pair H, which can be defined according to the target of the study, and β is the vector of corresponding regression coefficients. For example, if one wants to study the effect of a specific haplotype h^*, then one can set $x_H = 1_{(\delta_{h^*}(H)=2)}$ for a REC model, $x_H = 1_{(\delta_{h^*}(H)\geq 1)}$ for a DOM model and $x_H = \delta_{h^*}(H)$ for an ADD model. Similarly, if $\mathscr{H}$ is a set of haplotypes each of which is thought to have a similar effect on disease, for $H = (h, h')$ one can test its effect by defining $x_H = 1_{(h \in \mathscr{H} \text{ and } h' \in \mathscr{H})}$ under a REC model, $x_H = 1_{(h \in \mathscr{H} \text{ or } h' \in \mathscr{H})}$ under a DOM model, and $x_H = 1_{(h \in \mathscr{H})} + 1_{(h' \in \mathscr{H})}$ under an ADD model.

In what follows, we assume HWE holds in the control population, that is, for $H = (h, h')$, $\pi_H = 2p_h p_{h'}$ if $h \neq h'$ and $\pi_H = p_h^2$ if $h = h'$. We still use the notation $\mathbf{p}$ for the vector of frequencies of all haplotypes present in the sample. Incorporating (7.13) and the HWE assumption into (7.12), the retrospective likelihood function can be written as

$$L(\beta, \mathbf{p}) = \frac{\prod_{i=1}^{n} \{\sum_{H \in S_i} \pi_H \exp(x_H^T \beta)\}^{D_i} (\sum_{H \in S_i} \pi_H)^{1-D_i}}{\{\sum_H \pi_H \exp(x_H^T \beta)\}^r}, \qquad (7.14)$$

where r is the number of cases. Note that the intercept terms cancel out and do not appear in the likelihood function.

Expectation/Conditional Maximization Algorithm

To make inferences about β, one needs to compute the MLE of $\phi = (\mathbf{p}, \beta)^T$, and to do this, we apply a generalized EM algorithm, the so-called expectation/conditional maximization (ECM) algorithm. Let x_i denote the haplotype pair of individual i. Then the complete likelihood function is

$$L_c(\phi) = \prod_{i=1}^{n} \left(\prod_{H \in S_i} \rho_H^{1_{(x_i=H)}} \right)^{D_i} \left(\prod_{H \in S_i} \pi_H^{1_{(x_i=H)}} \right)^{1-D_i}.$$

In the E-step, given the current value $\phi^{(k)} = (\mathbf{p}^{(k)}, \beta^{(k)})^T$, we need to compute $\Pr(x_i = H | D_i, G_i, \phi^{(k)})$. For haplotype pair $H \in S_i = S(G_i)$,

$$u_i = \Pr(x_i = H | D_i = 0, G_i, \phi^{(k)}) = \frac{\pi_H^{(k)}}{\sum_{H' \in S_i} \pi_{H'}^{(k)}} 1_{(H \in S_i)},$$

$$v_i = \Pr(x_i = H | D_i = 1, G_i, \phi^{(k)}) = \frac{\theta_H^{(k)} \pi_H^{(k)}}{\sum_{H' \in S_i} \theta_{H'}^{(k)} \pi_{H'}^{(k)}} 1_{(H \in S_i)},$$

where $\pi_H^{(k)}$ and $\theta_H^{(k)}$ are calculated at $\phi = \phi^{(k)}$.

The M-step maximizes the conditional expectation of the log complete-data likelihood with respect to ϕ:

$$E(\log_c(\phi)|D, G, \phi^{(k)}) = \sum_{D_i=1} \sum_{H \in S_i} u_i \log \rho_H + \sum_{D_i=0} \sum_{H \in S_i} v_i \log \pi_H$$

$$= \sum_{D_i=1} \sum_{H \in S_i} u_i \log \left(\frac{\pi_H \exp(x_H^T \beta)}{\sum_{H^*} \pi_{H^*} \exp(x_{H^*}^T \beta)} \right) + \sum_{D_i=0} \sum_{H \in S_i} v_i \log(\pi_H),$$

$$(7.15)$$

which can be solved by the Newton-Raphson algorithm, but this may be unstable when the number of parameters is large for a large m. We suggest maximizing the objective function (7.15) by a conditional maximization strategy. That is, given $\mathbf{p}$, maximize (7.15) with respect to β; then given β, maximize (7.15) with respect to each element of $\mathbf{p}$ given the other elements.

Asymptotic Inference

We discuss the Score statistic (Sect. 1.2.4) for testing the null hypothesis $H_0 : \beta = 0$. Denote the number of haplotypes with non-zero estimates by J and their probabilities as $p_{h_1}, \ldots, p_{h_J}$, satisfying $\sum_{j=1}^{J} p_{h_j} = 1$. Reparameterize the haplotype frequencies using the new parameters $\tau = (\tau_1, \ldots, \tau_{J-1})$ given by

$$p_{h_j} = \frac{e^{\tau_j}}{1 + \sum_{k=1}^{J-1} e^{\tau_k}}, \quad j = 1, \ldots, J - 1$$

and $p_{h_J} = 1 - p_{h_1} - \cdots - p_{h_{J-1}} = 1/(1 + \sum_{k=1}^{J-1} e^{\tau_k})$. The reparameterization is not completely necessary, but it makes the computation more stable. The likelihood function (7.14) can then be written as a function of τ and β. Thus

$$U_\beta = \frac{\partial \log L(\beta, \mathbf{p})}{\partial \beta} = \sum_{i=1}^{n} D_i(\bar{X}_i - \bar{X}), \tag{7.16}$$

where

$$\bar{X}_i = \frac{\sum_{H \in S_i} \pi_H x_H \exp(x_H^T \beta)}{\sum_{H \in S_i} \pi_H \exp(x_H^T \beta)},$$

$$\bar{X} = \frac{\sum_H \pi_H x_H \exp(x_H^T \beta)}{\sum_H \pi_H \exp(x_H^T \beta)},$$

and

$$U_{\tau_j} = \frac{\partial \log L(\beta, \mathbf{p})}{\partial \tau_j} = 2 \sum_{i=1}^{n} (1 - D_i) p_{h_j} \left\{ \frac{\sum_{(h,h') \in S_i} p_{h'} I_{(h=h_j)}}{\sum_{(h,h') \in S_i} p_{h'}} - 1 \right\}$$

$$+ 2 \sum_{i=1}^{n} D_i p_{h_j} \left\{ \frac{\sum_{H=(h,h') \in S_i} p_{h'} \exp(x_H^T \beta) I_{(h=h_j)}}{\sum_{(h,h') \in S_i} p_{h'}} \right.$$

$$\left. - \frac{\sum_{H=(h,h')} p_{h'} \exp(x_H^T \beta) I_{(h=h_j)}}{\sum_{(h,h')} p_{h'}} \right\}, \tag{7.17}$$

where (h, h') denotes an ordered haplotype pair. Denote $U_\tau = (U_{\tau_1}, \ldots, U_{\tau_{J-1}})^T$ and the Score function as $U = U(\beta, \mathbf{p}) = (U_\beta^T, U_\tau^T)^T$, which can be written as $U = \sum_{i=1}^{n} U_i$. Evaluate U at $\beta = 0$ and $\widehat{\tau}_0$, where $\widehat{\tau}_0$ is the MLE of τ under $H_0 : \beta = 0$. Estimate the Fisher information matrix or the covariance matrix of U by $i_n = \sum_{i=1}^{n} U_i U_i^T$, also evaluated at $\beta = 0$ and $\widehat{\tau}_0$. Partition i_n according to β and τ as follows

$$i_n = \begin{bmatrix} i_{\beta\beta} & i_{\beta\tau} \\ i_{\tau\beta} & i_{\tau\tau} \end{bmatrix}.$$

Then the Score test is given by

$$\mathrm{ST} = U_\beta^T (i_{\beta\beta} - i_{\beta\tau} i_{\tau\tau}^{-1} i_{\tau\beta})^{-1} U_\beta,$$

where $(i_{\beta\beta} - i_{\beta\tau} i_{\tau\tau}^{-1} i_{\tau\beta})^{-1}$ is the $(1,1)$th submatrix of i_n^{-1} corresponding to β. This test asymptotically follows a chi-squared distribution with R (the length of β) degrees of freedom.

7.3.3 Haplotype Similarity

We have introduced association analysis methods based on comparing haplotype frequencies between cases and controls. A different yet related method is to test association through comparing haplotype similarities between cases and controls. This approach is based on the idea that for a disease mutation of recent origin, haplotypes from cases should share longer stretches of allele sequence around the disease locus than haplotypes from controls. A difference in the length of haplotype sharing between the two samples can result from a shorter coalescence time of a recent mutation in the case sample relative to the normal allele in the control sample. The coalescence time is the number of generations since an allele first occurred in the population. Therefore, any excessive sharing of haplotypes in cases may indicate the existence of association.

For two haplotypes h and h' with lengths m, which are two binary sequences, a similarity measure $M_{hh'}$ is defined to quantify the degree of similarity between h and h'. There are various ways to define such a measure. For example, a commonly used measure is the counting measure, which counts the number of common alleles shared in the two sequences or, equivalently, $M_{hh'} = m - d(h, h') = m - ||h - h'||_1$, where $d(h, h') = ||h - h'||_1$ is the hamming distance—the number of positions that the two sequences differ. Another commonly used measure is the length measure, which is the maximum number of adjacent loci that the two haplotypes share.

Define the total similarity measure of a haplotype block in controls as the weighted sum of similarity measures of every pair of haplotypes weighted by the probability of the pair, i.e.,

$$S_{\text{control}} = \sum_h \sum_{h'} q_h q_{h'} M_{hh'},$$

where q_h is the frequency of haplotype h in controls. The total similarity measure in cases is similarly defined as

$$S_{\text{case}} = \sum_h \sum_{h'} p_h p_{h'} M_{hh'},$$

where p_h is the frequency of haplotype h in cases.

To compare the haplotype similarity patterns between cases and controls, we can define the test statistic

$$T = |\widehat{S}_{\text{case}} - \widehat{S}_{\text{control}}|,$$

where $\widehat{S}_{\text{control}}$ and $\widehat{S}_{\text{case}}$ are the estimates of S_{control} and S_{case}, obtained by plugging in the estimated haplotype frequencies $\widehat{p}_h, \widehat{q}_h$ in S_{case} and S_{control}, respectively. The significance of T can be evaluated by a permutation method. Specifically, one can permute the case and control labels N times. Each time, the haplotype frequencies are estimated and the permuted versions of $\widehat{S}_{\text{control}}, \widehat{S}_{\text{case}}$ and the test statistic T are calculated. Let the N tests be T_i, $i = 1, \ldots, N$. Then the p-value of the test T can be computed as the proportion of T_i, $i = 1, \ldots, N$ that exceeds the observed T. If the cases are thought to be more similar than the controls, then one can apply a one-sided test by defining $T = \widehat{S}_{\text{case}} - \widehat{S}_{\text{control}}$ and applying the same permutation procedure.

7.4 Linkage Disequilibrium Contrast Tests

LD is essential for genetic association studies. The extent of LD varies between cases and controls and the comparison of LD patterns between the two groups can provide insight into multi-locus associations. In order to compare LD coefficients between the two groups, the haplotype frequencies within each group need to be estimated but the HWE assumption may be problematic. A different approach is to contrast the LD patterns based on the composite LD coefficient, application of which does not require estimating haplotype frequencies and does not rely on HWE. We discuss two methods of doing this in Sect. 7.4.1 and Sect. 7.4.2.

7.4.1 Composite LD Measure

For two loci with alleles A, a and B, b, the LD coefficient is given by

$$D_{AB} = p_{AB} - p_A p_B,$$

where p_{AB} is the frequency of haplotype AB and p_A and p_B are the frequencies of alleles A and B. Estimating the LD coefficient involves estimating haplotype frequency p_{AB} from genotype data under the HWE assumption. A composite measure of LD, which is the sum of the LD coefficient and a non-gametic LD coefficient, was proposed as a substitute of the LD coefficient. The alleles A and B at two loci can associate in an individual either by being together on the same haplotype (gametic) or by being together on the different (maternal and paternal) haplotypes (non-gametic). The non-gametic LD coefficient represents the inter-locus allelic dependence on the two haplotypes. Estimation of the composite measure does not require phase information and can therefore be appropriately estimated from observed unphased genotypes without the assumption of HWE.

Table 7.5 Probabilities of genotypes

	BB	Bb	bb	Total
AA	P^{AB}_{AB}	P^{AB}_{Ab}	P^{Ab}_{Ab}	P^A_A
Aa	P^{AB}_{aB}	$P^{AB}_{ab} + P^{Ab}_{aB}$	P^{Ab}_{ab}	P^A_a
aa	P^{aB}_{aB}	P^{aB}_{ab}	P^{ab}_{ab}	P^a_a
Total	P^B_B	P^B_b	P^b_b	1

Define the non-gametic LD coefficient as

$$D_{A/B} = p_{A/B} - p_A p_B,$$

where $p_{A/B}$ is the joint frequency of alleles A and B on a person's two different homologous chromosomes, indicted by the slash. The composite LD coefficient is then

$$\Delta_{AB} = D_{AB} + D_{A/B} = p_{AB} + p_{A/B} - 2p_A p_B.$$

The probabilities p_{AB} and $p_{A/B}$ cannot be separately estimated from counting genotypes without assuming HWE. However, the composite measure Δ_{AB} can be directly estimated from counting two-locus genotypes regardless of HWE.

We now show how the composite measure relates to the genotype frequencies. The genotype probabilities are given in Table 7.5, where $P^{h'}_h$ is the probability of the two haplotypes for an individual with the superscript and subscript representing haplotypes on the two homologous chromosomes, respectively. Then the haplotype frequencies can be written as

$$p_{AB} = P^{AB}_{AB} + \frac{1}{2}\left(P^{AB}_{Ab} + P^{AB}_{aB} + P^{AB}_{ab}\right),$$

$$p_{A/B} = P^{AB}_{AB} + \frac{1}{2}\left(P^{AB}_{Ab} + P^{AB}_{aB} + P^{Ab}_{aB}\right).$$

These probabilities are not estimable without assuming HWE. It can be shown that the composite LD coefficient can be written as

$$\Delta_{AB} = 2P^{AB}_{AB} + P^{AB}_{Ab} + P^{AB}_{aB} + \frac{1}{2}\left(P^{AB}_{ab} + P^{aB}_{Ab}\right) - 2p_A p_B.$$

Under HWE, it can be verified that $\Delta_{AB} = D_{AB}$ (Problem 7.6). Therefore, the composite LD measure is an extension of D_{AB}. Unlike D_{AB}, however, Δ_{AB} is a function of the genotype probabilities and allele probabilities in Table 7.5 and therefore can be directly estimated from the genotype counts. Using the data in Table 7.2, the

MLE of Δ_{AB} can be written as

$$\widehat{\Delta}_{AB} = \frac{2n_{11} + n_{12} + n_{21} + n_{22}/2}{n}$$
$$- 2\left(\frac{n_{1+} + n_{2+}/2}{n}\right)\left(\frac{n_{+1} + n_{+2}/2}{n}\right) \tag{7.18}$$

and, omitting high order terms, its variance is given by (see Weir [299])

$$\mathrm{Var}(\widehat{\Delta}_{AB}) \approx \{p_A(1 - p_A) + D_A\}\{p_B(1 - p_B) + D_B\}/n, \tag{7.19}$$

where $D_A = p_{AA} - p_A^2$ and $D_B = p_{BB} - p_B^2$ are the HWD coefficients at the two loci. To test $H_0 : \Delta_{AB} = 0$, we can apply the composite LD test

$$X_{\mathrm{CLD}}^2 = \widehat{\Delta}_{AB}^2 / \widehat{\mathrm{Var}}(\widehat{\Delta}_{AB}), \tag{7.20}$$

where $\widehat{\mathrm{Var}}(\widehat{\Delta}_{AB}) = \{\widehat{p}_A(1 - \widehat{p}_A) + \widehat{D}_A\}\{\widehat{p}_B(1 - \widehat{p}_B) + \widehat{D}_B\}/n$. This test has an asymptotic χ_1^2 distribution under H_0.

The composite LD measure is in fact half the covariance of the genotype scores at the two loci. Code genotypes AA, Aa, aa as scores $\xi = 2, 1, 0$ (the number of A alleles in a genotype at the first locus) and genotypes Bb, Bb, bb as scores $\eta = 2, 1, 0$ (the number of B alleles in a genotype at the second locus), and it can be shown that

$$\Delta_{AB} = \mathrm{Cov}(\xi, \eta)/2. \tag{7.21}$$

This fact can be verified as follows. Let ξ_1, η_1 be indicators of alleles A, B on one specific chromosome and ξ_2, η_2 of those on the other chromosome. Then

$$\mathrm{E}(\xi_1\eta_1) = \mathrm{E}(\xi_2\eta_2) = p_{AB}, \qquad \mathrm{E}(\xi_1\eta_2) = \mathrm{E}(\xi_1\eta_2) = p_{A/B},$$

and $\mathrm{E}(\xi_1) = \mathrm{E}(\xi_2) = p_A$, $\mathrm{E}(\eta_1) = \mathrm{E}(\eta_2) = p_B$. Therefore,

$$D_{AB} = \mathrm{Cov}(\xi_1, \eta_1) = \mathrm{Cov}(\xi_2, \eta_2),$$
$$D_{A/B} = \mathrm{Cov}(\xi_1, \eta_2) = \mathrm{Cov}(\xi_2, \eta_1).$$

Then, we have

$$\mathrm{Cov}(\xi, \eta) = \mathrm{E}(\xi_1\eta_1) + \mathrm{E}(\xi_2\eta_2) + \mathrm{E}(\xi_1\eta_2) + E(\xi_2\eta_1)$$
$$- \{\mathrm{E}(\xi_1) + \mathrm{E}(\xi_2)\}\{\mathrm{E}(\eta_1) + \mathrm{E}(\eta_2)\}$$
$$= 2p_{AB} + 2p_{A/B} - 4p_A p_B = 2\Delta_{AB}.$$

Furthermore, $\mathrm{Var}(\xi) = \mathrm{Var}(\xi_1 + \xi_2) = \mathrm{Var}(\xi_1) + \mathrm{Var}(\xi_2) + 2\,\mathrm{Cov}(\xi_1, \xi_2) = 2(p_A - p_A^2 + D_A)$ and $\mathrm{Var}(\xi) = 2(p_B - p_B^2 + D_B)$. Therefore, the correlation coefficient

$$r_{AB} = \frac{\mathrm{Cov}(\xi, \eta)}{\sqrt{\mathrm{Var}(\xi)\mathrm{Var}(\xi)}} = \frac{\Delta_{AB}}{\sqrt{(p_A - p_A^2 + D_A)(p_B - p_B^2 + D_B)}}.$$

Denote the sample correlation coefficient by $\widehat{r}_{AB}$. Then the LD test given in (7.20) can be written as

$$X_{\mathrm{CLD}}^2 = n(\widehat{r}_{AB})^2.$$

Table 7.6 Two-locus genotype counts for cases and controls

	Case			Total		Control			Total
	BB	*Bb*	*bb*			*BB*	*Bb*	*bb*	
AA	r_{11}	r_{12}	r_{13}	r_{1+}	*AA*	s_{11}	s_{12}	s_{13}	s_{1+}
Aa	r_{21}	r_{22}	r_{23}	r_{2+}	*Aa*	s_{21}	s_{22}	s_{23}	s_{2+}
aa	r_{31}	r_{32}	r_{33}	r_{3+}	*aa*	s_{31}	s_{32}	s_{33}	s_{3+}
Total	r_{+1}	r_{+2}	r_{+3}	r	Total	s_{+1}	s_{+2}	s_{+3}	s

7.4.2 Contrasting LD Measures

The LD contrast test for testing association between the disease and the two loci can be written as

$$X^2 = \frac{(\widehat{D}_1 - \widehat{D}_0)^2}{\widehat{\mathrm{Var}}(\widehat{D}_1 - \widehat{D}_0)}, \tag{7.22}$$

where $\widehat{D}_1$ and $\widehat{D}_0$ are the estimated LD coefficients of the cases and controls, respectively,

$$\widehat{\mathrm{Var}}(\widehat{D}_1 - \widehat{D}_0)$$
$$= \left(\frac{1}{2r} + \frac{1}{2s}\right)\{\widehat{p}_A(1 - \widehat{p}_A)\widehat{p}_B(1 - \widehat{p}_B) + (1 - 2\widehat{p}_A)(1 - 2\widehat{p}_B)\widehat{D}_{AB} - \widehat{D}_{AB}^2\}$$

is the estimated variance of the LD difference under the null hypothesis, where r and s are the numbers of cases and controls. The LD coefficients can be estimated from haplotype frequency estimates obtained from the EM algorithm. However, since HWE is assumed to hold in cases and controls in the maximum likelihood approach, which would not be expected to hold for a case-control sampling design, the above LD contrast test is biased. A different method is to contrast the composite LD measures between cases and controls.

Suppose the genotype counts for cases and controls are as given in Table 7.6 with a total of $n = r + s$ individuals. Let the composite LD coefficients for cases and controls be $\widehat{\Delta}_1$ and $\widehat{\Delta}_0$, respectively. Then

$$\widehat{\Delta}_1 = \frac{2r_{11} + r_{12} + r_{21} + r_{22}/2}{r} - 2\left(\frac{r_{1+} + r_{2+}/2}{r}\right)\left(\frac{r_{+1} + r_{+2}/2}{r}\right),$$
$$\widehat{\Delta}_0 = \frac{2s_{11} + s_{12} + s_{21} + s_{22}/2}{s} - 2\left(\frac{s_{1+} + s_{2+}/2}{s}\right)\left(\frac{s_{+1} + s_{+2}/2}{s}\right).$$

The composite LD contrast test can then be defined as follows

$$X_{\mathrm{CLDC}}^2 = \frac{rs}{n} \frac{(\widehat{\Delta}_1 - \widehat{\Delta}_0)^2}{\{\widehat{p}_A(1 - \widehat{p}_A) + \widehat{D}_A\}\{\widehat{p}_B(1 - \widehat{p}_B) + \widehat{D}_B\}}, \tag{7.23}$$

where the estimated allele frequencies $\widehat{p}_A$, $\widehat{p}_B$ and HWD coefficients $\widehat{D}_A, \widehat{D}_B$ are calculated under the null hypothesis H_0 of no association from the pooled sample $n_{ij} = r_{ij} + s_{ij}$, $i = 1, 2, 3$ and $j = 1, 2, 3$. Thus, $\widehat{p}_A = (n_{1+} + n_{2+}/2)/n$,

Table 7.7 Observed counts at the R990G (A) and A986S (B) loci in the CASR gene in the disease population (reproduced from Hamilton and Cole [113])

	BB	Bb	bb	Total
AA	109	50	10	169
Aa	34	4	0	38
aa	14	0	0	14
Total	157	54	10	221

$\widehat{p}_B = (n_{+1}+n_{+2}/2)/n$, $\widehat{D}_A = n_{1+}/n - \widehat{p}_A^2$, $\widehat{D}_B = n_{+1}/n - \widehat{p}_B^2$. Under H_0, X_{CLDC}^2 follows χ_1^2 asymptotically.

7.5 Examples

Example 1 We use a two-locus real dataset to illustrate the use of the EM algorithm. Table 7.7 shows the genotype counts for the 9 genotype combinations.

Starting from the initial values $p_{AB} = p_{Ab} = p_{aB} = p_{ab} = 0.25$, the unobserved quantities x and y can be predicted from (7.1) as $x = 4p_{AB}p_{ab}/(p_{AB}p_{ab} + p_{Ab}p_{aB}) = 2$ and $y = 2$. Plugging these values into (7.2), we have $p_{AB} = (2 \times 109 + 50 + 34 + x)/442 = 0.68778$, $p_{Ab} = (50 + 2 \times 10 + y + 0)/442 = 0.16290$, $p_{aB} = (34 + y + 2 \times 14 + 0)/442 = 0.14480$, $p_{ab} = 1 - p_1 - p_2 - p_3 = 0.00452$, which are the updated estimates of the haplotype frequencies. Calculating the expected values using (7.1), we obtain the new predictions $x = 4p_{AB}p_{ab}/(p_{AB}p_{ab} + p_{Ab}p_{aB}) = 0.46579$ and $y = 3.53421$, which are again plugged into (7.2) to obtain the updated estimates $p_{AB} = 0.68431$, $p_{Ab} = 0.16637$, $p_{aB} = 0.14827$, $p_{ab} = 0.00105$.

After repeating the above procedure 5 times, the haplotype frequencies converge to $\widehat{p}_{AB} = 0.6833$, $\widehat{p}_{Ab} = 0.1674$, $\widehat{p}_{aB} = 0.1493$, and $\widehat{p}_{ab} = 0$.

Example 2 We compute the LD coefficients using the same dataset as in Example 1. Clearly, $\widehat{D}_{AB} = 0$ and $\widehat{D}'_{AB} = 0$, since $\widehat{p}_{bb} = 0$. Using the formula in (7.18) and the variance formula, we have $\widehat{\Delta}_{AB} = -0.0409$ and its standard error $\sqrt{\mathrm{Var}(\widehat{\Delta}_{AB})} = 0.011$. The chi-squared test for $H_0 : \Delta_{AB} = 0$ is $X_{\mathrm{CLD}}^2 = 14.08$, which indicates high significance of LD.

7.6 Bibliographical Comments

The haplotype is an important concept and has been widely recognized as a useful tool in dissecting the genetic basis of complex diseases (The International HapMap Consortium [268, 269]). Although molecular haplotyping methods do exist (Michalatos-Beloin et al. [183], Eitan and Kashi [69], Hurley et al. [128], Konfortov et al. [149]), they are costly and are only applicable for obtaining phase information of haplotypes with short lengths. Therefore, in most population-based association analysis, the phase information is usually unknown to the researchers and the available data are unphased genotypes. There have been many methods in haplotype inference and haplotype-based association analysis. Niu [197] presented a comprehensive review of algorithms for inferring haplotypes from genotype data, and Liu et al. [174]. comprehensively reviewed methods for haplotype analysis.

Based on unphased genotype data, many efforts have been made to recover haplotypes or to estimate haplotype frequencies. The earliest phasing algorithm is Clark's parsimony method (Clark [37]), which resolves the minimum number of haplotypes that can explain the observed genotype data. The combinatorial algorithms were also investigated and improved by many researchers. Gusfield [110] showed that the parsimony algorithm can be cast into the framework of a maximum resolution (MR) problem and can be solved by an integer linear programming method. Gusfield [111] proposed an alternative combinatorial algorithm, the pure-parsimony method, which minimizes the number of haplotypes that can resolve all genotypes. It was shown that for a small dataset, say with less than 50 individuals and 30 SNPs, the pure-parsimony approach correctly infers 80–95% of the haplotype pairs. Brown and Harrower [22, 23] improved the efficiency of the Inductive Logic Programming (ILP) algorithm by including additional constraints.

The EM algorithm is a powerful method for finding MLEs with incomplete data (Dempster et al. [58]). Under the assumption of HWE, Excoffier and Slatkin [80], Hawley and Kidd [119], and Long et al. [175] proposed the EM algorithm for finding the MLEs of haplotype frequencies using unphased genotypes. Although HWE is assumed in the EM algorithm, Niu et al. [196] showed that its performance is not strongly affected by departures from HWE, particularly when the direction of departure is towards an excess of homozygosity. One drawback of the EM algorithm is that it may converge to a local maximum and different choices of initial values of the parameters may lead to different converged values. To avoid trapping at a local maximum, one useful strategy is to try different initial values of haplotype frequencies, another way is to use a stochastic-EM algorithm (Tregouët et al. [274]). For pooled DNA data, Ito et al. [130], Wang et al. [290], and Yang et al. [312] studied the EM algorithm for haplotype inference. The EM algorithm is computationally inefficient when the number of individuals in each pool is large. Zhang et al. [322] and Kuk et al. [154] proposed an approximate EM algorithm for estimating haplotype frequencies from large DNA pools. Generally, the EM-based methods are computationally infeasible when the number of loci is relatively large (say, greater than 15 to 20), even for unpooled data. Niu et al. [196] and Qin et al. [209] used a divide-and-conquer-combine algorithm, the partition-ligation (PL) method, to handle a large number of loci. Bayesian methods have been studied in haplotype inference. Stephens et al. [257, 258] proposed the coalescence-based Markov Chain Monte Carlo (MCMC) method using a pseudo-Gibbs sampler, and Niu et al. [196] proposed a prior annealing and partition-ligation (PL) strategy to handle a large number of loci. Xing et al. [307] proposed a method based on a nonparametric prior known as the Dirichlet process.

LD is a fundamental concept in genetic studies. Reviews of various measures of LD or gametic phase disequilibrium can be found in Devlin and Risch [59],

Jorde [138], McVean [182], Li [171]. Empirical studies have shown that the human genome demonstrates a blocklike LD structure (Daly et al. [54], Gabriel et al. [93] etc.). Wall and Pritchard [287] proposed haplotype block models aimed at capturing the underlying LD structure. Within a haplotype block, the LD coefficients are high and there may be only a few haplotypes that can occur. Consequently, tight LD information may be captured by a subset of haplotype-tagging SNPs (htSNPs) (Johnson et al. [132]). Zhang et al. [320], Stram et al. [263] proposed the certainty measure R_h^2 for each haplotype h when only a subset of SNPs are used; the subset of SNPs that maximizes the minimum certainty measures of all haplotypes comprises the htSNPs. Ke and Cardon [141], and Sebastiani et al. [237] investigated different methods for tagging haplotypes.

Haplotype-based association analysis needs to take account of the phase uncertainty. An intuitive approach is to separate the analysis into two stages: at the first stage the most likely haplotype pair for each individual is recovered, and at the second stage cases and controls are compared using these deduced haplotypes. This approach may substantially lose information and the results may be seriously biased (Schaid [229, 230]). A more powerful approach is to estimate haplotype frequencies and their effects simultaneously by introducing a regression model. Prospective likelihood methods based on logistic regression or generalized linear models (GLM) are investigated by Zaykin et al. [318], Schaid et al. [229] and others. These methods treat unobserved haplotypes as covariates in a regression model and compute the conditional expectation of the covariates given genotype observations under the null hypothesis with a HWE assumption in the pooled sample of cases and controls. Zhao et al. [328] proposed a prospective estimating equation approach that only requires HWE in control samples. Stram et al. [262] investigated the bias incurred by applying prospective likelihood methods in a case-control design and introducing the HWE assumption, and developed an approach incorporating the sampling proportions of case and control samples. To account for sample ascertainment, retrospective likelihood inference can be applied in studying haplotype-disease association in a case-control design. Epstein and Satten [78], Satten and Epstein [224], and Spinka et al. [256] investigated retrospective likelihood inferences of haplotype association. To guard against deviation from HWE, Satten and Epstein [224] introduced a fixation index to account for departure from HWE. In Sect. 7.3.2, we introduced the retrospective regression method of Epstein and Satten [78] and Satten and Epstein [224], but we have used an approximation to the Fisher information matrix for all parameters by using the Score function. Lin and Zeng [173] fully investigated the GLM haplotype regression models for various study designs, in which environmental factors can also be included. Zhang et al. [321] studied the haplotype-based regression method for a matched case-control design. To overcome the high-dimensionality problem in haplotype-association analysis, Tzeng et al. [276, 277] proposed to cluster similar haplotypes and thereby increase the power of haplotype-based association tests. They derived the variance estimate of the difference of counting measures of haplotype similarity between case and control groups, and proposed the following z-test $z = (\widehat{S}_{\text{case}} - \widehat{S}_{\text{control}})/\sqrt{\widehat{\text{var}}(S_{\text{case}}) + \widehat{\text{var}}(S_{\text{control}})}$, which has a standard normal distribution under the null hypothesis. For other similarity measures, bootstrap or a permutation method was recommended.

Contrasting LD patterns between cases and controls can be more powerful than the haplotype-based or single-locus approached. Abecasis and Cookson [2] provided a graphical representation method for contrasting pairwise LD matrices between cases and control. Nielsen et al. [194] proposed a LD contrasting method for two diallelic loci when phase is known. For unphased genotype data, most algorithms estimate haplotype frequencies by assuming HWE, which produces biased estimates and thus comparison of LD coefficients between cases and controls using the EM algorithm is not strictly appropriate. Alternatively, the composite LD measure (Weir [298], Weir and Cockerham [300]) had been used in contrasting LD. The composite LD coefficients can be directly estimated from genotype counts without requiring the HWE assumption. Weir [299] presented the MLE of the composite LD coefficient and its variance. Zaykin et al. [319] and Wang et al. [292] proposed association tests based on contrasting LD matrices between cases and controls. Nielsen et al. [194] investigated a two-SNP situation and found that a test comparing LD coefficients can be more powerful than a single-locus or a haplotype test and this is a promising addition to existing methods of characterizing multi-locus associations.

7.7 Problems

7.1 For the two-locus data shown in Table 7.2, verify that under the HWE assumption the likelihood function (7.4) is

$$L(\mathbf{p}) = (p_1^2)^{n_{11}} (2p_1 p_2)^{n_{12}} (p_2^2)^{n_{13}} (2p_1 p_3)^{n_{21}} (2p_1 p_4 + 2p_2 p_3)^{n_{22}} (2p_2 p_4)^{n_{23}}$$
$$\times (p_3^2)^{n_{31}} (2p_2 p_4)^{n_{32}} (p_4^2)^{n_{33}},$$

where $p_1 = p_{AB}$, $p_2 = p_{Ab}$, $p_3 = p_{aB}$, $p_4 = p_{ab}$ are haplotype frequencies, and the complete likelihood function (7.5) is

$$L_c(\mathbf{p}) = (p_1^2)^{n_{11}} (2p_1 p_2)^{n_{12}} (p_2^2)^{n_{13}} (2p_1 p_3)^{n_{21}} (2p_1 p_4)^{x} (2p_2 p_3)^{n_{22}-x} (2p_2 p_4)^{n_{23}}$$
$$\times (p_3^2)^{n_{31}} (2p_2 p_4)^{n_{32}} (p_4^2)^{n_{33}},$$

where x is the (unobserved) number of haplotype pairs $\{AB, ab\}$ among the n_{22} individuals with genotype combination (Aa, Bb).

7.2 For the dataset given in Table 7.7:

1) Starting from the initial values $p_{AB} = p_{Ab} = 0.2$, $p_{aB} = p_{ab} = 0.3$, use the algorithm in (7.1) and (7.2) to compute the MLEs of the haplotype frequencies.
2) Using the likelihood function given in Problem 7.1, verify that the log-likelihood function calculated within each iteration always increases.
3) Use the Newton-Raphson algorithm to maximize the likelihood function and compare with the results from the EM algorithm.

7.3 For two diallelic loci with alleles A, a and B, b, respectively, assuming HWE, show that the probability that an individual has haplotype pair $\{h, h'\} = \{AB, ab\}$ conditional on observing genotypes $G_1 = Aa$, $G_2 = Bb$ is given by

Table 7.8 Two-locus genotype data

	Case				Control		
	BB	*Bb*	*bb*		*BB*	*Bb*	*bb*
AA	51	42	8	*AA*	50	47	8
Aa	40	46	0	*Aa*	36	29	10
aa	5	0	13	*aa*	7	13	0

$$P(h = AB, h' = ab | G_1 = Aa, G_2 = Bb) = \frac{p_{AB} p_{ab}}{p_{AB} p_{ab} + p_{Ab} p_{aB}}.$$

7.4 Prove Eq. (7.11).

7.5 Prove Eq. (7.10) (hint: $\mathrm{E}(\widehat{\delta}_h) = \mathrm{E}\{\mathrm{E}(\delta_h | G)\} = \mathrm{E}(\delta_h)$, $\mathrm{E}(\widehat{\delta}_h \delta_h) = \mathrm{E}(\widehat{\delta}_h \times \mathrm{E}(\delta_h | G)) = \mathrm{E}(\widehat{\delta}_h^2))$.

7.6 Prove that $\Delta_{AB} = D_{AB}$ when HWE holds (hint: when HWE holds, $P_h^{h'} = 2 p_h p_{h'}$ for $h \neq h'$ and $P_h^h = p_h^2$).

7.7 Verify that the MLE $\widehat{\Delta}_{AB}$ of the composite LD measure is given by (7.18) and, using the Delta method, prove that the variance of $\widehat{\Delta}_{AB}$ is as presented in (7.19).

7.8 Use the composite LD contrast test (7.23) to analyze the dataset in Table 7.8.

Chapter 8
Gene-Gene Interactions

Abstract Chapter 8 discusses gene-gene interactions. The focus is on two-locus interactions. Different genetic models are incorporated in the two-locus models. The expressions of odds ratios for the main genetic effects and the gene-gene interaction are given. A saturated logistic regression model is also studied. Different test statistics for the two-locus interaction model are discussed. Their relation to contrasting log-odds ratios and contrasting LD measures are given. Their relation to the log-linear model is also discussed. For higher order gene-gene interactions, the multifactor dimensionality reduction method and logic regression are briefly discussed.

Gene-gene interaction plays an important role in dissecting complex diseases. It is known that for complex diseases a single gene may have a small or moderate effect and that multiple genes and/or environmental factors may act jointly, known as interaction or epistasis, to have a large effect on a disease. This chapter introduces some methods for analysis of gene-gene interactions. Gene-environment interactions will be discussed in Chap. 10.

In a statistical sense, gene-gene interaction describes the non-additivity of single-factor effects on the distribution of a response variable. Additivity of factors $\mathbf{x} = (x_1, \ldots, x_k)^T$ on a response variable y refers to

$$h(\mathrm{E}(y|x)) = \alpha + \beta^T \mathbf{x},$$

for some link function h, e.g., for a normal distribution model $h(u) = u$, the identity function, and for a logistic regression model $h(u) = \mathrm{logit}(u) = \log\{u/(1 - u)\}$. Existence of gene-gene interaction can be expressed as the deviation $\gamma(\mathbf{x})$ from the additivity model:

$$h(\mathrm{E}(y|x)) = \alpha + \beta^T \mathbf{x} + \gamma(\mathbf{x}),$$

where $\gamma(\mathbf{x})$ is nonlinear in $\mathbf{x}$, capturing interactions of the genetic factors, and the elements of β are known as main effects.

When the number of loci is small, the logistic regression model is an appropriate approach for the analysis of gene-gene interaction. Two-locus association analysis using a logistic regression model will be discussed in Sect. 8.1. However, when many loci and their interactions are considered, the classical statistical modeling approach may lack power due to high dimensionality of the covariates and many data

G. Zheng et al., *Analysis of Genetic Association Studies*,
Statistics for Biology and Health,
DOI 10.1007/978-1-4614-2245-7_8, © Springer Science+Business Media, LLC 2012

mining and machine learning approaches have been proposed. These include the restricted logistic regression approach, in which the number of regression parameters is reduced by restrictions on the effects, such as the logic regression method, and the combinatorial partitioning approach such as the multifactor dimensional reduction (MDR). Section 8.2 introduces the logic regression and MDR methods.

This chapter also introduces some statistical characterizations of gene-gene interaction effects, mainly for the two-locus case. We show that the gene-gene interaction effect can be regarded as a quantification of a differential inter-locus dependence structure between cases and controls, followed by some brief discussion on tests for detecting the existence of gene-gene interactions. Section 8.3 discusses a representation of some gene-gene interaction effects in a logistic regression model, then several gene-gene interaction tests contrasting dependence measures between cases and controls are discussed. It should be noted that the gene-gene interactions that we consider in this chapter are statistical interactions rather than biological interactions.

8.1 Two-Locus Association Analysis with Interactions

8.1.1 Saturated Logistic Regression Model

In order to apply a logistic regression model to analyze gene-gene interaction using case-control data, the genotypes of two loci and their interaction are added into the regression model as covariates. For three genotypes at a single locus, if there is no scientific knowledge about the underlying genetic model, two indicator (dummy) variables are often used to code the genotypes. Denote the genotypes of the first locus $G^{(1)}$ as $(G_0^{(1)}, G_1^{(1)}, G_2^{(1)}) = (aa, aA, AA)$ and of the second locus $G^{(2)}$ as $(G_0^{(2)}, G_1^{(2)}, G_2^{(2)}) = (bb, bB, BB)$. Code genotype $G^{(i)}$ as $c(G^{(i)}) = (I_{i1}, I_{i2})^T$, where $I_{i1} = I_{i2} = 0$ if $G^{(i)} = G_0^{(i)}$, $I_{i1} = 1$ and $I_{i2} = 0$ if $G^{(i)} = G_1^{(i)}$, and $I_{i1} = I_{i2} = 1$ if $G^{(i)} = G_2^{(i)}$, where $i = 1, 2$. The gene-gene interaction $G^{(1)} \times G^{(2)}$ is coded by $c(G^{(1)} \times G^{(2)}) = (I_{11}I_{21}, I_{11}I_{22}, I_{12}I_{21}, I_{12}I_{22})^T$.

Let $f = \Pr(\text{case}|G^{(1)}, G^{(2)})$ be a penetrance given the genotypes of the two loci. Then, the logistic regression model can be represented as

$$
\begin{aligned}
\text{logit}(f) &= \alpha_0 + \alpha_1 I_{11} + \alpha_2 I_{12} + \beta_1 I_{21} + \beta_2 I_{22} \\
&\quad + \gamma_{11} I_{11} I_{21} + \gamma_{12} I_{11} I_{22} + \gamma_{21} I_{12} I_{21} + \gamma_{22} I_{12} I_{22} \\
&= \alpha_0 + \alpha^T c(G^{(1)}) + \beta^T c(G^{(2)}) + \gamma^T c(G^{(1)} \times G^{(2)}),
\end{aligned} \tag{8.1}
$$

where $\alpha = (\alpha_1, \alpha_2)^T$ is the main effect for the first locus, $\beta = (\beta_1, \beta_2)^T$ is the main effect for the second locus, and $\gamma = (\gamma_{11}, \gamma_{12}, \gamma_{21}, \gamma_{22})^T$ is the interaction effect of the two loci.

If we are interested in detecting any main or interaction effects, we can test a global null hypothesis $H_0 : \alpha_1 = \alpha_2 = \beta_1 = \beta_2 = \gamma_{11} = \gamma_{12} = \gamma_{21} = \gamma_{22} = 0$. On the other hand, if the interaction alone is of interest, we can test $H_0 : \gamma_{11} = \gamma_{12} =

Table 8.1 Two-locus genotype counts for cases (controls)

Case (control)	bb	Bb	BB	Total
aa	R_{00} (S_{00})	R_{01} (S_{01})	R_{02} (S_{02})	$R_{0\cdot}$ ($S_{0\cdot}$)
Aa	R_{10} (S_{10})	R_{11} (S_{11})	R_{12} (S_{12})	$R_{1\cdot}$ ($S_{1\cdot}$)
AA	R_{20} (S_{20})	R_{21} (S_{21})	R_{22} (S_{22})	$R_{2\cdot}$ ($S_{2\cdot}$)
Total	$R_{\cdot 0}$ ($S_{\cdot 0}$)	$R_{\cdot 1}$ ($S_{\cdot 1}$)	$R_{\cdot 2}$ ($S_{\cdot 2}$)	r (s)

Table 8.2 ORs for a general two-locus model

ORs	bb	Bb	BB
aa	1	$\exp(\beta^T c_{\cdot 1})$	$\exp(\beta^T c_{\cdot 2})$
Aa	$\exp(\alpha^T c_{1\cdot})$	$\exp(\alpha^T c_{1\cdot} + \beta^T c_{\cdot 1} + \gamma^T c_{11})$	$\exp(\alpha^T c_{1\cdot} + \beta^T c_{\cdot 2} + \gamma^T c_{12})$
AA	$\exp(\alpha^T c_{2\cdot})$	$\exp(\alpha^T c_{2\cdot} + \beta^T c_{\cdot 1} + \gamma^T c_{21})$	$\exp(\alpha^T c_{2\cdot} + \beta^T c_{\cdot 2} + \gamma^T c_{22})$

$\gamma_{21} = \gamma_{22} = 0$. The LRT, Score test and Wald test can be used to test either H_0. The three tests are asymptotically equivalent and follow an asymptotic chi-squared distribution with 8 degrees of freedom for a global H_0, or with 4 degrees of freedom for only the gene-gene interaction. Note that the Score test is in fact Pearson's chi-squared test, which compares the nine two-locus genotype counts (cell counts R_{ij} and S_{ij} in Table 8.1) between cases and controls. More details are given later.

Rewrite the penetrance f in (8.1) as

$$p_1(G_i, G_j) = \Pr(\text{case} \,|\, G^{(1)} = G_i^{(1)}, G^{(2)} = G_j^{(2)})$$

and $p_0(G_i, G_j) = 1 - p_1(G_i, G_j)$. From model (8.1), we have

$$\exp(\alpha_i) = \left\{ \frac{p_1(G_i, G_0)}{p_0(G_i, G_0)} \right\} \Big/ \left\{ \frac{p_1(G_{i-1}, G_0)}{p_0(G_{i-1}, G_0)} \right\}, \tag{8.2}$$

$$\exp(\beta_i) = \left\{ \frac{p_1(G_0, G_i)}{p_0(G_0, G_i)} \right\} \Big/ \left\{ \frac{p_1(G_0, G_{i-1})}{p_0(G_0, G_{i-1})} \right\}, \tag{8.3}$$

$$\exp(\gamma^T c_{ij}) = \frac{\{\frac{p_1(G_i, G_j)}{p_0(G_i, G_j)}\} / \{\frac{p_1(G_0, G_0)}{p_0(G_0, G_0)}\}}{\exp(\alpha^T c_{i\cdot} + \beta^T c_{\cdot j})}, \tag{8.4}$$

where $c_{i\cdot} = c(G^{(1)})$ when $G^{(1)} = G_i^{(1)}$, $c_{\cdot j} = c(G^{(2)})$ when $G^{(2)} = G_j^{(2)}$, and $c_{ij} = c(G^{(1)}, G^{(2)})$ when $G^{(1)} = G_i^{(1)}$ and $G^{(2)} = G_j^{(2)}$. In (8.4), $\exp(\alpha^T c_{i\cdot})$ is the OR of $G^{(1)} = G_i^{(1)}$ over $G^{(1)} = G_0^{(1)} = aa$ given $G^{(2)} = G_0^{(2)} = bb$, and $\exp(\beta^T c_{\cdot i})$ is the OR of $G^{(2)} = G_i^{(2)}$ over $G^{(2)} = G_0^{(2)} = bb$ given $G^{(1)} = G_0^{(1)} = aa$. The numerator of (8.4) is the OR of $(G^{(1)}, G^{(2)}) = (G_i^{(1)}, G_j^{(2)})$ over $(G^{(1)}, G^{(2)}) = (G_0^{(1)}, G_0^{(2)}) = (aa, bb)$. The ORs of association for the two-locus model are given in Table 8.2.

Table 8.3 ORs for the two-locus model with the main effects of two loci coded by $(0, x, 1)$ and $(0, y, 1)$ and the gene-gene interaction effect coded by $(0, x, y, 1)$

ORs	bb	Bb	BB
aa	1	$\exp(y\beta)$	$\exp(\beta)$
Aa	$\exp(x\alpha)$	$\exp(x\alpha + y\beta + xy\gamma)$	$\exp(x\alpha + \beta + x\gamma)$
AA	$\exp(\alpha)$	$\exp(\alpha + y\beta + y\gamma)$	$\exp(\alpha + \beta + \gamma)$

8.1.2 Incorporating Two-Locus Genetic Models

The ORs and models can be simplified if genetic models, e.g., REC, ADD/MUL or DOM, can be incorporated into the framework of logistic regression models by appropriately assigning scores to two-locus genotype combinations. We consider a general model by coding the genotypes of two loci treating the genotypes as ordinal. First, we code genotypes differently from those used in Sect. 8.1.1. If the genotypes at both loci are ordinal, we code $c(G^{(1)}) = x_i$ if $G^{(1)} = G_i^{(1)}$ $(i = 0, 1, 2)$, $c(G^{(2)}) = y_j$ if $G^{(2)} = G_j^{(2)}$ $(j = 0, 1, 2)$, and $c(G^{(1)} \times G^{(2)}) = z_{ij}$ for $(G^{(1)}, G^{(2)}) = (G_i^{(1)}, G_j^{(2)})$ $(i, j = 0, 1, 2)$. For comparison, without a genetic model, $G^{(1)}$ and $G^{(2)}$ are coded with two indicator variables, respectively. $\mathbf{x} = (x_0, x_1, x_2)$, $\mathbf{y} = (y_0, y_1, y_2)$ and $\mathbf{z} = (z_{11}, z_{12}, z_{21}, z_{22})$ are the scores for the main and gene-gene interaction effects. Hence the logistic regression model with these specified scores can be written as

$$\mathrm{logit}(f) = \alpha_0 + \alpha c(G^{(1)}) + \beta c(G^{(2)}) + \gamma c(G^{(1)} \times G^{(2)}). \tag{8.5}$$

This model is much simpler than that given in (8.1), with only four scalar parameters $(\alpha_0, \alpha, \beta, \gamma)$. The null hypothesis of no gene-gene interaction can be written as a global null hypothesis $H_0 : \alpha = \beta = \gamma = 0$, or the gene-gene interaction only $H_0 : \gamma = 0$. The LRT, Score test, or Wald test derived from model (8.5) have an asymptotic chi-squared distribution with 3 degrees of freedom for a global null hypothesis or 1 degree of freedom for testing only the interaction. However, it requires specifying all the values of x_i, y_i and z_{ij}.

Choice of the scores relies on the underlying genetic model for each of the two loci as well as the two-locus interaction model, which, however, are usually unknown. Since linear transformations of the scores $\mathbf{x}$ and $\mathbf{y}$ do not affect the null hypothesis H_0 and test statistics (Problem 8.1), we can simply assume $(x_0, x_1, x_2) = (0, x, 1)$ and $(y_0, y_1, y_2) = (0, y, 1)$ for the main effects, where only x and y need to be specified. A simple choice of z_{ij} is $z_{ij} = x_i y_j$ so that $\mathbf{z} = (0, x, y, 1)$. The ORs corresponding to (8.5) with scores $\mathbf{x} = (0, x, 1)$, $\mathbf{y} = (0, y, 1)$ and $\mathbf{z} = (0, x, y, 1)$ are given in Table 8.3.

Some special two-locus models can be obtained from Table 8.3. For example, three two-locus models in the literature are (i) "MUL within and between loci", (ii) "two-locus interaction MUL effects", and (iii) "two-locus interaction threshold effects", which are present in Table 8.4. The MUL model is used in both (i) and (ii), while the DOM model is used in (iii). If we set $x = y = 1/2$, $\exp(x\alpha) = 1 + \delta_1$, $\exp(y\beta) = 1 + \delta_2$, and $\gamma = 0$, we obtain model (i), which has no gene-gene

Table 8.4 ORs for the three special two-locus genetic models

(i)	bb	Bb	BB
aa	1	$(1+\delta_2)$	$(1+\delta_2)^2$
Aa	$(1+\delta_1)$	$(1+\delta_1)(1+\delta_2)$	$(1+\delta_1)(1+\delta_2)^2$
AA	$(1+\delta_1)^2$	$(1+\delta_1)^2(1+\delta_2)$	$(1+\delta_1)^2(1+\delta_2)^2$

(ii)	bb	Bb	BB
aa	1	1	1
Aa	1	$(1+\delta)$	$(1+\delta)^2$
AA	1	$(1+\delta)^2$	$(1+\delta)^4$

(iii)	bb	Bb	BB
aa	1	1	1
Aa	1	$(1+\delta)$	$(1+\delta)$
AA	1	$(1+\delta)$	$(1+\delta)$

interaction. If we set $\alpha = \beta = 0$, $\exp(xy\gamma) = 1 + \delta$, and $x = y = 1/2$, we obtain model (ii), which has only gene-gene interaction effects (no main effects). If we set $\alpha = \beta = 0$, $\exp(xy\gamma) = 1 + \delta$, and $x = y = 1$, we obtain model (iii), which has only one gene-gene interaction effect. Other models similar to the three models presented in Table 8.4 can be obtained by choosing other values of x and y in Table 8.3 or by directly modifying the models in Table 8.4. For example, in Table 8.4 (ii), we can replace $(1+\delta)^2$ by $(1+2\delta)$ and $(1+\delta)^4$ by $(1+4\delta)$ to obtain a two-locus genetic model with "two-locus interaction ADD effects".

8.2 Association Analysis with Higher-Order Interactions

The logistic regression model (8.1) is easy to use for detecting association with lower-order interactions, but may lose power when higher-order interactions exist because a lot more parameters are involved in modeling higher-order interaction effects. There are generally two classes of approaches to overcome the curse of dimensionality. One is to reduce the number of parameters in a logistic regression model by assigning scores to the genotypes under proper genetic models, for example (8.5). However, since gene-gene interaction models are generally unknown, this approach is not robust to model misspecification and therefore subject to substantial power loss when the models are misspecified. Another approach is to use a machine learning method such as the tree method or a combinatorial partitioning method. Existing methods include the MDR, the combinatorial partitioning method, and the restricted partitioning method. The logic regression method in some sense combines the last two approaches. It reduces the dimensionality of the parameter space by introducing logical combinations of predictors, which are put into the framework of a logistic regression model. This section introduces the MDR method and the logic regression method.

8.2.1 Multifactor Dimensionality Reduction

Recognizing the limitation of the logistic regression method to deal with a large number of gene-gene interactions, the MDR approach was proposed in order to reduce the dimensionality of the multi-locus genotype space. The MDR approach is a model-free method and has been shown to have good power to identify high-order gene-gene interactions.

The central idea of the MDR is to collapse multi-locus genotypes with similar risks into a single factor for the purpose of reducing the dimensionality of the risk factors. For m loci each with 3 possible genotypes, there is a total of 3^m genotype combinations. Denote these genotype combinations by $G_1, \ldots, G_{3^m}$. Then the genotype counts in a case-control study can be summarized in a 2×3^m table. Let r_i and s_i be the genotype counts of G_i, $i = 1, 2, \ldots, 3^m$, for cases and controls, respectively. Let $f_i = r_i/s_i$. Note that f_i is an estimate of

$$\frac{\Pr(G_i \mid \text{case})}{\Pr(G_i \mid \text{control})} = \frac{\Pr(\text{case} \mid G_i)}{\Pr(\text{control} \mid G_i)} \times \frac{\Pr(\text{control})}{\Pr(\text{case})},$$

which is proportional to the odds (or risk) of disease, $\Pr(\text{case} \mid G_i)/\Pr(\text{control} \mid G_i)$. Define the genotype combinations (columns of the 2×3^m table) to be "high risk" if the ratio f_i exceeds some pre-specified threshold C (e.g., $C = r/s$), and "low-risk" otherwise. Then the "low-risk" columns and "high-risk" columns are separately collapsed, resulting in a 2×2 table. Hence the dimension of the risk factors (number of levels of genotype risk) is reduced from 3^m to 2. For the reduced table, the case:control ratio, $R_{2\times2}$, of the counts within the "high-risk" category can be computed as a measure of significance. An alternative approach is to apply Pearson's chi-squared statistic to the reduced table.

For example, for two diallelic loci with alleles A/a and B/b, respectively, there are nine genotype combinations (aa, bb), (aa, Bb), (aa, BB), (Aa, bb), (Aa, Bb), (Aa, BB), (AA, bb), (AA, Bb), (AA, BB), as shown in Table 8.1. Using two digits to represent each genotype, the first (second) digit counts the number of A (B) alleles in genotype G_1 (G_2). For example, (AA, Bb) is represented by 21 and (AA, BB) by 22. Then we can summarize the data in Table 8.1 into a 2×9 table (Table 8.5).

If, for example, we take the threshold as $C = r/s$, where r and s are the total numbers of cases and controls, and only f_{02}, f_{11}, f_{12} are greater than C, we then collapse genotypes 00, 11, 12 into a high-risk group and other genotypes into a low-risk group, leading to a 2×2 table (Table 8.6). The measure of association for this table is $R_{2\times2} = (R_{02} + R_{11} + R_{12})/(S_{02} + S_{11} + S_{12})$.

Table 8.5 Two-locus genotype counts

Genotype	00	01	**02**	10	**11**	**12**	20	21	22	Total
Case	R_{00}	R_{01}	$\mathbf{R_{02}}$	R_{10}	$\mathbf{R_{11}}$	$\mathbf{R_{12}}$	R_{20}	R_{21}	R_{22}	r
Control	S_{00}	S_{01}	$\mathbf{S_{02}}$	S_{10}	$\mathbf{S_{11}}$	$\mathbf{S_{12}}$	S_{20}	S_{21}	S_{22}	s
Risk ratio	f_{00}	f_{01}	$\mathbf{f_{02}}$	f_{10}	$\mathbf{f_{11}}$	$\mathbf{f_{12}}$	f_{20}	f_{21}	f_{22}	

Table 8.6 A collapsed 2×2 table with high-risk and low-risk groups

	High-risk	Low-risk	Total
Case	$\mathbf{R_{02} + R_{11} + R_{12}}$	$R_{00} + R_{01} + R_{10} + R_{20} + R_{21} + R_{22}$	r
Control	$\mathbf{S_{02} + S_{11} + S_{12}}$	$S_{00} + S_{01} + S_{10} + S_{20} + S_{21} + S_{22}$	s

The MDR method uses a K-fold cross-validation method to select the best subset of factors from a given set of M genetic factors. For example, a 10-fold cross-validation method randomly splits all samples into 10 sets of subsamples with the same or similar proportions of cases and controls as in the original samples. For each fold of cross-validation, we take one subsample (10%) as a testing dataset and the remaining nine subsamples (90%) as a training dataset. A total of 10 folds of cross-validations can be formed by taking each of the 10 subsamples as a testing dataset and the remaining nine subsamples as a training dataset.

In any fold of the cross-validation, for each subset of factors with size m ($m = 2, \ldots, M$), using only the training dataset, we collapse the 2×3^m table into a 2×2 table as described above. Then the m-factor collapsed table with the largest $R_{2 \times 2}$ is selected as the best m-factor model, which is used to calculate the prediction error on the testing dataset. For a balanced case-control design with the same number of cases and controls, we can simply predict the subjects with the "high-risk" factor as cases and the others as controls. This process is repeated 10 times, and the prediction errors are averaged. Finally, among all the best m-factor models ($m = 2, \ldots, M$), the one with the least averaged prediction error is selected as the final model or the MDR model. From the 10-fold cross-validations, in which the above process is repeated 10 times, the consistency of the selection of the final model across 10 cross-validations is recorded, which is defined as the number of times the same MDR model is identified in all 10 training datasets. The averaged cross-validation consistency measure over the 10 training datasets is reported. The significance of this averaged cross-validation consistency measure is evaluated by a permutation of the 10-fold cross-validations, and a p-value based on the permutation is used to assess the significance of the selected MDR model.

8.2.2 *Logic Regression*

Logic regression provides a way to search for high-order gene-gene interactions expressed as Boolean combinations of genetic variants that can best discriminate the case and control groups. We introduce briefly the logic regression method. Assuming that all covariates $\mathbf{X} = (X_1, \ldots, X_p)^T$ are binary, a logical expression (or Boolean expression) is a function of $X_1, \ldots, X_p$ with the logic operators *AND* ($\wedge$), *OR* ($\vee$) and *NOT* (c). For example, the logical expression

$$L = (X_1 \wedge X_2) \vee (X_3^c)$$

is 1 if and only if $X_1 = X_2 = 1$ or $X_3 = 0$. If X_1, X_2, X_3 are logical variables to denote homozygous genotypes at three loci, then $L = 1$ means "both loci 1 and 2 are homozygous or locus 3 is heterozygous". A single logical expression can be represented as a logic tree. Any logic tree can be obtained by simple operations such as growing branches, pruning branches, and substituting leaves (variables).

Figure 8.1 gives some examples, in which X_1^c is a branch and X_2 and X_3 are leaves. The initial logic tree $X_1^c \wedge (X_2 \vee X_3)$ is represented in (a) using diamonds. The covariates are indicated inside diamonds. If a diamond has dashed sides, it indicates the complement of the covariate inside the diamond, e.g. X_1^c and X_4^c. When the alternate operator $\wedge$ is used to replace $\vee$, the second logic tree (b) is obtained. Logic tree (c) is obtained by splitting the leaf X_3 to $X_3 \wedge X_4^c$. Logic tree (d) is obtained by pruning the branch X_1^c. Other operations not shown in Fig. 8.1 include "alternate a leaf", e.g. X_2 to X_2^c in $X_1^c \wedge (X_2^c \vee X_3)$; "grow a branch", e.g. X_4 in $X_1^c \wedge X_4 \wedge (X_2 \vee X_3)$; and "delete a leaf", e.g. $X_1^c \wedge X_2$, in which X_3 is deleted.

The logic regression method assumes that the linear predictors of a logistic regression model (or any other generalized linear model) are Boolean or logical combinations. A logic regression with one logical expression (or logic tree) is given by

$$\text{logit}(f) = \beta_0 + \beta_1 L. \tag{8.6}$$

The logic tree L can be selected adaptively by using the *simulated annealing algorithm*, which provides a stochastic search for an approximation of the global optimum in a large search space. In logic regression, the aim is to maximize the log-likelihood function specified by (8.6). The simulated annealing algorithm starts with $L = 0$. At each stage a new tree is selected at random among those that can be obtained by simple operations on the current tree. The new tree is accepted if it has a larger log-likelihood than the current one, otherwise it is accepted with a probability that depends on the difference of the current and the previous log-likelihoods and the stage of the algorithm. Allowing moving to a tree with a lower log-likelihood can avoid trapping around a local maximum. To overcome over-fitting, cross-validation or a permutation method can be used to control the sizes (number of leaves) of the trees.

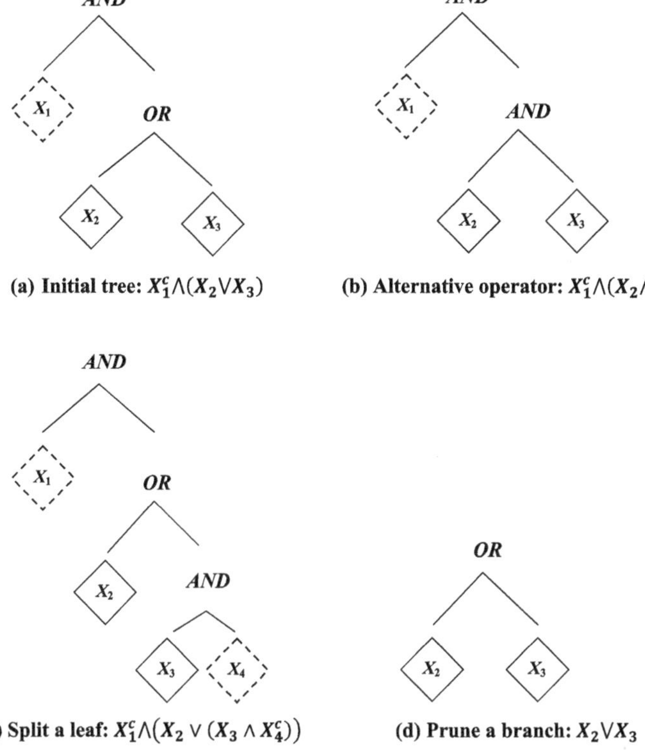

(a) Initial tree: $X_1^c \wedge (X_2 \vee X_3)$

(b) Alternative operator: $X_1^c \wedge (X_2 \wedge X_3)$

(c) Split a leaf: $X_1^c \wedge (X_2 \vee (X_3 \wedge X_4^c))$

(d) Prune a branch: $X_2 \vee X_3$

Fig. 8.1 Initial logic tree (**a**) $X_1^c \wedge (X_2 \vee X_3)$ with permissible moves to other logic trees: (**b**) $X_1^c \wedge (X_2 \wedge X_3)$ by using an alternate operator, (**c**) $X_1^c \wedge (X_2 \vee (X_3 \wedge X_4^c))$ by splitting a leaf, and (**d**) $X_2 \vee X_3$ by pruning a branch. A covariate is indicated inside a *diamond with dashed sides* to indicate the complement of the covariate inside

8.3 Test for Two-Locus Interactions

Testing the existence of a gene-gene interaction effect is important in association studies, especially when the marginal effects are small. Using the previous notation, the three genotypes (aa, aA, AA) of $G^{(1)}$ and (bb, bB, BB) of $G^{(2)}$ are denoted as $(G_0^{(1)}, G_1^{(1)}, G_2^{(1)})$ and $(G_0^{(2)}, G_1^{(2)}, G_2^{(2)})$, respectively. Let $f_{ij} = p_1(G_i^{(1)}, G_j^{(2)}) = \text{Pr}(\text{case}|G^{(1)} = G_i^{(1)}, G^{(2)} = G_j^{(2)})$ be the penetrance given in (8.1). Then the likelihood function using the data in Table 8.1 is given by

$$L(\theta) = L(\alpha_0, \alpha^T, \beta^T, \gamma^T) = \prod_{i,j} \{\text{logit}(f_{ij})\}^{r_{ij}} \{1 - \text{logit}(f_{ij})\}^{s_{ij}}, \qquad (8.7)$$

where $\theta = (\alpha_0, \alpha^T, \beta^T, \gamma^T)^T$. In some studies, only the gene-gene interaction is of interest. The null hypothesis is $H_0 : \gamma^T = 0$, i.e., $H_0 : \gamma_{11} = \gamma_{12} = \gamma_{21} = \gamma_{22} = 0$. The corresponding likelihood function under H_0 is

$$L_0(\theta) = L_0(\alpha_0, \alpha^T, \beta^T) = L(\alpha_0, \alpha^T, \beta^T, \gamma^T = 0), \qquad (8.8)$$

where $\theta = (\alpha_0, \alpha^T, \beta^T, 0)^T$. Let $\widehat{\theta} = (\widehat{\alpha}_0, \widehat{\alpha}^T, \widehat{\beta}^T, \widehat{\gamma}^T)^T$ and $\widetilde{\theta} = (\widetilde{\alpha}_0, \widetilde{\alpha}^T, \widetilde{\beta}^T, 0)^T$ be the MLEs that maximize the log-likelihood functions $l(\theta) = \log L(\theta)$ and $l_0(\theta) = \log L_0(\theta)$, respectively. Then they can be solved from

$$\partial l(\theta)/\partial\theta = 0 \quad \text{and}$$

$$\partial l_0(\theta)/\partial\theta = 0 \quad \text{or} \quad \partial l(\theta)/\partial\theta|_{H_0:\gamma^T=0} = 0. \tag{8.9}$$

Note that, in (8.9), $\theta = (\alpha_0, \alpha^T, \beta^T)^T$ in the first equation and $\theta = (\alpha_0, \alpha^T, \beta^T, \gamma^T)^T$ in the second equation. $\widehat{\theta}$ has a closed form solution but $\widetilde{\theta}$ does not, and has to be found numerically. We show an alternative simple approach to find $\widehat{\theta}$ in what follows.

From (8.2), (8.3) and (8.4), α^T, β^T and γ^T are all functions of ORs. Note that an OR under the retrospective distribution $\Pr(G|\text{disease status})$ is the same as that based on the prospective distribution $\Pr(\text{disease status}|G)$, for example,

$$\exp(\alpha_i) = \frac{\Pr(D = 1|G_i^{(1)}, G_0^{(2)})}{\Pr(D = 0|G_i^{(1)}, G_0^{(2)})} \bigg/ \frac{\Pr(D = 1|G_{i-1}^{(1)}, G_0^{(2)})}{\Pr(D = 0|G_{i-1}^{(1)}, G_0^{(2)})}$$

$$= \frac{\Pr(G_i^{(1)}, G_0^{(2)}|D = 1)}{\Pr(G_i^{(1)}, G_0^{(2)}|D = 0)} \bigg/ \frac{\Pr(G_{i-1}^{(1)}, G_0^{(2)}|D = 1)}{\Pr(G_{i-1}^{(1)}, G_0^{(2)}|D = 0)},$$

where $D = 1$ denotes cases and $D = 0$ controls. See also the discussion of ORs in Sect. 2.5.1. The probabilities in the latter expression for $\exp(\alpha_i)$ can be estimated easily using multinomial distributions and the data in Table 8.1 as follows. If we denote $p_{ij} = \Pr(G_i^{(1)}, G_j^{(2)}|D = 1)$ and $q_{ij} = \Pr(G_i^{(1)}, G_j^{(2)}|D = 0)$, then Table 8.7 gives all the probabilities for the observed genotype counts in Table 8.1. Then, using $(R_{ij}, i, j = 0, 1, 2) \sim Mul(r; p_{ij}, i, j = 0, 1, 2)$ and $(S_{ij}, i, j = 0, 1, 2) \sim Mul(s; q_{ij}, i, j = 0, 1, 2)$, the MLEs for p_{ij} and q_{ij} are $\widehat{p}_{ij} = R_{ij}/r$ and $\widehat{q}_{ij} = S_{ij}/s$. Thus,

$$\widehat{\alpha}_i = \log\left(\frac{R_{i0}S_{(i-1)0}}{S_{i0}R_{(i-1)0}}\right),$$

whose asymptotic variance can be obtained by the Delta method and the independence between R_{ij} and S_{ij}, and can thus be estimated by $\widehat{\text{Var}}(\widehat{\alpha}_i) = 1/R_{i0} + 1/S_{i0} + 1/S_{(i-1)0} + 1/R_{(i-1)0}$. Likewise,

$$\widehat{\beta}_i = \log\left(\frac{R_{0i}S_{0(i-1)}}{S_{0i}R_{0(i-1)}}\right),$$

$$\widehat{\text{Var}}(\widehat{\beta}_i) = 1/R_{0i} + 1/S_{0i} + 1/S_{0(i-1)} + 1/R_{0(i-1)}.$$

Denote $OR_{ij} = p_{ij}q_{00}/(q_{ij}p_{00})$. From Table 8.2, $\exp(\gamma^T c_{ij}) = OR_{ij}/\exp(\alpha^T c_{i\cdot} + \beta^T c_{\cdot j})$. Hence

$$\widehat{\gamma}^T c_{ij} = \log\left\{\frac{\widehat{OR}_{ij}}{\exp(\widehat{\alpha}^T c_{i\cdot} + \widehat{\beta}^T s c_{\cdot j})}\right\}.$$

An estimate of its asymptotic variance can be obtained by the Delta method (Problem 8.2). For α_0, we have $\widehat{\alpha}_0 = \widehat{p}_{00}/\widehat{q}_{00} = R_{00}/S_{00}$. Finally, the MLE $\widehat{\theta}$ and the

Table 8.7 Two-locus genotype probabilities for cases (controls)

Case (control)	bb	Bb	BB	Total
aa	$p_{00}\ (q_{00})$	$p_{01}\ (q_{01})$	$p_{02}\ (q_{02})$	$p_{0\cdot}\ (q_{0\cdot})$
Aa	$p_{10}\ (q_{10})$	$p_{11}\ (q_{11})$	$p_{12}\ (q_{12})$	$p_{1\cdot}\ (q_{1\cdot})$
AA	$p_{20}\ (q_{20})$	$p_{21}\ (q_{21})$	$p_{22}\ (q_{22})$	$p_{2\cdot}\ (q_{2\cdot})$
Total	$p_{\cdot 0}\ (q_{\cdot 0})$	$p_{\cdot 1}\ (q_{\cdot 1})$	$p_{\cdot 2}\ (q_{\cdot 2})$	$1\ (1)$

estimate of its asymptotic covariance matrix $\widehat{\mathrm{Var}}(\theta)$ can be obtained with closed forms (Problem 8.3). Further, we have asymptotically

$$\begin{bmatrix} \widehat{\alpha} \\ \widehat{\beta} \\ \widehat{\gamma} \end{bmatrix} - \begin{bmatrix} \alpha \\ \beta \\ \gamma \end{bmatrix} \approx N_8(0, \widehat{\Sigma})$$

in distribution, where $\widehat{\Sigma}$ is the estimate of the asymptotic covariance matrix and the dimension of $(\alpha^T, \beta^T, \gamma^T)^T$ is 8.

The above simple approach, however, cannot be used to find the MLE of θ under $H_0 : \gamma^T = 0$, which is $\widetilde{\theta}$, because $\gamma^T = 0$ places constraints on the probabilities p_{ij} and q_{ij}. For example, $\gamma_{11} = 0$ implies $\mathrm{OR}_{11} = \exp(\alpha_1 + \beta_1)$, that is, $p_{11}q_{10}q_{01}p_{00} = q_{11}p_{10}p_{01}q_{00}$. The usual MLEs of $\widehat{p}_{ij} = R_{ij}/r$ and $\widehat{q}_{ij} = S_{ij}/s$ do not necessarily satisfy this constraint. Hence, $\widetilde{\theta}$ is obtained numerically from (8.9).

To test $H_0 : \gamma^T = 0$, the LRT, Wald test and Score test with nuisance parameters can be applied (Sect. 1.2.4). The LRT is given by

$$\mathrm{LRT} = 2l(\widehat{\theta}) - 2l_0(\widetilde{\theta}). \tag{8.10}$$

Under H_0, it has an asymptotic χ_4^2 distribution. The Wald test is easier to use than the LRT because it only uses $\widehat{\theta}$ and $\widehat{\mathrm{Var}}(\widehat{\theta})$, not $\widetilde{\theta}$. To test the above H_0 using the Wald test, we decompose $\widehat{\mathrm{Var}}(\widehat{\theta})$ according to the parameter $\theta = (\alpha_0, \alpha^T, \beta^T, \gamma^T)^T$ as

$$\widehat{\mathrm{Var}}(\widehat{\theta}) = \begin{bmatrix} V_{\alpha_0\alpha_0} & V_{\alpha_0\alpha} & V_{\alpha_0\beta} & V_{\alpha_0\gamma} \\ V_{\alpha\alpha_0} & V_{\alpha\alpha} & V_{\alpha\beta} & V_{\alpha\gamma} \\ V_{\beta\alpha_0} & V_{\beta\alpha} & V_{\beta\beta} & V_{\beta\gamma} \\ V_{\gamma\alpha_0} & V_{\gamma\alpha} & V_{\gamma\beta} & V_{\gamma\gamma} \end{bmatrix}.$$

Then, under $H_0 : \gamma^T = 0$, from $\widehat{\gamma} \approx N_4(0, V_{\gamma\gamma})$, the Wald test is given by

$$\mathrm{WT} = \widehat{\gamma}^T V_{\gamma\gamma}^{-1} \widehat{\gamma} \sim \chi_4^2.$$

To derive the Score test for H_0, the Score function is given by

$$U(\widetilde{\theta}) = \frac{\partial l(\theta)}{\partial \gamma}\Big|_{\theta=\widetilde{\theta}}.$$

Compute the observed Fisher information matrix $i_n(\widetilde{\theta}) = -\partial^2 l(\theta)/\partial\theta\,\partial\theta^T|_{\theta=\widetilde{\theta}}$ and its inverse $i_n^{-1}(\widetilde{\theta})$. The 4×4 submatrix on the lower right diagonal of $i_n^{-1}(\widetilde{\theta})$ is denoted as $i^{\gamma\gamma}(\widetilde{\theta})$. Then the Score test is written as

$$ST = U(\widetilde{\theta})^T i^{\gamma\gamma}(\widetilde{\theta}) U(\widetilde{\theta}) \sim \chi_4^2 \quad \text{under } H_0.$$

The similar LRT, Wald test and Score test can also be derived for testing a global null hypothesis (Problem 8.4). Test statistics discussed above are derived under a general two-locus model. For some special models, e.g. a particular model in Table 8.3, these test statistics can also be derived (Problem 8.5).

8.3.1 A Representation of Two-Locus Interaction Effects

In this section, we first consider a representation of the two-locus interaction effects as the difference of inter-locus dependence measures between cases and controls using a logistic regression model. Then a general characterization of gene-gene interaction effects for the multi-locus situation is discussed. This motivates one to consider more general tests of gene-gene interactions by contrasting the dependence measures between case and control groups.

Using f_{ij}, p_{ij} and q_{ij} defined before and model (8.1), we have

$$\text{logit}(f_{ij}) = \alpha_0 + \alpha^T c_{i\cdot} + \beta^T c_{\cdot j} + \gamma^T c_{ij},$$

where $c_{i\cdot}$, $c_{\cdot j}$ and c_{ij} are given in Table 8.2. Denote $\Gamma_{ij} = \gamma^T c_{ij}$ for $i, j = 1, 2$. It follows that

$$\Gamma_{ij} = \log\left(\frac{p_{ij} p_{00}}{p_{i0} p_{0j}}\right) - \log\left(\frac{q_{ij} q_{00}}{q_{i0} q_{0j}}\right) = \log(\theta_{ij}) - \log(\psi_{ij}), \qquad (8.11)$$

where $\theta_{ij} = p_{ij} p_{00}/(p_{i0} p_{0j})$ is the OR of genotypes $(G_i^{(1)}, G_j^{(2)})$ relative to genotypes (aa, bb) among cases, and $\psi_{ij} = q_{ij} q_{00}/(q_{i0} q_{0j})$ is the OR of $(G_i^{(1)}, G_j^{(2)})$ relative to (aa, bb) among controls. These two quantities measure inter-locus dependence in the two groups. Equation (8.11) implies that, using logistic regression model (8.1), the gene-gene interaction effect can be represented as the difference of log-ORs between cases and controls.

8.3.2 Contrasting Log-Odds Ratios

Based on the representation (8.11), we can construct the Wald test for the gene-gene interaction effects, which is identical to the one obtained before. Note that $\Gamma_{ij} = 0$ for any i, j if and only if $\gamma = 0$. Thus, the gene-gene interaction can be tested under $H_0 : \Gamma_{ij} = 0$ for $i, j = 1, 2$.

Denote $\Gamma = (\Gamma_{11}, \Gamma_{12}, \Gamma_{21}, \Gamma_{22})^T$ and its MLE as $\widehat{\Gamma} = (\widehat{\Gamma}_{11}, \widehat{\Gamma}_{12}, \widehat{\Gamma}_{21}, \widehat{\Gamma}_{22})^T$, where

$$\widehat{\Gamma}_{ij} = \log\left(\frac{\widehat{p}_{ij}\,\widehat{p}_{00}}{\widehat{p}_{i0}\,\widehat{p}_{0j}}\right) - \log\left(\frac{\widehat{q}_{ij}\,\widehat{q}_{00}}{\widehat{q}_{i0}\,\widehat{q}_{0j}}\right) = \log(\widehat{\theta}_{ij}) - \log(\widehat{\psi}_{ij}),$$

and $\widehat{p}_{ij} = R_{ij}/r$ and $\widehat{q}_{ij} = S_{ij}/s$. By the Delta method, omitting the high order terms, the variances and covariances of $\widehat{\Gamma}_{ij}$, $i, j = 1, 2$, can be written as (Problem 8.1)

$$\mathrm{Cov}(\widehat{\Gamma}_{ij}, \widehat{\Gamma}_{kl}) = \begin{cases} \dfrac{1}{rp_{ij}} + \dfrac{1}{rp_{i0}} + \dfrac{1}{rp_{0j}} + \dfrac{1}{rp_{00}} \\ \qquad + \dfrac{1}{sq_{ij}} + \dfrac{1}{sq_{i0}} + \dfrac{1}{sq_{0j}} + \dfrac{1}{sq_{00}}, & \text{if } i = k, j = l \\[4pt] \dfrac{1}{rp_{00}} + \dfrac{1}{rp_{i0}} + \dfrac{1}{sq_{00}} + \dfrac{1}{sq_{i0}}, & \text{if } i = k, j \neq l \\[4pt] \dfrac{1}{rp_{00}} + \dfrac{1}{rp_{0j}} + \dfrac{1}{sq_{00}} + \dfrac{1}{Sq_{0j}}, & \text{if } i \neq k, j = l \\[4pt] \dfrac{1}{rp_{00}} + \dfrac{1}{sq_{00}}, & \text{if } i \neq k, j \neq l. \end{cases} \quad (8.12)$$

Denote the covariance matrix of $\widehat{\Gamma}$ as $\Sigma = \mathrm{Cov}(\widehat{\Gamma})$ and its estimate by $\widehat{\Sigma}$. Then the Wald test is given by

$$\mathrm{WT} = \widehat{\Gamma}^{T}\widehat{\Sigma}^{-1}\widehat{\Gamma} \sim \chi_4^2 \quad \text{under } H_0.$$

The LRT, Wald test, and Score test are asymptotically equivalent, but the Wald test has an advantage that it can be easily generalized to obtain more powerful tests by incorporating underlying genetic models. Consider a test $T_{\mathbf{a}} = \mathbf{a}^{T}\widehat{\Gamma}/(\mathbf{a}^{T}\widehat{\Sigma}\mathbf{a})^{1/2}$ for some prespecified weight vector $\mathbf{a}$. For a given $\mathbf{a}$, $T_{\mathbf{a}}^2$ has an asymptotic χ_1^2 and is presumably more powerful if the weight vector is properly constructed. Let $H = (c_{11}, c_{12}, c_{21}, c_{22})^{T}$. Thus, $\Gamma = H\gamma$ and H is given by

$$H = \begin{bmatrix} 1 & 0 & 0 & 0 \\ 1 & 1 & 0 & 0 \\ 1 & 0 & 1 & 0 \\ 1 & 1 & 1 & 1 \end{bmatrix}.$$

Then $\gamma = H^{-1}\Gamma$. If we construct a test based on $\mathbf{b}^{T}\gamma$ with the weight vector $\mathbf{b} = (xy, x, y, 1)^{T}$ corresponding to Table 8.3 and model (i), we can take $\mathbf{a} = (H^{T})^{-1}b$. Other weight vectors $\mathbf{b} = (1/4, 1/2, 1/2, 1)^{T}$ and $\mathbf{b} = (1, 1, 1, 1)^{T}$ can be used for models (ii) and (iii), respectively.

Another approach is to use maximum-type tests. Let $\mathbf{1}_k = (0, \ldots, 0, 1, 0, \ldots, 0)^{T}$ whose elements are 0 except for the kth position, which is 1 ($k = 1, 2, 3, 4$). Then, $T_{\mathrm{MAX}}^{(1)} = \max_{1 \le k \le 4} |T_{\mathbf{1}_k}|$. The weight vector $\mathbf{b} = (xy, x, y, 1)^{T}$ is a function of x and y, which may not be known in practice. Thus, we can consider $T_{\mathrm{MAX}}^{(2)} = \max_{0 \le x, y \le 1} |T_{\mathbf{b}}|$ or simply $T_{\mathrm{MAX}}^{(3)} = \max_{x, y = 0, 1/2, 1} |T_{\mathbf{b}}|$. These maximum tests are robust with respect to the weight vector. Using a single weight vector $\mathbf{a}$, test $T_{\mathbf{a}}$ is not robust when $\mathbf{a}$ is misspecified (cf. Sect. 6.3). The significance (p-value) of the three maximum tests can be assessed by a permutation method.

8.3.3 Relationship with the Log-Linear Model

The logistic regression model $\mathrm{logit}(f_{ij})$ can be linked to a log-linear model for the case and control genotype counts (r_{ij}, s_{ij}) given in Table 8.1. Let $c_{i\cdot}$, $c_{\cdot j}$ and c_{ij} be defined as before. Consider the following log-linear model for (r_{ij}, s_{ij}):

$$\log(q_{ij}) = \mu_0 + \tilde{\alpha}^T c_{i\cdot} + \tilde{\beta}^T c_{\cdot j} + \tilde{\gamma}^T c_{ij}, \tag{8.13}$$

$$\log(p_{ij}) = \mu_0 + \tilde{\alpha}^T c_{i\cdot} + \tilde{\beta}^T c_{\cdot j} + \tilde{\gamma}^T c_{ij} + \alpha_0 + \alpha^T c_{i\cdot} + \beta^T c_{\cdot j} + \gamma^T c_{ij}, \tag{8.14}$$

where p_{ij} and q_{ij} are given in Table 8.7. Equation (8.13) models the expected control genotype counts and Eq. (8.14) models the expected case genotype counts. From (8.14), we have

$$\log(p_{ij}) = \log(q_{ij}) + \alpha_0 + \alpha^T c_{i\cdot} + \beta^T c_{\cdot j} + \gamma^T c_{ij} = \log(q_{ij}) + \mathrm{logit}(f_{ij}).$$

Thus

$$\mathrm{logit}(f_{ij}) = \log(p_{ij}) - \log(q_{ij}). \tag{8.15}$$

Note that

$$\mathrm{logit}(f_{ij}) - \mathrm{logit}(f_{i0}) - \mathrm{logit}(f_{0j}) + \mathrm{logit}(f_{00}) = \gamma^T c_{ij} = \Gamma_{ij}.$$

Then, from (8.15),

$$\Gamma_{ij} = \log\left(\frac{p_{ij} p_{00}}{p_{i0} p_{0j}}\right) - \log\left(\frac{q_{ij} q_{00}}{q_{i0} q_{0j}}\right),$$

which is (8.11). Both the log-linear model and the logit model share the same parameters α, β and γ. However, the log-linear model can exploit the gene-gene independence or linkage equilibrium by setting $\tilde{\gamma}^T = 0$.

8.3.4 Contrasting LD Measures

We have discussed the LD contrast and composite LD contrast tests in Sect. 7.4. The two-locus representation (8.11) of the interaction effects enables us to view the two LD contrast tests (7.22) and (7.23) as two interaction tests. In addition to the LD contrast test discussed in Sect. 7.4, here we introduce interaction tests using other LD measures. We will show that the composite LD contrast test is in fact a test of comparing inter-locus covariances between cases and controls.

Let F be the inbreeding coefficient in cases. Then the probability of a case having the haplotype pair $\{h, h'\}$ is given by

$$P_h^{h'} = \begin{cases} p_h^2 + F p_h(1 - p_h), & h = h' \\ 2(1 - F) p_h p_{h'}, & h \neq h', \end{cases}$$

where p_h $(p_{h'})$ is the haplotype frequency of haplotype h (h') in cases. In controls, the probability having the haplotype pair is given by

$$Q_h^{h'} = q_h^2 I_{(h=h')} + 2q_h q_{h'} I_{(h \neq h')},$$

where q_h ($q_{h'}$) is the haplotype frequency of h (h') in controls. Define

$$d_1 = \frac{p_{AB} p_{ab}}{p_{Ab} p_{aB}}, \qquad d_0 = \frac{q_{AB} q_{ab}}{q_{Ab} q_{aB}},$$

for cases and controls, respectively, where $p_{AB}, p_{ab}, p_{Ab}, p_{aB}$ ($q_{AB}, q_{ab}, q_{Ab}, q_{aB}$) are two-locus haplotype frequencies in cases (controls). These two quantities are also measures of allele dependence or LD (see Eq. (7.8) in Sect. 7.2.1 where LD is measured by the difference of $p_{AB} p_{ab}$ and $p_{Ab} p_{aB}$, but here quotient is used).

Let $P_h^{h'}$ ($Q_h^{h'}$) be the probability of the haplotype pair $\{h, h'\}$ on the two homologous chromosomes for a case (control). From Table 7.5, we have the following representations of the interaction effects

$$
\begin{aligned}
\Gamma_{11} &= \log\left(\frac{(P_{ab}^{AB} + P_{aB}^{Ab}) P_{ab}^{ab}}{P_{ab}^{Ab} P_{ab}^{aB}}\right) - \log\left(\frac{(Q_{ab}^{AB} + Q_{aB}^{Ab}) Q_{ab}^{ab}}{Q_{ab}^{Ab} Q_{ab}^{aB}}\right) \\
&= \log\left(\frac{d_1 + 1}{2}\right) - \log\left(\frac{d_0 + 1}{2}\right) + O(F), \\
\Gamma_{12} &= \log\left(\frac{P_{aB}^{AB} P_{ab}^{ab}}{P_{ab}^{Ab} P_{aB}^{aB}}\right) - \log\left(\frac{Q_{aB}^{AB} Q_{ab}^{ab}}{Q_{ab}^{Ab} Q_{aB}^{aB}}\right) = \log(d_1) - \log(d_0) + O(F), \\
\Gamma_{21} &= \log\left(\frac{P_{Ab}^{AB} P_{ab}^{ab}}{P_{Ab}^{Ab} P_{ab}^{aB}}\right) - \log\left(\frac{Q_{Ab}^{AB} Q_{ab}^{ab}}{Q_{Ab}^{Ab} Q_{ab}^{aB}}\right) = \log(d_1) - \log(d_0) + O(F), \\
\Gamma_{22} &= \log\left(\frac{P_{AB}^{AB} P_{ab}^{ab}}{P_{Ab}^{Ab} P_{aB}^{aB}}\right) - \log\left(\frac{Q_{AB}^{AB} Q_{ab}^{ab}}{Q_{Ab}^{Ab} Q_{aB}^{aB}}\right) = 2\{\log(d_1) - \log(d_0)\} + O(F),
\end{aligned}
$$

where, in each expression, $O(F)$ contains the remaining terms and $O(F) = 0$ when $F = 0$. Because F is usually close to 0, all the interaction effects. Γ_{ij}, in the logistic regression model can be viewed as the difference of the LD coefficients d_1 and d_0 on the logarithmic scale. If, on the other hand, F is relatively large, then all the $O(F)$ terms cannot be omitted and the interaction effects measure the difference of the LD coefficients between cases and controls as well as the magnitude of the inbreeding coefficient. In this case, one should use the method contrasting log-ORs discussed in the previous section.

When $F \approx 0$, we can test for gene-gene interaction by using the following test

$$\chi^2 = \frac{\{\log(\widehat{d_1}) - \log(\widehat{d_0})\}^2}{\widehat{\text{Var}}\{\log(\widehat{d_1}) - \log(\widehat{d_0})\}},$$

where

$$\widehat{d_1} = \frac{\widehat{p}_{AB} \widehat{p}_{ab}}{\widehat{p}_{Ab} \widehat{p}_{aB}}, \qquad \widehat{d_0} = \frac{\widehat{q}_{AB} \widehat{q}_{ab}}{\widehat{q}_{Ab} \widehat{q}_{aB}},$$

and

$$\widehat{\text{Var}}\{\log(\widehat{d_1}) - \log(\widehat{d_0})\} = \frac{1}{\widehat{p}_{AB}} + \frac{1}{\widehat{p}_{Ab}} + \frac{1}{\widehat{p}_{aB}} + \frac{1}{\widehat{p}_{ab}} + \frac{1}{\widehat{q}_{AB}} + \frac{1}{\widehat{q}_{Ab}} + \frac{1}{\widehat{q}_{aB}} + \frac{1}{\widehat{q}_{ab}}.$$

This test is asymptotically equivalent to the LD contrast test given in (7.22) in Chap. 7 and, under the null hypothesis of no interaction, has a chi-squared distribution with 1 degree of freedom. But it has the same drawback as the LD contrast test that the haplotype frequencies need to be estimated separately for the cases and controls.

Alternatively, we can code the three genotypes at each locus as 0, 1, 2 by counting the minor alleles in the genotype, use the covariance between the two loci as a dependence measure, and contrast the covariances between cases and controls as a test of the gene-gene interaction (see Problem 8.7). Explicitly, let $(\xi_i^{(D)}, \eta_i^{(D)})$, $i = 1, 2, \ldots, n$ be the two-locus genotypes for all n individuals in group D ($D = 1$ for the case group and $D = 0$ for the control group). Then the sample covariances of the two loci are

$$\widehat{\Sigma}_D = \frac{1}{n-1} \sum_{i=1}^{n} (\xi_i^{(D)} - \bar{\xi}^{(D)})(\eta_i^{(D)} - \bar{\eta}^{(D)}), \quad D = 0, 1,$$

and the covariance contrast (CC) test is based on the Wald test

$$\chi_{CC}^2 = \frac{(\widehat{\Sigma}_1 - \widehat{\Sigma}_0)^2}{\widehat{\mathrm{Var}}(\widehat{\Sigma}_1) + \widehat{\mathrm{Var}}(\widehat{\Sigma}_0)}.$$

As we have noticed in Sect. 7.4.1, e.g. (7.21), the composite LD coefficient between two loci equals half the covariance, i.e., $\widehat{\Sigma}_D = 2\widehat{\Delta}_D$ and $\mathrm{Var}(\widehat{\Sigma}_D) = 4\,\mathrm{Var}(\widehat{\Delta}_D)$ for $D = 0, 1$. Thus, we have

$$\chi_{CC}^2 = \frac{(\widehat{\Delta}_1 - \widehat{\Delta}_0)^2}{\widehat{\mathrm{Var}}(\widehat{\Delta}_1) + \widehat{\mathrm{Var}}(\widehat{\Delta}_0)},$$

which is a composite LD contrast test. Therefore, contrasting covariances between cases and controls is equivalent to contrasting composite LD coefficients. Note that the margins of genotype counts in cases and controls in Table 7.6 use different notation from those in Table 8.1. In Table 7.6, for example, r_{1+} is used, but in Table 8.1, $r_{1.}$ is used. Using the notation in this chapter, we rewrite the composite LD contrast in (7.23) as follows:

$$\chi_{CC}^2 = \chi_{CLDC}^2 = \frac{rs}{n} \frac{(\widehat{\Delta}_1 - \widehat{\Delta}_0)^2}{\{\widehat{p}_A(1 - \widehat{p}_A) + \widehat{D}_A\}\{\widehat{p}_B(1 - \widehat{p}_B) + \widehat{D}_B\}},$$

where

$$\widehat{\Delta}_1 = \frac{2R_{22} + R_{21} + R_{12} + R_{11}/2}{r} - 2\left(\frac{R_{2.} + R_{1.}/2}{r}\right)\left(\frac{r_{.2} + r_{.1}/2}{r}\right),$$

$$\widehat{\Delta}_0 = \frac{2S_{22} + S_{21} + S_{12} + S_{11}/2}{s} - 2\left(\frac{S_{2.} + S_{1.}/2}{s}\right)\left(\frac{S_{.2} + S_{.1}/2}{s}\right),$$

$$\widehat{p}_A = (R_{2.} + S_{2.} + R_{1.}/2 + S_{1.}/2)/n,$$

$$\widehat{p}_B = (R_{.2} + S_{.2} + R_{.1}/2 + S_{.1}/2)/n,$$

$$\widehat{D}_A = (R_{2.} + S_{2.})/n - \widehat{p}_A^2,$$

$$\widehat{D}_B = (R_{.2} + S_{.2})/n - \widehat{p}_B^2.$$

Under the null hypothesis of no gene-gene interaction, $\chi^2_{\rm CC} = \chi^2_{\rm CLDC}$ and both follow χ^2_1 asymptotically under H_0.

8.3.5 Test for Second-Order Interactions for Multiple Loci

The gene-gene interaction effects can be treated as the difference of inter-locus dependence measures between cases and controls. The existence of gene-gene interactions can be tested using contrasting LD matrices, composite LD matrices, or any other dependence measures between cases and controls.

We illustrate the use of composite LD matrices for m loci. Let Ψ_1 and Ψ_0 be the composite LD matrices for cases and controls, respectively. They are half the variance-covariance matrices of genotypes when the genotypes are coded as 0, 1, 2 for the three genotypes at all loci. We can construct tests based on the contrasting matrices through $\Psi_1 \Psi_0^{-1}$ as follows

$$T = g(\Psi_1 \Psi_0^{-1}),$$

where typical choices of g function include the trace $g(A) = {\rm tr}(A)$, the determinant $g(A) = \det(A)$, or the largest eigenvalue $g(A) = \lambda_{\max}(A)$. Significance of T with these choices of g can be assessed by a permutation method. However, these tests may not be powerful since only eigenvalues are involved.

Note that any difference between Ψ_1 and Ψ_0 can be captured by the difference in the direction of the eigenvectors and the difference in their magnitudes (i.e., eigenvalues). Based on this observation, a test to contrast the first l principal components of the two matrices has been proposed, which compares the directions of the l principal vectors

$$Z_1 = {\rm tr}(E_1 E_1^T E_0 E_0^T),$$

where E_1 and E_0 are the matrices of the first l eigenvectors in cases and controls, respectively. It can be shown that Z_1 is the sum of squares of all pairwise inner products of the eigenvectors in E_1 and E_0. For example, if $l = 1$, $Z_1 = (E_1^T E_0)^2$. Another test is to compare the magnitudes of $\Psi_1 - \Psi_0$:

$$Z_2 = {\rm tr}\{(\Psi_1 - \Psi_0)^T (\Psi_1 - \Psi_0)\}.$$

These two tests can be used to test for gene-gene interactions among the m loci, and their significances (p-values) may be assessed by a permutation procedure.

8.3.6 Representation of Higher-Order Interactions

In a case-control study, let $\mathbf{x} = (x_1, \ldots, x_m)^T$ denote m binary genetic factors. For example, in an m-locus SNP study, $\mathbf{x}$ contains the indicator functions for presence of minor alleles on all m loci. Assume the distributions of $\mathbf{x}$ among cases ($D = 1$) and among controls ($D = 0$) are $f_1(\mathbf{x})$ and $f_0(\mathbf{x})$, respectively, i.e., $\mathbf{x}|_{D=1} \sim f_1(\mathbf{x})$

and $\mathbf{x}|_{D=0} \sim f_0(\mathbf{x})$. It follows that

$$\Pr(D=1|\mathbf{x}) = \frac{f_1(\mathbf{x})k}{f_1(\mathbf{x})k + f_0(\mathbf{x})(1-k)} = \frac{\exp\{\alpha + l(\mathbf{x})\}}{1 + \exp\{\alpha + l(\mathbf{x})\}}, \tag{8.16}$$

where $k = \Pr(D=1)$ is the disease prevalence, $l(\mathbf{x}) = \log\{f_1(\mathbf{x})/f_0(\mathbf{x})\}$ is the log-likelihood ratio, and $\alpha = \log\{k/(1-k)\}$ is the baseline odds. Generally, the null hypothesis of no gene-gene interaction means that there is no quadratic term or higher-order term in the log-likelihood ratio, i.e.,

$$l(\mathbf{x}) = \log\{f_1(\mathbf{x})/f_0(\mathbf{x})\} = h(a^T\mathbf{x} + b)$$

for some function h.

Denote the ORs of (u, v) among cases $(D=1)$ and controls $(D=0)$ as

$$OR_{u,v|D=d} = \frac{\Pr(u=1, v=1|D=d)\Pr(u=0, v=0|D=d)}{\Pr(u=1, v=0|D=d)\Pr(u=0, v=1|D=d)},$$

where $d = 0, 1$. We have used log-linear models to represent gene-gene interactions in Sect. 8.3.3. The following representations generalize the results in Sect. 8.3.3. The distribution of $\mathbf{x}$ can be represented by the following log-linear model

$$f_1(\mathbf{x}) = \exp\left\{\alpha_0 + \sum \alpha_i x_i + \sum_{i<j} \alpha_{ij} x_i x_j + \cdots + \alpha_{12\ldots m} x_1 x_2 \cdots x_m\right\},$$

$$f_0(\mathbf{x}) = \exp\left\{\beta_0 + \sum \beta_i x_i + \sum_{i<j} \beta_{ij} x_i x_j + \cdots + \beta_{12\ldots m} x_1 x_2 \cdots x_m\right\},$$

where, for $k \geq 2$, $\alpha_{i_1 i_2 \ldots i_l}$ and $\beta_{i_1 i_2 \ldots i_l}$ are measures of l-order dependence of components of $\mathbf{x}$. For example, for $i < j$,

$$\exp(\alpha_{ij}) = OR_{x_i,x_j|y=1,x_k=0,k\neq i,j,D=1} \quad \text{and}$$

$$\exp(\beta_{ij}) = OR_{x_i,x_j|y=0,x_k=0,k\neq i,j,D=0}$$

are the ORs of (x_i, x_j) given that other variables x_k, $k \neq i, j$, are 0 in cases and controls respectively and, for $i < j < k$,

$$\exp(\alpha_{ijk}) = \frac{OR_{x_i,x_j|D=1,x_k=1,x_l=0,l\neq i,j,k}}{OR_{x_i,x_j|D=1,x_k=0,x_l=0,l\neq i,j,k}},$$

$$\exp(\beta_{ijk}) = \frac{OR_{x_i,x_j|D=0,x_k=1,x_l=0,l\neq i,j,k}}{OR_{x_i,x_j|D=0,x_k=0,x_l=0,l\neq i,j,k}}.$$

Therefore

$$l(\mathbf{x}) = \alpha_0 - \beta_0 + \sum (\alpha_j - \beta_j) x_j$$
$$+ \sum_{i<j} (\alpha_{ij} - \beta_{ij}) x_i x_j + \cdots + (\alpha_{12\ldots m} - \beta_{12\ldots m}) x_1 x_2 \ldots x_m.$$

It follows that

$$\Pr(D = 1|\mathbf{x})$$

$$= \frac{\exp(\gamma_0 + \sum_j \gamma_j x_j + \sum_{i<j} \gamma_{ij} x_i x_j + \cdots + \gamma_{12\ldots m} x_1 x_2 \ldots x_m)}{1 + \exp(\gamma_0 + \sum_j \gamma_j x_j + \sum_{i<j} \gamma_{ij} x_i x_j + \cdots + \gamma_{12\ldots m} x_1 x_2 \ldots x_m)},$$

$$(8.17)$$

where $\gamma_{i_1 i_2 \ldots i_l} = \alpha_{i_1 i_2 \ldots i_l} - \beta_{i_1 i_2 \ldots i_l}$.

From (8.17), if $\alpha_{i_1 i_2 \ldots i_l} = \beta_{i_1 i_2 \ldots i_l}$ for all subscripts $i_1, \ldots, i_l$ and all $k \geq 2$, there is no gene-gene interaction. On the other hand, if for some $l \geq 2$, $\alpha_{i_1 i_2 \ldots i_l} \neq \beta_{i_1 i_2 \ldots i_l}$, then there exists l-order gene-gene interaction. This implies that the difference of dependence parameters between cases and controls represents gene-gene interaction effects.

8.4 Bibliographical Comments

Search for genetic factors in the etiology of complex diseases is one of the central objectives in most GWAS (Hoh and Ott [122], Wang et al. [295], Cordell [44], and Casci [26]). Success of such investigations relies on efficiency of analysis strategies in discovering marginal effects as well as joint effects of several interacting genetic markers. Single-locus analysis is widely used in GWAS, but this strategy may overlook the genes that have strong joint effects but small marginal effects. Therefore, analysis for multi-locus gene-gene interactions along with gene-environment interactions, to be discussed in Chap. 10, has been increasingly employed in GWAS.

Association analysis that incorporates multi-locus gene-gene interactions can be done using logistic regression models, which, however, may lose power if the number of loci is large or the sample size is small. Even for the case of two-locus interactions, four parameters are needed in capturing the gene-gene interaction effects, so that the LRT, Wald test, or Pearson's chi-squared test are all 8-degree-of-freedom tests for a global null hypothesis of no association. To increase the power to detect gene-gene interactions, two-locus genetic models can be incorporated. The three two-locus models in Table 8.4 can be found in Marchini et al. [179]. Alternatively, constraints can be placed on the parameters to restrict the parameter space. Song and Nicolae [252] studied models with a restricted parameter space for testing interactions.

Another approach is to use the logic regression method, in which logical combinations of genetic factors is used to reduce the number of predictors (Ruczinski et al. [221], Schwender and Ickstadt [236], Kooperberg et al. [151]). The logic regression model discussed in Sect. 8.2.2 is based on Ruczinski et al. [221] and the logic expression of $X_1^c \wedge (X_2 \vee X_3)$ with permissible moves can be found in Kooperberg and Ruczinski [152]. Machine learning methods provide another useful approach, including the MDR (Ritchie et al. [216, 217]), the combinatorial partitioning method (Nelson et al. [194] and Culverhouse et al. [50]) and the tree method (Chen et al. [34]), to reduce the dimensionality of the parameter space. Machine learning methods are similar to logic regression models in searching for combinations of genetic variants, but the former are model-free and easier to implement. We only briefly discussed machine learning methods; much research has been done in this area recently [160, 176, 189, 201].

There is no consensus on how interaction of multiple factors should be defined. Cox [47] defines statistical interaction as a deviation from additivity of single-factor effects. Let f_1 and f_2 be the probability distribution functions of the response variable y under factors 1 and 2, respectively, and $f_2(y) = f_1(y - \tau)$, where τ is the difference of the effects of the two factors. If τ depends on the initial level y, say, $\tau = \tau(y)$, of the response, then this implies a form of interaction. Otherwise, interaction of the two factors is absent and the two distributions have the same shape. Since examination of distributional shape may not be efficient with limited sample size, a common strategy is to consider variance only, that is, if the two variances of response y under factors 1 and 2 are different, then there exists an interaction with f_1 and f_2. If there exists a variance stabilizing transform of the response variable such that the variances are equal under the two factors, then the interaction is said to be removable. If such a transform does not exist, then the interaction is non-removable, which is also called "essential interaction" (Scheffé [227] and Wu et al. [305]).

For a case-control study, association analysis often compares the genotype probability distributions between cases and controls. We show in Sect. 8.3.6 that gene-gene interaction effects using a logistic regression model can be treated as the difference between inter-locus log-ORs in cases and controls. Therefore, detection of gene-gene interaction effects can be done by contrasting inter-locus dependence measures between cases and controls. Contrasting log-ORs between cases and controls is equivalent to the testing of gene-gene interaction effects using a logistic regression model. This idea can be extended to contrast other dependence measures such as the LD coefficients or composite LD coefficients. Zhao et al. [327] proposed to detect gene-gene interactions by testing the LD coefficient to be zero for two unlinked loci in the case group only. They noticed that for two unlinked loci in the population, the LD coefficient can be regarded as zero and their test is in fact an LD contrast test. Methods of association analysis by contrasting LDs can be found in Nielsen et al. [194], Zaykin et al. [319], and Wang et al. [292]. In particular, the test Z_1 using the first several principal components of the two matrices Ψ_1 and Ψ_0 in Sect. 8.3.5 is due to Zaykin et al. [319].

The log-linear model for gene-gene interactions using the expected genotype counts of cases and controls in Sect. 8.3.3 was used by Umbach and Weinberg [278] for detecting gene-environment interactions. The methods for testing gene-gene interactions are similar to those for detecting gene-environment interactions, especially if the environment has three exposure levels (factors). In this chapter, we did not discuss Bayesian methods for detecting gene-gene interactions, some of which can be found in Zhang and Liu [324], Wakefield et al. [286] and Ferreira et al. [85]. Other references with general discussions of gene-gene interactions include Moore et al. [184] and Foulkes [89].

We have focused on a discussion of statistical methods and models for detecting gene-gene interaction, which is basically statistical interaction, rather than biological interaction. The latter only requires that both genes have an effect, whether or not there is statistical interaction. It the two marginal effects exist, there must be a biological interaction; in that case the only reason to test for statistical interaction would be to determine the best way to quantify the effects. Wang et al. [293] and Wang et al. [294] provide a good review of various gene-gene interactions, including gene-environment interactions which we will discuss in Chap. 10, and discuss further how to best describe biological interaction.

8.5 Problems

8.1 Show that linear transformations of $\mathbf{x}$ from (x_0, x_1, x_2) to $(0, (x_1 - x_0)/(x_2 - x_0), 1)$ and $\mathbf{y}$ from (y_0, y_1, y_2) to $(0, (y_1 - y_0)/(y_2 - y_0), 1)$ do not affect the outcome of inference using a logistic regression model (8.5).

8.2 Let $p_{ij} = \Pr(\text{case}|G^{(1)} = G_i^{(1)}, G^{(2)} = G_j^{(2)})$, $q_{ij} = 1 - p_{ij}$, $\gamma = (\gamma_{11}, \gamma_{12}, \gamma_{21}, \gamma_{22})^T$ be log ORs for gene-gene interactions.

1) Using the logistic regression model

$$\text{logit}(p_{ij}) = \alpha_0 + \alpha^T c_{i\cdot} + \beta^T c_{\cdot j} + \gamma^T c_{ij},$$

show that

$$\exp(\gamma^T c_{ij}) = \frac{p_{ij}\, q_{00}\, p_{(i-1)0}\, q_{i0}\, p_{0(j-1)}\, q_{0j}}{q_{ij}\, p_{00}\, q_{(i-1)0}\, p_{i0}\, q_{0(j-1)}\, p_{0j}}$$

and

$$\exp(\gamma_{11}) = \exp(\gamma^T c_{11}),$$
$$\exp(\gamma_{12}) = \exp(\gamma^T c_{12}) / \exp(\gamma^T c_{11}),$$
$$\exp(\gamma_{21}) = \exp(\gamma^T c_{21}) / \exp(\gamma^T c_{11}),$$
$$\exp(\gamma_{22}) = \frac{\exp(\gamma^T c_{22}) \exp(\gamma^T c_{11})}{\exp(\gamma^T c_{12}) \exp(\gamma^T c_{21})}.$$

2) Derive the asymptotic variances and covariances for $\exp(\widehat{\gamma}^T c_{ij})$, $i, j = 1, 2$, using the Delta method.

8.3 Let $l(\theta)$ be the log-likelihood of (8.7) and $\widehat{\theta}$ be the MLE. Derive

$$\widehat{\text{Var}}(\widehat{\theta}) \approx -\left\{ \frac{\partial^2 l(\theta)}{\partial \theta\, \partial \theta^T}\Big|_{\widehat{\theta}} \right\}^{-1}.$$

8.4 Derive the LRT, Wald test and Score test for $H_0 : \alpha^T = 0, \beta^T = 0, \gamma^T = 0$. Note that the Wald test can be directly obtained using $\widehat{\theta}$ and its asymptotic covariance matrix from Problem 8.3.

8.5 Derive the LRT, Wald test and Score test for no gene-gene interaction $H_0 : \gamma = 0$ (γ is a scalar parameter) based on the model in Table 8.3.

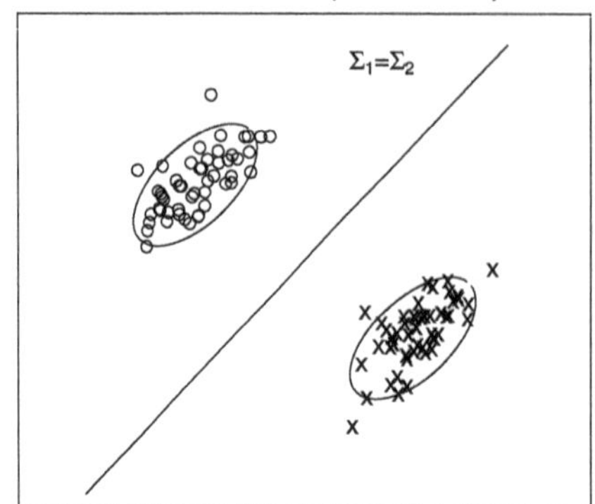

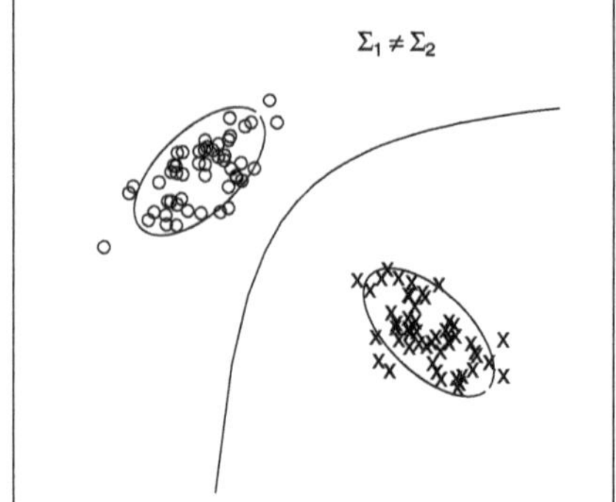

Fig. 8.2 Discriminating two normal populations

8.6 Derive the variance-covariance formulae in (8.12).

8.7 Interaction and quadratic discriminant function.

Suppose that $\mathbf{x}$ is a continuous random vector with $\mathbf{x}|_{D=1} \sim N(\mu_1, \Sigma_1)$ and $\mathbf{x}|_{D=0} \sim N(\mu_2, \Sigma_2)$. Use Eq. (8.16) to show that if $\Sigma_1 \neq \Sigma_2$, then there is an interaction using a logistic regression model and consequently, a quadratic discriminant function is needed to best discriminate between the two groups (see Fig. 8.2).

Part IV
Topics Related to Analysis of Case-Control Association

Chapter 9
Population Structure

Abstract Population stratification (PS) and correcting for PS are studied in Chap. 9. The chapter starts with an introduction to population structure and its impact on inference using the trend test. Different models of PS are given. Methods to correct for PS are discussed, including genomic control, structural association, principal component clustering , and multidimensional scaling plots. How to select marker loci to correct for PS is discussed. Comparison of the several methods is reported using simulations. How to simulate case-control data in the presence of PS is given.

In epidemiology studies aiming to establish the association between a disease and an exposure, confounding factors can often hinder establishing such an association correctly. Similarly, to test the association between a disease and a genetic variant in genetic epidemiology studies, confounding factors should be carefully addressed in order to infer a true association. The most important confounding factor in genetic epidemiology studies is the hidden population structure existing in a study sample (see Sect. 2.4). Such population structure often defines latent subpopulations, and allele (genotype) frequencies and disease prevalence may vary across the subpopulations and/or non-random mating may occur at the subpopulation level. Population structure can cause spurious association. If population structure is ignored in the analysis, association may be detected in a mixed population even if there is no association at the subpopulation level.

In this chapter, we begin with an introduction to population structure from a human genetics point of view, and a discussion of the effect of population structure in genetic association studies, followed by an introduction to methods for controlling the effect of population structure, including genomic control, association using STRUCTURE, principle components and clustering methods, and a multidimensional scaling method. Comparisons of some of these methods will also be discussed using simulations. Other methods will be briefly mentioned in the Bibliographical comments.

G. Zheng et al., *Analysis of Genetic Association Studies*,
Statistics for Biology and Health,
DOI 10.1007/978-1-4614-2245-7_9, © Springer Science+Business Media, LLC 2012

9.1 Population Structure

In humans, mating is often not random between subpopulations because of geographical and language barriers. As a result, the genetic variants have different allele frequencies across the subpopulations because of random drift. Such allele frequency differences at the subpopulation level result in population stratification. In contrast, genetic markers can be used to cluster a human population into subpopulations. The largest component of genetic structure in human populations falls along geographic/continental lines, as suggested by studies using either microsatellite markers or dense SNPs. It has been suggested that there are six major clusters detected by using genome-wide genetic markers. Among them are the five major geographic regions: Europeans/West Asians (whites), sub-Saharan Africans, East Asians, Pacific Islanders, and Native Americans. The correspondence between the self-reported racial/ethnic categories and the clusters defined by the genetic markers is near-perfect. Further studies using dense SNPs lead to similar conclusions, although the subpopulations often have mixed ancestries from major geographic regions. Figure 9.1 presents the worldwide human population structure based on 938 unrelated individuals from 51 populations analyzed using 650,000 SNPs. As suggested, mixed ancestries of the six founding populations can be observed for the samples from these 51 populations. Such mixed ancestry can be interpreted by either recent population admixture or shared ancestry before the divergence of two populations. A typical example of recent population admixture is provided by African Americans, whose admixture is mainly due to the recent admixture process between Africans and Europeans. In general, it has been consistently reported that African American genomes consist of around 80% African ancestry and 20% European ancestry, although much variation can be observed when samples are drawn from different regions in the United States. European Americans were usually considered as one homogenous population several years ago. With dense genetic markers available, population structure has been reported recently within European Americans, although such population structure is more difficult to detect than the population structure existing at the continental level. In fact, recent studies have clearly demonstrated that population structure can be detected among samples distanced by only several hundred kilometers.

Population subdivision results in inbreeding because the individuals in a subpopulation can share common ancestors even if random mating occurs in this subpopulation. Let F be Wright's inbreeding coefficient, which is defined as the reduction in heterozygosity expected in a population with random mating. Let p_i be the frequency of allele A_i in the population ($i = 1, 2$). The frequencies of genotypes are given by

$$\Pr(A_i A_j) = \begin{cases} F p_i + (1 - F) p_i^2 & \text{if } i = j \\ 2(1 - F) p_i p_j & \text{if } i < j. \end{cases} \tag{9.1}$$

In other words, population structure will result in HWD, or correlation of the two alleles in a genotype. Equation (9.1) can be used to describe either an inbreeding

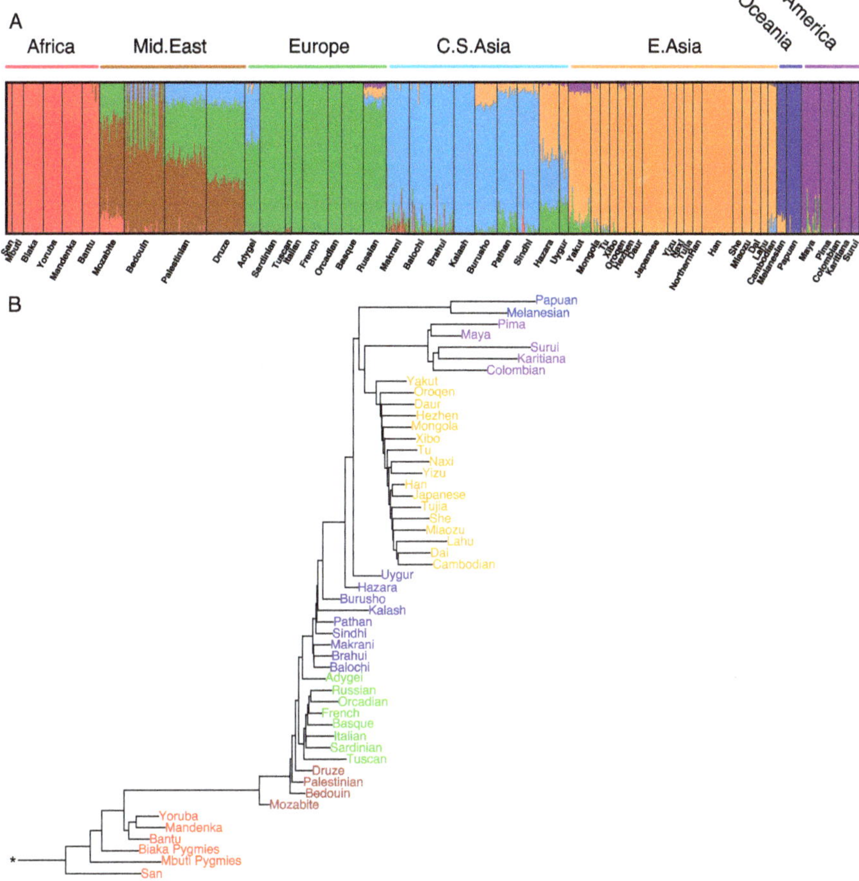

Fig. 9.1 Individual ancestry and a population dendrogram. (**A**) Region ancestry inferred by the frappe program. Each individual is represented by a vertical line. (**B**) Maximum likelihood tree of 51 populations (reproduced from Li et al. [166])

population or cryptic relatedness (Sect. 2.4). It can be shown that the correlation coefficient of the two alleles is F (Problem 9.1). Let X be the number of A alleles in an individual's genotype. Then $E(X) = 2p_1$, which is not dependent on F. However, the variance $\text{Var}(X) = 2p_1(1 - p_1)(1 + F)$ is inflated by a factor of $1 + F$, which is 1 when HWE holds ($F = 0$).

We consider population structure that arises from three models (Table 9.1): two models of population stratifications (PS-I and PS-II) and cryptic relatedness (CR), which can be described as follows. One population stratification (PS) model is denoted as PS-I, which does not require the disease prevalence to vary across the subpopulations. The other PS model, PS-II, requires both differential allele frequency and differential disease prevalence. Because PS is often hidden, it causes cases and controls to be sampled disproportionally with respect to the sizes of the subpopula-

Table 9.1 Population structure: population stratification (PS-I or PS-II) and cryptic relatedness (CR). J is the number of subpopulations

Population structure	At the subpopulation level			
	J	Allele frequency	Disease prevalence	HWE
PS-I	≥ 2	varies	–	Yes
PS-II	≥ 2	varies	varies	Yes
CR	1	–	–	No

tions. PS-II has more impact on the analysis of case-control data than PS-I. Thus, in the following, PS refers to PS-II. In PS, subpopulations are defined by a discrete variable with J distinct values. In the next section, we describe subpopulations that can be defined by a continuous variable. An admixed population is also denoted as PS, and then J refers to the number of discrete ancestral subpopulations. In both PS-I and PS-II, we assume HWE proportions hold in each subpopulation. On the other hand, HWE is not relevant if inference is genotype-based rather than allele-based. However, if we restrict attention to a single subpopulation, $F \neq 0$. This type of population structure is CR.

9.2 Impact of Population Stratification

9.2.1 A Model for Population Stratification

Because random mating may not be the case within the subpopulations, where culture is inherited as a result of different environmental effects, population structure can result in confounding effects in genetic association analysis. In Sect. 2.4, a simple model was introduced to describe the association between a genetic marker and a disease created by PS. Here we introduce a general population genetic model, which leads to spurious genotype-phenotype associations on account of PS.

Consider an association study in which individuals are sampled from a continuous geographical space Z, which is directly correlated with PS. We are interested in testing for association between a phenotype Y and a genotype G at a marker of interest. Suppose the phenotype is binary with $Y = 1$ as a case and 0 a control. We further assume that the genotype and phenotype of an individual are conditionally independent given that the individual is sampled at position $z \in Z$, that is, there is no direct or indirect association between Y and G for a fixed z. Mathematically, this is equivalent to

$$\Pr(G|z, Y = 1) = \Pr(G|z, Y = 0) = \Pr(G|z), \tag{9.2}$$

where $\Pr(G|z, Y = 1)$ and $\Pr(G|z, Y = 0)$ are the genotype frequencies at the point z for a case and a control, respectively, so the genotype and phenotype are independent conditional on the given region.

In an association study, we may not know where the cases and controls are sampled from. Thus, the null hypothesis H_0 can be written as

$$\Pr(G|Y = 1) = \Pr(G|Y = 0). \tag{9.3}$$

If H_0 is rejected based on (9.3) when (9.2) holds, the association is called spurious association. Note that if $z \in Z$ is a constant (both cases and controls are sampled from the same geographical region or from the same genetic background), (9.2) always guarantees (9.3) and spurious association will not occur.

To understand how spurious association can affect the analysis, we calculate the difference $\Delta = \Pr(G|Y=1) - \Pr(G|Y=0)$ when (9.2) holds. Let $\gamma(z)$ be the probability density function of sampling an individual at $z \in Z$. Denote the probability of observing Y at z as $\Pr(Y|z)$. Then the marginal distribution of Y is $\Pr(Y=y) = \int_z \Pr(Y=y|z)\gamma(z)dz$ for $y = 0, 1$. Using Bayes theorem,

$$\Pr(z|Y=y) = \frac{\Pr(Y=y|z)\gamma(z)}{\int_z \Pr(Y=y|z)\gamma(z)dz}. \tag{9.4}$$

Using (9.2) and (9.4), it can be shown that the difference Δ can be written as (Problem 9.2)

$$\Delta = \frac{\int_z \Pr(G|z)\Pr(Y=1|z)\gamma(z)dz - \{\int_z \Pr(Y=1|z)\gamma(z)dz\}\{\int_z \Pr(G|z)\gamma(z)dz\}}{\{\int_z \Pr(Y=1|z)\gamma(z)dz\}\{1 - \int_z \Pr(Y=1|z)\gamma(z)dz\}}, \tag{9.5}$$

which suggests that Δ is dependent on the sampling scheme $\gamma(z)$, and spurious association can occur if $\Pr(G|z)$ does not satisfy

$$\int_z \Pr(G|z)\Pr(Y=1|z)\gamma(z)dz = \left\{\int_z \Pr(Y=1|z)\gamma(z)dz\right\}\left\{\int_z \Pr(G|z)\gamma(z)dz\right\}.$$

In the above derivations, G stands for a genotype. The results still hold when G is an allele. In this case, the numerator in (9.5) is equivalent to the covariance between Y and G. Thus, (9.5) suggests that spurious associations can occur when Y and G are correlated with respect to the sampling scheme $\gamma(z)$.

The above results for a continuous Z can also be applied to a discrete population. Suppose that the space Z consists of J disjoint subpopulations denoted by $Z_1, Z_2, \ldots, Z_J$, respectively. The genotype frequency and disease prevalence are constant within the subpopulations, so that $\Pr(G|Z_j) = p_j$ and $\Pr(Y=1|Z_j) = k_j$, $j = 1, \ldots, J$. Denote $\gamma_j = \int_{Z_j} \gamma(z)dz$ with $\sum_{j=1}^J \gamma_j = 1$. Similar to (9.5), $\Delta_{\text{disc}} = \Pr(G|Y=1) - \Pr(G|Y=0)$ can be written as

$$\Delta_{\text{disc}} = \frac{\sum_{j=1}^J p_j k_j \gamma_j - (\sum_{j=1}^J k_j \gamma_j)(\sum_{j=1}^J k_j \gamma_j)}{(\sum_{j=1}^J k_j \gamma_j)(1 - \sum_{j=1}^J k_j \gamma_j)}.$$

Thus, there is no spurious association if and only if

$$\sum_{j=1}^J p_j k_j \gamma_j = \left(\sum_{j=1}^J p_j \gamma_j\right)\left(\sum_{j=1}^J k_j \gamma_j\right). \tag{9.6}$$

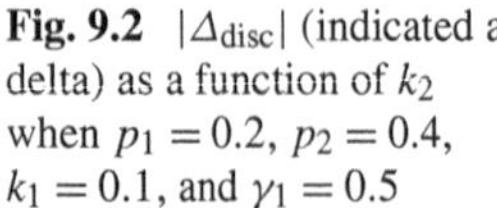

Fig. 9.2 $|\Delta_{\mathrm{disc}}|$ (indicated as delta) as a function of k_2 when $p_1 = 0.2$, $p_2 = 0.4$, $k_1 = 0.1$, and $\gamma_1 = 0.5$

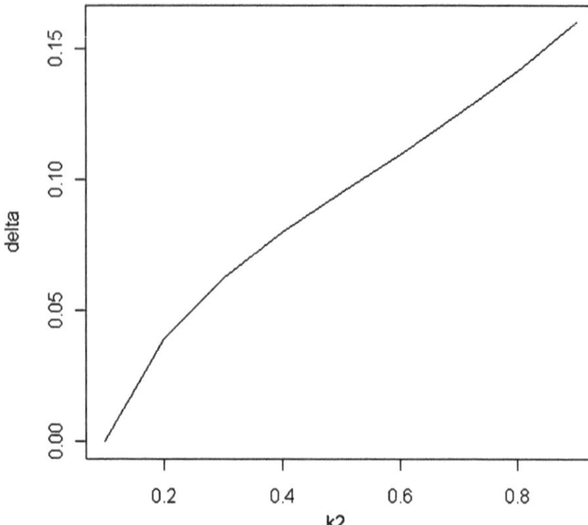

Fig. 9.3 $|\Delta_{\mathrm{disc}}|$ (indicated as delta) as a function of γ_1 (indicated as gamma1) when $p_1 = 0.2$, $p_2 = 0.4$, $k_1 = 0.1$, and $k_2 = 0.2$

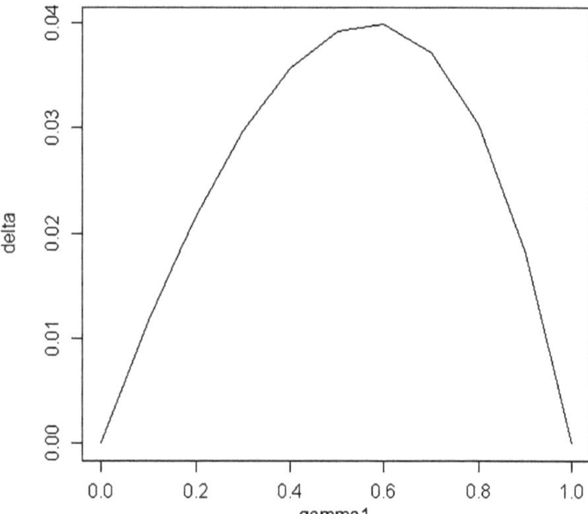

In the special case of $J = 2$, with $\gamma_1 \neq 0$ and $\gamma_2 \neq 0$, we have

$$(p_1 - p_2)(k_1 - k_2) = 0.$$

The above equation implies that, for $J = 2$, spurious association will occur if both genotypic frequency and disease prevalence vary across the subpopulations provided both subpopulations are sampled. For $J \geq 3$, varying allele genotype frequencies and disease prevalence across the subpopulations does not necessarily produce spurious association. For example, one may find values of p_i, k_i and γ_i that satisfy (9.6) for $J = 3$.

Table 9.2 Genotype counts of case-control samples for a single marker with alleles A and B. Genotypes are $(G_0, G_1, G_2) = (AA, AB, BB)$

	G_0	G_1	G_2	Total
Cases	r_0	r_1	r_2	r
Controls	s_0	s_1	s_2	s
Total	n_0	n_1	n_2	n

The absolute difference $|\Delta|$ or $|\Delta_{\mathrm{disc}}|$ can be used to measure the degree to which the null hypothesis is violated. From (9.4) and (9.6), the severity of the violation is dependent on the disease prevalence and allele (or genotype) frequencies in the subpopulations. For $J = 2$, Fig. 9.2 presents the relationship between $|\Delta_{\mathrm{disc}}|$ and the disease prevalence in the two subpopulations. It shows that the degree of violation increases as the difference of disease prevalence in the two subpopulations increases when the other parameters are fixed. The contribution of a subpopulation is presented in Fig. 9.3.

9.2.2 Impact on Trend Tests

The CATT (or the trend test) is commonly used to test association (Sect. 3.3). Let the case-control data at a diallelic marker be as displayed in Table 9.2.

The trend test can be in general written as a difference in weighted averages of the estimates of genotype frequencies between cases and controls

$$T_n = \sum_{i=0}^{2} \omega_i \widehat{p}_i - \sum_{i=0}^{2} \omega_i \widehat{q}_i,$$

where the weights ω_i $(i = 0, 1, 2)$ are known (often determined by the genetic model), and $\widehat{p}_i = r_i/r$ and $\widehat{q}_i = s_i/s$ are estimates of $p_i = \Pr(G_i|\text{case})$ and $q_i = \Pr(G_i|\text{control})$, respectively. Under the null hypothesis of no association H_0, we have $p_i = q_i = \Pr(G_i)$ for $i = 0, 1, 2$. Denote $\mu_n = \mathrm{E}_{H_0}(T_n)$ and $\sigma_n^2 = \mathrm{Var}_{H_0}(T_n)$ under H_0. Then, in the absence of PS,

$$\mu_n = \sum_{i=0}^{2} \omega_i p_i - \sum_{i=0}^{2} \omega_i q_i = 0, \tag{9.7}$$

$$\sigma_n^2 = (1/r + 1/s)\boldsymbol{\omega}^T \Omega \boldsymbol{\omega}, \tag{9.8}$$

where $\boldsymbol{\omega} = (\omega_0, \omega_1, \omega_2)^T$, and Ω is a 3×3 matrix with the (i, i)th element $p_i(1 - p_i)$ and the (i, j)th element $-p_i p_j$ $(i \neq j)$. Thus, asymptotically,

$$\frac{T_n - \mu_n}{\sigma_n} = \frac{T_n}{\sigma_n} \sim N(0, 1) \quad \text{under } H_0. \tag{9.9}$$

In the presence of PS, however, (9.7) and (9.8) are no longer valid, nor is the asymptotic distribution for the trend test (9.9). Given PS-II (Table 9.1), $\mu_n^* = E_{H_0}(T_n|PS) \neq \mu_n = 0$ and $\sigma_n^{*2} = \mathrm{Var}_{H_0}(T_n|PS) \neq \sigma_n^2$. Therefore, $T_n \approx N(\mu_n^*, \sigma_n^{*2})$ when n is large enough. Unfortunately, because the PS is hidden, μ_n^* and σ_n^* cannot be estimated using the data in Table 9.2.

9.3 Correcting for Population Stratification

We have observed that spurious associations can be obtained because of PS. Methods to eliminate spurious associations have been recently developed and this research area is still active. All the existing methods to correct for PS use genomic data to adjust a test statistic.

9.3.1 Genomic Control

One popular and simple approach to control for PS is the genomic control (GC) approach. For the data presented in Table 9.2, we use a simple trend test to illustrate the GC method. The trend test is given by

$$Z_{\mathrm{CATT}}^2 = \frac{n\{n(r_1 + 2r_2) - r(n_1 + 2n_2)\}^2}{r(n-r)\{n(n_1 + 4n_2) - (n_1 + 2n_2)^2\}}, \tag{9.10}$$

which asymptotically follows a χ_1^2 distribution under H_0 in the absence of PS.

Note that the numerator of (9.10) is proportional to the difference of the frequencies of allele B between cases and controls,

$$n(r_1 + 2r_2) - r(n_1 + 2n_2) = rs\{(r_1 + 2r_2)/r - (s_1 + 2s_2)/s\}. \tag{9.11}$$

In Sect. 3.4, we showed that Z_{CATT}^2 is asymptotically equivalent to the allele-based test, Z_{ABT}^2, which is based on the right hand side of (9.11). The trend test in (9.10) is also asymptotically optimal (most powerful) under the ADD model. Both Z_{CATT}^2 and Z_{ABT}^2 share the same numerator but have different denominators, where Z_{ABT}^2 estimates the variance of the numerator under HWE. The variance estimates in both Z_{CATT}^2 and Z_{ABT}^2 are often underestimated in the presence of population structure. Thus, they may have inflated Type I error rates under H_0. We focus on the numerator given by (9.11) and the trend test.

Following Sect. 9.2.2, given the PS, $Z_{\mathrm{CATT}} = T_n/\sigma_n \sim N(\mu_n^*/\sigma_n, (\sigma_n^*/\sigma_n)^2)$ when n is large enough and $r/n \neq 0$ or 1 as $n \to \infty$. Thus, $(Z_{\mathrm{CATT}} - \mu_n^*/\sigma_n)/(\sigma_n^*/\sigma_n) \sim N(0, 1)$, where μ_n^*/σ_n is the bias and σ_n^{*2}/σ_n^2 is the variance distortion or the variance inflation factor (VIF). Expressions for σ_n^* depends on the type of the population structure underlying the data (Table 9.1). To apply the GC method, however, one does not need to know the true type of structure. Of course, the GC method may work better for some types of population structure than others, which will be discussed later.

It is impossible to estimate the VIF using the data in Table 9.2. However, it can be estimated when a set of null markers that are unlinked to disease loci is available. In current GWAS, 500,000 to more than a million SNPs are genotyped, from which the null markers for controlling PS can be selected. We consider the ideal case that the VIF is a constant for all markers (the candidate marker and null markers). In general, several conditions are required for the VIF to be roughly constant: i) the markers under study have similar mutation rates; ii) there is no strong or subpopulation-specific selection; and iii) F should be close to a constant across the markers with respective to the underlying population structure. For modeling CR, the VIF is due to kinship coefficients, which are not dependent on individual loci. Thus, in this case, it is reasonable to assume a constant VIF.

Under the above assumptions, denote the values of the trend test at M unlinked markers as $Z^2_{\text{CATT},m}$, $m = 1, \ldots, M$. Then the VIF, denoted as λ, can be estimated by

$$\widehat{\lambda} = \text{median}\{Z^2_{\text{CATT},1}, \ldots, Z^2_{\text{CATT},M}\}/0.456,$$

the ratio of the sample median of the observed $Z^2_{\text{CATT},m}$, $m = 1, \ldots, M$ to that of the theoretical median of χ^2_1. When the sample size is large enough, under H_0, $\widehat{\lambda} \approx 1$ if there is no PS and $\widehat{\lambda} \approx \sigma_n^{*2}/\sigma_n^2$ when PS is present. If $\widehat{\lambda}$ is much larger (or smaller) than 1, the uncorrected trend test would have inflated (or deflated) Type I error rate under H_0, which affects the apparent power under H_1. To correct for PS, we re-scale the trend test to $Z^2_{\text{CATT}}/\widehat{\lambda}$, which asymptotically follows χ^2_1 under H_0. This adjustment process is referred to as GC. It has also been suggested that in estimating λ the median can be replaced by the mean. However, this can overestimate the VIF when there are multiple genetic variants contributing to a phenotypic variation.

Although applying the GC method does not need knowledge of the substructure of the population, an analytical expression for λ would help understand the impact of PS on the trend test. Consider PS-II given in Table 9.1. Let X_i $(i = 1, \ldots, r)$ be the number of B alleles in the ith case and Y_j $(j = 1, \ldots, s)$ the number of B alleles in the jth control. Assume there are J discrete subpopulations, as discussed in Sect. 9.2.1. Let $a_1, \ldots, a_J$ and $b_1, \ldots, b_J$ denote the sample sizes of cases and controls from each of the J subpopulations with $\sum_{j=1}^{J} a_j = r$ and $\sum_{j=1}^{J} b_j = s$. We assume $r = s$ for simplicity.

The trend test Z^2_{CATT} is proportional to the square of $T = \sum_i X_i - \sum_j Y_j$. Under H_0, the variance of T depends on whether or not the cases and controls are from the same subpopulation. Specifically,

$$\text{Var}(T) = \sum_{i=1}^{r} \text{Var}(X_i) + \sum_{j=1}^{s} \text{Var}(Y_j) + 2\sum_{i<l} \text{Cov}(X_i, X_l) + 2\sum_{j<l} \text{Cov}(Y_j, Y_l)$$
$$- 2\sum_{i}\sum_{j} \text{Cov}(X_i, Y_j).$$

From (9.1), we have $\text{Var}(X_i) = \text{Var}(Y_j) = 2p(1 - p)(1 + F)$, where p is the population frequency of allele B. We assume that there is no correlation for a pair of genotypes from two different subpopulations. $\text{Cov}(X_i, X_l) = \text{Cov}(Y_j, Y_l) = \text{Cov}(X_i, Y_j) = 4Fp(1 - p)$ for $i \neq l$ and $j \neq l$ when the samples are drawn from the same subpopulations. Then, taking into account the J subpopulations,

$$\text{Var}(T) = 4p(1 - p)\left[r(1 + F) \right.$$
$$\left. + 4F \sum_j \{a_j(a_j - 1) + b_j(b_j - 1) - 2a_j b_j\} \right]. \qquad (9.12)$$

It can be seen that $\text{Var}(T)$ reaches its maximum $4rp(1 - p)\{1 + F(2r - 1)\}$ when all cases are from one subpopulation and all controls are from another, and that it reaches its minimum $4rp(1 - p)(1 - F)$ when $a_j = b_j$ for all $j = 1, \ldots, J$ (Problem 9.4). In the trend test, when the PS is ignored, we estimate the variance as $\text{Var}(T) = \sum_i \text{Var}(X_i) + \sum_j \text{Var}(Y_j) = 4rp(1 - p)(1 + F)$. Thus, the VIF is given by

$$\lambda = \frac{\text{Var}(T)}{4rp(1 - p)(1 + F)}, \qquad (9.13)$$

where $\text{Var}(T)$ is given in (9.12), and is inflated most when cases and controls are from distinct subpopulations. In this case, λ can achieve its maximum $\{1 + F(2r - 1)\}/(1 + F)$. Alternatively, λ reaches its minimum $(1 - F)/(1 + F)$ when disease status is independent of the subpopulation membership.

The GC approach is computationally simple, does not need knowledge of the number of subpopulations J, and allows for a large J. It can work effectively with a small number of null markers. In some simulations and real examples, $M < 50$ can remove the impact of PS. It can also be used with pooled DNA samples instead of using individual genotypes, which can be substantially less expensive. However, there are some limitations of using the GC method, e.g., λ may be either overestimated or underestimated, resulting in either reducing statistical power or Type I error rate not being properly controlled. It re-scales the trend test but does not directly correct the bias due to PS.

When $J = 1$ and $F \neq 0$ (the CR in Table 9.1), VIF $\lambda \neq 1$ but the bias is 0. Therefore, the GC method is more effective in correcting for CR than for PS-II. Even though more popular methods to correct for PS have been developed lately, the VIF is still the most important simple measure to indicate whether or not there is PS, or if it has been corrected for either by the GC or an other method.

Note that the VIF given in (9.13) is independent of the allele frequency of the candidate marker (p cancels out). Thus, there is no restriction on the allele frequencies of the null markers. However, this is only true when the trend test for the ADD model is used. If the trend tests for other genetic models are used, e.g., the REC or DOM models, the VIF depends on p. Then, the GC method using null markers with arbitrary allele frequencies may not be effective. We assumed the same F for cases and controls. For the CR given in Table 9.1, if cases are more similar than controls, then one may use F_1 for cases and F_2 for controls with $F_1 \neq F_2$. Then, similarly to the calculations given before, it can be shown that (see Problem 9.5) when $r = s$

$$\text{Var}(T) = 2rp(1 - p)\{2 + (F_1 + F_2)(2r - 1)\}.$$

9.3.2 Structural Association

With several hundred thousand genetic markers genotyped across the genome, an individual's membership in a particular subpopulation can be inferred with high confidence. It is typically assumed that there is no population structure within each subpopulation. Therefore, after each individual membership has been inferred, any statistical method can be applied within each subpopulation to have a correct Type I error rate. This process is referred to as the Structural Association (SA) method. The subpopulation memberships of individuals can be inferred using a software called STRUCTURE, which is available free of charge (http://pritch.bsd.uchicago.edu/structure.html). Here we present the SA method for testing association. The SA method tests H_0 of no association between a candidate marker and a disease at the subpopulation level given in (9.2), rather than the overall H_0 indicated in (9.3). Thus, any association observed at the subpopulation level cannot be due to PS. After the subpopulations and the memberships have been inferred, the usual association test statistics, e.g., the trend test, can be applied at the subpopulation level.

Let G denote the set of genotypes of individuals at the candidate marker, P_0 and P_1 be the allele frequencies in the subpopulations under H_0 and H_1, respectively, and Q be a vector of genetic background measures of all individuals in the sample. Let $\text{Pr}_0(G; P_0, Q)$ and $\text{Pr}_1(G; P_1, Q)$ be the likelihoods for observing the genotypes under H_0 and H_1, respectively, given the genetic background Q. The likelihood ratio test statistic is given by

$$\Lambda(G) = \frac{\text{Pr}_1(G; \widehat{P}_1, \widehat{Q})}{\text{Pr}_0(G; \widehat{P}_0, \widehat{Q})},$$

where $\widehat{P}_0$, $\widehat{P}_1$ and $\widehat{Q}$ are the estimates of P_0, P_1 and Q, respectively. Note that the genetic background Q is estimated independently of the candidate marker.

Similar to the GC method, when a set of unlinked null markers have been genotyped, STRUCTURE, a Bayesian clustering method, or the EM algorithm can be applied to determine both the number of subpopulations J and the proportions of an observed individual's ancestry from the subpopulations. Specifically, assume that individuals inherit their marker alleles from a pool of J subpopulations (where J may be unknown). The allele frequencies at each locus within each subpopulation are assumed to be unknown and need to be estimated. Let q_{mj} denote the proportion of the mth genome ($m = 1, \ldots, M$) originating from the jth subpopulation. Based on the genotypes of all n individuals at the M unlinked null markers, either a MCMC approach or EM algorithm can be applied to estimate J and

$Q = \{q_{mj} : m = 1, \ldots, M; j = 1, \ldots, J\}$, and the allele frequency matrix in the sub-populations. Either microsatellite markers or SNPs can be used to produce reliable estimates of J and Q.

After the estimate of Q is obtained, denoted as $\widehat{Q}$, one estimates P_0 and P_1 under H_0 and H_1, respectively. An EM algorithm can be applied to estimate P_0 and P_1, denoted as $\widehat{P}_0$ and $\widehat{P}_1$, respectively. Let p_{jl}^d denote the lth allele frequency $(l = 1, 2)$ at the candidate marker in the jth subpopulation among individuals with disease status d. Under H_0, p_{jl}^d is not dependent on disease status d. Thus, the allele frequency matrix in all subpopulations is $P_0 = \{p_{jl} : j = 1, \ldots, J; l = 1, 2\}$. Let g_i^h denote the ith individual's hth allele at the candidate marker $(h = 1, 2)$. Here we assume the two alleles of an individual are independent and their order in a genotype is not distinguished. Then

$$\mathrm{Pr}_0(g_i^h = l | \widehat{P}_0, \widehat{Q}, d) = \sum_{j=1}^{J} \widehat{q}_{ij} \widehat{p}_{jl}, \quad l = 1, 2; \ h = 1, 2; \ i = 1, \ldots, n. \quad (9.14)$$

We further assume that HWE holds in each subpopulation and that the likelihood $\mathrm{Pr}_0(G; \widehat{P}_0, \widehat{Q})$ is proportional to the product of $\mathrm{Pr}_0(g_i^h = l; \widehat{P}_0, \widehat{Q}, d)$ for the alleles of all n individuals. Under H_1, the allele frequency matrix is dependent on the disease status d, and $P_1 = \{p_{jl}^d : j = 1, \ldots, J; l = 1, 2\}$, which has twice the number of parameters under H_0. Similarly,

$$\mathrm{Pr}_1(g_i^h = l | \widehat{P}_1, \widehat{Q}, d) = \sum_{j=1}^{J} \widehat{q}_{ij} \widehat{p}_{jl}^d, \quad l = 1, 2; \ h = 1, 2; \ i = 1, \ldots, n. \quad (9.15)$$

The likelihood $\mathrm{Pr}_1(G; \widehat{P}_1, \widehat{Q})$ is proportional to the product of $\mathrm{Pr}_1(g_i^h = l; \widehat{P}_1, \widehat{Q}, d)$ for all the alleles of n individuals. Given the estimated genetic backgrounds $\widehat{Q}$, the EM algorithm is applied to estimate P_0 and P_1 (Problem 9.6).

The p-value for testing H_0 using the SA method can be obtained by the following simulation procedure. Generate a new genotype at the candidate marker under H_0 for each individual as an independent random sample drawn from $\mathrm{Pr}_0(\cdot | \widehat{P}_0, \widehat{Q})$. Repeat this procedure L times and obtain genotype data sets $G^{(1)}, \ldots, G^{(L)}$. The empirical p-value is given by

$$\text{p-value} = \frac{1}{L} \#\{1 \leq l \leq L : \Lambda(G^{(l)}) > \Lambda(G)\},$$

where $\#\{A\}$ denotes the number of members in set $\{A\}$. Simulation studies show that this SA method can control the PS provided that the number of unlinked markers M is large enough, and that it is often more powerful than a family-based TDT, which is based on trio data (parents and a diseased offspring). One of the difficulties is the estimation of the number of subpopulations J, especially when there is a large number of subpopulations. Compared to the GC method, the SA method is much more computationally demanding, and it does not correct for CR (see Table 9.1).

The assumption of HWE, required for the independence of two alleles in a genotype, can be relaxed. The genetic background matrix Q is likely dependent on the disease status and incorporating this information may improve the performance of the SA method. The methods that we present in the next two sections would be more efficient than the SA method to correct for PS.

9.3.3 *Principal Components and Clustering*

Principal components (PCs) are often used to summarize high dimensional data without losing much information. PCs are ideal for summarizing the genetic markers across the genome and have been used for characterizing population differences. Studies suggest that the map produced by the first two PCs calculated from genomic data is highly correlated with latitudes and altitudes of worldwide populations. Thus the map produced by PCs may reflect the environmental and cultural variation in worldwide populations, as well as population migration. Recently, PCs have further been successfully applied to correcting PS in genetic association studies. The idea behind using PCs of genetic marker data is that an individual's genetic background can be represented by his/her genetic markers, which can be summarized using the principal components of marker data. In other words, individuals who have similar PC values likely come from the same subpopulation. A genetic association analysis conditional on PCs is equivalent to an analysis conditional on subpopulations, which will reduce the chance of producing spurious association.

A natural way to incorporate the PCs into a statistical model is based on a regression framework. For instance, we can model the association between a phenotype Y_i and genetic marker g_i for the ith individual using a generalized linear model

$$f(\mathrm{E}(Y_i)) = \beta_0 + \beta_1 g_i + \mu(T_i) = G_i^T \beta + \mu(T_i), \tag{9.16}$$

where $f(\mathrm{E}(y_i))$ is a link function, $\beta = (\beta_0, \beta_1)^T$ is the parameter vector, $G_i = (1, g_i)^T$, where g_i is a candidate marker to test, T_i is an individual's PCs obtained from the marker data, and $\mu(T_i)$ is a function of the PCs. Several methods have been proposed to model $\mu(T_i)$, including a mixture model in logistic regression, a semiparametric model using kernel smoothers, and a linear function of T_i. A common advantage of these models is that the effect of PS on a phenotype Y is taken care of by the function $\mu(T_i)$ in the logistic regression model.

Consider a case-control study with M unlinked null markers for controlling PS. Let $X_i = (x_{i1}, \ldots, x_{iM})^T$, $i = 1, \ldots, n = r + s$, be a vector of the ith individual's marker data, where x_{im} is the genotype value of the mth marker for the ith individual and its value is 0, 1 or 2, representing the number of A alleles in a genotype. The sample covariance matrix of marker data is

$$\Sigma = \mathrm{Cov}(X) = \sum_{i=1}^{n} (X_i - \bar{X})(X_i - \bar{X})^T, \tag{9.17}$$

Fig. 9.4 Histograms of the first two PCs when samples were simulated from two different populations (**A** and **B**) and when samples were simulated from an admixed population with two ancestral populations (**C** and **D**)

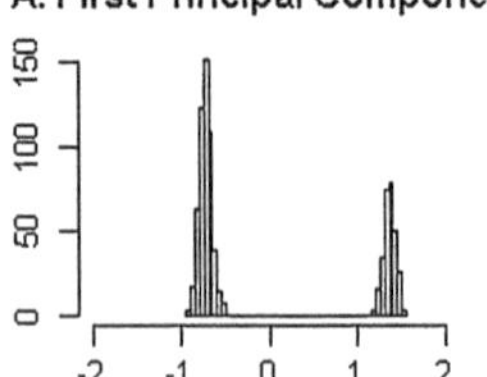

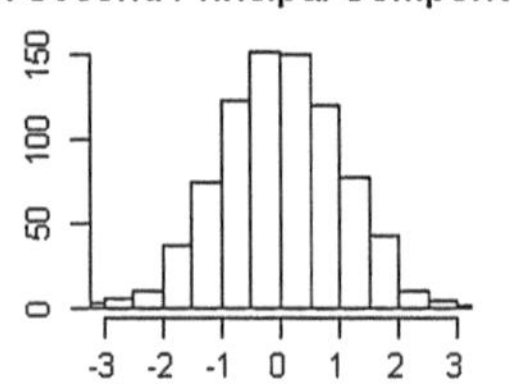

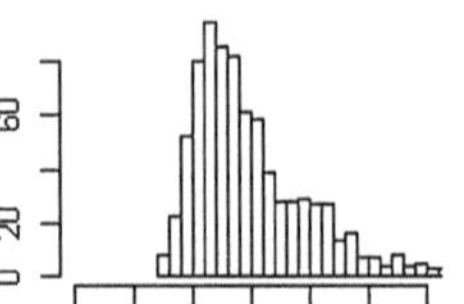

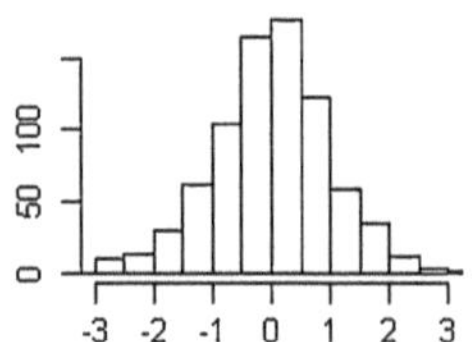

which is an $M \times M$ matrix. Let e_j be the jth eigenvector corresponding to the jth largest eigenvalue of Σ and denote the corresponding PC for the ith individual as $t_{ij} = (X_i - \bar{X})^T e_j$. Let $T_i = (t_{i1}, \ldots, t_{iq})$ be the first q PCs, where $q \leq M$. All the PC-based approaches are based on T_i. In the following sections, we discuss the PC-based approaches in detail.

Mixture Model

When a population consists of a mixture of subpopulations, it is natural to consider each PC of the marker data as coming from a mixture of several normal distributions. Figure 9.4 demonstrates the histograms of the first and second PCs when samples were simulated from two different populations (Fig. 9.4 A and B) and when samples were simulated from an admixed population with two parental populations (Fig. 9.4 C and D). It can be observed that the individuals from two different populations are clustered into two groups by the first PC. When individuals are sampled from an admixed population with two ancestral populations, the first PC can fit a mixture of two normal distributions. The second PC seems to fit a normal distribution well for both simulated datasets.

The distribution of PCs suggests we can use a mixture model to model population structure. Using the same notation as before, if there are J subpopulations, the PCs are assumed to follow approximately a mixture of J normal distributions. Because the PCs are independent, conditional on the jth subpopulation we can assume that the distribution of T_i is the product of q normal distributions, $f(T_i|j) = \prod_{l=1}^{q} \phi(t_{il}|\mu_{jl}, \sigma_{jl}^2)$, where $\phi(t_{il}|\mu_{jl}, \sigma_{jl}^2)$ is the density function $N(\mu_{jl}, \sigma_{jl}^2)$, and q is the number of PCs to use for controlling PS. The unconditional density function of T_i is

$$f(T_i) = \sum_{j=1}^{J} \lambda_j \prod_{l=1}^{q} \phi(t_{il}|\mu_{jl}, \sigma_{jl}^2),$$

where λ_j is the probability that an individual originates from the jth subpopulation, and $\sum \lambda_j = 1$.

Given an individual is from the jth subpopulation, a logistic regression model is applied:

$$\log\left\{\frac{\Pr(Y_i = 1|G_i, j)}{\Pr(Y_i = 0|G_i, j)}\right\} = G_i^T \beta + \delta_j, \tag{9.18}$$

where δ_j indicates the effect of the jth subpopulation subject to $\delta_J = 0$. It is assumed that the effect of the candidate gene is the same across subpopulations, but this is not necessary, because we can use a population specific β_j.

The likelihood for the observed data $Y_i = y_i$ is then

$$L = \prod_{i=1}^{n} f(y_i|G_i, T_i) = \prod_{i=1}^{n}\left\{\frac{\sum_{j=1}^{J} \lambda_j \Pr(y_i|G_i, j) f(T_i|j)}{f(T_i)}\right\},$$

where $\Pr(y_i|G_i, j)$ is specified by (9.18). To test the null hypothesis $H_0 : \beta_1 = 0$, the LRT can be applied. The Bayesian Information Criterion (BIC) can be used to estimate the number of subpopulations.

A question that arises from the PC analysis is how many PCs should be used in controlling for PS. This question can be modified to ask which PCs contribute ancestry information. From the analysis of the second PC, we observed that a PC distributes as a normal distribution if it does not contribute any ancestry information. We can thus test whether or not a PC deviates from a normal distribution by the Kolmogorov-Smirnov test.

Semi-parametric Approach

We use the same notation for a case-control design as in the previous section using the mixture model. A semi-parametric logistic model, denoted as QualSPT, can be used to model the relation between a trait and candidate gene locus with genetic background:

$$\log\left\{\frac{\Pr(y_i = 1|G_i, T_i)}{\Pr(y_i = 0|G_i, T_i)}\right\} = G_i^T \beta + \mu(T_i),$$

where $\mu(T_i)$ is a one-dimensional unknown smoothing function and T_i is q-dimensional. The model is semi-parametric because $\mu = \mu(T_i)$ is unspecified. Under this model, the null hypothesis of no association is written as $H_0 : \beta_1 = 0$.

The log-likelihood function is

$$l(\beta, \mu) = \sum_{i=1}^{n} l(\beta, \mu(T_i); G_i, y_i)$$

$$= \sum_{i=1}^{n} [y_i \{G_i^T \beta + \mu(T_i)\} - \log\{1 + \exp(G_i^T \beta + \mu(T_i))\}].$$

Several methods are available to estimate the parameter β and the non-parametric function $\mu(\cdot)$. The QualSPT statistic is based on the LRT statistic

$$\Lambda = \frac{L(\widehat{\beta}, \widehat{\mu}_1(T_i))}{L(0, \widehat{\mu}_0(T_i))},$$

where $\widehat{\mu}_0(T_i)$ and $\widehat{\mu}_1(T_i)$ are the MLEs of $\mu(\cdot)$ under H_0 and H_1, respectively, and $\widehat{\beta}$ is the MLE of β under H_1. Under H_0, the QualSPT LRT follows a chi-squared distribution with degrees of freedom equal to the length of the vector β.

For a given smoothing parameter h and a given kernel function $K(\cdot)$, an iterative estimation procedure for (β, μ) contains the following two steps:

Step 1. For a given $\widehat{\beta}^{(m)}$, η is solved from the following equation

$$\sum_{i=1}^{n} K\left(\frac{T_i - T}{h}\right) \frac{\partial}{\partial \eta} l(\widehat{\beta}^{(m)}, \eta; G_i, y_i) = 0.$$

Denote the solution of η at $T = T_i$ as $\widehat{\mu}^{(m)}(T_i)$ $(i = 1, \ldots, n)$.
Step 2. Solve β from the equation

$$\sum_{i=1}^{n} \frac{\partial}{\partial \beta} l(\beta, \widehat{\mu}^{(m)}(T_i); G_i, y_i) = 0,$$

which is denoted as an updated estimate $\widehat{\beta}^{(m+1)}$.

The algorithm repeats the above two-step process until convergence occurs. Different kernels can be used, although the choice of kernels has little effect on the estimation of β. For example, we can use the quadratic kernel $K(T_i) = \prod_{i=1}^{q} k(t_i)$, where

$$k(t_i) = (1 - t_i^2)^2, \quad \text{if } |t_i| \leq 1,$$
$$= 0, \quad \text{if } |t_i| > 1,$$

with $T_i = (t_{i1}, \ldots, t_{iq})$ representing the first q PCs for the ith individual.

We need to choose the smoothing parameter h. One way is to choose the h that minimizes a Kolmogorov test statistic. Specifically, for a given h, we perform QualSPT to M unlinked markers and obtain their corresponding p-values $p_1, \ldots, p_M$. Let F_n be the empirical distribution function of the M p-values, and F be a uniform distribution function. Define the Kolmogorov test as $L(h) = \max_x |F_n(x) - F(x)|$. The smoothing parameter h^* satisfies

$$h^* = \arg\min_h L(h).$$

The rationale for this method is that, if PS is well controlled, these p-values asymptotically follow a uniform distribution. Therefore, the best smoothing parameter h^* should be the one that minimizes the difference between the empirical distribution and the uniform distribution. This procedure also provides a method to check if the PS has been corrected by the set of unlinked markers. If the p-value of the Kolmogorov test with $h = h^*$ is greater than a pre-specified significance level, e.g. 0.05, we may consider that the PS has been well controlled. Otherwise, additional markers might be necessary to control the PS.

Linear Model Approach

In Eq. (9.16) we can replace $\mu(T)$ by a linear function of T, the PCs of genetic marker data, to account for the PS. This method first performs a regression analysis by regressing both phenotype and unlinked markers on the PCs. Association between the phenotype and the candidate marker is then tested using the residual correlation. This approach is simple and can be easily applied to test a large number of markers. To do this, one first fits the regression models using the first q PCs on the unlinked markers

$$y_i = \sum_{l=0}^{q} \beta_l t_{il} + \varepsilon_i,$$

$$g_i = \sum_{l=0}^{q} \alpha_l t_{il} + \tau_i,$$

where $t_{i0} = 1$ and ε_i and τ_i are random errors. Let $\widehat{\beta}_l$ and $\widehat{\alpha}_l$ $(l = 0, 1, \ldots, q)$ be the usual least squares estimators of β_l and α_l, respectively. Since the PCs are orthogonal, we have

$$\widehat{\beta}_l = \frac{\sum_{i=1}^{n} y_i t_{il}}{\sum_{i=1}^{n} t_{il}^2} \quad \text{and} \quad \widehat{\alpha}_l = \frac{\sum_{i=1}^{n} g_i t_{il}}{\sum_{i=1}^{n} t_{il}^2}.$$

We can then calculate the phenotype and genotype residuals for a particular candidate marker as

$$y_i^* = y_i - \sum_{l=0}^{q} \widehat{\beta}_l t_{il},$$

$$g_i^* = g_i - \sum_{l=0}^{q} \widehat{\alpha}_l t_{il},$$

where g_i $(i = 1, \ldots, n)$ is the genotype of the candidate marker of the ith individual. Let r be the sample correlation coefficient between y_i^* and g_i^*, $i = 1, \ldots, n$. Then a statistic to test association is given by

$$T = (N - q - 1)r^2,$$

which asymptotically follows a chi-squared distribution with one degree of freedom. Intuitively, y_i^* and g_i^* can be viewed as the trait and marker after removing the effect of PS. That is, we can consider y_i^* and g_i^* as if they were obtained from a homogenous population. Thus, any association test based on y_i^* and g_i^* will not be affected by the PS.

Calculating PCs

Current GWAS use 500,000 to more than a million SNPs. To calculate PCs, we usually have to calculate the eigenvalues and eigenvectors of the matrix given in (9.17), which is a high dimensional matrix. This computation requires huge computer memory space. However, PCs can be equivalently calculated from a matrix based on individuals. For example, let X be the $n \times M$ matrix, in which each row denotes an individual's marker genotype values for the M markers. Using the singular value decomposition, $X^T = USV^T$, where U is an $M \times n$ matrix whose kth column, denoted by U_k, corresponds to the kth eigenvector, S is a diagonal matrix of singular values and V is an $n \times n$ matrix whose kth column, denoted by V_k, corresponds to the ancestries along the kth axis. In the approach of traditional PCs, the kth PC is

$$XU_k = VSU^TU_k = s_k V_k,$$

where s_k is the kth singular value, because $U^T U_k$ is a vector whose components are 0 except for the kth, which is 1. Thus, PCs calculated based on individuals and the standard PCs analysis are the same up to a constant, which will have no effect in the regression modeling.

Using Family Data

Because of the simplicity of the linear regression method, it can be easily extended to using family data. For simplicity, we only consider using nuclear families. Assume that the data contain n_f nuclear families. The ith family has k_i members, with the first two being the father and mother ($j = 1, 2$). In addition to these families, we have r unrelated cases and s unrelated controls. The total number of individuals is $n_T = \sum_{i=1}^{n_f} k_i + r + s = \sum_{i=1}^{n_f} k_i + n$. We define each unrelated case or control as a family with a family size of 1 ($k_i = 1$ for each case or control). Thus, we have a total of $m = n_f + n$ families. Let y_{ij} and g_{ij} be the observed trait value and the marker genotype of the jth individual in the ith family ($j = 1, \ldots, k_i$). Although covariates can be incorporated, we do not consider covariates here. Let

$X_{ij} = (x_{ij1}, \ldots, x_{ijM})^T$ represent the marker genotypic values for the jth individual in the ith family.

Similar to case-control designs, we perform a PC analysis to summarize the marker data. Because the data now include both family and unrelated individuals, a standard PC analysis using all the available data will result in biased directions of the maximum variability for the data. Thus, we use the unrelated individuals (parents) in each family and the unrelated cases and controls to calculate the eigenvalues and eigenvectors. Then we calculate PCs for all individuals using the above eigenvectors.

Let t_{ijl} be the lth PC for the jth individual in the ith family ($l = 1, \ldots, q$, $j = 1, \ldots, k_i$, and $i = 1, \ldots, n$). We perform the linear regressions of phenotypes and candidate marker genotypes on the PCs for all individuals, ignoring the family structure. Denote the residuals of phenotypes and genotypes as y_{ij}^* and g_{ij}^*, respectively. The statistic for testing association between the phenotype and a candidate marker is given by

$$S^2 = \frac{T^2}{\widehat{\mathrm{Var}}(T)} = \frac{\{n_T^{-1} \sum_{i=1}^m \sum_{j=1}^{k_i} g_{ij}^* y_{ij}^*\}^2}{\widehat{\mathrm{Var}}(T)}.$$

To calculate $\mathrm{Var}(T)$, note that

$$\mathrm{Var}(T) = \mathrm{Var}\left(\sum_{i=1}^{n_f} T_i\right) + \mathrm{Var}\left(\sum_{i=n_f+1}^m T_i\right) = n_f \sigma_f^2 + n \sigma_u^2,$$

where σ_f^2 and σ_u^2 are estimated respectively by

$$\widehat{\sigma_f^2} = \frac{1}{n_f - 1} \sum_{i=1}^{n_f} (T_i - \bar{T}_f)^2,$$

$$\widehat{\sigma_u^2} = \frac{1}{n - 1} \sum_{i=n_f+1}^m (T_i - \bar{T}_u)^2,$$

where

$$T_i = \frac{1}{k_i} \sum_{j=1}^{k_i} g_{ij}^* y_{ij}^*, \quad \bar{T}_f = \frac{1}{n_f} \sum_{i=1}^{n_f} T_i, \quad \text{and} \quad \bar{T}_u = \frac{1}{n} \sum_{i=n_f+1}^m T_i.$$

An estimate of $\mathrm{Var}(T)$, $\widehat{\mathrm{Var}}(T)$, is obtained by replacing σ_f^2 and σ_u^2 by their estimates, respectively.

To examine whether or not we are able to calculate the children's PCs using the eigenvectors calculated from the genotypes of their parents and the unrelated cases and controls, we conducted simulations using 200 nuclear families, 200 cases and 200 controls, with 200 ancestry informative markers (AIMs). Two distinct mixture

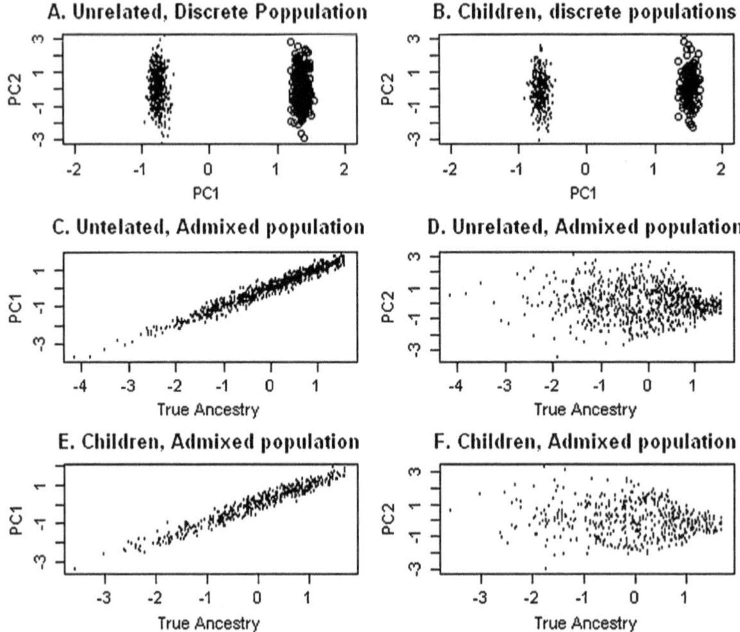

Fig. 9.5 Plots of the first two PCs when samples were drawn from (i) two discrete populations (**A** and **B**), and when samples were drawn from (ii) an admixture of two ancestral populations (**C–F**)

populations were simulated: (i) a discrete model that samples from two distinct populations, and (ii) an admixed population, with two ancestral populations, that mimics the formation of the African-American population. Figure 9.5 presents the first two PCs for the two different mixture populations.

The results indicate that, for both simulated samples, the PCs can well capture the variation of an individual's ancestry, and that a child's ancestry can also be estimated through the prediction of the PCs obtained from those of the unrelated individuals. Further, it can be seen that the first PC can distinguish individuals from the two subpopulations for both independent samples and children, but not the second PC (A and B). For samples from an admixed population, the first PC, but not the second, is highly correlated with the true ancestry (C-F).

9.3.4 Multidimensional Scaling Plots

Multidimensional Scaling (MDS) plots have been used as an important tool to analyze high dimensional data. Similar to PC analysis (PCA), MDS plots project the points in a high dimensional space to a lower dimensional space, but preserve the distances between points as much as possible. The coordinates of the points in the

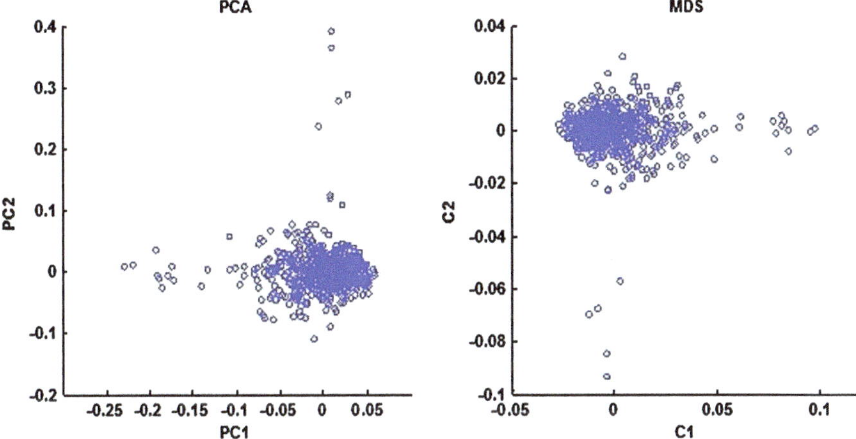

Fig. 9.6 PCA (*left panel*) and MDS (*right panel*) of the genotype data of 701 African-Americans sampled from Maywood, Illinois

lower dimensional space can be used in the association analysis to control for population structure. Figure 9.6 presents the first two PCs and the first two coordinates of MDS in African-American samples from Maywood, Illinois. Over 800,000 SNPs genotyped using the Affymetrix 6.0 platform were used in the analysis. We observe that the PCA and MDS result in almost identical plots.

9.4 Selection of Marker Loci

Ideally, the markers used to identify population structure should be unlinked to the disease loci. For GWAS, where over hundreds of thousands of SNPs are often genotyped, the selection of unlinked null SNPs can be achieved by thinning the SNPs according to their LD patterns. It has often been thought that AIMs are necessary for the first step. With a large number of markers available in association studies, using random SNPs should be better than selecting a limited number of AIMs. Figure 9.7 presents the correlations between the first PC and the true ancestry based on simulated African-American data for different sets of markers. We observe that using more random markers (b) is better than selecting a subset of AIMs (a). When more dense SNPs are used, we expect there to be many SNPs in strong LD (c). However, the LD affects the correlation very little. In fact, the best correlation between the first PC and the true ancestry is obtained on using all SNPs (about 2 million), rather than on using unlinked AIMs or independent SNPs. Therefore, as long as the SNPs are randomly distributed across the genome, we should use all the available genetic markers in the analysis.

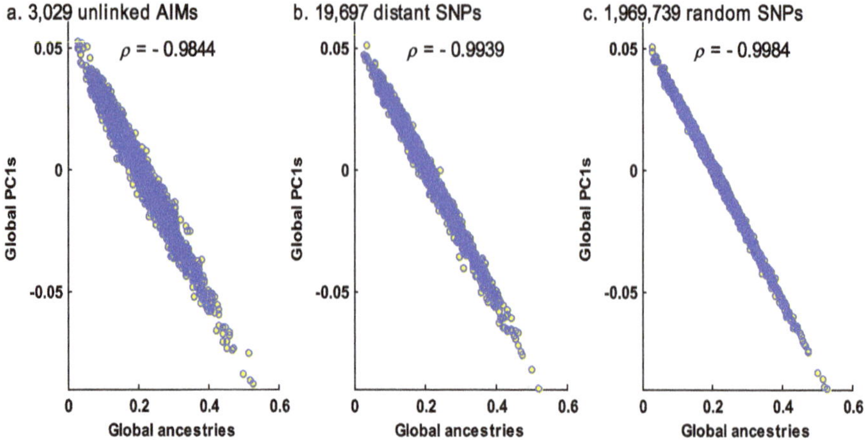

Fig. 9.7 Correlations between average true ancestry and the first PC based on different SNP sets: (**a**) The first PC based on 3,029 unlinked AIMs across the genome. (**b**) The first PC based on 19,697 distinct SNPs; many SNPs may be in LD. (**c**) The first PC based on dense SNPs; more SNPs may be in LD

9.5 Simulating Data in the Presence of Population Stratification

There are many ways to simulate case-control data in the presence of PS. A common method is the Balding-Nichols model. Suppose we simulate case-control data from a population with J subpopulations, in each of which HWE holds. We first discuss how to simulate markers not associated with a disease (null markers). Then we modify the algorithm to simulate disease markers.

To apply the Balding-Nichols model in a replicate, an ancestral allele frequency, denoted as p, is simulated from the uniform distribution $U(0.1, 0.9)$. Note that we exclude MAFs ≤ 0.1 as markers with MAF < 0.1 are often excluded from the analysis in GWAS. Then for the jth subpopulation, $j = 1, \ldots, J$, the allele frequency p_j of a marker is simulated from the Beta distribution $\text{Beta}(p(1 - F_{st})/F_{st}, (1 - p)(1 - F_{st})/F_{st})$, where F_{st} is Wright's inbreeding coefficient and specified *a priori* for all subpopulations and replicates. The parameter F_{st} here measures differentiation between the subpopulations. Under HWE in the jth subpopulation, the genotype frequencies of (G_0, G_1, G_2) for a null marker are given by $((1 - p_j)^2, 2p_j(1 - p_j), p_j^2)$. The genotype counts in cases and in controls in the jth subpopulation follow the same multinomial distribution with the probabilities $((1 - p_j)^2, 2p_j(1 - p_j), p_j^2)$. In this simulation, all p_j, $j = 1, \ldots, J$, follow the same Beta distribution and are independent. The mean and variance of a random variate from this Beta distribution are p and $p(1 - p)F_{st}$, respectively. Then, with the given proportions of cases and controls from the $j$the subpopulation, we can simulate genotype counts respectively for cases and for controls in this subpopulation. After all data are simulated for each subpopulation, we can pool the data to form a simple 2×3 table with one replicate.

In order to create PS in the data, the proportion of cases should not equal that of controls in all subpopulations. Otherwise, the simulation data can be regarded as a matched case-control design and PS has no impact on the analysis. The above procedure is used to simulate the null markers. To simulate a disease marker, we need to specify the prevalence $k_j = \Pr(\text{case}\,|\text{the } j\text{th subpopulation})$ and GRRs $(\lambda_{1j}, \lambda_{2j})$ in the jth subpopulation. For simplicity, one may assume GRRs are constant across the subpopulations. Thus, $(\lambda_{1j}, \lambda_{2j}) = (\lambda_1, \lambda_2)$. The simulation procedure is similar to that for the null marker. After $(g_{0j}, g_{1j}, g_{2j}) = ((1 - p_j)^2, 2p_j(1 - p_j), p_j^2)$ are calculated in the jth subpopulation, the genotype probabilities for controls and cases are given by $((1 - f_{0j})g_{0j}/(1 - k_j), (1 - \lambda_1 f_{0j})g_{1j}/(1 - k_j), (1 - \lambda_2 f_{0j})g_{2j}/(1 - k_j))$ and $(f_{0j}g_{0j}/k_j, \lambda_1 f_{0j}g_{1j}/k_j, \lambda_2 f_{0j}g_{2j}/k_j)$, respectively, where $f_{0j} = \Pr(\text{case}|G_0, \text{the } j\text{th subpopulation}) = (g_{0j} + \lambda_1 g_{1j} + \lambda_2 g_{2j})/k_j$ is the reference penetrance. If the disease is rare, we can use (g_{0j}, g_{1j}, g_{2j}) for controls and $(g_{0j}/R_j, \lambda_1 g_{1j}/R_j, \lambda_2 g_{2j}/R_j)$ for cases, where $R_j = k_j/f_{0j}$.

9.6 Comparison of Methods

Since both GC and PC analyses are computationally appealing, we compare them in this section by simulations. For PC analysis, we focus on QualSPT (the semi-parametric approach) and the linear regression method.

We used a panel of SNPs from a publicly available database that are AIMs across the genome for the African-American population. To form an admixed population, the allele frequencies of the SNPs and the marker map for both the African and European populations were downloaded from "http://www.journals.uchicago.edu". Briefly, at the first generation the marker genotypes of 10,000 unrelated individuals were simulated according to marker allele frequencies in the African population under HWE and independence of the markers. An admixed population was then formed by taking a proportion λ randomly selected from the African population to marry with people generated according to the marker allele frequencies in the European population, with the remaining proportion $1 - \lambda$ randomly mating among themselves. We drew λ from a uniform distribution between 0 and 0.08. The number of children produced by each marriage was assumed to follow a Poisson distribution with mean size 2. The number of crossovers between two marker loci at a distance d cM was assumed to follow a Poisson distribution with mean $d/100$. This process was repeated in the following generations. All the samples were drawn from the 5th generation, at which point the population was a mixture of approximately 80%/20% African and European ancestry.

We first simulated the data under the null hypothesis that no SNP is associated with the trait but the population structure contributes to the phenotypic variation. Hence, we assigned an individual's disease status with probability equal to his/her African ancestry. We simulated 500 cases and 500 controls respectively. In addition, we simulated 1,000 AIMs (SNPs) to correct for the population structure. We analyzed the association of the 1,000 SNPs using both QualSPT and linear regression with PCs. The CATT was also calculated for comparison. We used the first 10 PCs in the linear regression and the first PC in QualSPT.

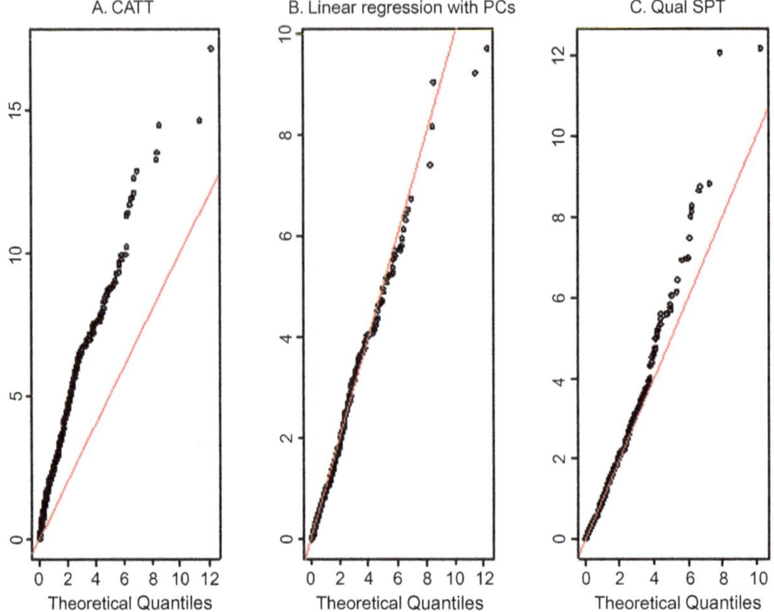

Fig. 9.8 Q-Q plots of three methods: (**A**) CATT. The plot is based on the test statistic values. GC VIF is 2.97; (**B**) Linear regression with the first 10 PCs. The plot is based on the test statistic values. GC VIF is 0.90; (**C**) QualSPT. The plot is based on $-\log 10$(p-value). GC VIF is 1.0

Table 9.3 P-values for testing association using different approaches to correct for population structure

Methods	CATT after GC	SA[*]	Mixture model	Linear regression	QualSPT
P-value	1.19×10^{-6}	$< 10^{-6}$	9.75×10^{-7}	1.29×10^{-6}	4×10^{-6}

[*]P-value is based on 1,000,000 permutations

Figure 9.8 presents the Q-Q plots of statistics to test for association using the simulated 1,000 SNPs with CATT, linear regression with PCs and QualSPT, respectively. Without proper correction for the population structure, the CATT apparently has large inflated Type I error rate, with a GC variance inflation factor value of 2.97. Both linear regression adjusting for the first 10 PCs and QualSPT have reasonable Type I error rates. The linear regression method seems to slightly over-correct the effect of the population structure using the simulated data.

We further simulated a disease variant. The penetrances of the disease genotypes were 0.20, 0.15 and 0.10 for genotypes carrying two, one and no risk alleles, respectively. The p-values using different approaches are reported in Table 9.3. For the CATT, we applied GC first. The results show that all p-values are similar after correcting for the population structure.

9.7 Bibliographical Comments

In this chapter, population structure is classified into PS-I, PS-II and CR (Table 9.1). An admixed population is regarded as a special case of PS. Classical definitions of PS and CR can be found in Crow and Kimura [49] and Elandt-Johnson [71]. Voight and Pritchard [282] defined a single population with CR, while Whittemore [302] considered population structure as a combination of PS and CR.

The worldwide population structure has been studied using various genetic markers, including microsatellite markers and dense SNPs [166, 220, 266]. The confounding effect of population structure in genetic association studies has been well documented in the study of type II diabetes mellitus and Gm3;5,13,14 in American Indians by Knowler et al. [148]. A general framework of how population structure produces confounding effects in case-control association studies was presented by Rosenberg et al. [219]. Population structure used to be considered a serious problem in admixed populations such as the African-American and Hispanic populations. Recently, it has been observed that population structure can also result in high type I error in association studies in the European American population, which was usually considered as a homogenous population [24]. In GWAS, the effects of population structure are often large [178], because the impact of population structure becomes stronger as the sample size increases.

The GC approach was first proposed by Devlin and Roeder [60], who suggested using the median of a one-degree-of-freedom chi-squared test statistic based on a set of unlinked markers to rescale the observed one-degree-of-freedom chi-squared test statistic. The power of GC, compared to that of the TDT, was studied by Bacanu et al. [11]. Extension of the GC to a robust chi-squared statistic with 2 degrees of freedom was studied by Zheng et al. [335], who also considered robustness of GC based on the trend tests with different genetic models. Using the mean of the test statistic based on a set of unlinked markers was also proposed [211]. Because the GC approach only corrects for the variance distortion of the trend test in the presence of population structure, directly correcting for bias using unlinked markers was considered by Gorroochurn et al. [104]. Their approach, however, requires matching allele frequencies of unlinked markers to that of the candidate marker at the subpopulation levels. This matching may not be achievable [341].

Although the methods to correct for PS presented in Sect. 9.3.3 and Sect. 9.3.4 are now more popularly used in practice, the GC approach is still the simplest method to examine whether or not the population structure is reasonably controlled. It is used in initial data analysis in most GWAS. A value of the VIF λ close to 1 indicates no PS effect, and $\lambda < 1.05$ is generally taken to suggest that any PS effect is not serious. Estimating the 95% CI for λ is also feasible by assuming that the markers are all independent. When there is no population structure, the estimate $\widehat{\lambda}$ asymptotically follows

$$\sqrt{M}(\widehat{\lambda} - 0.455) \sim N\left(0, \frac{1}{0.828 f(0.455)^2}\right),$$

where $f(0.455)$ is the value of the density function of the chi-squared distribution with 1 degree of freedom evaluated at 0.455 and M is the number of markers used

Fig. 9.9 The Q-Q plot of observed $-\log 10$(p-value) vs the expected value for a quantitative trait. 800,000 SNPs were simulated with sample size 2,000. There are 2,000 QTLs contributing 80% of the phenotypic variation. No PS is included. RegUa: linear regression analysis without including any PCs. GAPCC (global ancestry): linear regression analysis including the first 10 PCs calculated using all SNPs. LAPCC (local ancestry): linear regression analysis including the first 10 PCs calculated using only the SNPs in a local region where a tested SNP is located. The *shaded area* is the 95% confidence band

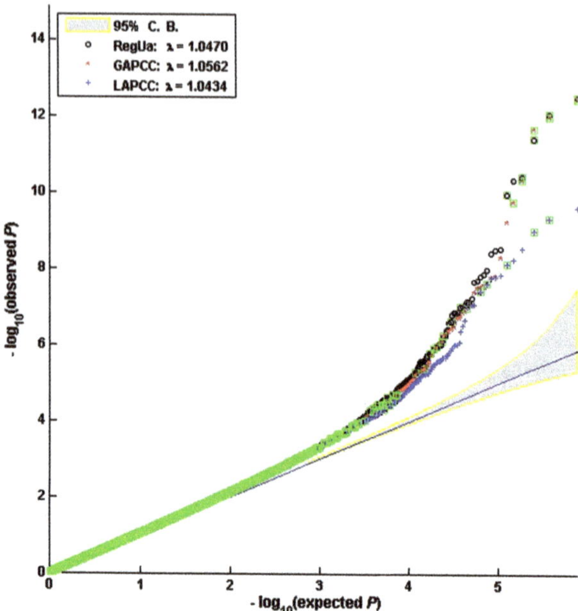

for controlling PS. We calculated a CI for $\widehat{\lambda}$ for 300,000 SNPs using this formula based on asymptotic theory and obtained the 95% CI (0.992, 1.008), which was also reported by [139]. However λ may be over-estimated when there are many genetic variants contributing to the phenotypic variation. For instance, in the simulation, if there were 2,000 quantitative trait loci (QTLs) contributing a total of 80% of the phenotypic variance across the genome, such as may occur for height, for example, we observed that the estimated values of λ can be outside the simulated 95% confidence band even if there is no PS (see Fig. 9.9). On the other hand, using PCs to correct PS has little negative impact. Thus, setting the GC inflation factor to 1 as a golden standard for controlling PS may be misleading, possibly resulting in loss of statistical power to detect true associations.

The SA approaches were studied by Pritchard et al. [207], who also developed the software STRUCTURE [82], based on Gibbs sampling, to cluster subpopulations. Satten et al. [225] studied a method of applying latent-class analysis to infer the population structure while simultaneously estimating the model parameters and testing for association. An EM based algorithm to cluster populations, which is computationally much faster and allows more markers than the Gibbs sampling approach, can be found in Tang et al. [265]. PC analysis of a set of marker genotypes was first used to characterize population differences by Cavalli-Sforza [28]. Using PCs to eliminate the effects of population structure was first studied in Zhu et al. [350], Zhang et al. [323] and Chen et al. [31], who also pointed out that a linear regression including the first PC can adequately control for population structure in an admixed population such as African-Americans. The PC mixture model can be computationally intensive and maximizing the likelihood function is challenging. The semi-parametric method is thus more attractive. Because a large number of markers are often available in GWAS, the PC-based linear regression method is more popular and computationally efficient, especially when the PCs are calculated from a matrix based on individuals [77, 205]. The PC-based linear regression method has also been extended to data comprising both family and unrelated samples [349].

When dense SNPs are available in GWAS, it is possible to estimate the degree of relationships among individuals in the absence of genealogical information. This can often be done by estimating the kinship matrix. The inferred relationships among individuals have been recently suggested for correcting the effect of both PS and CR in association studies via a variance component model [139, 206]. These methods decompose the variance into two parts, a component due to the sharing of genetic markers and a component of residual effects. However, whether population structure should be considered as a random or fixed effect is still under investigation [325]. Simulations suggested that mixed model approaches can perform well in general, but not for markers with very different allele frequencies in ancestral populations [325].

It has also been suggested in the literature that the GC approach works for both PS and CR, while PCs approaches can only control the confounding caused by PS, because CR could occur when there is a single population without random mating. Therefore, the GC approach should perform better in the presence of CR, as does the mixed model approach. When both PS and CR exist in the samples studied, including both PCs and variance components in a model should perform adequately well [325].

The Balding-Nichols method given in Sect. 9.5 is a common approach to simulate case-control data in the presence of PS [13]. This method was also referred to as a "random SNP" method in Price et al. [205], who also considered a "differentiated SNP" method, under which the allele frequencies in the subpopulations are specified. Then genotype frequencies are calculated under HWE. Other simulation procedures were given by Gorroochurn et al. [104, 105], Zheng et al. [335, 341]. See also discussion of different simulation procedures in Dadd et al. [53].

Finally, the methods that we discussed so far focus on adjusting global population structure, which is mainly caused by recent migration and random genetic drift. However, local genomic regions harboring functional variants may be subject to subtle forms of population structure as a result of not only demographic history but also natural selection and local random fluctuations of admixture [100, 264]. In addition, genetic phase disequilibrium can be present between a causal variant and a genetic marker whether they are close together or they are in different chromosomes when co-evolution has occurred. Thus, adjusting for local ancestry can be an appealing method to control the confounding caused by either global ancestry or local ancestry population structure (LAPCC in Fig. 9.9) [208].

9.8 Problems

9.1 Let the genotype frequencies in a population be given as in (9.1). Prove that the correlation of the two alleles in a genotype is F.

9.2 Show that $\Delta = \Pr(G|Y = 1) - \Pr(G|Y = 0)$ in Sect. 9.2.1 can be written as (9.5).

9.3 Give the values of p_j, k_j and γ_i $(j = 1, \ldots, J)$ that satisfy Eq. (9.6) when $J = 3$.

9.4 When does $\mathrm{Var}(T)$ given in (9.12) reach its maximum and minimum?

9.5 Let Wright's inbreeding coefficient in cases and controls be F_1 and F_2, respectively. Show that, when $r = s$, $\mathrm{Var}(T)$ in the CATT with the ADD model can be written as

$$\mathrm{Var}(T) = 2rp(1 - p)\{2 + (F_1 + F_2)(2r - 1)\}.$$

9.6 Assume that the genetic backgrounds are known. Using Eqs. (9.14) and (9.15), explain how P_0 and P_1 are estimated using the EM algorithm.

Chapter 10
Gene-Environment Interactions

Abstract Gene-environment interactions are considered in Chap. 10, which focuses on a $2 \times 2 \times 2$ table. The expressions of odds ratios for the genetic effect, the environmental factor effect, and the gene-environment interaction are given. More general cases for gene and environmental factors are briefly discussed. Three common tests for gene-environment interaction are studied, including the Score test, the likelihood ratio test (LRT) and the Wald test. Examples are given with detailed calculations.

We discuss gene-environment interactions and odds ratios for the association of the main genetic and environmental effects and gene-environment interactions under various models. Inference, including estimates and test statistics, for gene-environment interactions is studied. Maximum likelihood estimates and various test statistics, e.g., the likelihood ratio test, Score test and Wald test, for gene-environment interactions are presented. We focus on a binary exposure for the environmental factor and a binary genetic susceptibility. In this case, the data can be displayed in a $2 \times 2 \times 2$ table. A more general environmental factor and genetic susceptibility are also considered. We only consider gene-environment interactions for a single genetic marker. Some discussion of gene-environment interactions in the context of genome-wide association studies will be given in Chap. 12.

It should be understood that throughout this chapter we are only considering statistical interaction, not biological interaction. If two factors affect an outcome (phenotype), there must be biologic interaction at some level whether or not an additive statistical model is adequate to estimate actual effects.

10.1 Introduction

In Chap. 3, we studied a genetic association using a logistic regression model for case-control data. Covariates, including environmental factors, can be adjusted for by simply adding them to the logistic regression model so that the genetic effect and the effect of an environmental factor on the risk of development of a disease can be investigated separately. Gene-environment interaction, however, allows one to

G. Zheng et al., *Analysis of Genetic Association Studies*,
Statistics for Biology and Health,
DOI 10.1007/978-1-4614-2245-7_10, © Springer Science+Business Media, LLC 2012

study a joint genetic and environmental effect on the risk of development of a disease. Some rationales for studying gene-environment interaction are summarized in the literature, which include providing an accurate estimate of the population-attributable risk for genetic and environmental factors with gene-environment interaction, helping understand the disease mechanisms and biologic pathways, studying how the genetic effect would be modified by a change of environmental or risk factors, and helping design personalized treatment for a disease based on individual genetic susceptibility and levels of risk factors.

Although a case-control association study may be designed to have enough power to detect a main genetic effect and/or an environmental effect, it is known that there is less power to detect a gene-environment interaction. In epidemiology, one often does not test for a gene-environment interaction unless the main genetic and environmental effects are significant at a given level of significance. In genetic studies, however, we may expect a gene-environment interaction to be present in the absence of a main genetic or environmental effect. Besides the lower power to detect an interaction, testing gene-environment interaction may also involve an issue of multiple testing, especially for a $2 \times 3 \times k$ table, which contains case-control data with three genotypes and an environment with $k \geq 2$ levels. For example, for a $2 \times 3 \times 3$ table, an interaction can be defined in different ways in terms of the underlying genetic model (REC, ADD or DOM) and/or various models for the three exposure levels of an environment. Hence, it is important to report all the analyses under various models or appropriately correct for multiple testing.

We first describe gene-environment interactions using a binary environmental factor, such as exposed or not exposed, and a binary genetic susceptibility, such as with a genetic variant or without that genetic variant. This type of data can be presented in a $2 \times 2 \times 2$ table. ORs associated with the main genetic and environmental effects and gene-environment interactions are discussed. We focus on a multiplicative gene-environment interaction model for ORs. The ORs for the association of $2 \times 2 \times k$ and $2 \times 3 \times k$ tables are also considered. In the first table, the genetic susceptibility is binary but the environmental factor has k levels. In the second table, we consider three genotypes and an environmental factor with k levels.

In Chap. 8, we discussed gene-gene interactions and statistical methods to detect gene-gene interactions. Some of the methods described in that chapter are related to what we are presenting in this chapter.

10.2 Gene-Environment Interactions and Inference

10.2.1 A $2 \times 2 \times 2$ Table

Notation

Let D, G and E denote the binary disease status, a diallelic-allelic genetic marker, and an environment, respectively. Denote $D = 1$ for a case and $D = 0$ for a control.

The levels of a binary G are denoted as (G_0, G_1). More generally, $(G_0, G_1, G_2) = (AA, AB, BB)$ is used for the three genotypes of G with alleles A and B. A binary G may be of interest, for example, when B is the risk allele and the underlying genetic model is REC, G_0 is for AA or AB and G_1 is BB. Under the DOM model, G_0 is AA and G_1 is AB or BB. The levels of E are denoted as $(E_0, E_1, \ldots, E_{k-1})$ for $k \geq 2$. Although an environmental factor E can be continuous, we only focus on a qualitative one. We always denote G_0 and E_0 as the reference levels.

Let $c(G_i)$ and $c(E_j)$ be the coding values of G_i and E_j, respectively. For example, $c(G_1) = c(G_2) = 1$ and $c(G_0) = 0$ under the DOM model, and $c(E_1) = 1$ and $c(E_0) = 0$ for $k = 2$. In general, we code $c(G_i) = g_i$ ($i = 0, 1$ or $i = 0, 1, 2$) and $c(E_j) = e_j$ ($j = 0, 1, \ldots, k - 1$), where $g_0 = e_0 = 0$. We choose $g_i = i, i = 0, 1, 2$, for the ADD model by counting the number of B alleles in the genotype, and $e_j = j$, $j = 0, 1, \ldots, k - 1$, for an equal-spaced E. The above coding for G (or E) allows a linear relationship among the levels of G (or E).

Odds Ratios and Gene-Environment Interactions

Consider a binary G with $c(G_0) = g_0 = 0$ and $c(G_1) = g_1 = 1$ and a binary E with $c(E_0) = e_0 = 0$ and $c(E_1) = e_1 = 1$. Denote $p_1(G, E) = \Pr(D = 1|G, E)$ and $p_0(G, E) = 1 - p_1(G, E) = \Pr(D = 0|G, E)$. Using a logistic regression model, we have

$$\mathrm{logit}(p_1(G, E)) = \beta_0 + \beta_G c(G) + \beta_E c(E) + \beta_{GE} c(G) c(E). \qquad (10.1)$$

Then

$$\mathrm{OR}_{G|E_0} = \mathrm{OR}_{G:D|E=E_0} = \exp(\beta_G) = \frac{p_1(G_1, E_0)}{p_0(G_1, E_0)} \Big/ \frac{p_1(G_0, E_0)}{p_0(G_0, E_0)}$$

is the OR relating D to G given $E = E_0$,

$$\mathrm{OR}_{E|G_0} = \mathrm{OR}_{E:D|G=G_0} = \exp(\beta_E) = \frac{p_1(G_0, E_1)}{p_0(G_0, E_1)} \Big/ \frac{p_1(G_0, E_0)}{p_0(G_0, E_0)}$$

is the OR relating D to E given $G = G_0$, and

$$\exp(\beta_{GE}) = \frac{\mathrm{OR}_{E|G_1}}{\mathrm{OR}_{E|G_0}}$$

$$= \left\{ \frac{p_1(G_1, E_1)}{p_0(G_1, E_1)} \Big/ \frac{p_1(G_1, E_0)}{p_0(G_1, E_0)} \right\} \Big/ \left\{ \frac{p_1(G_0, E_1)}{p_0(G_0, E_1)} \Big/ \frac{p_1(G_0, E_0)}{p_0(G_0, E_0)} \right\}$$

$$= \frac{\mathrm{OR}_{G|E_1}}{\mathrm{OR}_{G|E_0}}$$

$$= \left\{ \frac{p_1(G_1, E_1)}{p_0(G_1, E_1)} \Big/ \frac{p_1(G_0, E_1)}{p_0(G_0, E_1)} \right\} \Big/ \left\{ \frac{p_1(G_1, E_0)}{p_0(G_1, E_0)} \Big/ \frac{p_1(G_0, E_0)}{p_0(G_0, E_0)} \right\}$$

Table 10.1 ORs for the association of D with a binary G and a binary E. Part (a) and part (b) are equivalent

Part (a)		E	
		E_0	E_1
G	G_0	1.0	$\mathrm{OR}_{E|G_0}$
	G_1	$\mathrm{OR}_{G|E_0}$	$\mathrm{OR}_{E|G_0} \times \mathrm{OR}_{G|E_0} \times \exp(\beta_{GE})$

Part (b)		E	
		E_0	E_1
G	G_0	1.0	$\exp(\beta_E)$
	G_1	$\exp(\beta_G)$	$\exp(\beta_G + \beta_E + \exp(\beta_{GE}))$

Table 10.2 RRs for the association of D with a binary G and a binary E under an additive interaction model

		E	
		E_0	E_1
G	G_0	0.0	$\mathrm{RR}_{E|G_0}$
	G_1	$\mathrm{RR}_{G|E_0}$	$\mathrm{RR}_{E|G_0} + \mathrm{RR}_{G|E_0} + \mathrm{RR}_{G,E}$

is the ratio of two ORs both relating D to E given $G = G_1$ and $G = G_0$, respectively, or, equivalently, the ratio of two ORs both relating D to G given $E = E_1$ and $E = E_0$, respectively. This interaction model is often referred to as a *multiplicative interaction model*. If $\beta_{GE} = 0$, $\mathrm{OR}_{E|G_1} = \mathrm{OR}_{E|G_0}$ or, equivalently, $\mathrm{OR}_{G|E_1} = \mathrm{OR}_{G|E_0}$. Hence, there is no gene-environment interaction. ORs and the multiplicative interaction model are natural choices when the logistic regression model (10.1) is used. An *additive interaction model* (i.e., an additive model with an interaction term) can be considered if one is interested in differences in risks instead of ORs. In the following, we only consider the multiplicative interaction model and ORs.

Note that the above $\exp(\beta_{GE})$ can also be expressed as

$$\exp(\beta_{GE}) = \frac{\frac{p_1(G_1,E_1)}{p_0(G_1,E_1)} \big/ \frac{p_1(G_0,E_0)}{p_0(G_0,E_0)}}{\mathrm{OR}_{E|G_0} \times \mathrm{OR}_{G|E_0}} = \frac{\mathrm{OR}_{G,E}}{\mathrm{OR}_{E|G_0} \times \mathrm{OR}_{G|E_0}},$$

where $\mathrm{OR}_{G,E} = \mathrm{OR}_{G,E:D}$ is the OR relating D to both G and E. Thus, we have

$$\mathrm{OR}_{G,E} = \mathrm{OR}_{E|G_0} \times \mathrm{OR}_{G|E_0} \times \exp(\beta_{GE}).$$

If $\beta_{GE} = 0$, $\mathrm{OR}_{G,E}$ is the product of the two ORs, $\mathrm{OR}_{E|G_0}$ and $\mathrm{OR}_{G|E_0}$, and there is no gene-environment interaction. All ORs for the association are given in Table 10.1. If an additive interaction model is of interest, the relative risks (RRs) for the association can be represented as in Table 10.2.

Table 10.3 Case (control) data with a binary G and a binary E

			E		Total
			E_0	E_1	
Cases (controls) G	G_0		R_{00} (S_{00})	R_{01} (S_{01})	$R_{0\cdot}$ ($S_{0\cdot}$)
	G_1		R_{10} (S_{10})	R_{11} (S_{11})	$R_{1\cdot}$ ($S_{1\cdot}$)
	Total		$R_{\cdot 0}$ ($S_{\cdot 0}$)	$R_{\cdot 1}$ ($S_{\cdot 1}$)	r (s)

Data and Inference

A dataset with r cases and s controls can be displayed in a $2 \times 2 \times 2$ table (Table 10.3). Each cell of Table 10.3 contains the number of cases (or controls) with the given levels of G and E. Using $c(G_0) = 0$, $c(G_1) = 1$, $c(E_0) = 0$ and $c(E_1) = 1$, the likelihood function for the data in the table can be written as

$$L(\beta) = \frac{\exp(r\beta_0 + R_{1\cdot}\beta_G + R_{\cdot 1}\beta_E + R_{11}\beta_{GE})}{\prod_{k=1}^{4}\{1 + \exp(\beta^T \mathbf{1}_k)\}^{N_k}}, \tag{10.2}$$

where $\beta = (\beta_0, \beta_G, \beta_E, \beta_{GE})^T$, $\mathbf{1}_1 = (1, 0, 0, 0)^T$, $\mathbf{1}_2 = (1, 1, 0, 0)^T$, $\mathbf{1}_3 = (1, 0, 1, 0)^T$, $\mathbf{1}_4 = (1, 1, 1, 1)^T$, $N_1 = n_{00} = R_{00} + S_{00}$, $N_2 = n_{10} = R_{10} + S_{10}$, $N_3 = n_{01} = R_{01} + S_{01}$, and $N_4 = n_{11} = R_{11} + S_{11}$.

Let $l(\beta)$ be the log-likelihood function. The MLEs of β_0, β_G, β_E and β_{GE}, denoted as $\widehat{\beta}_0$, $\widehat{\beta}_G$, $\widehat{\beta}_E$ and $\widehat{\beta}_{GE}$, can be solved from $\partial l(\beta)/\partial \beta^T = 0$. From Problem 10.1, we have

$$\exp(\widehat{\beta}_0) = \frac{R_{00}}{S_{00}},$$

$$\exp(\widehat{\beta}_G) = \frac{R_{10}}{S_{10}} \Big/ \frac{R_{00}}{S_{00}} = \frac{R_{10} S_{00}}{S_{10} R_{00}},$$

$$\exp(\widehat{\beta}_E) = \frac{R_{01}}{S_{01}} \Big/ \frac{R_{00}}{S_{00}} = \frac{R_{01} S_{00}}{S_{01} R_{00}},$$

$$\exp(\widehat{\beta}_{GE}) = \left(\frac{R_{11}}{S_{11}} \Big/ \frac{R_{10}}{S_{10}}\right) \Big/ \left(\frac{R_{01}}{S_{01}} \Big/ \frac{R_{00}}{S_{00}}\right) = \frac{R_{11} S_{10} S_{01} R_{00}}{S_{11} R_{10} R_{01} S_{00}}. \tag{10.3}$$

The asymptotic variances of the MLEs can be approximated by

$$-\{\partial^2 l(\beta)/\partial \beta \partial \beta^T |_{\widehat{\beta}}\}^{-1}.$$

Denote $a = (R_{00}^{-1} + S_{00}^{-1})^{-1}$, $b = (R_{01}^{-1} + S_{01}^{-1})^{-1}$, $c = (R_{10}^{-1} + S_{10}^{-1})^{-1}$ and $d = (R_{11}^{-1} + S_{11}^{-1})^{-1}$. From Problem 10.2, we have

$$-\frac{\partial^2 l(\beta)}{\partial \beta \partial \beta^T}\Big|_{\widehat{\beta}} = \begin{bmatrix} a+b+c+d & c+d & b+d & d \\ c+d & c+d & d & d \\ b+d & d & b+d & d \\ d & d & d & d \end{bmatrix}. \tag{10.4}$$

The $(2,2)$th, $(3,3)$th and $(4,4)$th elements of the inverse of the above matrix are estimates of the asymptotic variances of $\widehat{\beta}_G$, $\widehat{\beta}_E$ and $\widehat{\beta}_{GE}$, respectively. From Problem 10.2, they are respectively $1/a + 1/c$, $1/a + 1/b$ and $1/a + 1/b + 1/c + 1/d$. Thus, the MLE of β_{GE} is $\widehat{\beta}_{GE} = \log\{R_{11}S_{10}S_{01}R_{00}/(S_{11}R_{10}R_{01}S_{00})\}$ and the estimate of its asymptotic variance is $\widehat{\text{Var}}(\widehat{\beta}_{GE}) = 1/R_{11} + 1/S_{10} + 1/S_{01} + 1/R_{00} + 1/S_{11} + 1/R_{10} + 1/R_{01} + 1/S_{00}$. When the sample size $n = R + S$ is large enough,

$$\widehat{\beta}_{GE} - \beta_{GE} \approx N(0, \widehat{\text{Var}}(\widehat{\beta}_{GE})),$$

in distribution, where β_{GE} is the true value. This approximation can be used to give a 95% CI for β_{GE}.

Note that in (10.3) the MLEs of $\widehat{\beta}$ are solved from the Score equations (see Problem 10.1). In Chap. 8, an alternative simple approach to find similar MLEs was to use multinomial distributions and the fact that ORs using prospective and retrospective distributions are equivalent. That method can be applied here to find the MLEs and their asymptotic variances and covariances (see Problem 10.5).

Two special cases of (10.1) are $\beta_G = 0$ or $\beta_E = 0$, under which respectively

$$\exp(\beta_{GE}) = \frac{p_1(G_1, E_1)}{p_0(G_1, E_1)} \Big/ \frac{p_1(G_0, E_1)}{p_0(G_0, E_1)},$$

$$\text{or} \quad \exp(\beta_{GE}) = \frac{p_1(G_1, E_1)}{p_0(G_1, E_1)} \Big/ \frac{p_1(G_1, E_0)}{p_0(G_1, E_0)}.$$

The first one is the OR relating D to G among those with $E = E_1$ (samples with $E = E_0$ have no information for the interaction) and the second one is the OR relating D to E among those with $G = G_1$ (samples with $G = G_0$ have no information for the interaction). The MLEs and their asymptotic variances under these two special cases are different (Problem 10.4).

10.2.2 An Example

As an example, we consider the case-control study of a genetic susceptibility to a lung cancer with a binary smoking exposure: light ($E = E_0$) versus at least moderate ($E = E_1$). The data are given in Table 10.4.

Fitting the data in Table 10.4 with the logistic regression model given in (10.1), we obtain the MLE for the OR relating the cancer to the genetic susceptibility among light smokers as

$$\exp(\widehat{\beta}_G) = 5 \times 79/(9 \times 6) = 7.315$$

or the log OR as $\log(7.315) = 1.9899$. The estimate of the asymptotic variance of $\widehat{\beta}_G$ is

$$\widehat{\text{Var}}(\widehat{\beta}_G) = 1/5 + 1/79 + 1/9 + 1/6 = 0.4903.$$

Table 10.4 Case-control data of a genetic susceptibility to a lung cancer with smoking

			Smoking		Total
			E_0	E_1	
Cancer	G	G_0	6	27	33
		G_1	5	7	12
		Total	11	34	45
Normal	G	G_0	79	40	119
		G_1	9	7	16
		Total	88	47	135

Thus the 95% CI for the log OR, β_G, is

$$1.9899 \pm 1.96 \times 0.4903^{1/2} = (0.6173, 3.3625),$$

and the 95% CI for the OR, $\exp(\beta_G)$, is $(\exp(0.6173), \exp(3.3625)) = (1.854, 28.861)$.

Similarly, the MLE for the OR relating the cancer to light smoking among those without the genetic susceptibility is

$$\exp(\widehat{\beta}_E) = 27 \times 79/(40 \times 6) = 8.887.$$

Hence the log OR is $\log(8.887) = 2.185$ and

$$\widehat{\mathrm{Var}}(\widehat{\beta}_E) = 1/27 + 1/79 + 1/40 + 1/6 = 0.2414.$$

The 95% CI for the log OR, β_E, is

$$2.185 \pm 1.96 \times 0.2414^{1/2} = (1.222, 3.148),$$

and the 95% CI for the OR, $\exp(\beta_E)$, is $(\exp(1.222), \exp(3.148)) = (3.394, 23.289)$.

To examine if the ORs relating the cancer to the genetic susceptibility vary across smoking status, we compute the MLE for $\exp(\beta_{GE})$ as

$$\exp(\widehat{\beta}_{GE}) = 7 \times 9 \times 40 \times 6/(7 \times 5 \times 27 \times 79) = 0.2025.$$

The estimate of the asymptotic variance of $\widehat{\beta}_{GE}$ is

$$\widehat{\mathrm{Var}}(\widehat{\beta}_{GE}) = 1/7 + 1/9 + 1/40 + 1/6 + 1/7 + 1/5 + 1/27 + 1/79 = 0.8382.$$

The 95% CI for β_{GE} is

$$\log(0.2025) \pm 1.96 \times 0.8382^{1/2} = (-3.39, 0.1974),$$

which covers 0, or the 95% CI for $\exp(\beta_{GE})$ is $(0.034, 1.218)$, which covers 1. Thus, there is no significant evidence to support the gene-environment interaction at the 5% significance level. Other test statistics for gene-environment interactions will be discussed later.

10.2.3 More General G and E

In the previous section, both $G = (G_0, G_1)$ and $E = (E_0, E_1)$ are binary. We coded G as $(g_0, g_1) = (c(G_0), c(G_1)) = (0, 1)$ and E as $(e_0, e_1) = (c(E_0), c(E_1)) = (0, 1)$. In fact, inference is invariant to linear transformations of the coding values of G and E when they are binary. For example, we can code G by any (g_0, g_1) with $g_1 > g_0$ and E by any (e_0, e_1) with $e_1 > e_0$ (Problem 10.6). Thus, the coding values themselves have no meaning. This, however, is not true when G and E have more than two levels because the coding values themselves imply a relationship of the levels. For example, for the ADD model, $(g_0, g_1, g_2) = (0, 1, 2)$ is used for (AA, AB, BB), which specifies $\mathrm{OR}_{G_2|E_0} = \{\mathrm{OR}_{G_1|E_0}\}^2$, while $(g_0, g_1, g_2) = (0, 1, 4)$ specifies a different genetic model, under which $\mathrm{OR}_{G_2|E_0} = \{\mathrm{OR}_{G_1|E_0}\}^4$. Although G has three levels, its main effect is determined by a single parameter when $(g_0, g_1, g_2) = (0, 1, 2)$ is used. To avoid establishing a linear relationship among the three genotypes because we may not know the true relationship, we can code them by $c(G_0) = (0, 0)^T$, $c(G_1) = (1, 0)^T$ and $c(G_2) = (1, 1)^T$. In this case, two parameters $\beta_G = (\beta_{G_1}, \beta_{G_2})^T$ are used to determine the main genetic effect. This argument can also be applied to E with more than two levels.

Data and ORs for a $2 \times 2 \times k$ Table

Consider a binary G and an E with k levels. The data can be displayed in a $2 \times 2 \times k$ table (Table 10.5). Denote $p_1(G_i, E_j) = \Pr(D = 1 | G = G_i, E = E_j)$ and $p_0(G_i, E_j) = 1 - p_1(G_i, E_j)$, where

$$\mathrm{logit}(p_1(G_i, E_j)) = \beta_0 + \beta_G c(G_i) + \beta_E^T c(E_j) + \beta_{GE}^T c(G_i)c(E_j), \quad (10.5)$$

and $\beta_E = (\beta_{E_1}, \ldots, \beta_{E_{k-1}})^T$, $\beta_{GE} = (\beta_{GE_1}, \ldots, \beta_{GE_{k-1}})^T$, $c(E_0) = (0, \ldots, 0)^T$, $c(E_j) = (1, \ldots, 1, 0, \ldots, 0)^T$ (the first $j \geq 1$ elements are 1), $c(G_0) = 0$, and $c(G_1) = 1$. Then the ORs relating D to $G = G_i$ given $E = E_j$ and relating D to $E = E_j$ given $G = G_i$, denoted as $\mathrm{OR}_{G_i|E_j}$ and $\mathrm{OR}_{E_j|G_i}$, respectively, are given by

$$\mathrm{OR}_{G_i|E_j} = \exp\{\beta_G c(G_i) + \beta_{GE}^T c(G_i)c(E_j)\},$$

$$\mathrm{OR}_{E_j|G_i} = \exp\{\beta_E^T c(E_j) + \beta_{GE}^T c(G_i)c(E_j)\}.$$

ORs of the association for the $2 \times 2 \times k$ table are given in Table 10.6. Thus, the main effect of G is determined by β_G, the main environmental effect is determined by β_E, and the gene-environment interaction is determined by β_{GE}. If $\beta_{GE_1} = \cdots = \beta_{GE_{k-1}} = 0$, there is no gene-environment interaction, which is equivalent to $\beta_{GE}^T c(E_1) = \cdots = \beta_{GE}^T c(E_{k-1}) = 0$.

Table 10.5 Case-control data with a binary G and a k-level E

			E				Total
			E_0	E_1	$\cdots$	E_{k-1}	
Cases	G	G_0	R_{00}	R_{01}	$\cdots$	$R_{0(k-1)}$	$R_{0\cdot}$
		G_1	R_{10}	R_{11}	$\cdots$	$R_{1(k-1)}$	$R_{1\cdot}$
		Total	$R_{\cdot 0}$	$R_{\cdot 1}$	$\cdots$	$R_{\cdot(k-1)}$	r
Controls	G	G_0	S_{00}	S_{01}	$\cdots$	$S_{0(k-1)}$	$S_{0\cdot}$
		G_1	S_{10}	S_{11}	$\cdots$	$S_{1(k-1)}$	$S_{1\cdot}$
		Total	$S_{\cdot 0}$	$S_{\cdot 1}$	$\cdots$	$S_{\cdot(k-1)}$	s

Table 10.6 ORs for the association of D with a binary G and a k-level E. Part (a) and part (b) are equivalent

Part (a)		E			
		E_0	E_1	$\cdots$	E_{k-1}
G	G_0	1.0	$OR_{E_1\mid G_0}$	$\cdots$	$OR_{E_{k-1}\mid G_0}$
	G_1	$OR_{G_1\mid E_0}$	$OR_{E_1\mid G_0}\times$	$\cdots$	$OR_{E_{k-1}\mid G_0}\times$
			$OR_{G_1\mid E_0}\times\exp\{\beta_{GE}^T c(E_1)\}$	$\cdots$	$OR_{G_1\mid E_0}\times\exp\{\beta_{GE}^T c(E_{k-1})\}$

Part (b)		E			
		E_0	E_1	$\cdots$	E_{k-1}
G	G_0	1.0	$\exp(\beta_E^T c(E_1)$	$\cdots$	$\exp(\beta_E^T c(E_{k-1})$
	G_1	$\exp(\beta_G)$	$\exp(\beta_G)\times$	$\cdots$	$\exp(\beta_G)\times$
			$\exp\{\beta_E^T c(E_1)+\beta_{GE}^T c(E_1)\}$	$\cdots$	$\exp\{\beta_E^T c(E_{k-1})+\beta_{GE}^T c(E_{k-1})\}$

Inference for a 2 × 2 × k Table

The likelihood function for the data in Table 10.5 is given by

$$
L(\beta_0, \beta_G, \beta_E^T, \beta_{GE}^T)
$$

$$
= \prod_{i=0}^{1}\prod_{j=0}^{k-1}\{p_1(G_i, E_j)\}^{R_{ij}}\{p_0(G_i, E_j)\}^{S_{ij}}
$$

$$
= \exp\left[r\beta_0 + R_{1\cdot}\beta_G + \sum_{j=1}^{k-1}(R_{\cdot j}\beta_E^T + R_{1j}\beta_{GE}^T)c(E_j) \right]
$$

$$
\times \left[\prod_{j=0}^{k-1}\{1 + \exp(\beta_0 + \beta_E^T c(E_j))\}^{n_{0j}} \right]^{-1}
$$

$$\times \left[\prod_{j=0}^{k-1} \{1 + \exp(\beta_0 + \beta_G + \beta_E^T c(E_j) + \beta_{GE}^T c(E_j))\}^{n_{0j}} \right]^{-1}, \quad (10.6)$$

where $n_{ij} = R_{ij} + S_{ij}$, $p_1(G_i, E_j)$ is given in (10.5), and $p_0(G_i, E_j) = 1 - p_1(G_i, E_j)$. Denote the log-likelihood as $l(\beta)$ and $\beta = (\beta_0, \beta_G, \beta_E^T, \beta_{GE}^T)^T$. The MLE of β can be obtained from the Score equations $\partial l(\beta)/\partial \beta^T = 0$, which has a closed form solution. The MLEs of the parameters in β and their asymptotic variances and covariances can be obtained using multinomial distributions and the independence of cases and controls, as in the $2 \times 2 \times 2$ table. In the following, we show how to solve the Score equations to find the MLEs.

In $l(\beta)$, instead of considering β_E^T and β_{GE}^T, we first treat $\beta_E^T c(E_j)$ and $\beta_{GE}^T c(E_j)$ as parameters for $j = 1, \ldots, k - 1$. For a given j, from

$$\frac{\partial l(\beta)}{\partial \{\beta_{GE}^T c(E_j)\}} = 0, \qquad \frac{\partial l(\beta)}{\partial \{\beta_E^T c(E_j)\}} = 0,$$

we have

$$\sum_{j=1}^{k-1} n_{1j} \frac{\exp\{\beta_0 + \beta_G + (\beta_E + \beta_{GE})^T c(E_j)\}}{1 + \exp\{\beta_0 + \beta_G + (\beta_E + \beta_{GE})^T c(E_j)\}} = \sum_{j=1}^{k-1} R_{1j},$$

$$\sum_{j=1}^{k-1} n_{0j} \frac{\exp\{\beta_0 + \beta_E^T c(E_j)\}}{1 + \exp\{\beta_0 + \beta_E^T c(E_j)\}} = \sum_{j=1}^{k-1} R_{0j}.$$

Substituting them into $\partial l(\beta)/\partial \beta_0 = 0$ and $\partial l(\beta)/\partial \beta_G = 0$, we have $\exp(\beta_0)/\{1 + \exp(\beta_0)\} = R_{00}/n_{00}$ and $\exp(\beta_0 + \beta_G)/\{1 + \exp(\beta_0 + \beta_G)\} = R_{10}/n_{10}$, from which we have

$$\exp(\beta_0) = R_{00}/S_{00},$$

$$\exp(\beta_G) = R_{10} S_{00}/(S_{10} R_{00}).$$

Thus $\widehat{\beta}_0 = \log(R_{00}/S_{00})$ and $\widehat{\beta}_G = \log\{R_{10} S_{00}/(S_{10} R_{00})\}$. Next, we consider β_E^T and β_{GE}^T as parameters. From $\partial l(\beta)/\partial \beta_{GE} = 0$ and $\partial l(\beta)/\partial \beta_E = 0$, we have

$$\sum_{j=1}^{k-1} n_{1j} \frac{\exp\{\beta_0 + \beta_G + (\beta_E + \beta_{GE})^T c(E_j)\}}{1 + \exp\{\beta_0 + \beta_G + (\beta_E + \beta_{GE})^T c(E_j)\}} c(E_j) = \sum_{j=1}^{k-1} R_{1j} c(E_j),$$

$$\sum_{j=1}^{k-1} n_{0j} \frac{\exp\{\beta_0 + \beta_E^T c(E_j)\}}{1 + \exp\{\beta_0 + \beta_E^T c(E_j)\}} c(E_j) = \sum_{j=1}^{k-1} R_{0j} c(E_j).$$

It follows, for any j,

$$\exp\{\beta_0 + \beta_G + (\beta_E + \beta_{GE})^T c(E_j)\} = R_{1j}/S_{1j},$$

Table 10.7 Case-control data of a binary genetic susceptibility to a lung cancer with smoking (light E_0, moderate E_1 and heavy E_2)

			Smoking E_0	E_1	E_2	Total
Cancer	G	G_0	6	11	16	33
		G_1	5	4	3	12
		Total	11	15	19	45
Normal	G	G_0	79	22	18	119
		G_1	9	4	3	16
		Total	88	26	21	135

$$\exp\{\beta_0 + \beta_E^T c(E_j)\} = R_{0j}/S_{0j}.$$

Thus,

$$\exp\{\beta_E^T c(E_j)\} = R_{0j} S_{00}/(S_{0j} R_{00}),$$

$$\exp\{\beta_{GE}^T c(E_j)\} = \frac{R_{1j} S_{10} S_{0j} R_{00}}{S_{1j} R_{10} R_{0j} S_{00}},$$

from which we obtain the MLEs of $\beta_E^T c(E_j)$ and $\beta_{GE}^T c(E_j)$. Using these results, the ORs in Table 10.6 can be estimated using $\mathrm{OR}_{E_j|G_0} = \exp\{\beta_E^T c(E_j)\}$ and $\mathrm{OR}_{E_j|G_1} = \exp\{\beta_E^T c(E_j) + \beta_{GE}^T c(E_j)\}$. Their asymptotic variances can be directly obtained from multinomial distributions and the independence of cases and controls (see Problem 10.5). Although we can obtain MLEs of β_E^T and β_{GE}^T, to estimate the ORs we only need the MLEs of $\beta_E^T c(E_j)$ and $\beta_{GE}^T c(E_j)$ for $j = 1, \ldots, k - 1$.

An Example

To illustrate, the example given in Table 10.4 is represented with three categories for smoking (Table 10.7): light (E_0), moderate (E_1) and heavy (E_2).

Using the results presented before, we have $\mathrm{OR}_{G_1|E_0} = \exp(\beta_G) = 5 \times 79/(9 \times 6) = 7.315$, which is the same as $\mathrm{OR}_{G_1|E_0}$ estimated using the data in Table 10.4. The asymptotic variance of $\log(\mathrm{OR}_{G_1|E_0})$ and the 95% CI for $\mathrm{OR}_{G_1|E_0}$ are also the same as before, e.g., the 95% CI for $\mathrm{OR}_{G_1|E_0}$ is $(1.854, 28.861)$. To obtain the OR relating D to (G_1, E_1), we have

$$\mathrm{OR}_{G_1,E_1} = \exp\{\beta_G + \beta_E^T c(E_1) + \beta_{GE}^T c(E_1)\} = \frac{R_{11} S_{00}}{R_{00} S_{11}} = \frac{4 \times 79}{6 \times 4} = 13.17.$$

The log OR is $\log(13.17) = 2.578$ and the estimate of its asymptotic variance is $1/R_{11} + 1/S_{00} + 1/R_{00} + 1/S_{11} = 0.6793$. Hence the 95% CI for OR_{G_1,E_1} is

$$(\exp(2.578 - 1.96 \times 0.6793^{1/2}), \exp(2.578 + 1.96 \times 0.6793^{1/2})) = (2.618, 66.249).$$

Table 10.8 ORs for the association of D with a binary G and a equal-spaced k-level E. $\theta = \exp(\beta_{GE_1})$

		E			
		E_0	E_1	$\cdots$	E_{k-1}
G	G_0	1.0	$\mathrm{OR}_{E_1\mid G_0}$	$\cdots$	$\mathrm{OR}_{E_1\mid G_0}^{k-1}$
	G_1	$\mathrm{OR}_{G_1\mid E_0}$	$\mathrm{OR}_{E_1\mid G_0} \times \mathrm{OR}_{G_1\mid E_0} \times \theta$	$\cdots$	$\mathrm{OR}_{E_1\mid G_0}^{k-1} \times \mathrm{OR}_{G_1\mid E_0} \times \theta^{k-1}$

Restricted Models

The number of parameters can be reduced with some additional assumptions. For example, we can assume a MUL effect for E as $\mathrm{OR}_{E_j\mid G_0} = (\mathrm{OR}_{E_1\mid G_0})^j$, i.e. $e_j = j$ for all j. Hence, $\exp\{\beta_E^T c(E_j)\} = [\exp\{\beta_E^T c(E_1)\}]^j = \exp(j\beta_{E_1})$ for $j \geq 1$. The $k - 1$ parameters for the main effect of E can then be expressed in terms of a single parameter $\exp(\beta_{E_1})$. For the gene-environment interaction, if we assume a "top-to-bottom quantile" interaction effect as $\exp\{\beta_{GE}^T c(E_j)\} = [\exp\{\beta_{GE}^T c(E_1)\}]^j = \exp(j\beta_{GE_1})$ for $j \geq 1$, then each of the $k - 1$ interaction parameters can be expressed as a power of a single parameter $\theta = \exp\{\beta_{GE}^T c(E_1)\} = \exp(\beta_{GE_1})$. Table 10.6 presents all ORs for the association with these additional model assumptions. However, these model assumptions may not generally hold. For example, one may assume $\mathrm{OR}_{E_j\mid G_0} = j\mathrm{OR}_{E_1\mid G_0}$ for $j \geq 1$.

The likelihood function for the data in Table 10.5 under the model in Table 10.8 is given by

$$L(\beta) = \prod_{i=0}^{1} \prod_{j=0}^{k-1} \{p_1(G_i, E_j)\}^{R_{ij}} \{p_0(G_i, E_j)\}^{S_{ij}}$$

$$= \exp\left\{ r\beta_0 + R_1.\beta_G + \sum_{j=1}^{k-1} jR_{.j}\beta_{E_1} + \sum_{j=1}^{k-1} jR_{1j}\beta_{GE_1} \right\}$$

$$\times \left[\prod_{j=0}^{k-1} \{1 + \exp(\beta_0 + j\beta_{E_1})\}^{n_{0j}} \right]^{-1}$$

$$\times \left[\prod_{j=0}^{k-1} \{1 + \exp(\beta_0 + \beta_G + j\beta_{E_1} + j\beta_{GE_1})\}^{n_{1j}} \right]^{-1},$$

where $\beta = (\beta_0, \beta_G, \beta_{E_1}, \beta_{GE_1})^T$. This likelihood can be obtained from (10.6) by setting $\beta_{E_1} = \cdots = \beta_{k-1}$ and $\beta_{GE_1} = \cdots = \beta_{GE_{k-1}}$. When $k = 2$, the above likelihood $L(\beta)$ becomes the one in (10.2), and the MLE of β_{GE_1}, $\widehat{\beta}_{GE_1}$, has a closed form solution as before. For $k > 2$, however, $\widehat{\beta}_{GE_1}$ has no closed form solution, but can be obtained numerically. Its asymptotic variance can also be obtained numerically. When $\theta = 1$, there is no gene-environment interaction.

Table 10.9 ORs for the association of D with an ADD model for G and a equal-spaced k-level E. $\theta = \exp(\beta_{G_1 E_1})$

		E				
		E_0	E_1		$\cdots$	E_{k-1}
G	G_0	1.0	$\mathrm{OR}_{E_1|G_0}$		$\cdots$	$\mathrm{OR}_{E_1|G_0}^{k-1}$
	G_1	$\mathrm{OR}_{G_1|E_0}$	$\mathrm{OR}_{E_1|G_0} \times \mathrm{OR}_{G_1|E_0} \times \theta$		$\cdots$	$\mathrm{OR}_{E_1|G_0}^{k-1} \times \mathrm{OR}_{G_1|E_0} \times \theta^{k-1}$
	G_2	$\mathrm{OR}_{G_1|E_0}^2$	$\mathrm{OR}_{E_1|G_0} \times \mathrm{OR}_{G_1|E_0}^2 \times \theta^2$		$\cdots$	$\mathrm{OR}_{E_1|G_0}^{k-1} \times \mathrm{OR}_{G_1|E_0}^2 \times \theta^{2(k-1)}$

A $2 \times 3 \times k$ Table

For a $2 \times 3 \times k$ table, in which G has three levels, ORs for the association are given in Table 10.9. $\mathrm{OR}_{G_2|E_0} = \{\mathrm{OR}_{G_1|E_0}\}^2$ is assumed, and the other models for E and the interaction used in Table 10.8 are also assumed. The likelihood function for a $2 \times 3 \times k$ table using the model in Table 10.9 can be obtained as before and the MLEs for the parameters can be found numerically. When $\theta = 1$, there is no gene-environment interaction.

A $2 \times 3 \times k$ table is used for G with three genotypes, which is useful for an ADD model. In this case, one can also consider a $2 \times 2 \times k$ table in which G is based on alleles. The first part of Table 10.10 is a genotype-based $2 \times 3 \times 2$ table and the second part is an allele-based $2 \times 2 \times 2$ table. In the first table, the gene-environment interaction is defined by two parameters $\beta_{G_1 E}$ and $\beta_{G_2 E}$ or a single parameter $\beta_{G_1 E}$ under the ADD model. In the second table, it is defined by a single parameter β_{GE}. Inference for the gene-environment interaction using the data in the second part of Table 10.10 may be subject to allelic correlation. However, it is not clear if such a potential impact due to allelic correlation can be ignored if HWE holds in the population. If so, it is not clear if inferences for $\beta_{G_1 E}$ using the data from the first table and β_{GE} using the data from the second table are asymptotically equivalent. Similar issues are discussed in Sect. 3.4.2.

10.2.4 Gene-Environment Independence

The independence between gene and environment in the population with a rare disease is often assumed in the context of gene-environment interaction. Under this assumption, the OR relating to the gene-environment interaction can be estimated using cases only. To illustrate, we use the $2 \times 2 \times 2$ table in Table 10.3. Denote D for $D = 1$ and $\bar{D}$ for $D = 0$. From Sect. 10.2.1, we have

$$\exp(\beta_{GE}) = \frac{\Pr(D|G_1, E_1)\Pr(\bar{D}|G_1, E_0)\Pr(\bar{D}|G_0, E_1)\Pr(D|G_0, E_0)}{\Pr(\bar{D}|G_1, E_1)\Pr(D|G_1, E_0)\Pr(D|G_0, E_1)\Pr(\bar{D}|G_0, E_0)}$$

$$= \frac{\Pr(E_1|D, G_1)\Pr(E_0|\bar{D}, G_1)\Pr(E_1|\bar{D}, G_0)\Pr(E_0|D, G_0)}{\Pr(E_1|\bar{D}, G_1)\Pr(E_0|D, G_1)\Pr(E_1|D, G_0)\Pr(E_0|\bar{D}, G_0)}$$

Table 10.10 Case-control data with a binary E and a genotype-based G or an allele-based G

			E		Total
			E_0	E_1	
Cases	G	AA	R_{00}	R_{01}	$R_{0\cdot}$
		AB	R_{10}	R_{11}	$R_{1\cdot}$
		BB	R_{20}	R_{21}	$R_{2\cdot}$
		Total	$R_{\cdot 0}$	$R_{\cdot 1}$	r
Controls	G	AA	S_{00}	S_{01}	$S_{0\cdot}$
		AB	S_{10}	S_{11}	$S_{1\cdot}$
		BB	S_{20}	S_{21}	$S_{2\cdot}$
		Total	$S_{\cdot 0}$	$S_{\cdot 1}$	s

			E		Total
			E_0	E_1	
Cases	G	A	$2R_{00} + R_{10}$	$2R_{01} + R_{11}$	$2R_{0\cdot} + R_{1\cdot}$
		B	$2R_{20} + R_{10}$	$2R_{21} + R_{11}$	$2R_{2\cdot} + R_{1\cdot}$
		Total	$2R_{\cdot 0}$	$2R_{\cdot 1}$	$2r$
Controls	G	A	$2S_{00} + S_{10}$	$2S_{01} + S_{11}$	$2S_{0\cdot} + S_{1\cdot}$
		B	$2S_{20} + S_{10}$	$2S_{21} + S_{11}$	$2S_{2\cdot} + S_{1\cdot}$
		Total	$2S_{\cdot 0}$	$2S_{\cdot 1}$	$2s$

$$= \frac{\Pr(E_1|D, G_1)\,\Pr(E_0|D, G_0)}{\Pr(E_0|D, G_1)\,\Pr(E_1|D, G_0)}$$

$$\times \frac{\Pr(E_0|\bar{D}, G_1)\,\Pr(E_1|\bar{D}, G_0)}{\Pr(E_1|\bar{D}, G_1)\,\Pr(E_0|\bar{D}, G_0)} \tag{10.7}$$

$$\approx \frac{\Pr(E_1|D, G_1)\,\Pr(E_0|D, G_0)}{\Pr(E_0|D, G_1)\,\Pr(E_1|D, G_0)}, \tag{10.8}$$

where the second factor in (10.7) is approximately 1 under the assumptions of gene-environment independence and a rare disease (Problem 10.7).

Note that (10.8) shows that $\exp(\beta_{GE})$ can be approximated by the OR relating E to G among cases because it does not involve $\bar{D}$ (controls). However, even when the assumption holds, under the logistic regression model (10.1) the gene-environment independence cannot be incorporated and both cases and controls are used to estimate $\exp(\beta_{GE})$. An equation similar to (10.7) is also obtained for gene-gene interactions (Sect. 8.11).

10.3 Test Statistics for Gene-Environment Interaction

The LRT, Score test and Wald test will be discussed to test for a gene-environment interaction. The general formulas of these three tests in the presence of nuisance parameters given in Sect. 1.2.4 can be used. Four parameters, β_0, β_G, β_E and β_{GE}, appear in the logistic regression model (10.1). The parameters β_G and β_E are for the main genetic and environmental effects, respectively, and the last parameter is for the gene-environment interaction. To test for β_{GE}, the null hypothesis H_0 should be specified explicitly. For example, in $H_0 : \beta_{GE} = 0$, the parameters β_G and β_E are not specified, while in $H_0 : \beta_G = \beta_E = \beta_{GE} = 0$ (a global null hypothesis), all parameters of the main effects and the gene-environment interaction are specified. The test statistics corresponding to different H_0 are often different.

To illustrate these three tests, we consider the $2 \times 2 \times 2$ table with a binary G and a binary E given in Table 10.3. The likelihood for the data is given in (10.2). The log-likelihood, denoted as $l(\beta)$, can be written as

$$
\begin{aligned}
l(\beta) = r\beta_0 &+ R_{1.}\beta_G + R_{.1}\beta_E + R_{11}\beta_{GE} - n_{00}\log\{1 + \exp(\beta_0)\} \\
&- n_{10}\log\{1 + \exp(\beta_0 + \beta_G)\} - n_{01}\log\{1 + \exp(\beta_0 + \beta_E)\} \\
&- n_{11}\log\{1 + \exp(\beta_0 + \beta_G + \beta_E + \beta_{GE})\},
\end{aligned}
\tag{10.9}
$$

where $\beta = (\beta_0, \beta_G, \beta_E, \beta_{GE})^T$. The MLE, $\widehat{\beta} = (\widehat{\beta}_0, \widehat{\beta}_G, \widehat{\beta}_E, \widehat{\beta}_{GE})^T$, is given in (10.3) in Sect. 10.2.

10.3.1 Likelihood Ratio Test

Consider testing $H_0 : \beta_{GE} = 0$ against $H_1 : \beta_{GE} \neq 0$ without specifying β_G and β_E. Replacing β in $l(\beta)$ by $\widehat{\beta}$, we obtain $l(\widehat{\beta})$.

Under H_0, $l(\beta)$ is denoted as $l_0(\beta)$ and is given by

$$
\begin{aligned}
l_0(\beta) = r\beta_0 &+ R_{1.}\beta_G + R_{.1}\beta_E - n_{00}\log\{1 + \exp(\beta_0)\} \\
&- n_{10}\log\{1 + \exp(\beta_0 + \beta_G)\} - n_{01}\log\{1 + \exp(\beta_0 + \beta_E)\} \\
&- n_{11}\log\{1 + \exp(\beta_0 + \beta_G + \beta_E)\},
\end{aligned}
\tag{10.10}
$$

where $\beta = (\beta_0, \beta_G, \beta_E, 0)^T$. The estimate $\widetilde{\beta} = (\widetilde{\beta}_0, \widetilde{\beta}_G, \widetilde{\beta}_E, 0)^T$ that maximizes $l_0(\beta)$, or $l(\beta)$ under H_0, has no closed form solution. It can be found numerically. Then we compute $l_0(\widetilde{\beta})$. The LRT is given by

$$
\text{LRT} = 2l(\widehat{\beta}) - 2l_0(\widetilde{\beta}) \sim \chi_1^2 \quad \text{under } H_0.
$$

Consider testing $H_0 : \beta_G = \beta_E = \beta_{GE} = 0$, where $\beta = (\beta_0, \beta_G, \beta_E, \beta_{GE})^T$ without any restriction and $\beta = (\beta_0, 0, 0, 0)^T$ under H_0. In this case, $l(\widehat{\beta})$ is the same as before. However, $l_0(\theta) = r\beta_0 - n\log\{1 + \exp(\beta_0)\}$, which has a maximum value $l_0(\tilde{\beta}) = r \log r + s \log s - n \log n$, where $n = r + s$ is the total sample size. Hence, the LRT is given by

$$\text{LRT} = 2l(\hat{\beta}) - 2l_0(\tilde{\beta}) = 2l(\hat{\beta}) - 2(r \log r + s \log s - n \log n) \sim \chi_3^2 \quad \text{under } H_0.$$

10.3.2 Score Test

To obtain the Score test for $H_0 : \beta_{GE} = 0$, the restricted MLE of β under H_0, $\tilde{\beta}$, is given in (10.10). Hence the Score function is given by

$$U(\tilde{\beta}) = \frac{\partial l(\beta)}{\partial \beta_{GE}}\Big|_{\beta=\tilde{\beta}} = R_{11} - (R_{11} + S_{11})\frac{\exp(\tilde{\beta}_0 + \tilde{\beta}_G + \tilde{\beta}_E)}{1 + \exp(\tilde{\beta}_0 + \tilde{\beta}_G + \tilde{\beta}_E)}. \quad (10.11)$$

The observed Fisher information matrix is given by

$$i_n(\tilde{\beta}) = -\frac{\partial^2 l(\beta)}{\partial \beta \partial \beta^T}\Big|_{\beta=\tilde{\beta}}. \quad (10.12)$$

Then compute the inverse $i_n^{-1}(\tilde{\beta})$. Denote the $(4, 4)$th element of $i_n^{-1}(\tilde{\beta})$ as $i^{\beta_{GE}\beta_{GE}}$. Its inverse is also the estimate of the asymptotic variance of $U(\tilde{\beta})$. Finally, the Score test is given by

$$\text{ST} = U^T(\tilde{\beta}) i^{\beta_{GE}\beta_{GE}} U(\tilde{\beta}) \sim \chi_1^2 \quad \text{under } H_0.$$

To test a global hypothesis $H_0 : \beta_G = \beta_E = \beta_{GE} = 0$, β_0 is a nuisance parameter and estimated under H_0, which yields $\tilde{\beta}_0 = \log(r/s)$. Thus, $\tilde{\beta} = (\tilde{\beta}_0, 0, 0, 0)^T$. Then the Score function is given by

$$U(\tilde{\beta}) = \begin{bmatrix} \frac{\partial l(\beta)}{\partial \beta_G} \\ \frac{\partial l(\beta)}{\partial \beta_E} \\ \frac{\partial l(\beta)}{\partial \beta_{GE}} \end{bmatrix}\Bigg|_{\beta=\hat{\beta}} = \frac{rs}{n}\begin{bmatrix} R_{1.}/r - S_{1.}/s \\ R_{.1}/r - S_{.1}/s \\ R_{11}/r - S_{11}/s \end{bmatrix},$$

and

$$i_n(\tilde{\beta}) = -\frac{\partial^2 l(\beta)}{\partial \beta \partial \beta^T}\Big|_{\beta=\hat{\beta}}$$

$$= \frac{rs}{n^2}\begin{bmatrix} n & R_{1.} + S_{1.} & R_{.1} + S_{.1} & R_{11} + S_{11} \\ R_{1.} + S_{1.} & R_{1.} + S_{1.} & R_{11} + S_{11} & R_{11} + S_{11} \\ R_{.1} + S_{.1} & R_{11} + S_{11} & R_{.1} + S_{.1} & R_{11} + S_{11} \\ R_{11} + S_{11} & R_{11} + S_{11} & R_{11} + S_{11} & R_{11} + S_{11} \end{bmatrix}. \quad (10.13)$$

Let $a = rs(R_{00} + S_{00})/n^2$, $b = rs(R_{01} + S_{01})/n^2$, $c = rs(R_{10} + S_{10})/n^2$, and $d = rs(R_{11} + S_{11})/n^2$. Then the above matrix is identical in format to the one given in (10.4). Its inverse is given in Problem 10.3. That is,

$$
i_n^{-1}(\tilde{\beta}) =
\begin{bmatrix}
\frac{1}{a} & -\frac{1}{a} & -\frac{1}{a} & \frac{1}{a} \\
-\frac{1}{a} & \frac{1}{a}+\frac{1}{c} & \frac{1}{a} & -\frac{1}{a}-\frac{1}{c} \\
-\frac{1}{a} & \frac{1}{a} & \frac{1}{a}+\frac{1}{b} & -\frac{1}{a}-\frac{1}{b} \\
\frac{1}{a} & -\frac{1}{a}-\frac{1}{c} & -\frac{1}{a}-\frac{1}{b} & \frac{1}{a}+\frac{1}{b}+\frac{1}{c}+\frac{1}{d}
\end{bmatrix}.
$$

Define the submatrix corresponding to $(\beta_G, \beta_E, \beta_{GE})^T$ as

$$
\Sigma =
\begin{bmatrix}
\frac{1}{a}+\frac{1}{c} & \frac{1}{a} & -\frac{1}{a}-\frac{1}{c} \\
\frac{1}{a} & \frac{1}{a}+\frac{1}{b} & -\frac{1}{a}-\frac{1}{b} \\
-\frac{1}{a}-\frac{1}{c} & -\frac{1}{a}-\frac{1}{b} & \frac{1}{a}+\frac{1}{b}+\frac{1}{c}+\frac{1}{d}
\end{bmatrix}. \tag{10.14}
$$

Then the Score test can be written as $\mathrm{ST} = U^T(\tilde{\beta})\Sigma U(\tilde{\beta}) \sim \chi_3^2$ under H_0.

10.3.3 Wald Test

The Wald test is based on the asymptotic distribution of the MLE. To test $H_0 : \beta_{GE} = 0$, the MLE of β_{GE} is given by $\widehat{\beta}_{GE} = \log\{(R_{11}S_{10}S_{01}R_{00})/(S_{11}R_{10}R_{01}S_{00})\}$ and $\widehat{\mathrm{Var}}(\widehat{\beta}_{GE}) = 1/R_{11}+1/S_{10}+1/S_{01}+1/R_{00}+1/S_{11}+1/R_{10}+1/R_{01}+1/S_{00}$ (see Sect. 10.2.1). When the sample size n is large enough,

$$
\widehat{\beta}_{GE} - \beta_{GE} = \widehat{\beta}_{GE} \approx N(0, \widehat{\mathrm{Var}}(\widehat{\beta}_{GE})),
$$

where $\beta_{GE} = 0$ under H_0. Thus, the Wald test is given by

$$
\mathrm{WT} = \widehat{\beta}_{GE}^2 / \widehat{\mathrm{Var}}(\widehat{\beta}_{GE}) \sim \chi_1^2 \quad \text{under } H_0.
$$

To test $H_0 : \beta_G = \beta_E = \beta_{GE} = 0$, the MLEs of $(\beta_G, \beta_E, \beta_{GE})^T$ are given in (10.3). Denote the estimate of the asymptotic covariance matrix of the MLEs $(\widehat{\beta}_G, \widehat{\beta}_E, \widehat{\beta}_{GE})^T$ as Σ. Then,

$$
\Sigma =
\begin{bmatrix}
\frac{1}{a}+\frac{1}{c} & \frac{1}{a} & -\frac{1}{a}-\frac{1}{c} \\
\frac{1}{a} & \frac{1}{a}+\frac{1}{b} & -\frac{1}{a}-\frac{1}{b} \\
-\frac{1}{a}-\frac{1}{c} & -\frac{1}{a}-\frac{1}{b} & \frac{1}{a}+\frac{1}{b}+\frac{1}{c}+\frac{1}{d}
\end{bmatrix},
$$

where $a = (R_{00}^{-1} + S_{00}^{-1})^{-1}$, $b = (R_{01}^{-1} + S_{01}^{-1})^{-1}$, $c = (R_{10}^{-1} + S_{10}^{-1})^{-1}$ and $d = (R_{11}^{-1} + S_{11}^{-1})^{-1}$. Thus, the Wald test is given by

$$
\mathrm{WT} = (\widehat{\beta}_G, \widehat{\beta}_E, \widehat{\beta}_{GE})\Sigma^{-1}(\widehat{\beta}_G, \widehat{\beta}_E, \widehat{\beta}_{GE})^T \sim \chi_3^2 \quad \text{under } H_0,
$$

where

$$\Sigma^{-1} = \begin{bmatrix} \frac{(a+b)(c+d)}{a+b+c+d} & \frac{ad-bc}{a+b+c+d} & \frac{(a+b)d}{a+b+c+d} \\[2mm] \frac{ad-bc}{a+b+c+d} & \frac{(a+c)(b+d)}{a+b+c+d} & \frac{(a+c)d}{a+b+c+d} \\[2mm] \frac{(a+b)d}{a+b+c+d} & \frac{(a+c)d}{a+b+c+d} & \frac{(a+b+c)d}{a+b+c+d} \end{bmatrix}. \tag{10.15}$$

10.3.4 Examples

Using the data presented in Table 10.4, $R_{00} = 6$, $R_{01} = 27$, $R_{10} = 5$, $R_{11} = 7$, $S_{00} = 79$, $S_{01} = 40$, $S_{10} = 9$, and $S_{11} = 7$. Hence $R_{1.} = R_{10} + R_{11} = 12$, $R_{.1} = R_{01} + R_{11} = 34$, $S_{1.} = S_{10} + S_{11} = 16$, $S_{.1} = S_{01} + S_{11} = 47$. $n_{00} = R_{00} + S_{00} = 85$, $n_{01} = R_{01} + S_{01} = 67$, $n_{10} = R_{10} + S_{10} = 14$ and $n_{11} = R_{11} + S_{11} = 14$. The total numbers of cases and controls are $r = 45$ and $s = 135$, respectively, and $n = r + s = 180$.

Testing $H_0 : \beta_G = \beta_E = \beta_{GE} = 0$

We first consider testing the global null hypothesis $H_0 : \beta_G = \beta_E = \beta_{GE} = 0$. The log-likelihood functions are

$$l(\beta) = 45\beta_0 + 12\beta_G + 34\beta_E + 7\beta_{GE} - 85\log\{1 + \exp(\beta_0)\}$$
$$- 14\log\{1 + \exp(\beta_0 + \beta_G)\} - 67\log\{1 + \exp(\beta_0 + \beta_E)\}$$
$$- 14\log\{1 + \exp(\beta_0 + \beta_G + \beta_E + \beta_{GE})\}, \tag{10.16}$$
$$l_0(\beta_0) = 45\beta_0 - 180\log\{1 + \exp(\beta_0)\}.$$

The MLEs for $\beta = (\beta_0, \beta_G, \beta_E, \beta_{GE})^T$ based on $l(\beta)$ are given by

$$\widehat{\beta}_0 = \log(R_{00}/S_{00}) = -2.5777,$$
$$\widehat{\beta}_G = \log\{R_{10}S_{00}/(S_{10}R_{00})\} = 1.9899,$$
$$\widehat{\beta}_E = \log\{R_{01}S_{00}/(S_{01}R_{00})\} = 2.1847,$$
$$\widehat{\beta}_{GE} = \log\{R_{11}S_{10}S_{01}R_{00}/(S_{11}R_{10}R_{01}R_{00})\} = -1.5969. \tag{10.17}$$

The MLE for β_0 based on $l_0(\beta_0)$ is $\widetilde{\beta}_0 = \log(r/s) = -1.0986$. Hence, $-2l(\widehat{\beta}) = 171.377$ and $-2l_0(\widetilde{\beta}) = -2l_0(\widetilde{\beta}_0) = 202.441$. Thus, LRT $= 2l(\widehat{\beta}) - 2l_0(\widetilde{\beta}) = 202.441 - 171.377 = 31.064$. The p-value is 8.2×10^{-7}.

For the Score test, the Score function $U(\widetilde{\beta})$ and Σ given in (10.14) are

$$U(\widetilde{\beta}) = \frac{rs}{n} \begin{bmatrix} R_{1.}/r - S_{1.}/s \\ R_{.1}/r - S_{.1}/s \\ R_{11}/r - S_{11}/s \end{bmatrix} = \begin{bmatrix} 5 \\ 13.75 \\ 3.5 \end{bmatrix},$$

$$\Sigma = \begin{bmatrix} 0.4437 & 0.06275 & -0.4437 \\ 0.06275 & 0.14235 & -0.14235 \\ -0.4437 & -0.14235 & 0.90425 \end{bmatrix}.$$

Thus, $ST = U^T(\widetilde{\beta})\Sigma U(\widehat{\beta}) = 28.479$ with p-value 2.9×10^{-6}.

To compute the Wald test, the MLEs $(\widehat{\beta}_G, \widehat{\beta}_E, \widehat{\beta}_{GE})^T$ are given in (10.17). Σ^{-1} given in (10.15) is

$$\Sigma^{-1} = \begin{bmatrix} 5.1275 & -1.1367 & 2.6728 \\ -1.1367 & 6.0707 & 1.0830 \\ 2.6728 & 1.0830 & 3.0688 \end{bmatrix}.$$

Thus, $WT = (\widehat{\beta}_G, \widehat{\beta}_E, \widehat{\beta}_{GE})\Sigma^{-1}(\widehat{\beta}_G, \widehat{\beta}_E, \widehat{\beta}_{GE})^T = 22.676$ with p-value 4.7×10^{-5}.

Testing $H_0 : \beta_{GE} = 0$

We next consider only testing the gene-environment interaction $H_0 : \beta_{GE} = 0$. For the LRT, the log-likelihood function $l(\beta)$ is given by (10.16). So $\widehat{\beta}$ given in (10.17) can be used. Hence, $-2l(\widehat{\beta}) = 171.377$. Under H_0, $l_0(\beta)$ is obtained from (10.10):

$$l_0(\beta) = 45\beta_0 + 12\beta_G + 34\beta_E - 85\log\{1 + \exp(\beta_0)\}$$
$$- 14\log\{1 + \exp(\beta_0 + \beta_G)\} - 67\log\{1 + \exp(\beta_0 + \beta_E)\}$$
$$- 14\log\{1 + \exp(\beta_0 + \beta_G + \beta_E)\},$$

where $\beta = (\beta_0, \beta_G, \beta_E, 0)^T$. The estimates, $\widetilde{\beta}_0$, $\widetilde{\beta}_G$ and $\widetilde{\beta}_E$, can be solved from the equation $\partial l_0(\beta)/\partial \beta^T = 0$. The numerical results show that $\widetilde{\beta}_0 = -2.2857$ $\widetilde{\beta}_G = 1.0498$ and $\widetilde{\beta}_E = 1.7765$. Hence $-2l_0(\widetilde{\beta}) = 174.373$ and $LRT = 2l(\widehat{\beta}) - 2l_0(\widetilde{\beta}) = 174.373 - 171.377 = 2.996$ with p-value 0.0835.

For the Score test, the Score function from (10.11) is

$$U(\widetilde{\beta}) = 7 - 14\frac{\exp(\widetilde{\beta}_0 + \widetilde{\beta}_G + \widetilde{\beta}_E)}{1 + \exp(\widetilde{\beta}_0 + \widetilde{\beta}_G + \widetilde{\beta}_E)} = -1.8471.$$

Then, from (10.12),

$$i_n(\widetilde{\beta}) = \begin{bmatrix} 28.5302 & 5.6986 & 18.9657 & 3.2563 \\ 5.6986 & 5.6986 & 3.2563 & 3.2563 \\ 18.9657 & 3.2563 & 18.9657 & 3.2563 \\ 3.2563 & 3.2563 & 3.2563 & 3.2563 \end{bmatrix}.$$

The $(4, 4)$th element of $i_n^{-1}(\widetilde{\beta})$ is $\Sigma = 0.9206$. Hence $ST = U^2\Sigma = 3.1409$ with p-value 0.0764.

To apply the Wald test for $H_0 : \beta_{GE} = 0$, we have $\widehat{\beta}_{GE} = -1.5969$ and $\widehat{\text{Var}}(\widehat{\beta}_{GE}) = 0.8382$. Thus, $\text{WT} = \widehat{\beta}^2_{GE}/\widehat{\text{Var}}(\widehat{\beta}_{GE}) = 3.042$ with p-value 0.0811.

Remarks

The results show that, although different test statistics may have different p-values, they lead to the same conclusions. That is, the overall model is significant at the 0.05 level but the gene-environment interaction is not significant at that level. The Wald test is relatively easy to use as it has closed forms for either $H_0 : \beta_{GE} = 0$ or the global null hypothesis $H_0 : \beta_G = \beta_E = \beta_{GE}$. Computation of the LRT needs one to evaluate the log-likelihood functions but does not require computation of the Fisher information matrix or its inverse, while the Score test needs them. Both the LRT and Score test also require finding the MLEs numerically. The three test statistics are output from most statistical software.

When G and/or E have greater than 2 levels, the degrees of freedom of the chi-squared distribution for each of the three test statistics for $H_0 : \beta_{GE} = 0$ would be greater than 1. For example, for a binary G and a three-level E, the number of degrees of freedom is 2. However, if the top-to-bottom quantile interaction model is assumed (Sect. 10.2.3), the number of degrees of freedom is still 1 as only a single parameter is used, which may improve the power if the model assumption is valid.

Whether or not $\beta_{GE} = 0$ is of relevance to fitting a parsimonious model, but is irrelevant regarding the presence of biological interaction. If two factors (e.g., gene and environment) are involved in a disease, this in itself implies some kind of biological interaction.

10.4 Bibliographical Comments

We focus on gene-environment interaction of a single genetic marker and a discrete environmental factor. Gene-environment interactions in the context of genome-wide association studies will be discussed in Chap. 12 [126, 271]. Different definitions of gene-environment interactions were discussed by Smith and Day [249], Khouri et al. [142] and Hunter [126]. Hunter [126] also summarized the benefits of studying gene-environment interactions, some of which are also discussed in Sect. 10.1. A general discussion of interactions, including statistical interactions and biological interactions, can be found in Wang et al. [293]. This chapter is focused on statistical gene-environment interactions. Cordell [44] discussed how to model statistical interaction if one is interested in biological interaction. Wang et al. [294], on the other hand, briefly discussed how to infer biological interaction when statistical interaction is not significant.

Gene-environment independence was studied by Piegorsch et al. [203], who showed that, under this assumption and for a rare disease, gene-environment interaction can be tested by the association between genetic susceptibility and an environmental factor using cases only. However, using the logistic regression model for case-control data cannot exploit this assumption for the analysis. This concept was further exploited by Umbach and Weinberg [278]. They showed also that for a rare disease the logistic regression model for testing gene-environment interaction is equivalent to using a log-linear model and that the independence of gene and environment can be incorporated in the analysis using the log-linear model. Hence, using the logistic regression model is not appropriate when the independence between gene and environment holds in the population [278]. However, the log-linear model of Umbach and Weinberg [278] contains a large number of parameters to be estimated. A similar log-linear model was also used for gene-gene interactions (Sect. 8.3.3). In this chapter, we only consider a logistic regression model for testing gene-environment interactions. Chatterjee and Carrol [30] studied a retrospective model for case-control data and converted it to the logistic regression model with a joint distribution of a gene factor and an environmental factor. Hence, exploiting the independence of gene and environment, they could handle the joint distribution by writing them as two marginal distributions of gene and environment and estimated each of them nonparametrically. This approach allows a more general environmental factor to be tested, while not needing a large number of parameters to be estimated, as in Umbach and Weinberg [278]. Although the independence of gene and environment is a natural assumption in some situations, Albert et al. [7] showed that inference can be biased when this assumption is violated.

Inference of gene-environment interactions when an environmental factor has multiple exposure levels is not efficient due to the large number of degrees of freedom. The top-to-bottom interaction model of Foppa and Spiegelman [87] can be used to reduce the number of parameters for the gene-environment interaction and hence the number of degrees of freedom of test statistics. This interaction model is also used for calculating sample size and power for gene-environment interactions, which is discussed in the next chapter. The data in Table 10.4 and Table 10.7 used in the examples were originally reported by Nakachi et al. [188] and were used by Piegorsch et al. [203].

10.5 Problems

10.1 Using the notation of Sect. 10.2.1, let $u_1(\beta) = \exp(\beta_0)/\{1 + \exp(\beta_0)\}$, $u_2(\beta) = \exp(\beta_0 + \beta_G)/\{1 + \exp(\beta_0 + \beta_G)\}$, $u_3(\beta) = \exp(\beta_0 + \beta_E)/\{1 + \exp(\beta_0 + \beta_E)\}$, and $u_4(\beta) = \exp(\beta_0 + \beta_G + \beta_E + \beta_{GE})/\{1 + \exp(\beta_0 + \beta_G + \beta_E + \beta_{GE})\}$. Show that:

$$\partial l(\beta)/\partial \beta_0 = r - \sum_{k=1}^{4} N_k u_k(\beta) = 0,$$

$$\partial l(\beta)/\partial \beta_G = R_{1.} - N_2 u_2(\beta) - N_4 u_4(\beta) = 0,$$

$$\partial l(\beta)/\partial \beta_E = R_{.1} - N_3 u_3(\beta) - N_4 u_4(\beta) = 0,$$

$$\partial l(\beta)/\partial \beta_{GE} = R_{11} - N_4 u_4(\beta) = 0,$$

from which the MLEs of β_G, β_E and β_{GE} can be obtained.

10.2 Show that $-\partial^2 l(\beta)/\partial\beta\partial\beta^T$ can be expressed as (10.4), whose determinant is $abcd$.

10.3 Verify that the inverse of (10.4) is

$$
\left\{ -\frac{\partial^2 l(\beta)}{\partial\beta\partial\beta^T}\Big|_{\tilde{\beta}} \right\}^{-1} =
\begin{bmatrix}
\frac{1}{a} & -\frac{1}{a} & -\frac{1}{a} & \frac{1}{a} \\
-\frac{1}{a} & \frac{1}{a}+\frac{1}{c} & \frac{1}{a} & -\frac{1}{a}-\frac{1}{c} \\
-\frac{1}{a} & \frac{1}{a} & \frac{1}{a}+\frac{1}{b} & -\frac{1}{a}-\frac{1}{b} \\
\frac{1}{a} & -\frac{1}{a}-\frac{1}{c} & -\frac{1}{a}-\frac{1}{b} & \frac{1}{a}+\frac{1}{b}+\frac{1}{c}+\frac{1}{d}
\end{bmatrix}.
$$

10.4 Derive the MLE of $\exp(\beta_{GE})$ and its asymptotic variance under the two special cases of (10.1) with $\beta_G = 0$ and $\beta_E = 0$, respectively. See Sect. 10.2.

10.5 The asymptotic variance of $\widehat{\beta}_{GE}$ can be directly obtained using multinomial distributions,

$$(R_{00}, R_{01}, R_{10}, R_{11}) \sim Mul(r;\, p_1(0,0),\, p_1(0,1),\, p_1(1,0),\, p_1(1,1)),$$

$$(S_{00}, S_{01}, S_{10}, S_{11}) \sim Mul(s;\, p_0(0,0),\, p_0(0,1),\, p_0(1,0),\, p_0(1,1)),$$

and the fact that cases and controls are independent.

10.6 In Sect. 10.2.1, the binary G and binary E both take values 0 and 1. Suppose G takes values g_0 and g_1, $g_1 > g_0$ and E takes values e_0 and e_1, $e_1 > e_0$. The logistic regression model is given by $\mathrm{logit}(p_1(G, E)) = \beta_0 + \beta_G G + \beta_E E + \beta_{GE} GE$. Let $\tilde{G} = (G - g_0)/(g_1 - g_0)$ and $\tilde{E} = (E - e_0)/(e_1 - e_0)$ be linear transformations. Denote $\tilde{\beta}_0 = \beta_0 + \beta_G g_0 + \beta_E e_0 - \beta_{GE} g_0 e_0$, $\tilde{\beta}_{\tilde{G}} = (\beta_G + \beta_{GE} e_0)(g_1 - g_0)$, $\tilde{\beta}_{\tilde{E}} = (\beta_E + \beta_{GE} g_0)(e_1 - e_0)$, and $\tilde{\beta}_{\tilde{G}\tilde{E}} = \beta_{GE}(g_1 - g_0)(e_1 - e_0)$. Show that, under the above reparameterization, $\mathrm{logit}(p_1(\tilde{G}, \tilde{E})) = \tilde{\beta}_0 + \tilde{\beta}_{\tilde{G}}\tilde{G} + \tilde{\beta}_{\tilde{E}}\tilde{E} + \tilde{\beta}_{\tilde{G}\tilde{E}}\tilde{G}\tilde{E}$, where $\tilde{G}$ and $\tilde{E}$ both take values 0 and 1.

10.7 Show that, under the assumption of gene-environment independence and a rare disease,

$$\Pr(E_0|\bar{D}, G_1)\Pr(E_1|\bar{D}, G_0) \approx \Pr(E_1|\bar{D}, G_1)\Pr(E_0|\bar{D}, G_0).$$

Chapter 11
Power and Sample Size Calculations

Abstract Chapter 11 covers sample size and power calculations for testing genetic association, gene-environment interaction, and gene-gene interaction. Asymptotic power for testing a single marker association using the trend test is derived. The power calculations are discussed under perfect linkage disequilibrium or under imperfect linkage disequilibrium. The asymptotic power for Pearson's test is also given. Asymptotic power is presented using either genotype relative risks or odds ratios. How to use an existing Power Program to calculate sample size and power for single marker association is illustrated. A general approach is described for testing interactions. Then testing gene-environment and gene-gene interactions are treated as special cases. The same Power Program is used to calculate the asymptotic power/sample size for testing gene-gene and gene-environment interactions. Examples are used to illustrate the use of the Power Program.

In the design of genetic association studies, power and sample size calculations are required in order to avoid an under-powered study. For most common designs, it is often required that the power to detect a single association is at least 80% given the significance level 0.05 and a particular GRR or OR under a specific genetic model. To calculate the power or sample size, other parameters need to be specified, which include, but are not limited to, the allele frequency, the disease prevalence, and the proportion of cases in the sample. If HWE proportions hold in the study population, genotype frequencies can be calculated using the allele frequency. Otherwise, Wright's inbreeding coefficient is specified and used to compute genotype frequencies given the allele frequency. If the sample size and power are calculated for a marker locus rather than a disease locus, the LD parameter also needs to be specified. With so many parameters varying, sample sizes could range from less than a thousand to more than ten thousand to detect an association with 80% power.

In this chapter, we focus on association studies using unrelated cases and controls. For a single marker analysis, sample size and power calculations are considered for both disease and marker loci. For testing interactions, we only consider a disease locus. A general approach to test for interactions is considered. Then gene-environment and gene-gene interactions are treated as special cases. A program to calculate power and sample size for single marker analysis, gene-environment

G. Zheng et al., *Analysis of Genetic Association Studies*,
Statistics for Biology and Health,
DOI 10.1007/978-1-4614-2245-7_11, © Springer Science+Business Media, LLC 2012

interaction and gene-gene interaction is discussed. The use of this program is illustrated with examples.

11.1 Single Marker Analysis Using Trend Tests

11.1.1 Power and Sample Size Formulas

The trend test studied in Sect. 3.3.1 can be written as

$$Z_{\mathrm{CATT}}(x) = \frac{U_x}{\{\widehat{\mathrm{Var}}(U_x)\}^{1/2}}, \tag{11.1}$$

where

$$U_x = n\psi_0\psi_1\mathbf{x}^T(\widehat{\mathbf{P}} - \widehat{\mathbf{Q}}),$$
$$\widehat{\mathrm{Var}}(U_x) = n\psi_0\psi_1[(\mathbf{x}^2)^T(\psi_1\widehat{\mathbf{P}} + \psi_0\widehat{\mathbf{Q}}) - \{\mathbf{x}^T(\psi_1\widehat{\mathbf{P}} + \psi_0\widehat{\mathbf{Q}})\}^2], \tag{11.2}$$

in which $\psi_0 = s/n$ and $\psi_1 = r/n$, $\mathbf{x} = (x_0, x_1, x_2)^T = (0, x, 1)^T$, $\mathbf{x}^2 = (0, x^2, 1)^T$, $\widehat{\mathbf{P}} = (\widehat{p}_0, \widehat{p}_1, \widehat{p}_2)^T$, $\widehat{\mathbf{Q}} = (\widehat{q}_0, \widehat{q}_1, \widehat{q}_2)^T$, $\widehat{p}_i = r_i/r$ and $\widehat{q}_i = s_i/s$ $(i = 0, 1, 2)$. Here $x = 0, 1/2, 1$ is an indicator for the underlying genetic model of REC, ADD (or MUL), and DOM, respectively. For sample size and power calculation using trend tests, we assume x is given. Under the null hypothesis H_0, for a given x, $Z_{\mathrm{CATT}}(x) \sim N(0, 1)$ asymptotically.

To calculate sample size and power, we use the asymptotic distribution of $Z_{\mathrm{CATT}}(x)$ under the alternative hypothesis H_1, which can be obtained from Slutsky's theorem. First, denote

$$\mu_{1x} = \psi_0\psi_1\mathbf{x}^T(\mathbf{P} - \mathbf{Q}), \tag{11.3}$$
$$\widetilde{\sigma}_{1x}^2 = \psi_0\psi_1[(\mathbf{x}^2)^T(\psi_1\mathbf{P} + \psi_0\mathbf{Q}) - \{\mathbf{x}^T(\psi_1\mathbf{P} + \psi_0\mathbf{Q})\}^2], \tag{11.4}$$

where $\mathbf{P} = (p_0, p_1, p_2)^T$ and $\mathbf{Q} = (q_0, q_1, q_2)^T$, and

$$p_i = \Pr(G_i|\mathrm{case}) \quad \text{and} \quad q_i = \Pr(G_i|\mathrm{control})$$

for the given genotype G_i $(i = 0, 1, 2)$. Then

$$\mathrm{E}(U_x|H_1) = n\mu_{1x},$$
$$\mathrm{Var}(U_x|H_1) = n^2\psi_0^2\psi_1^2\mathbf{x}^T(\Sigma_P/r + \Sigma_Q/s)\mathbf{x} = n\sigma_{1x}^2,$$

where

$$\sigma_{1x}^2 = \psi_0^2\psi_1\mathbf{x}^T\Sigma_P\mathbf{x} + \psi_0\psi_1^2\mathbf{x}^T\Sigma_Q\mathbf{x}, \tag{11.5}$$

and Σ_P and Σ_Q are 3×3 matrices with respectively the (i, i)th element $p_i(1 - p_i)$ and $q_i(1 - q_i)$ $(i = 0, 1, 2)$, and the (i, j)th element $-p_ip_j$ and $-q_iq_j$ $(i \neq j)$. Thus, under H_1, $n^{-1}\widehat{\mathrm{Var}}(U_x) \to \widetilde{\sigma}_{1x}^2$ as $n \to \infty$ and $\psi_0 \in (0, 1)$, and, when n is large enough,

$$\{U_x - \mathrm{E}(U_x|H_1)\}/\{\mathrm{Var}(U_x|H_1)\}^{1/2} \sim N(0, 1). \tag{11.6}$$

Next, under H_1, we have (Problem 11.1)

$$\Pr(Z_{\text{CATT}}(x) < t \mid H_1) = \Phi\left(\frac{t\tilde{\sigma}_{1x} - n^{1/2}\mu_{1x}}{\sigma_{1x}}\right). \tag{11.7}$$

Given the above result, following the discussions in Sect. 1.6, the asymptotic power of the trend test for the significance level α is given by

$$\text{Power} = \Pr(|Z_{\text{CATT}}(x)| > z_{1-\alpha/2} \mid H_1) = 1 - \Phi\left(\frac{z_{1-\alpha/2}\tilde{\sigma}_{1x} - n^{1/2}\mu_{1x}}{\sigma_{1x}}\right)$$
$$+ \Phi\left(-\frac{z_{1-\alpha/2}\tilde{\sigma}_{1x} + n^{1/2}\mu_{1x}}{\sigma_{1x}}\right), \tag{11.8}$$

where $z_{1-\alpha} = \Phi^{-1}(1-\alpha)$ is the upper 100αth percentile of $N(0,1)$.

Denote the power as $1 - \beta$. Then, from (11.8), the sample size n to have at least $1 - \beta$ power can be approximated by

$$\frac{z_{1-\alpha/2}\tilde{\sigma}_{1x} - n^{1/2}\mu_{1x}}{\sigma_{1x}} \leq \Phi^{-1}(\beta) = z_\beta,$$

from which

$$n \geq \left(\frac{z_{1-\alpha/2}\tilde{\sigma}_{1x} - z_\beta\sigma_{1x}}{\mu_{1x}}\right)^2. \tag{11.9}$$

In the two subsequent subsections, we discuss how to compute $\mathbf{P}$ and $\mathbf{Q}$ for a disease locus and a marker. Then, using the prespecified $\mathbf{x}$ and ψ_1, μ_{1x}, $\tilde{\sigma}_{1x}^2$ and σ_{1x}^2 can be calculated from (11.3), (11.4) and (11.5), respectively. Finally, the asymptotic power and sample size can be obtained from (11.8) and (11.9), respectively.

An alternative approach to derive the asymptotic power is to use a non-centrality chi-squared distribution. Denote $\delta = \mathrm{E}(U_x \mid H_1)/\{\mathrm{Var}(U_x \mid H_1)\}^{1/2}$. From (11.6), as n is large,

$$T_x = Z_{\text{CATT}}(x)\frac{\tilde{\sigma}_{1x}}{\sigma_{1x}} \sim N(\delta, 1).$$

Thus, under H_1, $T_x^2 \sim \chi_1^2(\delta^2)$, a chi-squared distribution with 1 degree of freedom and non-centrality parameter δ^2. The asymptotic power can also be obtained using the above result as

$$\text{Power} = \Pr(Z_{\text{CATT}}^2(x) > c_1 \mid H_1) = \Pr\left(T_x^2 > c_1\left\{\frac{\tilde{\sigma}_{1x}}{\sigma_{1x}}\right\}^2 \mid H_1\right)$$
$$= 1 - \text{Probchi}(c_1^*, 1, \delta^2),$$

where c_1 is the $100(1-\alpha)$th percentile of a central $\chi_1^2(0)$, $c_1^* = c_1\{\tilde{\sigma}_{1x}/\sigma_{1x}\}^2$, and $\text{Probchi}(\cdot, 1, \delta^2)$ is the cumulative distribution of a chi-squared distribution with 1 degree of freedom and a non-centrality parameter δ^2. Note that $c_1^* = c_1$ under H_0 but $c_1^* \neq c_1$ under H_1, because $\widehat{\mathrm{Var}}(U_x)$ in (11.2) is estimated under H_0 by pooling cases and controls while $\mathrm{Var}(U_x \mid H_1)$ is computed under H_1. An alternative approach is to consider a trend test whose denominator is given by

$\widehat{\mathrm{Var}}^*(U_x) = n^2\psi_1^2\psi_0^2\mathbf{x}^T(\widehat{\Sigma}_P + \widehat{\Sigma}_Q)\mathbf{x}$, where $\widehat{\Sigma}_P$ ($\widehat{\Sigma}_Q$) is estimated by replacing p_i (q_i) with $\widehat{p}_i$ ($\widehat{q}_i$). Then the asymptotic power can be written as $1 - \mathrm{Probchi}(c_1, 1, \delta^2)$, because $c_1^* = c_1$ under H_1.

When using this last approach, there is no closed-form formula for sample size calculation. It can be approximated by varying the sample size until the asymptotic power is close to the target one.

11.1.2 Perfect Linkage Disequilibrium

Under the assumption of perfect LD, we consider a disease locus. Assume the alleles of the disease locus are B and b. Denote the genotypes as $(G_0, G_1, G_2) = (BB, Bb, bb)$ and $g_i = \mathrm{Pr}(G_i)$. Let the disease prevalence be $k = \mathrm{Pr}(\mathrm{case}) = \sum_{i=0}^{2} g_i f_i = f_0(g_0 + g_1\lambda_1 + g_2\lambda_2)$, where f_i is the penetrance (Sect. 2.1) and $\lambda_i = f_i/f_0$, $i = 1, 2$, are the GRRs (Sect. 2.2). Denote the frequency of allele b as p.

The following steps can be used to compute sample size and power for a disease locus:

1) Specify k, p, a genetic model $\mathbf{x}$, GRR λ_2, ψ_1, and the significance level α;
2) Specify the power $1 - \beta$ for computing the sample size;
3) Or specify the sample size n for computing the power;
4) Compute g_i assuming HWE;
5) Compute GRR λ_1 using λ_2 and the genetic model;
6) Compute $f_0 = k/(g_0 + g_1\lambda_1 + g_2\lambda_2)$, $f_1 = \lambda_1 f_0$, and $f_2 = \lambda_2 f_0$;
7) Compute $p_i = g_i f_i/k$ and $q_i = g_i(1 - f_i)/(1 - k)$ for $i = 0, 1, 2$;
8) Compute μ_{1x}, $\widetilde{\sigma}_{1x}$ and σ_{1x};
9) Compute the power using (11.8) or the sample size using (11.9).

Example

Let $k = 0.1$, $p = 0.3$, $x = 0.5$, $\lambda_2 = 1.5$, $\psi = 0.5$, $\alpha = 0.05$, and $1 - \beta = 0.80$. Then, under HWE, $(g_0, g_1, g_2) = (0.49, 0.42, 0.09)$. Given $x = 0.5$ (the ADD model), $\lambda_1 = (1 + \lambda_2)/2 = 1.25$. Hence, the penetrances are given by $(f_0, f_1, f_2) = (0.0870, 0.1087, 0.1304)$. It follows $\mathbf{P} = (0.4261, 0.4565, 0.1174)^T$ and $\mathbf{Q} = (0.4971, 0.4159, 0.0870)^T$. Applying (11.3), (11.4) and (11.5), we have $\mu_{1x} = 0.0127$, $\widetilde{\sigma}_{1x}^2 = 0.0272$ and $\sigma_{1x}^2 = 0.0270$, respectively. Given $n = 500$, the power given by (11.8) is 0.4052, and given the target power $1 - \beta = 0.8$, the sample size given by (11.9) is $n = 1,324$ ($r = s = 662$).

Results

Tables 11.1 and 11.2 report the sample sizes given the target power $1 - \beta = 0.8$ and the power given the sample size $n = 1,000$, respectively. The values of other

Table 11.1 Sample sizes for testing association using the trend test for a disease locus with $\alpha = 0.05$, $\lambda_2 = 1.5$ and $1 - \beta = 0.80$

k	p	Model	ψ_1		
		(x)	0.3	0.5	0.7
0.1	0.1	REC	14,466	12,620	15,530
		ADD	3,160	2,696	3,256
		DOM	1,032	886	1,074
	0.3	REC	1,832	1,586	1,940
		ADD	1,566	1,324	1,584
		DOM	754	632	748
	0.5	REC	876	748	902
		ADD	1,508	1,266	1,502
		DOM	1,134	936	1,090
0.2	0.1	REC	11,042	9,694	11,988
		ADD	2,462	2,106	2,548
		DOM	798	688	836
	0.3	REC	1,408	1,226	1,504
		ADD	1,230	1,042	1,246
		DOM	598	500	592
	0.5	REC	680	584	706
		ADD	1,192	1,000	1,188
		DOM	912	750	874

parameters required in calculating sample size and power are also given in the tables. The results show that when $\psi_1 = 0.5$, i.e. $r = s$, the design has highest power given the total sample size, on fixing the other parameters, or requires the smallest sample size to achieve 80% power. The results also show that there is less power to detect a REC disease with small allele frequency, while there is less power to detect a DOM disease with a larger allele frequency. The power (sample size) increases (decreases) with the disease prevalence. The power or sample size vary substantially across the three genetic models and different allele frequencies.

11.1.3 Imperfect Linkage Disequilibrium

A marker locus, which is in LD with the disease locus, is often used. Denote the alleles of the disease locus as B and b as before, and the alleles of the marker as A and a. Let $\Pr(a) = p$ and $\Pr(b) = q$. Denote the genotypes at the disease locus as $(G_0^*, G_1^*, G_2^*) = (BB, Bb, bb)$ and at the marker as $(G_0, G_1, G_2) = (AA, Aa, aa)$.

Denote the penetrances at the disease and marker loci as f_i^* and f_i, respectively $(i = 0, 1, 2)$. Following Sect. 2.2.1, let

Table 11.2 Asymptotic power (%) for testing association using the trend test for a disease locus with $\alpha = 0.05$, $\lambda_2 = 1.5$ and $n = 1,000$

k	p	Model	ψ_1		
		(x)	0.3	0.5	0.7
0.1	0.1	REC	14.2	12.4	8.5
		ADD	36.2	40.0	33.0
		DOM	78.8	84.6	77.1
	0.3	REC	55.8	60.4	50.4
		ADD	61.2	68.2	60.2
		DOM	89.8	94.2	89.7
	0.5	REC	84.9	90.0	84.0
		ADD	62.6	70.2	62.8
		DOM	74.7	82.6	76.6
0.2	0.1	REC	16.8	14.7	9.8
		ADD	44.2	48.8	40.6
		DOM	87.8	92.2	86.8
	0.3	REC	66.5	71.6	61.5
		ADD	71.6	78.4	70.7
		DOM	95.3	97.8	95.4
	0.5	REC	92.2	95.7	91.9
		ADD	72.8	80.0	73.0
		DOM	83.7	89.9	84.9

$$F_1 = 1 - q + D/(1 - p), \qquad F_2 = 1 - q - D/p,$$
$$F_3 = q - D/(1 - p), \qquad F_4 = q + D/p,$$

where p, q and D are given in Table 2.1 in Sect. 2.2.1, and D is the LD parameter. The standardized D' is used here, which is given by

$$D' = \frac{D}{\min((1 - q)p, (1 - p)q)}, \quad \text{if } D > 0,$$
$$= \frac{D}{\min((1 - q)(1 - p), pq)}, \quad \text{if } D \leq 0.$$

Note that $0 \leq D' \leq 1$. When $D' = 0$, the marker and the disease locus are in linkage equilibrium. We assume $0 < D' < 1$. See Sect. 2.2.1 for a discussion of the signs of D' and D. Denote the GRRs at the disease and marker loci as $\lambda_i^* = f_i^*/f_0^*$ and $\lambda_i = f_i/f_0$, respectively, for $i = 1, 2$. Then, from (2.2)–(2.4),

$$f_0 = f_0^*(F_1^2 + 2F_1F_3\lambda_1^* + F_3^2\lambda_2^*),$$
$$f_1 = f_0^*(F_1F_2 + F_1F_4\lambda_1^* + F_2F_3\lambda_1^* + F_3F_4\lambda_2^*),$$
$$f_2 = f_0^*(F_2^2 + 2F_2F_4\lambda_1^* + F_4^2\lambda_2^*).$$

The following steps can be used to compute sample size and power for a marker locus:

1) Specify k, p, q, D', a genetic model $\mathbf{x}$ at the disease locus, GRR λ_2^*, ψ_1, and the significance level α;
2) Specify the power $1 - \beta$ to compute the sample size;
3) Or specify the sample size n to compute the power;
4) Compute D, F_1, F_2, F_3 and F_4;
5) Compute $g_i^* = \Pr(G_i^*)$ and $g_i = \Pr(G_i)$ assuming HWE ($i = 0, 1, 2$);
6) Compute GRR λ_1^* using λ_2^* and the genetic model and

$$f_0^* = k/(g_0^* + g_1^*\lambda_1^* + g_2^*\lambda_2^*);$$

7) Compute f_i for $i = 0, 1, 2$ at the marker, and

$$p_i = g_i f_i/k \quad \text{and} \quad q_i = g_i(1 - f_i)/(1 - k) \quad (i = 0, 1, 2);$$

8) Compute μ_{1x}, $\tilde{\sigma}_{1x}$ and σ_{1x};
9) Compute the power using (11.8) or the sample size using (11.9).

Example

Let $k = 0.1$, $p = 0.3$ (for the marker), $q = 0.2$ (for the disease locus), $x = 0.5$ (the ADD model), $D' = 0.95$, $\lambda_2^* = 1.5$, $\psi = 0.5$, $\alpha = 0.05$, $n = 1,000$, and $1 - \beta = 0.80$. Then $D = 0.133$ and $(F_1, F_2, F_3, F_4) = (0.99, 0.35667, 0.01, 0.64333)$. Under HWE, $(g_0^*, g_1^*, g_2^*) = (0.64, 0.32, 0.04)$ and $(g_0, g_1, g_2) = (0.49, 0.42, 0.09)$. Given the ADD model at the disease locus, $\lambda_1^* = (1 + \lambda_2^*)/2 = 1.25$. Hence, $f_0^* = 0.09091$ and $(f_0, f_1, f_2) = (0.0914, 0.1058, 0.1202)$, which still forms an ADD model at the marker ($f_1 = (f_0 + f_2)/2$). It follows that $\mathbf{P} = (0.4477, 0.4442, 0.1081)^T$ and $\mathbf{Q} = (0.4947, 0.4173, 0.0880)^T$. Applying (11.3), (11.4) and (11.5), we have $\mu_{1x} = 0.0084$, $\tilde{\sigma}_{1x}^2 = 0.02688$ and $\sigma_{1x}^2 = 0.02681$, respectively. Given $n = 1,000$, the power given by (11.8) is 36.68%, and given the power $1 - \beta = 0.8$, the sample size given by (11.9) is $n = 2,990$.

Results

Tables 11.3 and 11.4 report the sample size given the target power $1 - \beta = 0.8$ and the power given the sample size $n = 1,000$ for a marker locus, respectively. The values of other parameters required in calculating sample size and power are also given in the tables. With the other parameters being fixed, the required sample size to achieve 80% power decreases (the power for the given sample size increases) when $D' > 0$ increases. Since the allele frequency of the risk allele at the disease locus is fixed at $q = 0.2$, the results change significantly when the frequency of the risk allele p at the marker varies. Overall, a better design is obtained when p is closer to q. For example (Table 11.3), the required sample size for the REC model

Table 11.3 Sample size for testing association using the trend test for a marker locus with $\alpha = 0.05$, $\lambda_2 = 1.5$, $\psi_1 = 0.5$, and $1 - \beta = 0.80$. p is the allele frequency of the risk allele at the marker locus, while the frequency of the risk allele at the disease locus is fixed at $q = 0.2$

k	p	Model	D'		
		(x)	0.8	0.8	1.0
0.1	0.1	REC	27,038	18,908	13,716
		ADD	5,714	4,544	3,704
		DOM	2,518	1,984	1,604
	0.3	REC	13,558	9,626	7,054
		ADD	4,204	3,328	2,702
		DOM	1,848	1,426	1,128
	0.5	REC	40,056	29,564	22,426
		ADD	9,610	7,592	6,148
		DOM	5,162	3,966	3,124
0.2	0.1	REC	20,946	14,594	10,548
		ADD	4,476	3,556	2,896
		DOM	1,970	1,550	1,252
	0.3	REC	10,623	7.530	5,510
		ADD	3,312	2,622	2,128
		DOM	1,462	1,128	892
	0.5	REC	31,586	23,306	17,671
		ADD	7,594	5,998	4,858
		DOM	4,104	3,156	2,488

is 13,716 when $k = 0.1$, $D' = 1$ and $p = 0.1$, but 7.054 when $p = 0.3$ and the other parameters are the same, because p is closer to $q = 0.2$.

Compared to the results when the marker and the disease locus are in LD, the required sample size (power) is much larger (smaller) when $D' \leq 1$ and $p \neq q$. Other patterns of sample size and power in terms of genetic models and k are similar to those in Tables 11.1 and 11.2.

11.2 Pearson's Chi-Squared Test

In the previous section, trend tests $Z_{\text{CATT}}(x)$ are used to calculate power and sample size when the genetic model is known. The closed forms for power and sample size for a marker and a disease locus are given based on (11.8) and (11.9). The power and sample size vary substantially across the genetic models. When the true genetic model is unknown, $Z_{\text{CATT}}(0.5)$ is often used. On the other hand, Pearson's test is also commonly used, being robust to the genetic model. We consider the power and sample size calculation using Pearson's test. We only consider computations for a disease locus, which can be readily modified for a marker.

Table 11.4 Asymptotic power (%) for testing association using the trend test for a marker locus with $\alpha = 0.05$, $\lambda_2^* = 1.5$, $\psi_1 = 0.5$, and $n = 1,000$. p is the allele frequency of the risk allele at the marker locus while the frequency of the risk allele at the disease locus is fixed at $q = 0.2$

k	p	Model (x)	D'		
			0.8	0.8	1.0
0.1	0.1	REC	8.3	9.9	11.8
		ADD	21.6	26.0	30.7
		DOM	42.3	51.1	59.9
	0.3	REC	11.8	14.7	18.4
		ADD	27.7	33.6	39.9
		DOM	54.0	65.0	75.1
	0.5	REC	7.3	8.1	9.1
		ADD	14.7	17.4	20.4
		DOM	23.4	29.0	35.4
0.2	0.1	REC	9.4	11.3	13.9
		ADD	26.3	31.8	37.7
		DOM	51.4	61.4	70.7
	0.3	REC	13.8	17.5	22.2
		ADD	33.7	40.9	48.4
		DOM	63.9	75.1	84.3
	0.5	REC	7.9	8.9	10.2
		ADD	17.4	20.8	24.6
		DOM	28.2	35.1	42.7

It has been shown (see Bibliographical Comments) that, under H_1, Pearson's test $T_{\chi_2^2}$ follows a chi-squared distribution with 2 degrees of freedom with a non-centrality parameter δ^2, which can be written as

$$\delta^2 = n\psi_0\psi_1 \sum_{i=0}^{2} \frac{(p_i - q_i)^2}{\psi_1 p_i + \psi_0 q_i},$$

where p_i and q_i are calculated for cases and controls at the disease locus. Let c_2 be the $100(1 - \alpha)$th percentile of a central chi-squared distribution with 2 degrees of freedom. Then the power with sample size n to detect H_1 specified by GRRs can be written as

$$\text{Power} = \Pr(T_{\chi_2^2} > c_2 | H_1) = 1 - \text{Probchi}(c_2, 2, \delta^2), \tag{11.10}$$

where $\text{Probchi}(\cdot, 2, \delta^2)$ is the cumulative distribution of a chi-squared distribution with 2 degrees of freedom and a non-centrality parameter δ^2. While (11.10) can be used to compute the power given n and the significance level α, an explicit formula to compute the sample size n given power $1 - \beta$ is not available. But the sample size n can be approximated by varying n in (11.10) until, say, 80% power is reached.

Table 11.5 Asymptotic power (%) for testing association using the trend test $Z_{\text{CATT}}(0.5)$ and Pearson's test for the disease locus with $\alpha = 0.05$, $k = 0.1$, and $\psi_1 = 0.5$

p	Model	$n = 1000$, $\lambda_2 = 1.5$		$n = 3000$, $\lambda_2 = 1.2$	
	(x)	$Z_{\text{CATT}}(0.5)$	Pearson's	$Z_{\text{CATT}}(0.5)$	Pearson's
0.1	REC	6.5	10.0	5.8	7.6
	ADD	40.0	31.3	23.8	18.3
	DOM	82.5	76.3	58.8	50.6
0.3	REC	35.2	49.9	20.9	29.6
	ADD	68.2	58.0	45.5	36.0
	DOM	88.7	89.3	70.6	69.7
0.5	REC	77.2	83.4	52.7	58.8
	ADD	70.2	60.0	49.9	40.0
	DOM	73.7	73.8	47.2	54.2

11.2.1 Example

We compute the sample size to reach 80% power for the disease locus using $T_{\chi_2^2}$ with $k = 0.1$, $p = 0.3$ (the frequency of the risk allele), $\alpha = 0.05$, and $\lambda_2 = 1.5$. The results are also compared to those obtained using $Z_{\text{CATT}}(0.5)$. When the true model is REC, ADD and DOM, the total sample size for $Z_{\text{CATT}}(0.5)$ is 3138, 1324 and 782, respectively. The total sample size for using $T_{\chi_2^2}$ is given by 1950 (80.0% power under the REC model), 1624 (80.1% power under the ADD model) and 780 (80.1% power under the DOM model). The asymptotic power with those sample sizes is given in parentheses. Although Pearson's test is robust to the genetic model, sample size calculations depend on GRRs under H_1, which depends on a genetic model. Thus, sample sizes vary across the genetic models for using either test. Both tests have a similar sample size under the DOM model, but the trend test requires a much larger sample size under the REC model, while Pearson's test requires a relatively larger sample size under the ADD model.

11.2.2 Asymptotic Power of Pearson's Chi-Squared Test and the Trend Test

The asymptotic power of $T_{\chi_2^2}$ and $Z_{\text{CATT}}(0.5)$ for $n = 1,000$, $\alpha = 0.05$, $k = 0.1$, and $\psi_1 = 0.5$ are reported in Table 11.5. It shows that the trend test and Pearson's test have different asymptotic power given n under the REC and ADD models.

11.3 Using Odds Ratios

In sample size and power calculations discussed before, GRRs (λ_1, λ_2) are specified, and the penetrances (f_0, f_1, f_2) are calculated. When the genetic model is known, only a single GRR λ_2 is required, and $\lambda_1 = 1 - x + x\lambda_2$ is obtained for $x = 0$, $1/2$ and 1 under the REC, ADD and DOM models, respectively.

The ORs can also be used (Sect. 2.5.1). Given the penetrance f_i, the ORs can be computed using

$$\mathrm{OR}_i = \frac{f_i(1 - f_0)}{f_0(1 - f_i)}, \quad i = 1, 2.$$

If the ORs are specified in the calculations, the GRRs can be obtained if the other specified parameters are given. First, we have

$$f_i = \frac{\mathrm{OR}_i\, f_0}{\mathrm{OR}_i\, f_0 + 1 - f_0}. \tag{11.11}$$

For the REC model, $f_0 = f_1$. Then, given OR_2, using $k = f_0(g_0 + g_1) + f_2 g_2$, we have (Problem 11.5)

$$f_0 = \frac{-(1 + a) + \sqrt{(1 + a)^2 + 4kb}}{2b}, \tag{11.12}$$

where $a = (g_2 - k)(\mathrm{OR}_2 - 1)$ and $b = (1 - g_2)(\mathrm{OR}_2 - 1)$. For the DOM model, $f_1 = f_2$ and $k = f_0 g_0 + f_2(1 - g_0)$. Thus,

$$f_0 = \frac{-(1 + c) + \sqrt{(1 + c)^2 + 4kd}}{2d}, \tag{11.13}$$

where $c = (1 - g_0 - k)(\mathrm{OR}_2 - 1)$ and $d = g_0(\mathrm{OR}_2 - 1)$.

Under the REC model, $\lambda_1 = 1$ and $\mathrm{OR}_1 = 1$ are equivalent; and under the DOM model, $\lambda_1 = \lambda_2$ and $\mathrm{OR}_1 = \mathrm{OR}_2$ are equivalent. However, this is not true for the ADD model, under which $\lambda_1 = (1 + \lambda_2)/2$ does not imply $\mathrm{OR}_1 = (1 + \mathrm{OR}_2)/2$ and vice versa (Problem 11.5). In general, given OR_1 and OR_2, we can substitute f_i, $i = 1, 2$, in $k = g_0 f_0 + g_1 f_1 + g_2 f_2$ with (11.11) and obtain

$$k = f_0 \left\{ g_0 + g_1 \frac{\mathrm{OR}_1}{(\mathrm{OR}_1 - 1)f_0 + 1} + g_2 \frac{\mathrm{OR}_2}{(\mathrm{OR}_2 - 1)f_0 + 1} \right\}. \tag{11.14}$$

Hence f_0 can be solved from the above equation numerically and f_i can be obtained from (11.11).

Table 11.6 reports f_0 solved from (11.12) and (11.13) and GRR λ_2 under the REC and DOM models given $\mathrm{OR}_2 = 1.5$ and values of p and k. When OR is fixed, GRR changes with p and k. When k is small, $\mathrm{GRR}_2 \approx \mathrm{OR}_2$, but all values of $\mathrm{GRR}_2 < \mathrm{OR}_2$, which indicates that specifying GRRs and ORs are different in calculating sample size and power. However, (11.12), (11.13) and (11.14) show that one only needs to specify either GRRs (or ORs), and then ORs (or GRRs) are determined by the GRRs (or ORs, p and k).

Table 11.6 Penetrances and GRRs given $OR_2 = 1.5$ under the REC and DOM models. HWE holds in the population

p	k	REC		DOM	
		f_0	λ_2	f_0	λ_2
0.1	0.01	0.0099	1.493	0.0091	1.493
	0.05	0.0498	1.464	0.0728	1.466
	0.10	0.0996	1.429	0.1423	1.434
	0.25	0.2492	1.333	0.3324	1.342
0.3	0.01	0.0099	1.493	0.0080	1.494
	0.05	0.0480	1.465	0.0403	1.470
	0.10	0.0963	1.431	0.0816	1.441
	0.25	0.2426	1.338	0.2115	1.357
0.5	0.01	0.0089	1.493	0.0073	1.495
	0.05	0.0448	1.467	0.0369	1.473
	0.10	0.0902	1.435	0.0749	1.446
	0.25	0.2301	1.345	0.1962	1.366

11.4 Using a Power Program

A Power Program (V3.0) was developed by the National Cancer Institute (see Bibliographical Comments in Sect. 11.6) for sample size and power calculations. The program can also be used to calculate sample size and power for interactions, which will be described later. The software can be downloaded from http://dceg.cancer.gov/tools/design/power. Here we describe how to use it for single marker analysis.

11.4.1 Specifications

To enter the parameter values, a user can choose "Default Values" for a new computation or "Previous Run" to repeat the previous computation with different parameter values. The program can also read a parameter file. "Case-Control" is then chosen as the study design and a control to case ratio needs to be specified. This ratio, in terms of our notation, is $s/r = \psi_0/\psi_1$. Up to two exposure variables can be used. For single marker analysis, only one exposure variable is used (treating it as a candidate gene). The exposure level is from 2 to 10, which is chosen by the user. For the REC or DOM models, two-level is chosen with score 0 and 1, and for the ADD model, three-level is used with scores 0, 1, and 2. The significance level α (type I error) is entered and a two-sided test is chosen (do not choose this if a one-sided alternative hypothesis is to be used). The program does not allow the user to specify the frequency of the risk allele or the minor allele frequency.

Instead, it asks for probabilities for all exposure levels. Note that the three genotypes are denoted as $(G_0, G_1, G_2) = (BB, Bb, bb)$. Under the REC model, the score for genotypes BB and Bb is 0 and for genotype bb is 1 (if b is a risk allele). The probabilities entered in the program are the sum of genotype frequencies for BB and Bb for level (score) 0 and the genotype frequency for bb for level (score) 1. For example, if the allele frequency for b is 0.3, then 0.09 is entered for score 1 and $1 - 0.09 = 0.91$ (or $0.42 + 0.49 = 0.91$) is entered for score 0. The baseline disease probability $\Pr(\text{case} \,|\, G_0)$ is specified, which is the reference penetrance f_0. The OR is specified. For exposure with more than two levels, the OR is specified for the top-to-bottom (bb versus BB). Only a single OR is specified. Thus, the program assumes that one knows the genetic model. The user then decides the objective of the calculation by choosing "Sample Size" with a target power, or "Power" with a given sample size (the number of cases). After clicking "Finish", results are output in a new window.

11.4.2 Examples

We illustrate the use of the Power Program with several examples.

```
Example 1 (REC model with two levels): Default Values

Study Design
Case-Control Control to Case Ratio: 1

Exposures
Number: one
Exposure 1 Levels (2-10): 2

Type I Error
Alpha-Level: 0.05 Two-Sided

Exposure Scores Probabilities

Scores Total
0 0.91
1 0.09
Total 1.00

Probability of Disease at Baseline: 0.1

Single Exposure Odds Ratios:
Odds Ratio Under the Alternative Hypothesis
Exposure 1
0: 1
1: 1.5

Calculations
Calculate
Sample Size
Given: Power: 0.8
Finish
```

The program outputs sample sizes along with the parameter values entered. The sample sizes are reported as:

```
No. cases = 1035.5 No. controls = 1035.5 No. subjects = 2071.0
```

We know that a REC model can also be specified as three-level with scores 0, 0 and 1. This is not allowed in the Power Program because strictly increasing scores are required. Thus, we chose scores 0, 0.001 and 1 as an approximation (note that the scores only allow three decimal places in the program), and obtained the total sample size of 2073.2, which is very close to the original 2071.0.

```
No. cases = 1036.6 No. controls = 1036.6 No. subjects = 2073.2
```

To calculate the power given the sample size (the number of cases), we only need to change a portion of the entries of Example 1 as follows:

```
......
Calculations
Calculate
Power
Given: Sample size: 1000
Finish
```

Then the power is 78.6%.

```
No. cases = 1000.0 No. controls = 1000.0 No. subjects = 2000.0
Study Power = 0.786
```

In the first example, the choice of scores, 0 and 1, has no impact on the sample size and power calculations. For example, we can use scores 0 and 2 and obtain the same sample size and power. This is not true, however, if a three-level score is considered, which will be demonstrated below. In the second example, we also change some parameter values and compute the power given the sample size.

```
Example 2 (ADD model with three levels): Default Values

Study Design
Case-Control Control to Case Ratio: 1.5

Exposures
Number: one
Exposure 1 Levels (2-10): 3

Type I Error
Alpha-Level: 0.05 Two-Sided

Exposure Scores Probabilities

Scores Total
0 0.49
1 0.42
2 0.09
Total 1.00


Probability of Disease at Baseline: 0.01

Single Exposure Odds Ratios:
Odds Ratio Under the Alternative Hypothesis
Exposure 1
0: 1
```

```
1: 1.5

Calculations
Calculate
Power
Given: Sample Size: 1000
Finish
```

The program outputs the study power 90.6% along with the parameter values entered. The original sample sizes and the calculated power are reported as:

```
No. cases = 1000.0 No. controls = 1500.0 No. subjects = 2500.0
Study Power = 0.906
```

If we change the scores from 0, 1, 2 to 0, 1, 3, the power becomes 85.1%. However, as long as equally spaced scores are used, the power does not change after a linear transformation of the scores. For example, the power is still 90.6% if the scores 0, 2 and 4 are used.

In the next example, we still consider the ADD model but specify two levels (allele b versus allele B under HWE) using the same parameter values. Note that the allele-based penetrances will be different from the genotype-based ones, and that the OR is for b versus B, which is different from the OR for bb versus BB. Thus, the power is expected to be different.

```
Example 3 (ADD model with two levels): Default Values

Study Design
Case-Control Control to Case Ratio: 1.5

Exposures
Number: one
Exposure 1 Levels (2-10): 2

Type I Error
Alpha-Level: 0.05 Two-Sided

Exposure Scores Probabilities

Scores Total
0 0.70
1 0.30
Total 1.00

Probability of Disease at Baseline: 0.01

Single Exposure Odds Ratios:
Odds Ratio Under the Alternative Hypothesis
Exposure 1
0: 1
1: 1.5

Calculations
Calculate
Power
Given: Sample Size: 1000
Finish
```

The power becomes 99.7%, which is much higher than that with three levels, because the ORs refer to different comparisons in the two examples.

11.4.3 Limitations

The Power Program is very easy to use. However, it has some limitations for genetic association studies. First, because the program was not developed specifically for genetic association studies, it does not allow one to specify the allele frequency. Instead, the probability of susceptibility has to be specified. Thus, the user has to compute this with or without HWE and enter the results into the program. Second, when the score has three levels, only strictly increasing scores may be used. This only works for the ADD model. For the REC or DOM models, one can only choose two levels. A more flexible program would allow a REC model to be entered with scores 0, 0 and 1, so that the genotype frequencies for the three genotypes could be entered. To examine the performance of sample size and power calculation when the genetic model is misspecified, the program should allow one to enter two ORs, not just the top-to-bottom one. Currently, the program assumes that the true genetic model is known. Third, it can only calculate power or sample size for a candidate-gene, which assumes perfect LD between the susceptibility and disease loci. If the LD between the marker and disease locus is measured as D' (Sect. 11.1.3), the sample size n when $|D'|$ is not equal to 1 can be obtained from the results presented in Sect. 11.1.3. Based on the results in Table 11.3, for the ADD model, one can first calculate the sample size n under $|D'| = 1$ using the Power program. Then the actual sample size with $|D'| < 1$ is approximately equal to n divided by $|D'|^2$. This is not true, however, for the REC or DOM models.

11.5 Testing Interactions

Sample size and power calculations for testing gene-environment and gene-gene interactions are considered here. They are often discussed in terms of ORs in the literature. Either interaction can be tested in a logistic regression model. We consider testing a general interaction, and then treat gene-environment exposure interaction and gene-gene interaction as special cases.

11.5.1 Score Statistic for an Interaction

Score Statistic

Let V_1 and V_2 be two binary variables. A logistic regression model is commonly used for testing an interaction of V_1 and V_2, given by

$$\text{logit}\{p_1(\mathbf{V})\} = \text{logit}\{\text{Pr}(\text{case}|V_1, V_2)\} = \beta_0 + \beta_1 V_1 + \beta_2 V_2 + \beta_{12} V_1 V_2, \quad (11.15)$$

Table 11.7 ORs for main effects and the interaction between V_1 and V_2

	$V_1 = 0$	$V_1 = 1$
$V_2 = 0$	1.0	$\mathrm{OR}_{V_1=1|V_2=0}$
$V_2 = 1$	$\mathrm{OR}_{V_2=1|V_1=0}$	OR_{V_1,V_2}

where $\mathbf{V} = (V_1, V_2)$ and $V_1, V_2 = 0, 1$. In (11.15), β_i $(i = 1, 2)$ is the log OR for the main effect of V_i and $\beta_{12} = \log \mathrm{OR}_{12}$ is the log OR for the interaction. Let $p_0(\mathbf{V}) = 1 - p_1(\mathbf{V})$. Then

$$\beta_1 = \ln \mathrm{OR}_{V_1=1|V_2=0} = \ln\left\{ \frac{p_1(\mathbf{V} = (1,0))}{p_0(\mathbf{V} = (1,0))} \Big/ \frac{p_1(\mathbf{V} = (0,0))}{p_0(\mathbf{V} = (0,0))} \right\},$$

$$\beta_2 = \ln \mathrm{OR}_{V_2=1|V_1=0} = \ln\left\{ \frac{p_1(\mathbf{V} = (0,1))}{p_0(\mathbf{V} = (0,1))} \Big/ \frac{p_1(\mathbf{V} = (0,0))}{p_0(\mathbf{V} = (0,0))} \right\}.$$

Note that this definition of interaction assumes the main effects are additive on the logistic scale. In the case of a rare disease, $\mathrm{logit}(p) \approx \log(p)$, i.e. the main effects are additive on a log scale, so that we are testing for multiplicative interaction. All the ORs are summarized in Table 11.7, where we denote

$$\mathrm{OR}_{V_1,V_2} = \mathrm{OR}_{V_1=1|V_2=0} \times \mathrm{OR}_{V_2=1|V_1=0} \times \mathrm{OR}_{12}.$$

The null hypothesis of no interaction is $H_0 : \beta_{12} = 0$ and the alternative hypothesis is $H_1 : \beta_{12} \neq 0$ (two-sided), where the main effects β_1 and β_2 are not specified under either H_0 or H_1. Denote the parameters $\theta_0 = (\beta_0, \beta_1, \beta_2)^T$ and $\theta_1 = (\beta_0, \beta_1, \beta_2, \beta_{12})^T$.

Denote the counts of cases and controls with $V_1 = i$ and $V_2 = j$ as R_{ij} and S_{ij}, respectively $(i, j = 0, 1)$, and $n_{ij} = R_{ij} + S_{ij}$. The total sample size is $n = \sum_{i,j} N_{ij}$, the total number of cases is $r = \sum_{i,j} R_{ij}$, and the total number of controls is $s = \sum_{i,j} S_{ij}$. Then the log-likelihood function can be written as

$$\begin{aligned}
l(\theta_1) = {} & r\beta_0 + (R_{10} + R_{11})\beta_1 + (R_{01} + R_{11})\beta_2 + R_{11}\beta_{12} \\
& - n_{00} \log\{1 + \exp(\beta_0)\} - n_{01} \log\{1 + \exp(\beta_0 + \beta_2)\} \\
& - n_{10} \log\{1 + \exp(\beta_0 + \beta_1)\} \\
& - n_{11} \log\{1 + \exp(\beta_0 + \beta_1 + \beta_2 + \beta_{12})\}.
\end{aligned} \tag{11.16}$$

When testing $H_0 : \beta_{12} = 0$, θ_0 is treated as a set of nuisance parameters. The MLE of θ_0 under H_0, denoted as $\widehat{\theta}_0$, can be solved from (Problem 11.6)

$$\frac{\partial l(\theta_1)}{\partial \theta_0}\Big|_{H_0} = 0. \tag{11.17}$$

Let

$$i_n(\widehat{\theta}_0) = -\frac{\partial^2 l}{\partial \theta_1 \theta_1^T}\Big|_{H_0, \theta_0 = \widehat{\theta}_0},$$

which is a 4×4 observed Fisher information matrix evaluated under H_0 with $\widehat{\theta}_0$. The second order partial derivatives are given in Problem 11.6. Denote its inverse as

$i_n^{-1}(\widehat{\theta}_0)$, whose $(4,4)$th element is denoted as $i_n^{\beta_{12}\beta_{12}}(\widehat{\theta}_0)$. The Score function under H_0 is given by

$$U_{12} = \frac{\partial l(\theta_1)}{\partial \beta_{12}}\Big|_{H_0,\theta_0=\widehat{\theta}_0} = R_{11} - n_{11}p_1(\mathbf{V} = (1,1))|_{H_0,\widehat{\theta}_0},$$

whose asymptotic variance under H_0 is $V_0(U_{12}) = 1/i_n^{\beta_{12}\beta_{12}}(\widehat{\theta}_0)$. Thus, the Score statistic for testing $H_0 : \beta_{12} = 0$ is given by

$$Z_{12} = \frac{U_{12}}{\{V_0(U_{12})\}^{1/2}}, \tag{11.18}$$

which follows $N(0,1)$ under H_0 when n is large enough. The null hypothesis is rejected at the level α if $|Z_{12}| > z_{1-\alpha/2}$.

Asymptotic Power and Sample Size

The power and sample size for the interaction can be calculated in a similar manner as in Sect. 11.1.1 when the trend test is used, because (11.1) and (11.18) have similar patterns. Denote

$$\frac{1}{n}V_0(U_{12}) \xrightarrow{H_1} \widetilde{\sigma}_{12}^2,$$

$$E(U_{12}|H_1) = n\mu_{12},$$

$$\frac{1}{n}\mathrm{Var}(U_{12}) = \sigma_{12}^2.$$

Then the asymptotic power for a given significance level α is given by

$$\text{Power} = \Pr(|Z_{12}| > z_{1-\alpha/2}|H_1) = 1 - \Phi\left(\frac{z_{1-\alpha/2}\widetilde{\sigma}_{12} - n^{1/2}\mu_{12}}{\sigma_{12}}\right)$$

$$+ \Phi\left(-\frac{z_{1-\alpha/2}\widetilde{\sigma}_{12} + n^{1/2}\mu_{12}}{\sigma_{12}}\right), \tag{11.19}$$

while the sample size n to achieve $1 - \beta$ power is given by

$$n \geq \left(\frac{z_{1-\alpha/2}\widetilde{\sigma}_{12} - z_\beta\sigma_{12}}{\mu_{12}}\right)^2. \tag{11.20}$$

Although (11.19) and (11.20) are similar to (11.8) and (11.9), computations of $\widetilde{\sigma}_{12}$, σ_{12} and μ_{12} are more complex. The Power Program that we described in Sect. 11.4 can be used for calculations of sample size and power for both gene-environment and gene-gene interactions.

11.5.2 Gene-Environment Interactions

Various test statistics for gene-environment interactions have been studied in Sect. 10.3. To test the interaction between a genetic susceptibility locus and a two-level environment exposure, the Score statistic derived in the previous section can

Table 11.8 Case-control data classified by a two-level exposure variable without specifying a genetic model. The total number of cases (controls) is r (s)

		$G_0 = BB$	$G_1 = Bb$	$G_2 = bb$
cases	$E = 0$	R_{00}	R_{01}	R_{02}
	$E = 1$	R_{10}	R_{11}	R_{12}
controls	$E = 0$	S_{00}	S_{01}	S_{02}
	$E = 1$	S_{10}	S_{11}	S_{12}

Table 11.9 Case-control data with a two-level exposure variable under the REC model, when b is the risk allele

	$E = 0$		$E = 1$	
	$G = 0$	$G = 1$	$G = 0$	$G = 1$
cases	$\widetilde{R}_{00} = R_{00} + R_{01}$	$\widetilde{R}_{10} = R_{02}$	$\widetilde{R}_{01} = R_{10} + R_{11}$	$\widetilde{R}_{11} = R_{12}$
controls	$\widetilde{S}_{00} = S_{00} + S_{01}$	$\widetilde{S}_{10} = S_{02}$	$\widetilde{S}_{01} = S_{10} + S_{11}$	$\widetilde{S}_{11} = S_{12}$

Table 11.10 Case-control data with a two-level exposure variable under the ADD model, when b is the risk allele

	$E = 0$		$E = 1$	
	$G = 0$	$G = 1$	$G = 0$	$G = 1$
cases	$\widetilde{R}_{00} = 2R_{00} + R_{01}$	$\widetilde{R}_{10} = R_{01} + 2R_{02}$	$\widetilde{R}_{01} = 2R_{10} + R_{11}$	$\widetilde{R}_{11} = R_{11} + 2R_{12}$
controls	$\widetilde{S}_{00} = 2S_{00} + S_{01}$	$\widetilde{S}_{10} = S_{01} + 2S_{02}$	$\widetilde{S}_{01} = 2S_{10} + S_{11}$	$\widetilde{S}_{11} = S_{11} + 2S_{12}$

be applied with V_1 replaced by G and V_2 by E (see Sect. 10.3.2 for more discussion on applying the Score statistic to test for gene-environment interactions).

Data and Genetic Model

The observed case-control data with the exposure variable E can be displayed as in Table 11.8 without specifying a genetic model. Given a genetic model (REC, ADD and DOM), the data in Table 11.8 can be displayed in a $2 \times 2 \times 2$ table. Tables 11.9, 11.10 and 11.11 are $2 \times 2 \times 2$ tables for the three genetic models, respectively. For the ADD model, the data can also be displayed as in Table 11.8 with scores $0, 1, 2$. Thus, the environment exposure has two levels, while the gene has either two or three levels depending on the genetic models. Assigning scores to the three levels is not easy without knowing the genetic model. Using Table 11.10 for the ADD model would lead to different sample size and power calculations compared to using Table 11.8 with scores $0, 1, 2$ because the specifications of ORs are different in the two tables. Examples are presented to illustrate the use of the Power Program.

Table 11.11 Case-control data with a two-level exposure variable under the DOM model, when b is the risk allele

	$E = 0$		$E = 1$	
	$G = 0$	$G = 1$	$G = 0$	$G = 1$
cases	$\widetilde{R}_{00} = R_{00}$	$\widetilde{R}_{10} = R_{01} + R_{02}$	$\widetilde{R}_{01} = R_{10}$	$\widetilde{R}_{11} = R_{11} + R_{12}$
controls	$\widetilde{S}_{00} = S_{00}$	$\widetilde{S}_{10} = S_{01} + S_{02}$	$\widetilde{S}_{01} = S_{10}$	$\widetilde{S}_{11} = S_{11} + S_{12}$

Specifications

To apply the Power Program, the following parameters are specified.

1) Control to case ratio (s/r);
2) A significance level α;
3) A one-sided or two sided alternative hypothesis;
4) The marginal probabilities of exposure levels and susceptibility;
5) Probability of disease at the baseline $f_0 = \Pr(\text{case} \,|\, G_0)$;
6) Three ORs: two for the main effects (or marginal effects) of the exposure and gene, and one for the interaction;
7) A sample size (the number of cases) for power calculation or a target power for sample size calculation.

In the above specifications, the main effect for the environment refers to the OR of exposure in the control group, while the main effect for the gene refers to the OR of gene susceptibility in the non-exposed group. The marginal effects refer to the ORs of susceptibility and exposure in the general population.

Examples

```
Example 1 (REC model with two levels): Default Values

Study Design
Case-Control Control to Case Ratio: 1

Exposures
Number: two
Exposure 1 Levels (2-10): 2
Exposure 2 Levels (2-10): 2

Type I Error
Alpha-Level: 0.05 Two-Sided

Exposure Scores Probabilities
(Only specify the margins. The cells in the center
are obtained as the products of the margins under the
null hypothesis.)

Scores 0 1 Total
```

```
0 0.455 0.045 0.50
1 0.455 0.045 0.50
Total 0.91 0.09 1.00

Probability of Disease at Baseline: 0.1
Model: multiplicative (logistic)

Odds Ratio Under the Alternative Hypothesis
Specify: Main Effect
Exposure 1: 1.5
Exposure 2: 1.5
Interaction: 2

Calculations
Calculate
Power
Given: Sample Size: 1000
Finish
```

The output for power to detect gene-environment interaction given the sample sizes is given by

```
No. cases = 1000.0 No. controls = 1000.0 No. subjects = 2000.0
Study Power = 0.642
```

If we change the genetic model to ADD (Table 11.8) with three levels and scores 0, 1, 2, and keep the same margins for the exposure, then the margins for the gene become 0.49, 0.42, and 0.09 for scores 0, 1, and 2. On re-running the program, we obtain the new study power for interaction as 0.697 with the same sample sizes. For the DOM model with two-level exposures, the new margins for the gene are 0.49 and $0.51 (= 0.42 + 0.09)$. With other parameters fixed the same, the study power becomes 0.955. The results show that the power depends on the underlying genetic model.

```
Example 2 (REC model with two levels): Default Values

Study Design
Case-Control Control to Case Ratio: 1

Exposures
Number: two
Exposure 1 Levels (2-10): 2
Exposure 2 Levels (2-10): 2

Type I Error
Alpha-Level: 0.05 Two-Sided

Exposure Scores Probabilities
(Only specify the margins. The cells in the center are
obtained as the products of the margins under the null
hypothesis.)

Scores 0 1 Total
0 0.637 0.063 0.70
1 0.273 0.027 0.30
Total 0.91 0.09 1.00
```

```
Probability of Disease at Baseline: 0.1
Model: multiplicative (logistic)

Odds Ratio Under the Alternative Hypothesis
Specify: Marginal
Exposure 1: 1.5
Exposure 2: 1.5
Interaction: 4

Calculations
Calculate
Power
Given: Sample Size: 1000
Finish
```

The output for power to detect gene-environment interaction given the sample sizes is given by

```
No. cases = 1000.0 No. controls = 1000.0 No. subjects = 2000.0
Study Power = 0.993
```

11.5.3 Gene-Gene Interactions

The approach discussed in Sect. 11.5.1 can be used to test gene-gene interaction. Thus, the power and sample size formulas given before can be used but both exposure variables are genetic susceptibility. The probabilities are more complicated for two susceptibility genes due to genetic model uncertainty. If three genetic models are plausible for each candidate-gene, then there are 9 different combinations of models for gene-gene interaction: REC-REC, REC-ADD, REC-DOM, ADD-REC, ADD-ADD, ADD-DOM, DOM-REC, DOM-ADD, and DOM-DOM. For more discussion of using genetic models and different test statistics for gene-gene interactions, see Chap. 8. For illustration, we consider the following example, assuming a REC-ADD model, using the Power Program.

Example

```
Example (G1 = REC and G2 = ADD): Default Values

Study Design
Case-Control Control to Case Ratio: 1

Exposures
Number: two
Exposure 1 Levels (2-10): 2
Exposure 2 Levels (2-10): 3

Type I Error
Alpha-Level: 0.05 Two-Sided

Exposure Scores Probabilities
```

```
(Only specify the margins. The cells in the center are
obtained as the products of the margins under the null
hypothesis.)

Scores 0 1 2 Total
0 0.5824 0.2912 0.0364 0.91
1 0.0576 0.0288 0.0036 0.09
Total 0.64 0.32 0.04 1.00

Probability of Disease at Baseline: 0.1
Model: multiplicative (logistic)

Odds Ratio Under the Alternative Hypothesis
Specify: Main Effect
Exposure 1: 1.5
Exposure 2: 1.5
Interaction: 4

Calculations
Calculate
Power
Given: Sample Size: 1000
Finish
```

The output for power to detect gene-gene interaction given for the REC-ADD model and the sample sizes is:

```
No. cases = 1000.0 No. controls = 1000.0 No. subjects = 2000.0
Study Power = 0.774
```

11.6 Bibliographical Comments

We considered power and sample size calculations for genetic association studies using case-control data. The focus is on single marker analysis, for which several methods have been discussed. The power and sample size calculations for gene-environment and gene-gene interactions are unified. Use of the Power Program is illustrated.

The formulas for sample size and power calculations under perfect LD for a single marker analysis can be found in Friedlin et al. [91]. Extensions of these to the LD situation are discussed by Pfeiffer and Gail [202] and Hanson et al. [114]. All these approaches assume a known genetic model. However, the sample size and power vary substantially when the genetic model changes from the REC model to the DOM model. Li et al. [169] consider some power calculations for robust tests, including a maximum robust test studied in Friedlin et al. [91] and Pearson's test. Statistical analysis of case-control data is affected by both genotyping errors and phenotyping errors. Ahn et al. [6] study how genotyping error can affect the power of trend tests, while Zheng and Tian [346] and Edwards et al. [68] study the impact when phenotypes (cases/controls) are diagnosed with errors. Zheng and Tian [346] focus on the trend test while Edwards et al. [68] also consider Pearson's test. The impact of different estimates of the variance of the trend test on the asymptotic power is considered by Zheng and Gastwirth [337].

A general approach to test interactions is presented by Lubin and Gail [177], which can be used to test case-control association in single marker analysis and gene-environment and gene-gene interactions. The Power Program is developed to calculate sample size and power based on this approach. How to test gene-gene interaction and calculate sample size and power, however, are not explicitly explained. The approach also assumes a known genetic model. How to deal with an unknown genetic model in interactions for sample size and power calculations is not discussed. Some special cases are considered by Foppa and Spiegelman [87] and Hwang et al. [129]. The former assume that the ORs for the main effects due to the exposure and gene are known, while the latter assume that there is no genetic main effect in the absence of an environmental factor [94]. These special cases put constraints on the parameter spaces under the null and alternative hypotheses, which lead to an under-powered study when these parameters are actually estimated in testing gene-environment interaction. In Sect. 11.5.1, we did not give explicit expressions for $\widetilde{\sigma}_{12}^2$, μ_{12} and σ_{12}^2, which can be found in Lubin and Gail [177]. We only focused on a binary environmental factor. For general categorical environment variables, see Foppa and Spiegelman [87] and Garcia-Closas and Lubin [94].

In this chapter, we did not discuss power and sample size calculations for haplotype analysis. Readers can refer to Schaid [231] for some discussion. This is often more complicated than calculating power and sample size for single marker analysis and interactions, owing to the unknown phases of halotypes and specification of genotype/haplotype frequencies. A case-only study for gene-environment interaction is an efficient design to study disease etiology that assumes HWE in the population. Sample size and power calculations to detect gene-environment interaction using case-only designs have been studied in the literature. Readers can refer to Yang et al. [311] and Clarke and Morris [38] for more details. We focused on sample size and power calculations for an unmatched case-control study. Gauderman [98] discussed sample size calculations for detecting gene-environment interaction for a matched case-control design (Chap. 4). In particular, he used sample size requirements to compare the matched case-control design with some family-based designs, including case-parent and case-sibling designs. A software program, "Quanto", that implements his method can be freely downloaded from "http://hydra.usc.edu/gxe". This program can also compute sample sizes for genes and gene-gene interactions using the matched case-control design, case-parents design, case-sibling design, and case-only design.

11.7 Problems

11.1 For a given x, derive the asymptotic distribution of $Z_{\mathrm{CATT}}(x)$, given in (11.7), under H_1.

11.2 For a given x, prove that $\widetilde{\sigma}_{1x}^2 = \sigma_{1x}^2 + \mu_{1x}^2$.

11.3 Prove that the asymptotic power using the trend test with the denominator $\{\widehat{\mathrm{Var}}^*(U_x)\}^{1/2}$ is always higher than that using the trend test with $\{\widehat{\mathrm{Var}}(U_x)\}^{1/2}$.

11.4 Compute the sample size n required to detect association with a disease locus given the allele frequency p and GRRs (λ_1, λ_2) (or λ_2 with a genetic model) based on the trend test $Z_{\mathrm{CATT}}(0.5)$ and Pearson's chi-squared test $T_{\chi_2^2}$. Let $\alpha = 0.05$ and the target power be 80%. Then conduct simulations to compare the empirical power to the theoretical one.

11.5 Relationship between ORs and GRRs

(a) Prove (11.12) and (11.13).
(b) Show that the DOM model defined using the GRRs and ORs are equivalent.
(c) Show that the REC model defined using the GRRs and ORs are equivalent.
(d) Show that if $\lambda_1 = (1+\lambda_2)/2$, then $\mathrm{OR}_1 < (1+\mathrm{OR}_2)/2$. Hence, the ADD model defined using the GRRs is not equivalent to that defined using the ORs.

11.6 Show that $\partial l(\theta_1)/\partial \theta_0^T$ in (11.17) can be written as

$$\frac{\partial l}{\partial \beta_0} = \sum_{i,j=0}^{1} \{R_{ij} - n_{ij} p_1(\mathbf{V} = (i, j))\},$$

$$\frac{\partial l}{\partial \beta_1} = \sum_{j=0}^{1} \{R_{1j} - n_{1j} p_1(\mathbf{V} = (1, j))\},$$

$$\frac{\partial l}{\partial \beta_2} = \sum_{i=0}^{1} \{R_{i1} - n_{i1} p_1(\mathbf{V} = (i, 1))\}.$$

Denote $p_0(\mathbf{V}) = 1 - p_1(\mathbf{V})$. Then show that

$$-\frac{\partial^2 l}{\partial \beta_0^2} = \sum_{i,j=0}^{1} n_{ij} p_0(\mathbf{V} = (i, j)) p_1(\mathbf{V} = (i, j)),$$

$$-\frac{\partial^2 l}{\partial \beta_0 \beta_1} = -\frac{\partial^2 l}{\partial \beta_1^2} = \sum_{j=0}^{1} n_{1j} p_0(\mathbf{V} = (1, j)) p_1(\mathbf{V} = (1, j)),$$

$$-\frac{\partial^2 l}{\partial \beta_0 \beta_2} = -\frac{\partial^2 l}{\partial \beta_2^2} = \sum_{i=0}^{1} n_{i1} p_0(\mathbf{V} = (i, 1)) p_1(\mathbf{V} = (i, 1)),$$

$$-\frac{\partial^2 l}{\partial \beta_1 \beta_2} = -\frac{\partial^2 l}{\partial \beta_{12}^2} = -\frac{\partial^2 l}{\partial \beta_0 \beta_{12}} = -\frac{\partial^2 l}{\partial \beta_1 \beta_{12}} = -\frac{\partial^2 l}{\partial \beta_2 \beta_{12}}$$
$$= n_{11} p_0(\mathbf{V} = (1, 1)) p_1(\mathbf{V} = (1, 1)).$$

Part V
Introduction to Genome-Wide Association Studies

Chapter 12
Genome-Wide Association Studies

Abstract Test statistics that have been discussed in previous chapters can be used in the analysis of genome-wide association studies (GWAS). However, in addition to association analysis, GWAS contain other aspects. We give a brief introduction to GWAS in this chapter, including some aspects of quality control, genome-wide ranking, testing gene-environment and gene-gene interactions in GWAS, and replication studies. A short introduction to GWAS is first given. Some details of quality control, including testing HWE, are discussed next. For the analysis of GWAS, we consider genome-wide ranking with the trend test, Pearson's test and two robust tests. Strategies for testing gene-environment and gene-gene interactions in GWAS are discussed. Finally, we review replication studies to confirm significant findings in GWAS.

Test statistics that have been discussed in previous chapters can be used in the analysis of genome-wide association studies (GWAS). However, in addition to association analysis, GWAS contain other aspects. We give a brief introduction to GWAS in this chapter, including some aspects of quality control, genome-wide ranking, testing gene-environment and gene-gene interactions in GWAS, and replication studies. A short introduction to GWAS is first given. Some details of quality control, including testing HWE, are discussed next. For the analysis of GWAS, we consider genome-wide ranking with the trend test, Pearson's test and two robust tests. Strategies for testing gene-environment and gene-gene interactions in GWAS are discussed. Finally, we review replication studies to confirm significant findings in GWAS.

12.1 Introduction

GWAS are designed to detect common genetic variants that could influence a variety of diseases and disorders. A common genetic variant often refers to a marker with MAF no less than 1% in the population. Population-based study designs using unrelated individuals are commonly employed in GWAS, but family-based or community-based study designs with related samples are also used. Phenotypes

G. Zheng et al., *Analysis of Genetic Association Studies*,
Statistics for Biology and Health,
DOI 10.1007/978-1-4614-2245-7_12, © Springer Science+Business Media, LLC 2012

studied in GWAS include binary, quantitative or ordinal traits. We focus on case-control data in this chapter, although most discussions also apply to other types of traits. The number of markers tested in GWAS has increased from 100,000 SNPs in 2005 to more than 1 million SNPs at present, plus additional imputed SNPs.

The genotyping technology currently used by Affymetrix, Inc. for GWAS is "Genome-Wide Human SNP Array 6.0", which consists of more than 906,000 SNPs, where 482,000 SNPs were selected unbiasedly from "Genome-Wide Human SNP Array 5.0", and an additional 424,000 SNPs were selected using tag SNPs, for chromosomes X and Y, and mitochondrial SNPs, etc. On the other hand, Illumina, Inc. provides a variety of whole-genome genotyping arrays, including "Human Omni5 BeadChip" with over 4 million SNPs and arrays with up to 500,000 custom SNPs.

Before conducting analyses of association in GWAS, quality control is first carried out. In Sect. 12.2, we discuss some aspects of quality control. After quality control filtering, in which low-quality SNPs are removed, the remaining SNPs are tested for association. Regardless of the type of trait, each SNP is tested for association at a prespecified significance level (e.g., 5E−08) or a level adjusted by the Bonferroni correction. Test statistics discussed before can be used for association analysis. Once the candidate SNPs are obtained from the analysis, one can check information about the SNPs by using the SNP rs number to search the dbSNP Home Page (http://www.ncbi.nlm.nih.gov/SNP/). The search outcomes include some details about the SNP and its alleles, neighboring SNPs, its chromosome and physical location for a given genome build, whether or not the SNPs are covered by genes, and the name and reference of the genes, etc. In Sect. 12.3.1, we discuss genome-wide ranking and show how the ranks of SNPs with true association depend on the choice of test statistics.

In addition to the above single-marker analysis, haplotype association and gene-environment and gene-gene interactions may also be analyzed. Some discussion of these analyses in GWAS is given in Sect. 12.3.2. Finally, a replication study is an essential step to confirm any significant findings in the initial study, and this is considered in Sect. 12.4.

12.2 Quality Control

GWAS data without any quality control are raw data. The initial quality control steps include some biological and technological quality checks. For example, contaminated DNA and low-quality SNPs are excluded. Genotypes are called using one of the genotype calling algorithms for each individual based on the signal intensities of alleles for each SNP. Low-quality genotype calls are also excluded. To conduct these quality control steps, special expertise in biology, technology and computing algorithms and high capacity computers are required. In some cases, however, the above quality control steps are done through collaborations. For example, if one accesses the GWAS data from the database of Genotypes and Phenotypes (dbGap) (http://www.ncbi.nlm.nih.gov/gap), both raw data and the data after initial quality control steps may be available.

The next steps of quality control involve calculations of the missing rate and call rate. The missing rate per SNP is the percentage of individuals whose genotypes are not called for a given SNP. SNPs with missing rates greater than 2% to 3% are usually removed from the analysis. The call rate per individual is the percentage of SNPs whose genotypes are called for a given individual. Individuals with call rates lower than 95% to 97% are also removed. Different GWAS may set slightly different thresholds for the missing rate and call rate. One can calculate the MAF for a SNP using either controls or the combined case-control samples. SNPs with MAFs less than 1%, including monomorphic SNPs, are also not analyzed because there is virtually no power in GWAS to detect association with such rare variants.

Deviation from HWE proportions in controls is tested for each SNP using either an asymptotic chi-squared test or an exact test (Sect. 2.3.2). Note that if family data are used, testing HWE is not trivial due to the relatedness in the data. The program FREQ in S.A.G.E. calculates the allele frequencies and departure from HWE for each SNP by maximum likelihood from family data assuming Mendelian inheritance. It does this by modeling the founder genotypic frequencies as a function of the allele frequencies and the locus specific inbreeding coefficient. So it will estimate these parameters even if none of the pedigree founders are typed. Dividing the inbreeding coefficient by its standard error can then be used to test HWE. Some references for other methods of testing HWE using family data are given in Sect. 12.5. SNPs with extremely significant deviation from HWE, based on a pre-specified significance level (or with the Bonferroni correction), are regarded as due to genotyping error, outliers from multiple testing and other quality-related issues, and are removed from the analysis. Certain genotyping error leads to deviation from HWE (see simulation results reported later in this section). However, association can also lead to deviation from HWE, especially deviation from HWE in cases. Thus, testing HWE is only done using controls.

We conducted a simulation with 10 SNPs with true association (two with the REC model, six with the ADD model and two with the DOM model), whose MAFs were simulated from the uniform distribution $U(0.1, 0.5)$ and GRRs were simulated from $U(1.2, 1.6)$ for the given genetic models. In the simulation, HWE held in the general population (Wright's inbreeding coefficient $F = 0$) and there was no genotyping error. The sample size was either 1,500 or 2,500 cases (controls). P-values for testing HWE using controls, cases or combined case-control samples were obtained and are reported in Table 12.1.

The results in Table 12.1 justify testing HWE using controls, but not cases nor combined samples, because the p-values using the cases or combined samples tend to be strongly significant when the sample size or the GRR is large enough, especially under the REC or DOM models. This is consistent with the results presented in Sect. 3.6 and Sect. 6.6.1, where deviation from HWE in cases is expected for SNPs with true association under the REC or DOM models. We used $1E-04$ significance level in Table 12.1. But if we apply the Bonferroni correction to the 0.05 level for testing 10 SNPs, no significant deviation from HWE in controls is observed.

Table 12.1 P-values for testing deviation from HWE using controls, cases or combined samples given that HWE holds in the general population. There is no genotype error. The disease prevalence is 0.15. P-values are in bold if they are less than 1E−04

$r = s$	Model	MAF	GRR	Controls	Cases	Combined
1,500	REC	0.32	1.43	8.07E−01	3.10E−03	4.49E−02
		0.28	1.30	8.66E−01	4.46E−03	2.91E−02
	ADD	0.39	1.20	7.90E−01	8.79E−01	8.00E−01
		0.43	1.60	5.59E−01	6.68E−01	6.69E−01
		0.19	1.45	7.44E−01	9.54E−01	6.55E−01
		0.18	1.46	3.61E−01	8.44E−01	5.10E−01
		0.26	1.28	8.36E−01	8.54E−01	8.36E−01
		0.33	1.54	2.83E−01	9.38E−01	3.48E−01
	DOM	0.40	1.24	6.93E−01	2.00E−02	2.25E−01
		0.22	1.31	6.92E−01	5.66E−03	1.04E−01
2,500	REC	0.41	1.30	6.80E−01	1.32E−04	1.26E−02
		0.41	1.55	2.26E−02	**4.84E−08**	1.54E−02
	ADD	0.43	1.46	5.80E−01	3.93E−01	9.21E−01
		0.50	1.38	6.88E−01	2.37E−01	3.11E−01
		0.40	1.27	4.59E−01	5.87E−01	4.34E−01
		0.33	1.23	7.37E−01	3.78E−02	9.32E−02
		0.30	1.56	5.17E−01	8.08E−01	3.73E−01
		0.35	1.56	3.64E−01	5.84E−01	6.21E−01
	DOM	0.49	1.57	1.31E−01	**3.67E−11**	**5.75E−08**
		0.15	1.25	2.46E−01	1.93E−01	9.90E−02

Next, we conducted a similar simulation but HWE did not hold in the population. We used Wright's inbreeding coefficient $F = -0.1$ or 0.1 to produce deviation from HWE. Results reported in Table 12.2 show that p-values for testing HWE using controls also tend to be significant. With the same MAFs as in Table 12.2, we also simulated 10 null SNPs and tested HWE. Similar patterns to those of the associated SNPs in Table 12.2 were also observed (the results are not reported here). Hence, when HWE does not hold, removing SNPs with extreme deviation from HWE in controls is likely to exclude some SNPs with true association as well as some null SNPs from GWAS analysis. On the other hand, we conducted similar simulations with $F = -0.05$ or 0.05. We did not observe significant deviation at the 1E−04 level among the 10 SNPs with true association.

In a further simulation, we considered genotyping error but assumed HWE proportions in the population. Two different models for genotyping error were considered. The first model, referred to as "error 1" model, assumes error occurs in calling alleles A and B:

$$\Pr(A \text{ allele is called as } B \text{ allele}) = \Pr(B \text{ allele is called as } A \text{ allele}) = e,$$

Table 12.2 P-values for testing deviation from HWE using controls, cases or combined samples given Wright's inbreeding coefficient F. There is no genotyping error. The disease prevalence is 0.15. 1,500 cases and 1,500 controls are used. P-values (using controls) are in bold if they are less than 1E−04

F	Model	MAF	GRR	Controls	Cases	Combined
−0.1	REC	0.42	1.29	**4.79E−05**	2.17E−03	5.48E−07
		0.18	1.34	**5.08E−05**	4.01E−04	7.90E−08
	ADD	0.27	1.22	**7.67E−07**	5.30E−03	5.02E−08
		0.20	1.52	**8.96E−09**	1.83E−05	8.93E−12
		0.32	1.29	**6.76E−08**	4.70E−05	2.89E−11
		0.24	1.58	2.48E−04	1.10E−05	3.98E−08
		0.44	1.33	**7.76E−05**	2.69E−05	1.08E−08
		0.22	1.53	1.55E−03	1.02E−10	1.44E−11
	REC	0.49	1.47	2.63E−02	1.62E−11	7.81E−10
		0.10	1.51	3.41E−04	1.33E−08	8.67E−11
0.1	REC	0.11	1.25	2.47E−03	1.96E−10	5.13E−12
		0.14	1.52	1.84E−02	7.77E−16	2.66E−14
	ADD	0.45	1.53	5.62E−03	2.60E−03	9.27E−06
		0.25	1.42	**9.14E−06**	1.17E−05	1.35E−10
		0.32	1.45	**7.61E−05**	1.73E−05	3.33E−09
		0.12	1.50	3.84E−02	6.18E−04	5.94E−05
		0.46	1.29	9.41E−04	3.74E−04	5.28E−07
		0.49	1.53	1.11E−03	1.39E−02	2.54E−05
	DOM	0.11	1.50	1.26E−03	2.90E−01	2.88E−03
		0.24	1.46	2.40E−03	4.26E−01	1.03E−01

where we chose $e = 0.2$, a quite large error rate. This is a special case of a more general genotyping error model allowing the above two probabilities to be unequal [103]. Therefore, given the true genotype frequencies (g_0, g_1, g_2) for (AA, AB, BB), the observed genotype frequencies with error are given by (p_0, p_1, p_2), where $p_0 = (1 - e)^2 g_0 + e(1 - e)g_1 + e^2 g_2$, $p_1 = 2e(1 - e)g_0 + \{e^2 + (1 - e)^2\}g_1 + 2e(1 - e)g_2$ and $p_2 = e^2 g_0 + e(1 - e)g_1 + (1 - e)^2 g_2$. The second model, referred to as "error 2" model, allows error directly in calling genotypes [62]. Assuming genotype AA is not likely to be called as BB and vice versa, the second model assumes the probability that a homozygous genotype is called as heterozygous is γ and the probability that a heterozygous genotype is called as homozygous is η. Then [103], $p_0 = (1 - \gamma)g_0 + (\eta/2)g_1$, $p_1 = \gamma g_0 + (1 - \eta)g_1 + \gamma g_2$ and $p_2 = (\eta/2)g_1 + (1 - \gamma)g_2$. When $e = \eta = \gamma = 0$, there is no genotyping error (referred to as "no error"), so $p_i = g_i$, $i = 0, 1, 2$. Similar simulations were conducted to test HWE with HWE proportions in the population. Three models were considered: no error, error 1 model and error 2 model. In each case we simulated 10 associated SNPs with genetic models specified as before and 10 null SNPs with the same MAFs as the associated SNPs. The p-values for testing HWE are reported in Table 12.3. The results show that, under error 1 model when there is allele call error with a 20% error rate, no significant deviation from HWE is observed. This is consistent with the analytical findings reported in the literature [355]. However, when there is genotype call error with $\eta = \gamma = 0.1$, strong deviation from HWE is observed for the associated SNPs as well as for the null SNPs, especially when the number of controls is 2,500.

The results in Tables 12.1, 12.2, 12.3 show that, when testing HWE for GWAS quality control, the control samples should be used, a small significance level such as the one based on Bonferroni correction can be used, and that deviation from HWE can be observed for SNPs with true association when there is genotyping error. SNPs that are removed from single-marker analysis due to departure from HWE can be analyzed later if necessary. For example, some SNPs removed may be in high LD with the candidate SNPs that show strong association in single marker analysis. Then, these removed SNPs can be re-analyzed with the candidate SNPs in haplotype analysis.

In Chap. 9, we discussed PS and methods to correct PS when it is present. In GWAS, a simple measure for PS is the variance over-dispersion measure, the VIF, discussed in Sect. 9.3, which is the ratio of the observed median of the trend test Z^2_{CATT} over that of the theoretical one (0.456). When there is no PS, under the null hypothesis of no association the VIF is 1. Thus, a large (or small) value of VIF implies PS. A large VIF would lead to identifying SNPs with spurious association. In practice, a VIF > 1.1 would be considered as inflated and an appropriate method to correct for PS needs to be applied. Using the self-reported ethnicity in GWAS analysis may not always control the VIF. For example, in the WTCCC [301], the VIFs for seven diseases before correcting for PS are 1.11, 1.07, 1.11, 1,06, 1.03, 1.05 and 1.08, while after correcting for PS using the PCA method they become 1.09, 1.06, 1.07, 1.07, 1.03, 1.05 and 1.06, respectively. Q-Q plots of the observed test statistics versus those simulated from the theoretical distribution under the null hypothesis are also helpful to visually examine the deviation of the observed statistics in the presence of PS.

12.3 Analysis of GWAS

12.3.1 Genome-Wide Scans and Ranking

Analysis of GWAS often starts with a simple single-marker analysis strategy, testing one SNP at a time. For genome-wide scans of a binary trait, test statistics to be used include, but are not limited to, the allele-based test comparing the frequency of an allele between cases and controls (Sect. 3.4), the trend test under the ADD model (Sect. 3.3.1), Pearson's chi-squared test (Sect. 3.3.3), or robust tests (e.g., MAX3 or MIN2) (Sect. 6.3.1 and Sect. 6.4). When the trait is quantitative, a linear regression model is often used.

Table 12.3 P-values of testing HWE in controls when there is no genotyping error (no error), error 1 (allele call error), or error 2 (genotype call error). $e = 0.2$ and $\eta = \gamma = 0.1$. The bold entries are p-values significant at the level 5E−03 with Bonferroni correction for testing 10 SNPs. The null SNPs have the same MAFs as the associated SNPs. The genetic models are for the associated SNPs

No. controls	Model	MAF	GRR	No error		Error 1		Error 2	
				Assoc.	Null	Assoc.	Null	Assoc.	Null
1,500	REC	0.33	1.43	2.80E−01	5.08E−01	5.04E−01	9.25E−01	1.24E−02	5.64E−02
		0.39	1.58	4.28E−01	9.34E−02	5.02E−01	6.69E−02	3.83E−01	9.50E−01
	ADD	0.16	1.43	7.55E−01	7.87E−01	3.65E−01	4.30E−01	1.64E−01	1.91E−01
		0.11	1.21	5.39E−01	6.01E−01	9.45E−01	9.25E−01	5.71E−01	4.27E−01
		0.44	1.36	3.82E−01	2.68E−01	1.56E−01	2.27E−01	**1.77E−03**	**4.87E−03**
		0.28	1.29	6.90E−01	5.04E−01	9.64E−01	9.77E−01	4.50E−02	1.24E−01
		0.18	1.53	6.88E−01	9.59E−01	9.72E−01	7.51E−01	5.19E−01	4.07E−01
		0.41	1.54	5.76E−01	6.86E−01	5.57E−01	4.53E−01	5.01E−02	1.51E−01
	DOM	0.35	1.30	3.68E−01	3.18E−01	6.67E−01	4.24E−01	5.24E−02	9.79E−03
		0.11	1.40	2.27E−01	3.37E−01	2.77E−01	5.07E−01	1.60E−01	2.81E−01
2,500	REC	0.38	1.24	7.92E−01	9.27E−01	6.37E−01	9.73E−01	9.97E−03	7.99E−02
		0.14	1.56	5.78E−01	6.85E−01	5.12E−02	2.79E−01	9.82E−03	6.08E−02
	ADD	0.46	1.56	3.10E−01	1.04E−01	6.78E−02	6.06E−02	**1.13E−04**	**1.90E−04**
		0.35	1.52	6.59E−01	5.49E−01	9.89E−01	8.02E−01	2.21E−02	2.64E−02
		0.29	1.40	8.52E−01	9.20E−01	8.83E−01	9.78E−01	1.09E−01	1.15E−01
		0.29	1.30	3.32E−01	5.15E−01	6.32E−01	4.02E−01	3.50E−02	8.15E−02
		0.45	1.23	5.72E−01	8.63E−01	9.75E−01	7.21E−01	**1.69E−03**	6.92E−03
		0.28	1.30	5.91E−01	4.39E−01	2.94E−01	3.90E−01	2.09E−01	6.58E−01
	DOM	0.19	1.30	2.63E−01	9.60E−02	3.68E−01	3.07E−01	5.63E−03	**2.57E−03**
		0.43	1.29	6.40E−01	2.84E−01	6.66E−01	7.52E−01	**1.93E−03**	**1.50E−03**

When the p-values of a test statistic are obtained for all SNPs, they are compared to a prespecified genome-wide significance level, e.g., 5E−08, or the conventional significance level adjusted for multiple testing using the Bonferroni correction. A SNP has significant association with the trait, subject to confirmation using independent samples, if its p-value is less than the genome-wide significance level. It is possible that, in GWAS, none of the SNPs has a p-value less than the significance level. In this case, all the SNPs can be ranked by their p-values (or the test statistics), and a small number of top-ranked SNPs can be selected as candidate SNPs for further consideration. SNPs with previously reported association may be confirmed, and some novel genes may also be identified.

One should not expect, in genome-wide scans or ranking, the SNPs with true association to have p-values less than 5E−08 or to be always ranked near the top. Many factors affect the order of the ranks for the SNPs with true association, e.g., MAFs, genetic models, the total number of SNPs with true association, genetic effects, and the sample size (or power). Under some assumptions, the probabilities of the ranks of SNPs with true association can be derived (Problem 12.1).

Let $Y_1, \ldots, Y_M$ be statistics for SNPs with true association, whose p-values are denoted as $q_1, \ldots, q_M$, and $X_1, \ldots, X_{N-M}$ be statistics for SNPs without association (i.e., null SNPs), whose p-values are denoted as $p_1, \ldots, p_{N-M}$, where N is the total number of SNPs in a GWAS. Rank $q_1, \ldots, q_M$ as $q_{(1:M)} < \cdots < q_{(M:M)}$, and $p_1, \ldots, p_{N-M}$ as $p_{(1:N-M)} < \cdots < p_{(N-M:N-M)}$. Then $\Pr(q_{(1:M)} < p_{(k:N-M)})$ measures how likely the most significant SNP with true association would have a better rank than the kth ranked null SNP. When $N = 500{,}000$, $M = 10$ and $k = 10$, it refers to the probability that at least one of the 10 SNPs with true association would be ranked in the top 10 among 500,000 SNPs. $\Pr(q_{(1:M)} < p_{(k:N-M)} \mid \min(q_{(1:M)}, p_{(1:N-M)}) < \alpha)$ has a similar interpretation except that it is conditional on at least one SNP having p-value smaller than α, where α is the genome-wide significance level. These theoretical probabilities depend on many factors, including M, N and the power to detect the SNPs with true association.

Tables 12.4 and 12.5 report simulation results in genome-wide ranking with equal number of cases r and controls s, and $n = r + s$. We simulated a single GWAS with 500,000 SNPs, where 10 SNPs had true association, among which the numbers of SNPs with the REC, ADD and DOM models were $2, 4, 2$, respectively. The other 499,990 SNPs were null. All MAFs were simulated from $U(0.1, 0.5)$ and the GRR for each of the 10 associated SNPs was simulated from $U(1.2, 1.6)$. All 500,000 SNPs were ranked separately for each of the test statistics considered. The ranks of the 10 associated SNPs were recorded and are reported in Tables 12.4 and 12.5. In Table 12.4 HWE holds in the population, and in Table 12.5 deviation from HWE occurs in the cases for the 4 SNPs with true association under the REC and DOM models (Wright's inbreeding coefficient is 0.2, which was made large to see an effect). In Table 12.4, the ranks of the 10 SNPs with association are similar by any of the methods. However, in Table 12.5, we see that deviation from HWE in cases for the two SNPs with the REC model and the two SNPs with the DOM model may have an impact on genome-wide ranking using the trend test. For example, the three

Table 12.4 Ranks of 10 SNPs with true association under different genetic models in a genome-wide ranking of 500,000 SNPs. The prevalence is 0.15 and the sample size n varies ($r = s$). HWE holds in the population

$r = s$	SNP	GRR	MAF	MIN2	MAX3	CATT	Pearson's
1,500	REC	1.37	0.28	40	57	24	57
		1.38	0.16	247,606	152,413	262,551	187,903
	ADD	1.44	0.30	3,626	3,631	2,279	5,736
		1.52	0.49	15	18	9	38
		1.39	0.32	1,200	1,788	753	2,968
		1.37	0.41	2,401	3,546	1,511	3834
		1.33	0.43	8,740	12,585	5,636	16,150
		1.35	0.30	39	56	23	78
	DOM	1.54	0.14	1	1	1	1
		1.31	0.49	1,664	560	3,402	1,027
2,500	REC	1.55	0.31	7	5	12	5
		1.49	0.38	8	4	38	6
	ADD	1.40	0.47	13	17	9	24
		1.53	0.14	3	3	3	3
		1.22	0.37	6	9	5	8
		1.28	0.42	4	6	4	9
		1.44	0.40	34	46	23	86
		1.45	0.36	2	2	2	2
	DOM	1.26	0.19	372	348	231	649
		1.38	0.29	1	1	1	1

SNPs (two with the REC model and one with the DOM model) in Table 12.5 with $r = s = 2,500$ have ranks 5463, 2956 and 8034 and would not be detected if the trend test is applied. Since the results were based on a single GWAS of 500,000 SNPs without any replication, actual results may vary when other GWAS data are used.

For the SNPs whose p-values are significant or that are top-ranked, BFs (Chap. 5) can be reported along with their p-values. The BFs are especially useful when the results are compared across GWAS, e.g., between the initial study and the confirmation study. P-values measure the significance of SNPs regardless of the power or sample size, while BFs incorporate both significance of the SNPs and the power (sample size) to detect significant association. If the p-value of the trend test under a genetic model is reported, we can report the BF under the same genetic model. However, when the p-value of a robust test is reported, we can report the three BFs under the REC, ADD and DOM models.

Table 12.5 Ranks of 10 SNPs with true association under different genetic models in a genome-wide ranking of 500,000 SNPs. The prevalence is 0.15 and the sample size n varies ($r = s$). Deviation from HWE occurs in the controls for the associated SNPs under the REC and DOM models

$r = s$	SNP	GRR	MAF	MIN2	MAX3	CATT	Pearson's
1,500	REC	1.43	0.45	1	2	547	1
		1.51	0.45	2	1	2	2
	ADD	1.30	0.20	5,744	2,520	3,713	3,671
		1.59	0.23	5	5	4	5
		1.55	0.31	4	4	3	4
		1.49	0.18	86	113	46	205
		1.30	0.43	2,079	1,293	1,281	2,091
		1.43	0.22	3,271	4,753	2,066	7,354
	DOM	1.56	0.32	3	3	1	3
		1.31	0.39	7	6	60	6
2,500	REC	1.33	0.21	2	2	5,463	2
		1.31	0.42	1	1	2,956	1
	ADD	1.24	0.28	37	51	24	55
		1.34	0.27	724	1,047	443	1,530
		1.41	0.39	267	398	169	720
		1.24	0.35	26,425	36,821	17,320	49,843
		1.58	0.34	3	3	1	3
		1.41	0.34	6	9	3	7
	DOM	1.34	0.22	4	4	2	4
		1.22	0.31	5	5	8,034	5

12.3.2 Haplotype Analysis and Interactions

A large number of haplotypes can be formed and tested in GWAS, which results in a large number of multiple tests. Hence, candidate SNPs (or candidate genes) can be first identified in single-marker analysis. Then the methods for haplotype analysis discussed in Chap. 7 can be applied to the haplotype formed by the candidate SNPs. Haplotype analysis can be more powerful than single-marker analysis for SNPs in LD with functional loci or when the variations in traits are inherited in haplotypes.

Unlike haplotype analysis, which tests association of SNPs in LD, gene-gene interaction tests association of a combination of SNPs on the same or different chromosomes on the assumption that they are not in gametic phase disequilibrium. However, there are more combinations of gene-gene interaction terms to be tested in GWAS. With 500,000 SNPs, there are more than 100 billion combinations of any two SNPs. In addition, it is known that the power to detect gene-gene interaction is often lower than to test marginal effects, even though the interaction may exist without the marginal effects. A two-step analysis strategy is helpful [151, 179]. First, candidate SNPs in single-marker analysis are selected at a given significance level, e.g., 0.01. Then we only test gene-gene interactions for these marginally significant SNPs, using the methods discussed in Chap. 8.

Recent GWAS show that only a small portion of the heritability has been explained by the identified genetic variants. This finding, along with the empirical evidence, suggests that some of the missing heritability could be due to gene-environment interactions. Lower power and multiple testing are challenges for testing gene-environment interaction in GWAS. Two strategies have been studied in the literature. Both relate to selecting a small number of SNPs to test for gene-environment interaction. The first approach is similar to that mentioned above in testing gene-gene interaction. That is, one tests gene-environment interaction only for the SNPs (and the environments if there is more than one risk factor) which show marginal effects at a prespecified significance level, e.g. 0.01 [150]. In the second approach, we test gene and environment association using the pooled case-control samples (n_0, n_1, n_2) and identify SNPs with most significant association. Then we test gene-environment interaction with these SNPs using the case-control data. It can be shown that the selection of SNPs and the procedure to test for the interaction are independent [187].

In haplotype analysis and testing interactions, we need to correct for multiple testing. One simple approach is to apply the Bonferroni correction for the actual number of hypotheses tested or apply other approaches such as controlling the false discovery rate.

12.4 Replication and Follow-Up

Replication is an important step in GWAS. It is often necessary to confirm the findings of the initial study using independent samples. A good design of a replication study, with careful choices of study population and trait, and with a large sample size, would increase the chance of replicating the SNPs with true association. The importance of replication and guidelines of how to conduct replication studies can be found in the literature [190, 191]. We emphasize a few points here.

A replication study should have enough power to separate true association from null association. However, if the study power for replication is calculated based on the observed effect of a significant SNP, the "winner's curse" may have an adverse effect on the power calculation [306]. In genetic association studies, the winner's curse refers to any bias related to estimating genetic effects based on selecting the most significant SNPs for replication. There is a tendency to overestimate the genetic effects so that the follow-up study would be under-powered.

A replication study should use independent case-control data, sampled from the same population as the initial study. Breaking the whole sample into independent testing and training sets is often less powerful [246]. Multi-stage sampling or meta-analysis can be applied to a replication study. Selecting the same phenotype is crucial in a replication study because the phenotype determines the underlying genetic model and the performance of test statistics depends on the genetic model. The same or similar phenotypes, along with similar covariates, should be used for both cases and controls. If case-control status is determined based on a quantitative trait with a threshold model, using more extreme traits for cases and controls would improve the power to replicate the findings. The same test statistic based on the same genetic model should be first used in a replication study, although using the same test is not always optimal. For example, if the initial study is tested based on a trend test optimal for the DOM model, the same test based on the DOM model is not optimal in a replication study, because, for complex traits, the true genetic model is not known and the optimal test also depends on the LD between the SNP and the functional loci.

Although some may argue there is no correction necessary when replicating multiple SNPs, it is still necessary to correct for multiple testing if multiple tests are applied to replicate each SNP, e.g., if both the trend test and Pearson's chi-squared test are applied to replicate each SNP. Furthermore, a combination of the p-values (or test statistics) of the initial and replication studies should be more significant than that of the initial study (Problem 12.2).

12.5 Bibliographical Comments

In this chapter, we provide a short review of GWAS. The WTCCC [301] and its online supplementary materials cover most of the procedures for the analysis of GWAS, including those we did not mention here. A comprehensive reference focusing on biostatistical aspects of GWAS is given in Ziegler et al. [352]. Strategies for analysis of gene-environment interaction in GWAS, referred to as "gene-environment-wide association studies", is reviewed by Thomas [271]. Other strategies and statistical methods for testing gene-gene and gene-environment interactions can be found in a review by Kooperberg et al. [151]. We mentioned selection bias due to the winner's curse in GWAS [306]. Many statistical methods have been proposed to correct for it (e.g., [101, 254, 353]). Other biases also exist as a result of genome-wide ranking [131], which we did not discuss here. The NCI-NHGRI [191] provided detailed descriptions of how to design, analyze and report replication studies, as well as general guidelines on how to report phenotype-genotype association.

Some topics related to GWAS are not discussed in this chapter, including testing untyped SNPs and imputing SNPs [172]. Analysis of copy number variants (CNVs) in GWAS is not covered here either [289, 354]. Other methods for analysis of GWAS can be found in the journal *Statistical Science*, which published a special issue on statistical methods for genome-wide association studies [342].

We mentioned that the program FREQ in S.A.G.E. (http://darwin.case.edu/sage/) can be used to test departure from HWE using family data. Other analytical approaches have also been developed to test HWE using family data. For example, Bourgain et al. [20] developed several tests for deviation from HWE not due to inbreeding, and noticed that the usual chi-squared test for HWE ignoring the relatedness within families would greatly inflate Type I error. Li and Graubard [167] considered testing HWE using data collected from a complex survey, which includes family data. Zou and Donner [355] showed that departure from HWE does not imply any allele call error, the first model discussed in Sect. 12.2. The results in Table 12.3, under error 1 model, also demonstrate this. They further argued that, although genotype call error leads to departure from HWE, the power to detect genotyping error is low. The cautionary note of Zou and Donner [355] on testing HWE as a quality control step was mostly for candidate-gene studies. With improved technology for genotyping and calling algorithms, genotyping error and call error are much reduced in GWAS. Hence, the purpose of checking deviation from HWE in GWAS quality control is not just to detect genotyping error.

12.6 Problems

12.1 In a GWAS of N SNPs, assume all SNPs are independent, and that the test statistics of the SNPs with true association $Y_1, \ldots, Y_M$ follow the same distribution $F_1(y)$ with density $f_1(y)$, and the test statistics for the null SNPs $X_1, \ldots, X_{N-M}$ follow the same distribution $F_0(x)$ with density $f_0(x)$. Let the ordered p-values be $q_{(i:M)}$, $1 \leq i \leq M$, and $q_{(k:N-M)}$, $1 \leq k \leq N - M$, as given in Sect. 12.3.1. Using the results in Sect. 1.1.4, derive the following results [317].

(a) Show that the densities of $q_{(1:M)}$ and $p_{(k:N-M)}$ are given respectively by

$$f_{1:M}(q) = M \frac{f_1(F_0^{-1}(1-q))}{f_0(F_0^{-1}(1-q))} F_1^{M-1}(F_0^{M-1}(1-q)),$$

$$f_{k:N-M}(p) = \frac{(N-M)!}{(k-1)!(N-M-k)!} p^{k-1}(1-p)^{N-M-k}.$$

(b) Show that the joint density of $(p_{1:N-M}, p_{k:N-M})$ $(k > 1)$ can be written as

$$f_{1k:N-M}(p_1, p_k) = \frac{(N-M)!}{(k-1)!(N-M-k)!} (p_k - p_1)^{k-1}(1-p_k)^{N-M-k}.$$

(c) Show that $\Pr(q_{1:M} < p_{k:N-M}) = \int_{p>q} f_{k:N-M}(p) f_{1:M}(q) dp\,dq$, and

$$\Pr(q_{1:M} < p_{k:N-M} \mid \min(q_{1:M}, p_{1:N-M}) < \alpha)$$
$$= \frac{\Pr(q_{1:M} < p_{k:N-M}) - \Pr(\alpha < q_{1:M} < p_{k:N-M}, p_{1:N-M} > \alpha)}{\int_{q>\alpha} f_{1:M}(q) dq \int_{p>\alpha} f_{1:N-M}(p) dp}.$$

(d) Derive $\Pr(\alpha < q_{1:M} < p_{k:N-M}, p_{1:N-M} > \alpha)$.

12.2 Let p_1 and p_2 be the p-values of the initial and replication studies, respectively. Since the data in the two studies are independent, Fisher's combination of the two p-values can be considered as a joint analysis, given by

$$T = -2\log(p_1) - 2\log(p_2) \sim \chi_4^2$$

under H_0. When is the p-value of T smaller than p_1?

Part VI
Introduction to Family-Based Association Studies

Chapter 13
Analysis of Family Data

Abstract Chapter 13 covers the analysis of family data, including linkage and association studies. Both model-free and model-based linkage analyses are discussed. For the former, estimating marker identity by descent, interval mapping, the Haseman-Elston regression method for a quantitative trait, and the likehood variance component method are studied. The transmission-Disequilibrium Test (TDT) is presented. Robust tests for linkage using affected sibpairs and for association using parent-offspring trio data are presented. Finally, family-based methods for linkage and association analysis (FBAT) are reviewed.

When two loci are close enough on the same chromosome that the alleles at the two loci tend to cosegregate to the next generation, the two loci are linked. In genetic studies, linkage analysis will test whether a marker locus and a disease locus are linked, whereas association analysis investigates the linkage disequilibrium between a marker and a disease locus in a population. Association analysis can be viewed as a linkage analysis in which an entire population is considered as a whole family and we can trace the flow of alleles from generation to generation. Linkage analysis can be model-based or model-free, which refers to the mode of inheritance assumed for the trait whose underlying chromosome locations are being tested. This chapter begins with an introduction to model-based linkage analysis, followed by model-free methods, variance component methods, and the transmission/disequilibrium test (TDT). For family-based association studies, we focus on a parent-offspring trio design using the TDT. Some robust procedures discussed in Chap. 6 will be applied to the trio design. A general family-based association test (FBAT) is introduced with applications to the trio design and some general pedigrees. Some of the advantages and disadvantages of these different methods will also be mentioned. Because we only give an introduction to the analysis of family data, some details are omitted. The references for the materials presented in this chapter are given in the Bibliographical Comments section (Sect. 13.6).

G. Zheng et al., *Analysis of Genetic Association Studies*,
Statistics for Biology and Health,
DOI 10.1007/978-1-4614-2245-7_13, © Springer Science+Business Media, LLC 2012

13.1 Model-Based Methods for Linkage Analysis

Model-based methods are also sometimes called "lod score" methods, or "parametric" analyses, and the use of lod scores for linkage analysis was developed by Newton Morton in his seminal article. In these methods, the mode of inheritance of the phenotype (a genetic model) is specified. These methods have been very successful in past decades in identifying disease genes for Mendelian diseases. We consider a dichotomous phenotype, either affected (cases) or unaffected (controls), and a diallelic trait locus. Denote the two alleles as D and d, and their corresponding allele frequencies as p and $1 - p$, respectively. Under the assumption of random mating, or HWE proportions, the genotype frequencies for DD, Dd and dd are p^2, $2p(1 - p)$ and $(1 - p)^2$, respectively. Let the penetrances of the three genotypes be f_{DD}, f_{Dd} and f_{dd}. Note that in this chapter we use a different notation for analyzing family data. For analyzing population-based case-control data, the three penetrances were denoted as f_0, f_1 and f_2. In this chapter, (f_0, f_1, f_2) are used to denote other probabilities (e.g., see Sect. 13.2.1) while we use f_{DD}, f_{Dd} and f_{dd} to denote penetrances. We previously used ϕ and Φ for the PDF and CDF of $N(0, 1)$. In this chapter, however, they are the kinship coefficient and matrix, respectively. Other differences in notation in this chapter will be pointed out when they appear. We further assume that the affection status of an individual is only dependent on his or her own genotype. Let $(Y_1, \ldots, Y_K)$ denote the phenotypes in a family of size K, and $(g_1, \ldots, g_K)$ denote their genotypes at the trait locus. We have

$$\Pr(Y_1, \ldots, Y_K | g_1, \ldots, g_K) = \prod_{k=1}^{K} \Pr(Y_k | g_k).$$

We assume a marker locus M with two alleles, A and a. Let θ denote the recombination fraction between the trait and marker loci, i.e. the proportion of offspring expected to inherit together the alleles at M and A that are on the same chromosome of a homologous pair a parent has. Let $(m_1, \ldots, m_K)$ denote the genotypes at the marker locus M. We usually do not observe the trait genotypes. The likelihood for observing the phenotypes and marker genotypes in a family is dependent on the parameters $(\theta, p, f_{DD}, f_{Dd}, f_{dd})$. That is, the likelihood of θ, the parameter of interest, for the data is given by

$$\Pr(\text{data} | \theta, p, f_{DD}, f_{Dd}, f_{dd})$$
$$= \Pr(Y_1, \ldots, Y_K, m_1, \ldots, m_K | \theta, p, f_{DD}, f_{Dd}, f_{dd})$$
$$= \sum_{g_1, \ldots, g_K} \prod_{k=1}^{K} \Pr(Y_k | g_k) \Pr(m_1, g_1; \ldots; m_K, g_K).$$

For illustration, we assume a nuclear family of size k and denote the father and mother as individuals 1 and 2. Then the above likelihood function becomes

$$\Pr(m_1) \Pr(m_2) \sum_{g_1} \Pr(Y_1 | g_1) \Pr(g_1) \sum_{g_2} \Pr(Y_2 | g_2) \Pr(g_2)$$

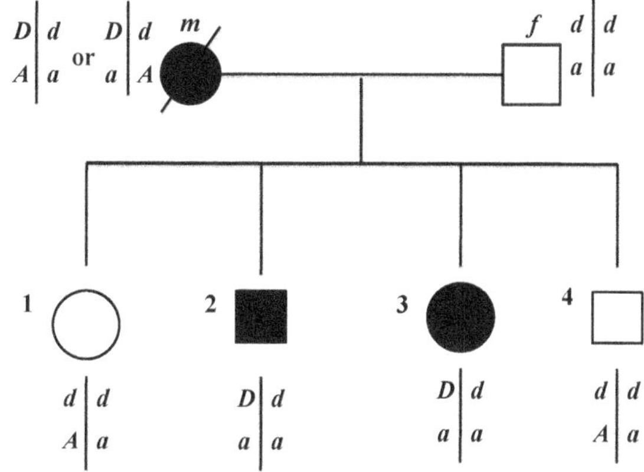

Fig. 13.1 A pedigree of 6 individuals with a rare DOM disease. A *filled circle* or *square* denotes a family member who is affected. A full penetrance model is assumed, i.e. $f_{DD} = f_{Dd} = 1$ and $f_{dd} = 0$

$$\times \prod_{k=3}^{K} \sum_{g_k} \Pr(Y_k|g_k)\,\Pr(m_k, g_k|m_1, g_1; m_2, g_2),$$

which is a function of $(\theta, p, f_{DD}, f_{Dd}, f_{dd})$, because $\Pr(m_k, g_k|m_1, g_1; m_2, g_2)$ is a function of the recombination fraction θ. For a general or large pedigree, the likelihood function can be efficiently calculated using the Elston-Stewart algorithm, which has been implemented in the Software packages LINKAGE (ftp://linkage.rockefeller.edu/software/linkage/), FASTLINK (http://www.ncbi.nlm.nih.gov/CBBresearch/Schaffer/fastlink.html) and the Statistical Analysis for Genetic Epidemiology (S.A.G.E.) (http://darwin.cwru.edu/sage).

In a linkage analysis between a trait and a marker locus, the null hypothesis (H_0) is free recombination, corresponding to $\theta = 1/2$, and the alternative hypothesis (H_1) is linkage, corresponding to $0 \le \theta < 1/2$. The logarithm to base 10 of the likelihood ratio,

$$Z(\theta) = \log_{10} \frac{\Pr(\text{data}|\theta, p, f_{DD}, f_{Dd}, f_{dd})}{\Pr(\text{data}|\theta = 1/2, p, f_{DD}, f_{Dd}, f_{dd})},$$

for various values of θ is termed a lod score, or lod. Let $Z(\widehat{\theta})$ be the value evaluated at the MLE of θ, $\widehat{\theta}$, or the maximized lod, which is a measure of support for linkage versus absence of linkage. Asymptotically, under H_0, $4.605 \times Z(\widehat{\theta})$ follows χ_1^2 because $2 \times \log 10 = 4.605$. Thus, a maximum lod score > 3 implies a p-value ~ 0.0001, because we have a one-sided alternative $H_1 : \theta < 1/2$.

Consider an autosomal DOM disease segregating in a family, as in Fig. 13.1. Assume all individuals have been genotyped at the marker locus, as shown in Fig. 13.1. We further assume an individual carrying the disease allele D is always affected. Since the mother is affected and she has both affected and unaffected children, her genotype at the disease locus must be heterozygous Dd, while the father, who is unaffected, must have genotype dd. Thus, the father always transmits the haplotype da to offspring. We can then infer the phased genotypes for all the offspring. Although we can easily infer the mother's genotype at the disease locus, we are not certain of her phase. The possible phased genotype for the mother is either DA/da

or Da/dA. Because we have the genotype information at both the marker and trait loci, the likelihood for the pedigree in Fig. 13.1 can be written as

$$
\begin{aligned}
&\Pr(\text{data}|\theta, p, f_{DD}, f_{Dd}, f_{dd}) \\
&= \Pr(Y_f, Y_m, \ldots, Y_4, m_f, m_m, \ldots, m_4, \\
&\quad g_f, g_m, \ldots, g_4|\theta, p, f_{DD} = 1, f_{Dd} = 1, f_{dd} = 0) \\
&= \Pr(m_f, g_f) P(m_m, g_m) \prod_{k=1}^{4} \Pr(m_k, g_k|m_f, g_f; m_m, g_m).
\end{aligned}
$$

If the mother's phased genotype is known, then the conditional probability of an offspring phased genotype given the parents' phased genotypes can be calculated by counting the number of recombinants and non-recombinants in the family. For example, given the mother's phased genotype is DA/da, there are four recombinants. The likelihood for this case is

$$
\Pr(m_f, g_f) \Pr(m_m, g_m) \times \left(\frac{1}{2}\theta\right)^4.
$$

Analogously, given the mother's phased genotype is Da/dA, there are four non-recombinants, so that the likelihood is

$$
\Pr(m_f, g_f) \Pr(m_m, g_m) \times \left\{\frac{1}{2}(1-\theta)\right\}^4.
$$

If we do not have the phase information for the mother, we let the two phased genotypes have equal probability to occur. Then the likelihood is

$$
\Pr(\text{data}|\theta, p, f_{DD}, f_{Dd}, f_{dd}) = \frac{1}{2^5} \Pr(m_f, g_f) \Pr(m_m, g_m)\{(1-\theta)^4 + \theta^4\}.
$$

The lod score is

$$
\begin{aligned}
Z(\theta) &= \log_{10} \frac{\Pr(\text{data}|\theta, p, f_{DD}, f_{Dd}, f_{dd})}{\Pr(\text{data}|\theta = \frac{1}{2}, p, f_{DD}, f_{Dd}, f_{dd})} \\
&= 3\log_{10}(2) + \log_{10}\{(1-\theta)^4 + \theta^4\},
\end{aligned}
$$

which reaches its maximum when $\theta = 0$.

A family or set of families is informative for linkage if the lod score $Z(\theta)$ is not equal to zero when $\theta < 1/2$. Similarly, offspring are called informative for linkage when their marker genotypes reveal linkage information. If there were only one offspring in the above example, we would have the lod score $Z(\theta) = 0$. Thus, there is no information for linkage in a nuclear family when there is only one offspring. In general, when there are at least two offspring in a family, the family provides linkage information.

When there are multiple independent families, it is straightforward to calculate the lod score for all the families together. Letting $Z_i(\theta)$ be the lod score for family i, the lod score for N independent families is

$$
Z(\theta) = \sum_{i=1}^{N} Z_i(\theta).
$$

When multiple studies are available, we can also sum the lod scores from the multiple studies. Traditionally, we publish lod score curves as a function of θ in every study, to allow the pooling of independent studies. Caution should be taken that we should add the lod score functions first, and then take the maximization of the sum for the estimation of θ and testing for linkage, rather than adding the maximum lods from different studies.

Traditionally, to control the probability of being in error when we declare linkage, a p-value of 10^{-4} is required for significance. In a linkage test of a marker, the usual significance level is defined as

$$\alpha = \Pr(\text{rejection of } H_0 \text{ given } \theta = 1/2),$$

and the power is defined as

$$1 - \beta = \Pr(\text{rejection of } H_0 \text{ given } \theta < 1/2).$$

The probability of being in error when we declare there is linkage, i.e., the posterior probability of Type I error, is a function of both the usual Type I error (i.e. the probability of error given H_0 is true) and the prior probability that H_0 is true. That is

$$\Pr(\theta < 1/2 | \text{rejection of } H_0) = \frac{(1 - \beta)\Pr(\theta < 1/2)}{(1 - \beta)\Pr(\theta < 1/2) + \alpha\Pr(\theta = 1/2)}.$$

Using the fact that two loci picked randomly from a genome have a small prior probability (approximately $\Pr(\theta < 1/2) = 0.05$) of being linked, it approximately follows that using a p-value of 10^{-4} before accepting linkage controls to 5% the probability of being in error when declaring there is linkage.

For large families, calculating lod scores is extremely tedious and may be impossible by hand. Even with the help of computers, the computation time can be intensive. The Elston-Stewart algorithm is a recursive method to calculate likelihoods for large families with a limited number of markers.

13.2 Model-Free Methods for Linkage Analysis

If a marker and trait loci are linked, then pairs of relatives who are similar with respect to the trait phenotype will also be similar with respect to the marker phenotype, and conversely. Thus, we can test the correlation between trait and marker similarity, which is the basis of model-free linkage analysis.

13.2.1 Estimating Marker Identity by Descent

Model-free methods of linkage analysis can be based on marker identity in state, or on marker identity by descent (IBD). Both methods measure the marker similarity and tend to be equivalent as a marker becomes more and more polymorphic.

Methods based on IBD are more powerful than those based on identity in state. We introduce the estimation of marker IBD for full siblings. But the same idea can be extended to any types of relative pairs in a pedigree. If we have enough information at a marker locus—for example, the sibs' parents are also genotyped for the marker or a sufficient number of sibs are genotyped—it is often possible to deduce the number of alleles a sibpair shares IBD. In general, the number of alleles shared IBD between a sibps cannot be counted unambiguously. Haseman and Elston proposed estimating the IBD allele sharing probabilities at a marker locus by utilizing the marker information available on the sibs and their parents. Let f_0, f_1 and f_2 now denote the prior probabilities that a relative pair share $i = 0$, 1 and 2 alleles IBD, respectively. For full sibs, $f_0 = 1/4$, $f_1 = 1/2$, $f_2 = 1/4$. By Bayes theorem, the estimated posterior probability that the sibs share i alleles IBD given the available marker information I_m, denoted as $\widehat{f_i}$, is simply

$$\widehat{f_i} = \Pr(i\,|\,I_m) = \frac{f_i\,\Pr(I_m\,|\,i)}{\Pr(I_m)} = \frac{f_i\,\Pr(I_m\,|\,i)}{\sum_{i=0}^{2} f_i\,\Pr(I_m\,|\,i)}.$$

In general, the estimate of $\widehat{f_i}$ is dependent on having accurate estimates of the marker genotype frequencies. However, $\widehat{f_i}$ is not dependent on the genotype frequencies when both parents and the sibs are genotyped. Let π be the proportion of alleles shared IBD by a sibpair, which can only take on values 0, $1/2$, or 1. π is estimated by $\widehat{\pi} = \widehat{f_2} + \widehat{f_1}/2$. It can be shown that π and $\widehat{\pi}$ have the highest correlation for a single marker.

When families whose structures are more extensive than just nuclear families are available, the IBD sharing probabilities can be estimated in a multipoint fashion with greater accuracy, using for example the Lander-Green algorithm—whose computation time increases linearly in the number of markers and exponentially in the size of the families. The computer program package MAPMAKER/SIBS implements the Lander-Green algorithm. The website is ftp://ftp-genome.wi.mit.edu/distribution/software/sibs/. The full speed version of the algorithm is implemented in the S.A.G.E. program GENIBD.

13.2.2 Interval Mapping

An alternative multipoint algorithm for estimating π_q, the proportion of alleles IBD at a location q, is calculated from the single point estimates of IBD at a set of m marker loci on the same chromosome. To illustrate, let L_1 and L_2 be the locations of two markers. A trait locus is at L_q between the two markers (Fig. 13.2). Let π_1 and π_2 be the proportions of alleles IBD at markers L_1 and L_2, respectively. Let the recombination fraction between L_1 and L_q, L_q and L_2, and L_1 and L_2 be θ_1, θ_2 and θ_{12}, respectively.

If π_1 and π_2 are known, the estimated proportion of alleles IBD for the trait locus can be calculated using a linear regression as

$$\pi_q = \alpha + \beta_1 \pi_1 + \beta_2 \pi_2, \tag{13.1}$$

Fig. 13.2 Schematic of a chromosome segment with 2 marker loci and one trait locus

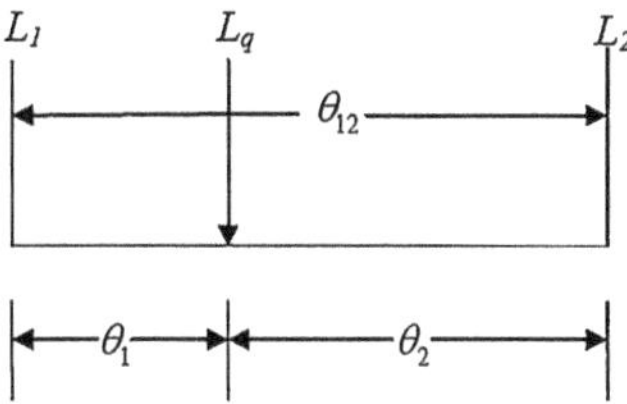

where the values of β_1 and β_2 are calculated using the equations

$$
\begin{bmatrix} \mathrm{Cov}(\pi_1, \pi_q) \\ \mathrm{Cov}(\pi_2, \pi_q) \end{bmatrix} = \begin{bmatrix} \mathrm{Var}(\pi_1) & \mathrm{Cov}(\pi_1, \pi_2) \\ \mathrm{Cov}(\pi_1, \pi_2) & \mathrm{Var}(\pi_2) \end{bmatrix} \begin{bmatrix} \beta_1 \\ \beta_2 \end{bmatrix}.
$$

Using the facts that (assuming no interference) $\mathrm{Var}(\pi_i) = 1/8$, $\mathrm{Cov}(\pi_1, \pi_2) = (1 - 2\theta_{12})^2/8$, and $\mathrm{Cov}(\pi_i, \pi_q) = (1 - 2\theta_i)^2/8$ for $i = 1, 2$, we have

$$
\beta_1 = \frac{(1 - 2\theta_1)^2 - (1 - 2\theta_2)^2(1 - 2\theta_{12})^2}{1 - (1 - 2\theta_{12})^4}, \tag{13.2}
$$

$$
\beta_2 = \frac{(1 - 2\theta_2)^2 - (1 - 2\theta_1)^2(1 - 2\theta_{12})^2}{1 - (1 - 2\theta_{12})^4}, \tag{13.3}
$$

$$
\alpha = (1 - \beta_1 - \beta_2)/2. \tag{13.4}
$$

Substituting Eqs. (13.2)–(13.4) into (13.1) will result in an estimate of the proportion of alleles IBD, $\widehat{\pi}_q$, for a trait locus. This algorithm can be extended to estimate π_q from the single point estimates of IBD at a set of m marker loci on a chromosome. Let $\widehat{\pi}_1, \ldots, \widehat{\pi}_m$ be the IBD estimates for m marker loci. The a linear regression of π_q is

$$
\widehat{\pi}_q = \alpha + \beta_1 \widehat{\pi}_1 + \cdots + \beta_m \widehat{\pi}_m.
$$

The regression coefficients can be estimated using the fact that for any two loci i and j with recombination fraction θ_{ij} between them,

$$
\mathrm{E}\{\mathrm{Cov}(\widehat{\pi}_i, \widehat{\pi}_j)\} = 8V(\widehat{\pi}_i)V(\widehat{\pi}_j)(1 - 2\theta_{ij})^2
$$

and

$$
\mathrm{E}\{\mathrm{Cov}(\widehat{\pi}_i, \widehat{\pi}_q)\} = V(\widehat{\pi}_i)(1 - 2\theta_i)^2,
$$

where $V(\widehat{\pi}_i)$ is the empirical estimate of the variance $\mathrm{Var}(\widehat{\pi}_i)$ at locus i. This multipoint algorithm gives an estimate of π_q at any location other than the locations for which marker information is available. Thus, the IBD sharing estimate at each marker location can be obtained, and the regression method can be applied to obtain a fast and good approximation to true multipoint estimates at all chromosomal locations, on the assumption of no interference.

13.2.3 The Original Haseman-Elston (HE) Regression
for a Quantitative Trait

When we have the IBD sharing information at a locus, we can essentially compare
the phenotype similarity and the IBD sharing between relative pairs. For example,
let Y_{1j} and Y_{2j} be the trait values for the jth sibpair, with the following model:

$$Y_{1j} = \mu + g_{1j} + e_{1j},$$
$$Y_{2j} = \mu + g_{2j} + e_{2j},$$

where μ is the overall mean and g_{ij} and e_{ij} are quantitative trait locus (QTL) and
environmental effects, respectively. Denote the variances of g_{ij} and e_{ij} as σ_g^2 and
σ_e^2, respectively. Let $\Delta Y_j = (Y_{1j} - Y_{2j})^2$ and π_j denote the proportion of alleles
that the jth sibpair shares IBD at a trait locus. Assuming no dominant effect, it can
be shown that

$$\mathrm{E}(\Delta Y_j | \pi_j) = (\sigma_e^2 + \sigma_g^2) - 2\sigma_g^2 \pi_j.$$

Let π_{mj} denote the proportion of alleles the jth sibpair shares IBD at a marker
locus m and $\widehat{\pi}_{mj}$ be the estimate of π_{mj}, $\widehat{\pi}_{mj} = \widehat{f}_{m2j} + 0.5\widehat{f}_{m1j}$, where $\widehat{f}_{mij}$ is the
estimated probability that the jth sibpair shares i alleles IBD ($i = 0$, 1, or 2) at the
marker locus, conditional on the marker information available on the sibpair and
their relatives. Under the assumption of linkage equilibrium between the marker
and trait loci, it can be shown that

$$\mathrm{E}(\Delta Y_j | \widehat{\pi}_{mj}) = \{\sigma_e^2 + 2(1 - 2\theta + 2\theta^2)\sigma_g^2\} - 2(1 - 2\theta)^2 \sigma_g^2 \widehat{\pi}_{mj},$$

which can be represented as a linear regression model that has been termed
Haseman-Elston (HE) regression:

$$\mathrm{E}(\Delta Y_j | \widehat{\pi}_{mj}) = \alpha - \beta \widehat{\pi}_{mj}.$$

Based on the above regression model, we can test the null hypothesis of no linkage $H_0 : \beta = 0$ by a one-sided t-test. There has been a concern that the regression
method requires the residuals to be normally distributed in order to have appropriate
type I error in the test. It has been shown that the HE regression is quite robust to deviations from normality for reasonable sample sizes. Because of its robustness and
simplicity, the HE regression has been extended to various situations, for example,
to a multivariate regression, two unlinked QTLs, parent-of-origin effects etc.

13.2.4 The New HE Regression

The original HE regression is less powerful than the full likelihood-based variance
component methods when trait normality holds approximately. It has been pointed
out that the full likelihood function for a sibpair can be written in terms of both
a sum and a difference of trait values. An extension of the HE method has been

Table 13.1 Definitions of the dependent variables for various forms of HE regression (reproduced from Wang and Elston [291])

Method	Acronym	Dependent variables
Original	oHE	$0.5(Y_{1j} - Y_{2j})^2$
Revisited	rHE	$(Y_{1j} - \bar{Y})(Y_{2j} - \bar{Y})$
Weighted	wHE	$\frac{1}{2}\{(1 - w)(Y_{1j} + Y_{2j} - 2\bar{Y})^2 - w(Y_{1j} - Y_{2j})^2\}$
Sibship sample mean	smHE	$(Y_{1j} - \bar{Y}_j)(Y_{2j} - \bar{Y}_j)$
Shrinkage mean	pmHE	$(Y_{1j} - \tilde{\mu}_j)(Y_{2j} - \tilde{\mu}_j)$

$\bar{Y}$ overall mean; $\bar{Y}_j$: sibship mean; $\tilde{\mu}$: shrinkage mean; w: weight

proposed that uses both the sibpair trait sum and difference as dependent variables, and estimates the slope by averaging the estimates from the two regressions, i.e., of the squared sum and squared difference, which is the best estimate when the residuals have the same variance for both the squared sum and difference. Based on the same idea, the overall mean-centered cross-product of sibpair traits was adopted as the trait similarity measure in the revisited HE regression. Table 13.1 lists the different trait similarity measurements that are implemented in the program SIBPAL of the S.A.G.E. program package.

It is known that the assumption of the same residual variance for the squared sum and difference can be violated, resulting in loss of statistical power for the revisited HE regression. To improve the power, different weighting methods have been proposed for the two slopes estimated from the squared sum and difference; these methods differ in how to estimate the weight of the two regression slopes using their estimated variances.

Regression-based linkage methods have also been extended for pairs in any type of pedigree structure, using generalized estimating equations (GEEs). It has been demonstrated that the different choices of the working covariance matrix in GEEs will correspond to the different HE and variance component methods. A two-level HE is also proposed for quantitative trait linkage analysis and general pedigrees under the framework of multiple level regression. The two-level HE can make use of all the information available in any general pedigree, simultaneously incorporating individual-level and pedigree effects, and feasibly modeling various complex genetic effects.

13.2.5 *Maximum Likelihood Variance Component Model*

Variance component model-based linkage analysis is also widely used in mapping QTLs. The variance component approach to linkage analysis has been extended to general pedigrees. Assuming a quantitative trait Y_i for the ith individual affected by n QTLs linearly,

$$Y_i = \mu + \sum_{j=1}^{n} g_{ij} + e_i,$$

where μ is the overall mean, g_{ij} is the effect for the jth QTL, and e_i is a random environmental effect. Similar to before, g_{ij} and e_i are independent variables with means 0. The variance of Y_i is $\mathrm{Var}(Y_i) = \sum_{j=1}^{n} \sigma_{g_j}^2 + \sigma_e^2$, where $\sigma_{g_j}^2$ is the variance for the jth QTL. Here we assume additive effects for all g_{ij}, i.e. all $g_{ij}, j = 1, \ldots, n$, are independent.

We can calculate the covariance between the trait values of any pair of relatives, Y_1 and Y_2, as

$$\mathrm{Cov}(Y_1, Y_2) = \mathrm{E}\{(Y_1 - \mu)(Y_2 - \mu)\} = \mathrm{E}\left\{ \left(\sum_{j=1}^{n} g_{1j} + e_1 \right) \left(\sum_{j=1}^{n} g_{2j} + e_2 \right) \right\}$$

$$= \mathrm{E}\left\{ \sum_{j=1}^{n} g_{1j} g_{2j} \right\} = \sum_{j=1}^{n} \mathrm{E}\{\mathrm{E}(g_{1j} g_{2j} | i)\}, \tag{13.5}$$

where i represents that individuals 1 and 2 share i alleles IBD at the jth QTL. Let f_{ij} be the probability of individuals 1 and 2 sharing i alleles IBD at the jth QTL, $i = 0, 1, 2$. From (13.5), we have

$$\mathrm{Cov}(Y_1, Y_2) = \sum_{j=1}^{n} \sum_{k=0}^{2} \mathrm{Pr}(i = k) \mathrm{E}(g_{1j} g_{2j} | i = k)$$

$$= \sum_{j=1}^{n} \{ \mathrm{Pr}(i = 1) \mathrm{E}(g_{1j} g_{2j} | i = 1) + \mathrm{Pr}(i = 2) \mathrm{E}(g_{1j} g_{2j} | i = 2) \}$$

$$= \sum_{j=1}^{n} \left\{ \frac{1}{2} \mathrm{Pr}(i = 1) \sigma_{g_j}^2 + \mathrm{Pr}(i = 2) \sigma_{g_j}^2 \right\} \tag{13.6}$$

$$= \sum_{j=1}^{n} \left(\frac{1}{2} f_{1j} + f_{2j} \right) \sigma_{g_j}^2. \tag{13.7}$$

Equation (13.6) is obtained as follows: $i = 2$ implies $g_{1j} \equiv g_{2j}$, so $\mathrm{E}(g_{1j} g_{2j} | i = 2) = \mathrm{E}(g_{1j}^2) = \sigma_{g_i}^2$. Then we use the results in Table 13.2 to derive $\mathrm{E}(g_{1j} g_{2j} | i = 1)$. From Table 13.2, $\mathrm{E}(g_{1j} g_{2j} | i = 1) = p(1 - p) = \frac{1}{2} \sigma_{g_j}^2$ (Problem 13.1). Hence, the phenotypic correlation between individuals 1 and 2 is given by

$$\rho(Y_1, Y_2) = \sum_{j=1}^{n} \left(\frac{1}{2} f_{1j} + f_{2j} \right) h_{g_j}^2,$$

Table 13.2 The possible genotype configuration of individuals 1 and 2 when they share 1 allele IBD. Allele A has frequency p

Individual 1's genotype	Individual 2's genotype	g_{1j}	g_{2j}	Probability
AA	AA	$2(1-p)$	$2(1-p)$	p^3
AA	Aa	$2(1-p)$	$1-2p$	$p^2(1-p)$
AA	aa	$2(1-p)$	$-2p$	0
Aa	AA	$1-2p$	$2(1-p)$	$p^2(1-p)$
Aa	Aa	$1-2p$	$1-2p$	$p(1-p)$
Aa	aa	$1-2p$	$-2p$	$p(1-p)^2$
aa	AA	$-2p$	$2(1-p)$	0
aa	Aa	$-2p$	$1-2p$	$p(1-p)^2$
aa	aa	$-2p$	$-2p$	$(1-p)^3$

where $h_{g_j}^2$ is the heritability contributed by the jth QTL, given by

$$h_{g_j}^2 = \frac{\sigma_{g_j}^2}{\sum_{j=1}^n \sigma_{g_j}^2 + \sigma_e^2}.$$

In linkage analysis, we do not have information for all the QTLs and usually use the expectation of f_{1j} and f_{2j} over the genome to obtain the approximation

$$\mathrm{Cov}(Y_1, Y_2) = 2\phi\sigma_g^2,$$

where $\sigma_g^2 = \sum_{j=1}^n \sigma_{g_j}^2$ is the total additive genetic variance and $\phi = \frac{1}{2}\mathrm{E}(f_{1j}/2 + f_{2j})$ is the kinship coefficient between individuals 1 and 2. In fact, this idea has been used for estimating the missing heritability for common variants using GWAS data. Since we are interested in an individual QTL (e.g., the jth QTL), we can rewrite Eq. (13.7) as

$$\mathrm{Cov}(Y_1, Y_2) = \pi_j\sigma_{g_j}^2 + 2\phi\sigma_g^{*2},$$

where $\pi_j = f_{1j}/2 + f_{2j}$ is the proportion of allele shared IBD by individuals 1 and 2 at a particular QTL of interest, as opposed to small background QTLs represented by ϕ and $\sigma_g^{*2} = \sigma_g^2 - \sigma_{g_j}^2$ is the total genetic variance after excluding the jth QTL. For any pair of members from a pedigree and all the n QTLs, Eq. (13.5) corresponds to the covariance matrix

$$\Omega = \hat{\Pi}_j\sigma_{g_j}^2 + 2\Phi\sigma_g^{*2} + I\sigma_e^2,$$

where $\hat{\Pi}_j$ is a matrix whose elements represent the proportion of alleles IBD at the jth QTL for the pairs of individuals, Φ is the kinship coefficient matrix, and I is the identity matrix. The matrix $\hat{\Pi}_j$ can be estimated using genetic markers.

Assuming the phenotypic vector Y follows a multivariate normal distribution, the log-likelihood for the data is

$$\log L(\mu, \sigma_{g_j}^2, \sigma_g^{*2}, \sigma_e^2 | Y) = -\frac{N}{2}\log(2\pi) - \frac{1}{2}\log|\Omega|(Y-\mu)^T\Omega^{-1}(Y-\mu),$$

where N is the number of individuals, and μ is an overall mean vector in which covariates can be modeled. The standard maximum likelihood theory can be applied to estimate the parameters $\theta = (\mu, \sigma_{g_j}^2, \sigma_g^{*2}, \sigma_e^2)^T$. In linkage analysis, the null hypothesis is $H_0 : \sigma_{g_j}^2 = 0$, which can be tested by the LRT

$$\mathrm{LRT} = 2\{\log L(\widehat{\theta}) - \log L(\widetilde{\theta})\},$$

where $\widehat{\theta} = (\widehat{\mu}, \widehat{\sigma}_{g_j}^2, \widehat{\sigma}_g^{*2}, \widehat{\sigma}_e^2)^T$ and $\widetilde{\theta} = (\widetilde{\mu}, 0, \widetilde{\sigma}_g^{*2}, \widetilde{\sigma}_e^2)^T$ are the estimates under H_1, no restriction, and H_0, respectively. The lod score can be defined as

$$\mathrm{Lod} = \log_{10} \frac{L(\widehat{\theta})}{L(\widetilde{\theta})} = 4.605 \times \mathrm{LRT}.$$

When the multivariate normality assumption holds, the LRT asymptotically follows a 0.5:0.5 mixture distribution of a χ_1^2 and a point mass at zero. Alternative test statistics, such as the Score test and Wald test, can be applied.

13.2.6 Qualitative Traits

We have mentioned the lod score method for analyzing qualitative traits at the beginning of this chapter. Linkage analysis can also be carried out by studying the IBD sharing conditional on the trait phenotypes. The idea is that individuals in a pedigree who have inherited disease alleles in common are likely to share genetic material in the region of the disease locus more often than expected by chance. There are advantages in conditioning on affected individuals only, including 1) removing one penetrance parameter reduces the degrees of freedom in statistical tests; 2) affected individuals often contribute most of the linkage information; 3) an affected individual is more likely to carry a disease susceptibility allele than an unaffected person, particularly for those with late ages of onset.

Under the null hypothesis H_0 that a marker is not linked to a disease locus, affected sibpairs will share 0, 1, or 2 alleles IBD at the marker with the probabilities $(\frac{1}{4}, \frac{1}{2}, \frac{1}{4})$. We can test linkage by testing whether the observed IBD sharing in the sample of affected sibpairs is consistent with the probabilities under H_0, against the alternative hypothesis H_1 that there is a skewing toward higher numbers of alleles shared IBD, as would be expected for the case of affected pairs if the marker is linked to the trait.

Let (z_0, z_1, z_2) be the true underlying probabilities that an affected sibpair shares 0, 1, 2 alleles IBD at a marker position. Several different test statistics have been developed to test $H_0 : (z_0, z_1, z_2) = (1/4, 1/2, 1/4)$ when we know exactly how many alleles are shared IBD by each sibpair. One method to test linkage is a goodness-of-fit test with two degrees of freedom:

$$\chi_2^2 = \sum \frac{(O_i - E_i)^2}{E_i},$$

where O_i and E_i represent the observed and expected number of sibpairs sharing i alleles IBD, respectively. Let $(\widehat{z}_0, \widehat{z}_1, \widehat{z}_2)$ be sample estimates of (z_0, z_1, z_2). That is, $\widehat{z}_i = n_i/n$ if n_i is the observed number of sharing i alleles IBD among n sibpairs ($i = 0, 1, 2$). The "mean" test is based on the mean number of alleles shared IBD:

$$T_{\text{mean}} = \frac{\widehat{z}_1 + 2\widehat{z}_2 - \mathrm{E}(\widehat{z}_1 + 2\widehat{z}_2|H_0)}{\sqrt{\mathrm{Var}(\widehat{z}_1 + 2\widehat{z}_2|H_0)}} = \sqrt{2n}(\widehat{z}_1 + 2\widehat{z}_2 - 1),$$

and the proportion test based on $\widehat{z}_2$ is

$$T_{\text{prop}} = \frac{\widehat{z}_2 - \mathrm{E}(\widehat{z}_2|H_0)}{\sqrt{\mathrm{Var}(\widehat{z}_2|H_0)}} = \sqrt{\frac{n}{3}}(4\widehat{z}_2 - 1),$$

where n is the number of affected sibpairs. Both T^2_{mean} and T^2_{prop} have an asymptotic χ^2_1 distribution under H_0. Among the three test statistics, χ^2_2, T_{mean} and T_{prop}, the "mean" test has been shown to be generally more powerful than the other two tests. Although the above methods are model-free, their power is dependent on the underlying genetic model. Hence, no single test is uniformly most powerful for any alternative hypothesis. It has been showed that T_{mean} is most powerful under a multiple monogenic mode of inheritance and is locally optimal otherwise. On the other hand, the maximum of T_{mean} and T_{prop} is suggested as a method that is more robust than either individual test.

Both T_{mean} and T_{prop} belong to a family of normally distributed tests of the following form

$$T(w) = \frac{\widehat{z}_2 + w\widehat{z}_1 - \mathrm{E}(\widehat{z}_2 + w\widehat{z}_1|H_0)}{\sqrt{\mathrm{Var}(\widehat{z}_2 + w\widehat{z}_1|H_0)}} = \frac{\sqrt{n}\{\widehat{z}_2 - \frac{1}{4} + w(\widehat{z}_1 - \frac{1}{2})\}}{\frac{1}{4}\sqrt{3 - 4 + 4w^2}}, \qquad (13.8)$$

where w is a weight parameter. Setting $w = 1/2$ results the mean test T_{mean}, while setting $w = 0$ results the proportion test T_{prop}. Later, we will show that the interesting range for w is $w \in [0, 1/2]$.

A test with the weight $w = 0.275$ is referred to as a "minmax" test, which is similar to the test using the midpoint $w = 1/4$ as a weight. The "minmax" test is more robust than T_{mean} and T_{prop} when the true value of w is unknown. See Sect. 13.4 for more discussion of robust procedures.

An alternative to the above one-degree-of-freedom tests $T^2(w)$ is a two-degree-of-freedom LRT, LRT_2, also called the maximum lod score (MLS), which is based on the likelihood ratio

$$\frac{\mathrm{Pr}(\text{data}\,|z_0, z_1, z_2)}{\mathrm{P}(\text{data}\,|\frac{1}{4}, \frac{1}{2}, \frac{1}{4})} = \frac{\mathrm{Pr}(\text{data}\,|z_0, z_1, z_2)}{\mathrm{P}(\text{data}\,|z_{00}, z_{10}, z_{20})},$$

where $(z_{00}, z_{10}, z_{20}) = (1/4, 1/2, 1/4)$. Denote f_{ij} as the probability of observing the markers of the ith sibpair, given they share j alleles IBD. The likelihood for the ith sibpair is $\sum_{j=0}^{2} z_j f_{ij}$. For n affected sibpairs, the lod score is

$$T(z) = \log_{10}\left\{\prod_{i=1}^{n} \frac{\sum_{j=0}^{2} z_j f_{ij}}{\sum_{j=0}^{2} z_{j0} f_{ij}}\right\} = \sum_{i=1}^{n} \log_{10} \frac{\sum_{j=0}^{2} z_j f_{ij}}{\sum_{j=0}^{2} z_{j0} f_{ij}}. \qquad (13.9)$$

The MLS can be estimated by maximizing (13.9) with respect to (z_0, z_1, z_2) under the constraint $z_0 + z_1 + z_2 = 1$ and $0 \le z_j \le 1$, $j = 0, 1, 2$. The estimates of

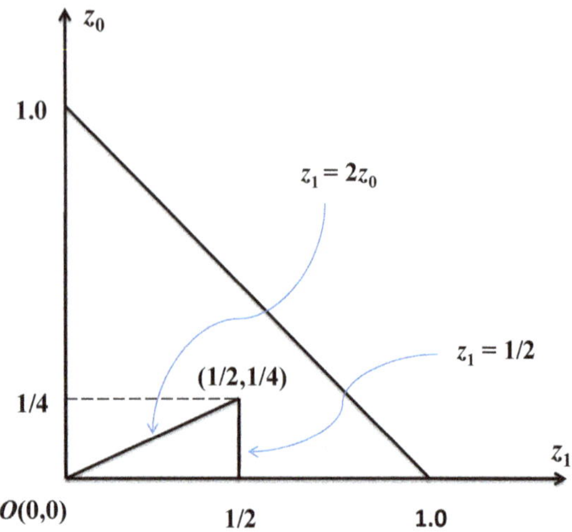

Fig. 13.3 The *large triangle* is the unrestricted search area for the MLEs of (z_0, z_1) and $z_2 = 1 - z_0 - z_1$. The *small triangle*, bounded by $z_1 = 2z_0$, $z_1 = 1/2$ and $z_0 = 0$, imposes the restrictions on the search area for the MLEs on the assumption that only Mendelian loci cause the trait

(z_0, z_1, z_2) obtained by maximizing (13.9) are equivalent to the MLEs because the denominator is a constant. The MLEs, denoted as $(\widehat{z}_0, \widehat{z}_1, \widehat{z}_2)$, can also be used in the one-degree-of-freedom tests. It has been shown that the power of LRT_2 can be increased by constraining the maximization so that $(\widehat{z}_0, \widehat{z}_1, \widehat{z}_2)$ lie in a "possible triangle" defined by $\widehat{z}_0 > 0, \widehat{z}_1 < 1/2, \widehat{z}_1 > 2\widehat{z}_0$, which corresponds to the values of $(\widehat{z}_0, \widehat{z}_1, \widehat{z}_2)$ that are consistent with simple Mendelian inheritance assuming monogenic inheritance (Fig. 13.3). LRT_2 can be converted into a one-degree-of-freedom LRT, LRT_1, by adding the further constraint $\widehat{z}_1 = 1/2$. In general, the power of LRT_2 is lower than LRT_1. However, LRT_2 has some advantages for extending to the case of multi-locus models, that is, saturation in which a single trait is caused by multiple disease loci that may themselves be linked or unlinked.

13.3 Transmission/Disequilibrium Test

Case-control association studies have been a powerful tool in genetic epidemiological studies, as demonstrated in many GWAS. However, one problem is that without genotyping many genetic markers it is difficult to know whether a significant result is biologically meaningful, or just a consequence of the case and control samples coming from populations with different genetic backgrounds. To avoid this problem, appropriate controls must be selected. A popular design is to sample one affected child with two parents. Consider a diallelic marker (e.g. SNP) with two alleles, A and B. For each family we are able to determine which of a parent's two alleles is transmitted to an affected offspring. Suppose we have a sample of n parent-offspring trios. For each family (trio), we consider the two transmitted parental alleles as a case and the two nontransmitted alleles as a control. Then we can examine whether allele A is present more frequently in cases than in controls by a matched or unmatched design.

Table 13.3 The counts of mating types and the offspring marker genotype, and the transmitted/nontransmitted alleles

Parental		Offspring		Transmitted	
Mating type (MT)	Count	Genotype	Count	Yes	No
MT1: $AA \times AA$	n_1	AA	n_1	A, A	A, A
MT2: $AA \times AB$	n_2	AA	n_{22}	A, A	A, B
		AB	n_{21}	A, B	A, A
MT3: $AA \times BB$	n_3	AB	n_3	A, B	A, B
MT4: $AB \times AB$	n_4	AA	n_{42}	A, A	B, B
		AB	n_{41}	A, B	A, B
		BB	n_{40}	B, B	A, A
MT5: $AB \times BB$	n_5	AB	n_{51}	A, B	B, B
		BB	n_{50}	B, B	A, B
MT6: $BB \times BB$	n_6	BB	n_6	B, B	B, B

Table 13.4 Counts of two transmitted alleles (cases), i.e., offspring genotypes, and two nontransmitted alleles (controls) for a single marker with alleles A and B in a matched pair design with n matched sets (trios)

Cases	Controls		
	AA	AB	BB
AA	n_1	n_{22}	n_{42}
AB	n_{21}	$n_3 + n_{41}$	n_{51}
BB	n_{40}	n_{50}	n_6

There are six different mating types if we ignore the parental order of the genotypes. Their counts among n trios are denoted as n_i, $i = 1, \ldots, 6$, respectively, and $\sum_i n_i = n$. Table 13.3 presents the counts of the six mating types and the offspring genotype with two transmitted/nontransmitted alleles. In Table 13.4, the counts are presented as a matched pair design (see Table 4.1). To analyze the data in Table 13.4, random mating is a necessary condition if the null hypothesis is no association, so two pairs of alleles (transmitted and nontransmitted) in each matched set are independent. If the null hypothesis is no linkage, random mating is not necessary. The counts in Table 13.4 are arranged in Table 13.5 with the A allele present or absent in the offspring genotype. This forms a two-level matched pair design and McNemar's test given in Sect. 4.3.1 can be applied. The test is referred to as the matched genotype relative risk (MGRR), given by

$$\text{MGRR} = \frac{(B' - C')^2}{B' + C'} = \frac{\{(n_{42} - n_{40}) + (n_{51} - n_{50})\}^2}{n_{42} + n_{40} + n_{51} + n_{50}} \sim \chi_1^2 \quad \text{under } H_0. \quad (13.10)$$

The null hypothesis H_0 refers to no association or linkage between a disease and a marker.

We can apply the MTT (4.4) to the matched pair data in Table 13.4. In Sect. 4.4, we also discussed the MDT test. The MTT is also the MDT under the 1:1 matching. The MTT uses the scores $(0, x, 1)$ for the three offspring genotypes (AA, AB, BB),

Table 13.5 Arrangement of the counts in Table 13.4 with allele A present or absent in the offspring genotype

Cases	Controls		Total
	A present	A absent	
A present	A'	B'	W
A absent	C'	D'	X
Total	Y	Z	n

$$A' = n_1 + n_2 + n_3 + n_{41}$$
$$B' = n_{42} + n_{51}$$
$$C' = n_{40} + n_{50}$$
$$D' = n_6$$

Table 13.6 Arrangement of the data in Table 13.5 without matching

	A present	A absent	Total
Cases	W	X	n
Controls	Y	Z	n
Total	$W + Y$	$X + Z$	$2n$

where $x \in [0, 1]$ is determined by the underlying genetic model. Using the data in Table 13.4, the MTT is given by

$$Z^2_{\mathrm{MTT}}(x) = \frac{\{x(n_{22} - n_{21}) + (n_{42} - n_{40}) + (1 - x)(n_{51} - n_{50})\}^2}{x^2(n_{22} + n_{21}) + (n_{42} + n_{40}) + (1 - x)^2(n_{51} + n_{50})} \sim \chi^2_1 \quad \text{under } H_0.$$

$$(13.11)$$

Comparing (13.10) and (13.11), MGRR $= Z^2_{\mathrm{MTT}}(0)$. Thus, the MGRR test is the MTT under the REC model with $x = 0$. This is not surprising as the data in Table 13.5 are obtained by pooling genotypes AA and AB in Table 13.4 which have the same risk of being a case under the REC model.

Table 13.5 can also be converted to a 2×2 unmatched table, as summarized in Table 13.6. The usual chi-squared statistic for testing independence can be applied to Table 13.6, which is often referred to as the genotype-based haplotype relative risk (GHRR) statistic and is given by

$$\text{GHRR} = \frac{2n(WZ - XY)^2}{(W + Y)(X + Z)n^2} = \frac{(B' - C')^2}{\frac{1}{2n}(2A' + B' + C')(B' + C' + 2D')}. \quad (13.12)$$

The difference between the MGRR and GHRR statistics is the estimate of $\mathrm{Var}(B' - C')$.

The above test statistics are based on the counts of transmitted/nontransmitted genotypes. We can also consider the counts of transmitted/nontransmitted alleles of each individual. In this case, the data can be summarized as in Table 13.7 and

Table 13.7 Counts for combinations of transmitted and nontransmitted marker alleles A and B among n parent-offspring trios ($2n$ parents)

Transmitted	Nontransmitted		Total
	A	B	
A	a	b	$w = a + b$
B	c	d	$x = c + d$
Total	$y = a + c$	$z = b + d$	$2n$

$$a = 2n_1 + n_2 + n_3$$
$$b = n_{22} + 2n_{42} + n_{41} + n_{51}$$
$$c = n_{21} + 2n_{40} + n_{41} + n_{50}$$
$$d = 2n_6 + n_3 + n_5$$

Table 13.8 Arrangement of the counts in Table 13.7 without matching

	A	B	Total
Transmitted	w	x	$2n$
Nontransmitted	y	z	$2n$
Total	$w + y$	$x + z$	$4n$

McNemar's test can be applied, which is referred to as the transmission/disequilibrium test (TDT) and is given by

$$\text{TDT} = \frac{(b - c)^2}{b + c} \sim \chi_1^2 \quad \text{under } H_0, \tag{13.13}$$

which has been used to test linkage when disease association has already been established. Similar to the genotype-based analysis, the unmatched analysis can also be applied here, as we can arrange the data as in Table 13.8. The haplotype-based haplotype relative risk (HHRR) statistic is proposed to test for independence in Table 13.8:

$$\text{HHRR} = \frac{4n(wz - xy)^2}{(w + y)(x + z)4n^2} = \frac{(b - c)^2}{(2a + b + c)(b + c + 2d)/4n}.$$

Thus, the distinction between the TDT and the HHRR test lies in the variances in the denominators. It has been shown that the HHRR test is more powerful for association than the TDT because the former uses the homozygous parents in addition to the heterozygous parents. However, the HHRR test needs the assumption that the allele frequency does not vary across the different families—a situation that can occur when there is population stratification. If we compare the MTT in (13.11) and the TDT in (13.13), we see $\text{TDT} = Z_{\text{MTT}}^2(1/2)$ with $x = 1/2$ (optimal for the ADD model) if $n_{42} + n_{40} = n_{41}$. Under H_0, given the mating type $AB \times AB$, $(n_{40}, n_{41}, n_{42}) \sim Mul(n_4; 1/4, 1/2, 1/4)$ based on Mendel's laws. Thus, $\text{E}(n_{42} + n_{40}) = n_4/2 = \text{E}(n_{41})$. It follows that $n_{42} + n_{40} \approx n_{41}$ under H_0 and the TDT can be related to the MTT under the ADD model.

Table 13.9 Probabilities of the counts in Table 13.7

Transmitted	Nontransmitted		Total
	A	B	
A	$q^2 + q\Delta/p$	$q(1-q) + (1-\theta-q)\Delta/p$	$q + (1-\theta)\Delta/p$
B	$q(1-q) + (\theta-q)\Delta/p$	$(1-q)^2 - (1-q)\Delta/p$	$1 - q - (1-\theta)\Delta/p$
Total	$q + \theta\Delta/p$	$1 - q - \theta\Delta/p$	1

Suppose a disease locus has two alleles D and d, with corresponding frequencies $1-q$ and q, respectively, and that the population frequency of A and B, the two alleles of a marker, are p and $1-p$, respectively. Let the coefficient of LD be Δ and the recombination fraction be θ between the disease and marker loci, respectively. Then the four haplotypes and their respective population frequencies can be calculated as follow: $\Pr(Ad) = pq + \Delta$, $\Pr(Bd) = (1-p)q - \Delta$, $\Pr(AD) = p(1-q) - \Delta$, and $\Pr(BD) = (1-p)(1-q) + \Delta$. For a REC disease, the probabilities corresponding to the four cells of Table 13.7 are as presented in Table 13.9, which suggests that, when $\theta = 1/2$ or $\Delta = 0$, we have $E(b) = E(c)$, whatever the values of p and q. Thus, the TDT tests the null hypothesis $\Delta(1 - 2\theta) = 0$, so it can clearly be considered either as a test of association (null hypothesis $\Delta = 0$ provided $\theta < 1/2$), a situation which is sometimes called a candidate-gene association study, or as a test of linkage (null hypothesis $\theta = 1/2$ provided $\Delta \neq 0$). When population structure exists, the TDT is a valid test of linkage, irrespective of the pedigree structure. However, the TDT is invalid as a test of association when multiplex sibships are present. The contingency statistics, GHRR and HHRR, are not valid tests for association in general because they require random mating in the population and no admixture for at least two generations before sampling the affected offspring.

General Score tests for testing association of genetic markers with disease, using trios, have been developed based on the conditional probabilities. One method is to consider a conditional logistic regression, in which a matched set consists of an observed case marker genotype (of offspring) and all three control marker genotypes that the parents could have produced. In this model, the TDT is a special case of the general Score tests corresponding to a binary indicator to code for genotypes or an ADD model (A presenting or absent).

Let the trait value be y, which is 1 if the individual is affected and 0 if not. The probability of the offspring marker genotype, conditional on the parents' marker genotypes and given that the offspring is affected, is

$$
\begin{aligned}
\Pr(g_o | g_m, g_f, y = 1) &= \frac{\Pr(y = 1, g_m, g_f, g_o)}{\Pr(y = 1, g_m, g_f)} \\
&= \frac{\Pr(y = 1 | g_m, g_f, g_o)\Pr(g_o | g_m, g_f)\Pr(g_m, g_f)}{\sum_{g_o^* \in G} \Pr(y = 1 | g_m, g_f, g_o^*)\Pr(g_o^* | g_m, g_f)\Pr(g_m, g_f)},
\end{aligned}
$$

(13.14)

where g_o, g_m, and g_f are the marker genotypes of the offspring, mother and father, the sum in the denominator is over all four possible marker genotypes that the parents can produce, and g_o^* is one of these genotypes. $\Pr(g_o|g_m, g_f)$ depends only on the usual transmission probabilities given by Mendel's laws and does not involve any parameter of interest. Thus, $\Pr(g_o^*|g_m, g_f)$ is equal to $1/4$. Assuming that $\Pr(y = 1|g_m, g_f, g_o) = \Pr(y|g_o)$, a penetrance, (13.14) reduces to

$$\Pr(g_o|g_m, g_f, y = 1) \propto \frac{\Pr(y = 1|g_o)}{\sum_{g_o^* \in G} \Pr(y = 1|g_o^*)}. \tag{13.15}$$

Consider two examples. If $g_m = g_f = AA$, $g_o = AA$ and $g_o^* = \{AA, AA, AA, AA\}$. It follows $\Pr(y = 1|g_o^*) \equiv \Pr(y = 1|AA)$. Hence, (13.15) becomes $\Pr(g_o|g_m, g_f, y = 1) \propto 1/4$, which does not contribute to the conditional likelihood. In other words, the mating type $AA \times AA$ is not informative. If $g_m = AB$ and $g_f = AB$, then $g_0^* = \{AA, AB, BA, BB\}$. If $g_0 = AA$, we have

$$\Pr(AA|g_m = g_f = AB, y = 1) \propto \frac{\Pr(y = 1|AA)}{\Pr(y = 1|AA) + 2\Pr(y = 1|AB) + \Pr(y = 1|BB)}$$

$$= \frac{1}{1 + 2\frac{\Pr(y=1|AB)}{\Pr(y=1|AA)} + \frac{\Pr(y=1|BB)}{\Pr(y=1|AA)}}. \tag{13.16}$$

The ratios of penetrances in (13.16) are called GRRs and denoted as $\lambda(g)$. Using our notation for the GRRs in previous chapters, we have $\lambda_1 = \lambda(AB)$ and $\lambda_2 = \lambda(BB)$, where AA is used as a reference genotype. Then Eq. (13.15) can be written as

$$\Pr(g_o|g_m, g_f, y = 1) \propto \frac{\lambda(g_o)}{\sum_{g_o^* \in G} \lambda(g_o^*)}.$$

The conditional probabilities as functions of the GRRs (λ_1, λ_2) are given in Table 13.10 for the informative mating types (MT2, MT4 and MT5).

The marker GRRs can be denoted as follows: $x = (2, 0)^T$ for AA, $x = (1, 1)^T$ for AB, and $x = (0, 2)^T$ for BB. Thus, the first element of x is the number of A alleles and the second element is the number of B alleles. The log-additive regression model is given by $\log(\lambda(g)) = x^T \beta$, where β models the genetic effects of the marker. If n trios are observed, the total conditional likelihood for matched data is given by

$$L(\beta) \propto \prod_{i=1}^{n} \frac{\exp(x_i^T \beta)}{\sum_{g_o^* \in G} \exp(x^{*T} \beta)}.$$

The null hypothesis of no association, $H_0 : \beta = 0$, can be tested by the Score statistic

$$\mathrm{ST} = U^T V^{-1} U \sim \chi_2^2 \quad \text{under } H_0,$$

where $U = \partial \log L / \partial \beta|_{H_0 : \beta = 0}$ and the elements of V are given by

$$V_{ij} = -\partial^2 \log L / \partial \beta_i \partial \beta_j|_{H_0 : \beta = 0}.$$

This Score test does not directly test the null hypothesis $H_0 : \lambda_1 = \lambda_2 = 1$ nor $H_0 : \lambda(g) = 1$ for any $g \in G$, which will be discussed in Sect. 13.4.

Table 13.10 From Table 13.3: the conditional probabilities (cond. prob.) of observing an affected (case) offspring marker genotype given the mating type. Only informative mating types are given

Parental		Offspring		Cond. prob.
Mating type (MT)	Count	Genotype	Count	
MT2: $AA \times AB$	n_2	AA	n_{22}	$1/(1+\lambda_1)$
		AB	n_{21}	$\lambda_1/(1+\lambda_1)$
MT4: $AB \times AB$	n_4	AA	n_{42}	$1/(1+2\lambda_1+\lambda_2)$
		AB	n_{41}	$2\lambda_1/(1+2\lambda_1+\lambda_2)$
		BB	n_{40}	$\lambda_2/(1+2\lambda_1+\lambda_2)$
MT5: $AB \times BB$	n_5	AB	n_{51}	$\lambda_1/(\lambda_1+\lambda_2)$
		BB	n_{50}	$\lambda_2/(\lambda_1+\lambda_2)$

13.4 Robust Methods

We first discuss linkage analysis using affected sibpairs. Then we consider testing for association between a marker and a disease using parent-offspring trios. In both, we focus on robust procedures based on Score statistics.

13.4.1 Linkage Analysis Using Affected Sibpairs

Following Sect. 13.2.6, let (z_0, z_1, z_2) be the probabilities that an affected sibpair shares $(0, 1, 2)$ alleles IBD. Under the null hypothesis of no linkage, $(z_0, z_1, z_2) = (1/4, 1/2, 1/4)$. In Fig. 13.3, the large triangle is the area of (z_0, z_1), in which the null point $(z_1, z_0) = (1/2, 1/4)$ is an inner point. The small triangle imposes constraints on the area for (z_0, z_1), for which the null point is on the boundary. As we have seen in Chap. 6, when the space for the alternative hypothesis is reduced, the power of a test statistic would increase. The smaller the space, the more power a test statistic will have. However, there is a trade-off between the power (or efficiency) and robustness. If the space is too small and the true parameter value lies outside the space, then test statistics based on the smaller space become less robust, i.e., the true model is misspecified.

The large and small triangles in Fig. 13.3 are denoted as Λ_L and Λ_S, respectively, and given by

$$\Lambda_L = \{(z_0, z_1) : 0 \le z_0, z_1 \le 1; z_0 + z_1 \le 1\},$$

$$\Lambda_S = \{(z_0, z_1) : 0 \le z_0, z_1 \le 1; 2z_0 \le z_1 \le 1/2\}.$$

The LRTs based on Λ_L and Λ_S have different asymptotic distributions. The former has a usual χ_2^2 distribution under H_0, and the latter has a mixture of three chi-squared distributions with different degrees of freedom. In this section, we focus on the Score test for Λ_S.

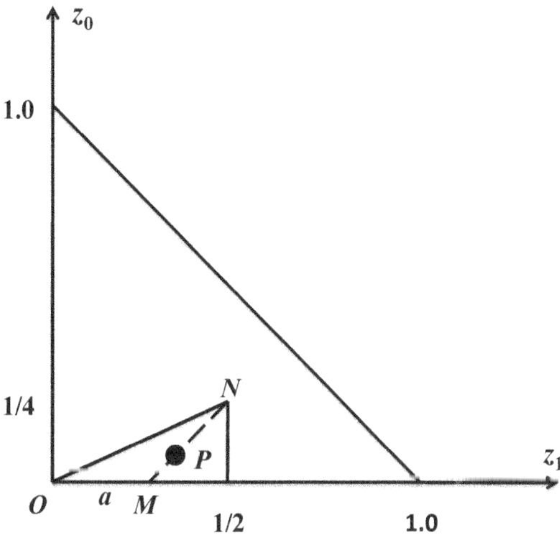

Fig. 13.4 The *point* N is the null point and the *point* P is a true point under the alternative hypothesis of linkage. The distance between O and M is denoted as $a \in [0, 1/2]$

Figure 13.4 plots the triangles Λ_L and Λ_S. Assume the true value of (z_1, z_0) is denoted as P in Fig. 13.4. Then we can connect the null point $N : (z_1, z_0) = (1/2, 1/4)$ and the point P, which crosses at the z_1-axis at point $M : (a, 0)$, where a is the distance between O and M. Note that a is not defined under H_0, under which P is N. Denote the distance between two points M and N as $|MN| = |NM|$. Let $\lambda = |PN|/|MN|$. Then $\lambda \in [0, 1]$. In other words, we reparameterize the null point N using two parameters (λ, a). Under H_0, $\lambda = 0$ but a is not defined and is only a nuisance parameter in this parameterization. The coordinates of P can be expressed as

$$z_0 = \frac{1-\lambda}{4}, \qquad z_1 = \frac{1-\lambda}{2} + \lambda a,$$

and $z_2 = 1 - z_0 - z_1$. It can also be expressed as a mixture of $(a, 0)$ and $(1/2, 1/4)$ for P, $(z_1, z_0) = \lambda(a, 0) + (1 - \lambda)(1/2, 1/4)$.

Assume we have n independent sibpairs and observe (n_0, n_1, n_2) sibpairs who share $(0, 1, 2)$ alleles IBD. The likelihood function is proportional to

$$L(\lambda, a) = \left(\frac{1-\lambda}{4}\right)^{n_0} \left(\frac{\lambda(2a-1)+1}{2}\right)^{n_1} \left(\frac{1+\lambda(3-4a)}{4}\right)^{n_2}$$
$$\propto (1-\lambda)^{n_0}\{\lambda(2a-1)+1\}^{n_1}\{1+\lambda(3-4a)\}^{n_2}.$$

To test $H_0 : \lambda = 0$ with the nuisance parameter a, the Score test given in Sect. 1.2.4 cannot be directly applied because the nuisance parameter a is not estimable under H_0. Thus, we assume a is known and apply the Score test in Sect. 1.2.3 without a nuisance parameter. Therefore, the Score test is a function of a, which can be written as (Problem 13.2)

$$Z_{\text{ST}}(a) = \frac{\sqrt{n}\{4(a-1)\widehat{z}_0 + (6a-4)\widehat{z}_1 + (3-4a)\}}{\sqrt{3 - 8a + 6a^2}} \sim N(0, 1) \quad \text{under } H_0,$$

$$(13.17)$$

where $\widehat{z}_i = n_i/n$ $(i = 0, 1, 2)$.

We have used a family of tests $T(w)$, $w \in [0, 1/2]$, given in (13.8) to test for linkage. In fact, $T(w)$ and $Z_{ST}(a)$ are identical if we use a one-to-one monotone mapping function $w = a/\{2(a-1)\}$, which maps $[0, 1/2]$ onto $[0, 1/2]$ (Problem 13.2). Thus, the mean and proportion tests correspond to $Z_{ST}(0)$ and $Z_{ST}(1/2)$, respectively. The "minmax" test with $w = 0.275$ corresponds to $Z_{ST}(a)$ with $a \approx 0.355$, and the test $T(w)$ with the midpoint $w = 1/4$ corresponds to $Z_{ST}(a)$ with $a = 1/3$.

Note that to apply $Z_{ST}(a)$, we need to know a unless a special value of a is chosen, e.g., $a = 0$ or $a = 1/2$. In practice, a is unknown. For a family of normally distributed Score statistics $\{Z_{ST}(a) : a \in [0, 1/2]\}$, we can apply the robust tests discussed in Chap. 6. The asymptotic null correlation of $Z_{ST}(a_1)$ and $Z_{ST}(a_2)$, $a_1 \neq a_2$, can be written as (Problem 13.2)

$$\rho_{a_1,a_2} = \frac{3 - 4(a_1 + a_2) + 6a_1a_2}{\sqrt{3 - 8a_1 + 6a_1^2}\sqrt{3 - 8a_2 + 6a_2^2}}. \tag{13.18}$$

It follows that, for any $a \in [0, 1/2]$, we have $\rho_{0,a} + \rho_{a,1/2} \geq 1 + \rho_{0,1/2}$, a sufficient condition under which $\rho_{0,1/2}$ is the minimum among all the correlations ρ_{a_1,a_2}, $0 \leq a_1, a_2 \leq a_2$; see (6.13) of Sect. 6.2.1. Thus, $Z_{ST}(0)$ and $Z_{ST}(1/2)$ is the extreme pair, and the MERT (Sect. 6.2.1) for the family $\{Z_{ST}(a) : a \in [0, 1/2]\}$ has the form

$$Z_{MERT} = \frac{Z_{ST}(0) + Z_{ST}(1/2)}{\sqrt{2(1 + \rho_{0,1/2})}} \sim N(0, 1),$$

where $\rho_{0,1/2} = 0.8165$.

Usually, the MERT does not belong to the family of normally distributed test statistics as the family is not closed to any convex linear combination. For testing linkage using $\{Z_{ST}(a) : a \in [0, 1/2]\}$, however, the MERT belongs to that family. That is, there is $a^* \in [0, 1/2]$ such that $Z_{MERT} = Z_{ST}(a^*)$. It can be shown that

$$a^* = \frac{3 - \sqrt{6}}{4 - \sqrt{6}} \approx 0.355.$$

In terms of the weight w used in $T(w)$, we have $w = (3 - \sqrt{6})/2 \approx 0.275$. Thus, the "minmax" test is the MERT. More discussion of these two tests will be given in the Bibliographical Comments (Sect. 13.6).

Other robust tests have also been discussed in Chap. 6, including maximum tests and the CLRT. Since the minimum null correlation is greater than 0.8, the ARE for using the MERT would be at least $(1 + \rho_{0,1/2})/2 = (1 + 0.8165)/2 \approx 90.8\%$ relative to the best test $Z_{ST}(a)$ with a correctly specified $a \in [0, 1/2]$. Therefore, the gain of power or efficiency using more complex robust tests would be limited, if any.

13.4.2   Association Analysis Using Trios

For association analysis using trios, instead of using the conditional likelihood method for the matched data as in Sect. 13.3, we use the conditional probabilities in

Table 13.10 directly. Since trios are independent, applying multinomial distributions to mating types 2, 4 and 5, the likelihood function is proportional to

$$L(\lambda_1, \lambda_2) = \frac{\lambda_1^{n_{21}}}{(1+\lambda_1)^{n_2}} \times \frac{\lambda_1^{n_{41}} \lambda_2^{n_{40}}}{(1+2\lambda_1+\lambda_2)^{n_4}} \times \frac{\lambda_1^{n_{51}} \lambda_2^{n_{50}}}{(\lambda_1+\lambda_2)^{n_5}}$$

$$= \frac{\lambda_1^{n_{21}+n_{41}+n_{51}} \lambda_2^{n_{40}+n_{50}}}{(1+\lambda_1)^{n_2}(1+2\lambda_1+\lambda_2)^{n_4}(\lambda_1+\lambda_2)^{n_5}}.$$

The LRT, Score test and Wald test discussed in Sect. 1.2.3 can be applied to test $H_0 : \lambda_1 = \lambda_2 = 1$. Each test has an asymptotic χ_2^2 distribution under H_0. The two-degree-of-freedom tests are robust because they do not rely on an underlying genetic model. However, the following approach often leads to a more robust test.

Let $\lambda_2 = \lambda$. Then $\lambda_1 = 1 - x + x\lambda_2$ for $x \in [0, 1]$, where x is determined by the genetic model; $x = 0$, $1/2$ and 1 for the REC, ADD and DOM models. We assume x is known. Then the likelihood function can be written as $L(\lambda|x)$. We focus on the Score test as a function of x because x is not estimable under $H_0 : \lambda = 1$. The Score test (Problem 13.3) can be written as

$$Z(x) = \frac{\frac{\partial \log L(\lambda|x)}{\partial \lambda}\big|_{H_0:\lambda=1}}{\sqrt{\mathrm{E}_{H_0}\{-\frac{\partial^2 \log L(\lambda|x)}{\partial \lambda^2}\big|_{H_0:\lambda=1}\}}}$$

$$= \frac{x\{(n_{21} + n_{41} + n_{51}) - (n_2 + n_4 + n_5)/2\} + (n_{40} - n_4/4) + (n_{50} - n_5/2)}{\sqrt{\frac{x^2}{4}n_2 + \frac{4x^2-4x+3}{16}n_4 + \frac{(x-1)^2}{4}n_5}}.$$

$$(13.19)$$

Under H_0, for a given x, $Z^2(x) \sim \chi_1^2$. When the underlying genetic model is REC (ADD or DOM), $Z(0)$ ($Z(1/2)$ or $Z(1)$) is asymptotically optimal, which is more powerful than the two-degree-of-freedom tests. On the other hand, when the genetic model is unknown, the latter are more robust than $Z^2(x)$ with a misspecified x.

In particular, for the ADD model with $x = 1/2$, we have

$$Z(1/2) = \frac{(n_{21} - n_{22}) + 2(n_{40} - n_{42}) + (n_{50} - n_{51})}{\sqrt{n_2 + 2n_4 + n_5}}.$$

The TDT given in (13.13), using the counts given in Table 13.7, can be written as

$$\mathrm{TDT} = \frac{\{(n_{22} - n_{21}) + 2(n_{42} - n_{40}) + (n_{51} - n_{50})\}^2}{n_2 + 2n_4 + n_5}.$$

Thus, $\mathrm{TDT} \equiv Z^2(1/2)$. We have also shown that the TDT is equivalent to the MTT under the ADD model. These results show that the TDT is optimal for testing association using trios under the ADD model. Therefore, it is expected that the TDT is sub-optimal under a non-additive model.

When the true genetic model is unknown, the optimal $Z(x)$ is not available. Robust procedures can be considered. The asymptotic null correlation ρ_{x_1,x_2} of $Z(x_1)$ and $Z(x_2)$, conditional on (n_2, n_4, n_5), can be directly obtained for any $0 \leq x_1, x_2 \leq 1$ using the multinomial distributions for genotype counts and the fact that the genotype counts across mating types are independent. It can be shown that

$(Z(0), Z(1))$ is the extreme pair with the minimum correlation $\rho_{0,1}$, which has an upper bound $1/3$. Thus, the MERT is less efficient than a maximum test if the minimum correlation is less than 0.5. A simple maximum test is given by

$$MAX3 = \max\{|Z(0)|, |Z(1/2)|, |Z(1)|\}.$$

Its asymptotic null distribution can be obtained from Monte-Carlo simulation conditional on the observed (n_2, n_4, n_5). Under H_0, $(n_{21}, n_{22}) \sim Mul(n_2; 1/2, 1/2)$, $(n_{40}, n_{41}, n_{42}) \sim Mul(n_4; 1/4, 1/2, 1/4)$, and $(n_{50}, n_{51}) \sim Mul(n_5; 1/2, 1/2)$. Thus, for each replicate, we can generate offspring genotypes using the above distributions and compute MAX3. After a large number of replicates have been simulated, an empirical distribution of MAX3 can be obtained to estimate the p-value of MAX3.

Other robust tests using trio data are also proposed, including the CLRT and an adaptive genetic model selection procedure. We do not discuss those tests here, but references are given in Sect. 13.6.

13.5 Family-Based Methods for Linkage and Association Analysis: FBAT

13.5.1 A General FBAT

A general approach to the analysis of family-based data has been proposed and is often called family-based association test (FBAT). We can classify the possible tests in a family design according to three possible hypotheses:

(i) H_0: There is no linkage and no association between a marker and a disease susceptibility locus;
(ii) H_0: There is linkage but no association between a marker and a disease susceptibility locus; and
(iii) H_0: There is association but no linkage between the marker and a disease susceptibility locus.

FBAT refers to testing the first or second null hypothesis, while the purpose of the TDT is to test the third null hypothesis. The general idea of the FBAT approach is to condition on the traits and on the parental genotypes, and then computes the distribution of the test statistic from the distribution of offspring genotypes under the null hypothesis. When parents' genotypes are missing, FBAT conditions on the sufficient statistic for the parental genotypes under the null hypothesis.

The test statistic in FBAT is based on

$$U = \sum_{i,j} Y_{ij}\{X_{ij} - E(X_{ij}|S_i)\}, \tag{13.20}$$

where i indexes the family, j indexes the nonfounders in the family, and S_i denotes the sufficient statistic for the parental genotypes and traits. Here, Y_{ij} denotes a coding function for the trait and X_{ij} is a coding function for a genotype. X_{ij} is centered around its expected value $E(X_{ij}|S_i)$, conditional on the sufficient statistic S_i under the null hypothesis. The distribution of U in (13.20) under the null hypothesis is obtained by treating the X_{ij} as a random variable, but conditioning on Y_{ij} and S_i. Under the null hypothesis, $E(U) = 0$. The FBAT test statistic is defined as

$$\chi^2_{\text{FBAT}} = \frac{U^2}{\text{Var}(U)},\tag{13.21}$$

where

$$\text{Var}(U) = \sum_i \sum_{j,j'} Y_{ij} Y_{ij'} \, \text{Cov}(X_{ij}, X_{ij'}|S_i, Y_{ij}, Y_{ij'}).$$

For large sample sizes, χ^2_{FBAT} is approximately distributed as χ^2_1. The conditional covariance in (13.21) only depends on S_i, and not on the traits, when the null hypothesis is no linkage. For testing no association in the presence of linkage, however, the conditional covariance will also depend on the traits. Algorithms have been developed to calculate the conditional distribution under the two null hypotheses: no linkage and no association in the presence of linkage. For trios, when the parental genotypes are known, it is straightforward to compute the distribution of X_{ij} given parental genotypes by using Mendel's first law. If there is no linkage and there are multiple offspring, transmissions to all offspring are independent and we can treat the offspring as if they come from different families. When linkage is present, the transmissions to different offspring in a family will be dependent on the unknown recombination fraction and the affection statuses of the offspring. To remove the dependence of the joint distribution on the unknown recombination fraction, FBAT conditions the distribution of the IBD observed among the offspring. This approach will result in discarding many families as noninformative when parental genotypes are unknown. Thus, calculating an empirical variance to estimate $\text{Var}(U)$ in (13.21) has been suggested. FBAT can be easily extended to the cases of either multiple alleles or multiple traits. In this case U is a vector referring to the multiple alleles or traits. Then the FBAT statistic is the quadratic form $U^T \text{Var}(U)^{-1}U$, where $\text{Var}(U)$ is a covariance matrix, and the FBAT statistic has an asymptotic χ^2_d distribution, where d equals the rank of $\text{Var}(U)$.

13.5.2 Application to Parent-Offspring Trios

As an application of FBAT, we consider a parent-offspring trio design. Let X_{ij} be the number of A alleles in the offspring, and X_{ij1} and X_{ij2} be the two alleles the offspring carries, with 1 representing A and 0 the other allele. Then $X_{ij} = X_{ij1} + X_{ij2}$. When the parental genotypes are available, the sufficient statistic S_i is the parental genotypes and the offspring trait value. Under either no linkage or no association, we have $X_{ij} - E(X_{ij}|S_{ij}) = 0$ when both the parents are homozygous. Thus, transmissions from homozygous parents do not contribution to the test statistic. When one parent is heterozygous, the offspring has 50% probability of being either homozygous or heterozygous, depending on which allele is transmitted from the heterozygous parent. Assume X_{ij1} is the allele transmitted from the heterozygous parent. We have

$$\mathrm{E}(X_{ij}|S_{ij}) = \mathrm{E}(X_{ij1}|S_{ij}) + \mathrm{E}(X_{ij2}|S_{ij}) = \frac{1}{2} + X_{ij2}$$

and $X_{ij} - \mathrm{E}(X_{ij}|S_{ij}) = X_{ij1} - \frac{1}{2}$, which is $1/2$ if A is transmitted and $-1/2$ if the other allele is transmitted from the heterozygous parent. Similarly, when both parents are heterozygous, we have $\mathrm{E}(X_{ij}|S_{ij}) = 1$, and $X_{ij} - \mathrm{E}(X_{ij}|S_{ij}) = 1, 0$ or -1, depending on the offspring genotype. Assume our data are parent-offspring trios and all the offspring are affected ($Y_{ij} = 1$). Further, assuming there are n heterozygous parents, then $U = \sum\{X_{ij} - \mathrm{E}(X_{ij}|S_i)\} = n_A - \frac{1}{2}n$, where n_A is the number of transmissions of the A allele from heterozygous parents to affected offspring, and $\mathrm{Var}(U)$ can be calculated as

$$\mathrm{Var}(U) = \sum_{i,j} \mathrm{Var}(X_{ij}|S_{ij}) = \frac{n}{4},$$

because each transmission from a heterozygous parent has variance equal to $1/4$. Thus,

$$\chi^2_{\mathrm{FBAT}} = \frac{4(n_A - \frac{n}{2})^2}{n} = \frac{(n_A - n_B)^2}{n_A + n_B},$$

where n_B is the number of transmissions of the other allele from heterozygous parents to affected offspring. We can observe that the FBAT statistic for trios is identical to the TDT derived in Sect. 13.3. Thus, FBAT can be viewed as a generalization of the TDT.

13.5.3 A General Pedigree

The idea of conditioning on parental genotypes can be extended to general pedigrees, where we now condition on all founders' genotypes, provided their genotypes are known. The power can be potentially increased when analyzing large pedigrees.

When parents' or founders' genotypes are unknown, FBAT evaluates the distribution of the test statistic using the conditional distribution of offspring genotypes conditional on a sufficient statistic for any nuisance parameter in the model. Let x denote the founders' genotypes and traits, which is a sufficient statistic for the nuisance parameters under the null hypothesis. When founders' genotypes are missing, the minimal sufficient statistic is a function of the outcome y, observed offspring and founder genotypes and traits. Two outcomes y and y' have the same value of the observed data minimal sufficient statistic if, and only if, for any value of the full data minimal sufficient statistic, x, either $\mathrm{Pr}(y|x)$ and $\mathrm{Pr}(y'|x)$ are both equal to zero, or the ratio $\mathrm{Pr}(y|x)/\mathrm{Pr}(y'|x)$ is invariant to the choice of x. The algorithm for computing the conditional distribution in a pedigree has the following steps. Following

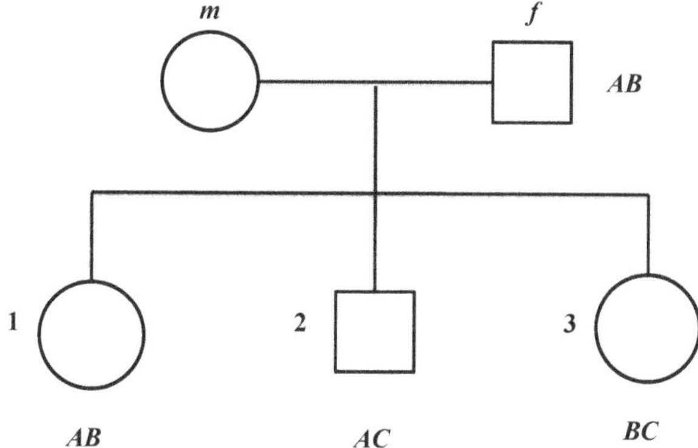

Fig. 13.5 A five-member nuclear family with the mother's genotype missing

each step, we will give an example of how to calculate the conditional distribution for a nuclear family of five members with the mother's genotype missing, under the null hypothesis of no linkage (Fig. 13.5).

(i) Find all the patterns of founders' marker genotypes that are compatible with the genotyped markers.

Example In Fig. 13.5, only the mother has a missing genotype. Given the observed genotypes in the pedigree, the compatible mother's genotypes are AC or BC.

(ii) For each of the compatible founders' genotypes obtained in Step 1, find the set of compatible's offspring genotypes. Find the intersection of the sets of compatible offspring genotypes. Calculate the probabilities of the offspring genotypes given the compatible founders' genotypes. Find the subset of the compatible offspring genotypes that has exactly the same compatible genotypes of founders' genotypes as the observed genotypes in the offspring.

Example (continued) Given the mother's genotype is AC, the possible offspring genotypes are AA, AB, AC and BC. Given mother's genotype is BC, the possible offspring genotypes are AB, AC, BB and BC. The intersection of these two sets of offspring genotypes contains AB, AC and BC. The conditional probabilities of the offspring genotypes given the mother's and father's genotypes are listed in Table 13.11. For the three offspring, the possibly genotypes are $\{AB\}$, $\{AC\}$, $\{BC\}$, $\{AB, AC\}$, $\{AB, BC\}$, $\{AC, BC\}$, and $\{AB, AC, BC\}$, where $\{g\}$ refers to all three offspring having the same genotype g, $\{g_1, g_2\}$ refers to at least one offspring having either g_1 or g_2, and $\{g_1, g_2, g_3\}$ refers to the three offspring genotypes being g_1, g_2, g_3, respectively. If the offspring genotypes are $\{AB\}$, the mother's genotype can be any of AA, AB or BB, which is not compatible with Step 1, and so we do not include $\{AB\}$. Similarly, we exclude $\{AC\}$, $\{BC\}$, and $\{AC, BC\}$. To be compatible with the mother's genotypes in Step 1, the offspring genotypes can be $\{AB, AC\}$, $\{AB, BC\}$, or $\{AB, AC, BC\}$. Thus, the final compatible offspring genotypes include $\{AB, AC\}$, $\{AB, BC\}$ and $\{AB, AC, BC\}$.

Table 13.11 Conditional probabilities of offspring genotypes given the mother's and father's genotypes

Mother, father	Offspring		
	AB	AC	BC
AC, AB	1/4	1/4	1/4
BC, AB	1/4	1/4	1/4

Table 13.12 Conditional probabilities of the compatible offspring genotypes given the mother's and father's genotypes

Mother, father	Offspring				
	$\{AB, AC, BC\}$	$\{AB, AB, AC\}$	$\{AB, AC, AC\}$	$\{AB, AB, BC\}$	$\{AB, BC, BC\}$
AC, AB	$(1/4)^3$	$(1/4)^3$	$(1/4)^3$	$(1/4)^3$	$(1/4)^3$
BC, AB	$(1/4)^3$	$(1/4)^3$	$(1/4)^3$	$(1/4)^3$	$(1/4)^3$

Table 13.13 Ratios of the conditional probability of compatible offspring genotypes to the conditional probability of the observed offspring genotypes

Mother, father	Offspring				
	$\{AB, AC, BC\}$	$\{AB, AB, AC\}$	$\{AB, AC, AC\}$	$\{AB, AB, BC\}$	$\{AB, BC, BC\}$
AC, AB	1	1	1	1	1
BC, AB	1	1	1	1	1

(iii) For every compatible founders' genotype found in Step 1 and for every possible offspring genotype found in Step 2, we compute the ratios of the conditional probability of possible (compatible) genotypes in the offspring to that of the observed genotypes in the offspring.

Example (continued) We calculate the conditional probabilities of the possible offspring genotypes given the mother's and father's genotypes, as listed in Table 13.12. Arrange for the first column to be the observed offspring genotypes $\{AB, AC, BC\}$. Compute the ratios by dividing the numbers in each column of Table 13.12 by the numbers in the first column (observed) of Table 13.12, resulting in Table 13.13.

(iv) For the offspring genotypes found in Step 2, the ratios found in Step 3 will be the same for all the compatible founders' genotypes found in Step 1. This is a basic requirement for a sufficient statistic. These offspring genotypes have positive conditional probabilities.

Example (continued) Since the numbers in each of the columns in Table 13.13 are the same, these offspring genotypes will have positive probabilities conditional on the sufficient statistic.

Table 13.14 Conditional distributions or probabilities P of offspring genotypes G given that one homozygous parent's genotype is AA

G	Conditional distribution
$\{AA\}$ or $\{AB\}$	$P = 1.$
$\{AA, AB\}$	Randomly assign equal $P = 1/2$ to AA and AB to each sib, discarding outcomes without at least one AA and one AB sib.
$\{AB, AC\}$	Randomly assign equal $P = 1/2$ to AB and AC to each sib, discarding outcomes without at least one AB and one AC sib.

(v) Compute the conditional probability of each offspring genotype found in Step 4. The conditional distribution is calculated by arbitrarily choosing any one of the compatible founders' genotypes found in Step 1 and computing the conditional probabilities of offspring genotypes given the chosen founders' genotypes and the genotypes found in Step 4.

Example (continued) For each of the five sets of offspring genotypes found in Step 4, listed in Table 13.12, we permute the genotypes. For $\{AB, AC, BC\}$, there are six ordered permutations, given by $\{AB, AC, BC\}$, $\{AB, BC, AC\}$, $\{AC, AB, BC\}$, $\{AC, BC, AB\}$, $\{BC, AB, AC\}$ and $\{BC, AC, AB\}$. For the other four sets, each has three ordered permutations. For example, for $\{AB, AB, AC\}$, we have the permutations $\{AB, AB, AC\}$, $\{AB, AC, AB\}$ and $\{AC, AB, AB\}$. The distribution of compatible offspring genotypes conditional on the sufficient statistic is given by all the permutations of the offspring genotypes found in Step 4. The conditional probability for the offspring genotypes $\{AB, AC, BC\}$ is thus calculated by

$$(1/4)^3/\{6 \times (1/4)^3 + 3 \times (1/4)^3 + 3 \times (1/4)^3 + 3 \times (1/4)^3 + 3 \times (1/4)^3\}$$
$$= 1/18,$$

where $(1/4)^3$ is the conditional probability from Table 13.12 and the integers $6, 3, 3, 3, 3$ in the denominator correspond to the number of different ordered permutations of genotypes for the offspring. The conditional probabilities for the other genotype patterns are also $1/18$. These probabilities can also be obtained by randomly assigning AB, AC and BC with probabilities $1/3, 1/3, 1/3$ to each offspring independently, discarding the outcomes without AB assigned at least once or without at least one of AC and BC at least once.

In general, the conditional distributions for different offspring genotypes are given conditional on the parental genotype. These conditional probabilities are given in Tables 13.14, 13.15, 13.16.

Given the conditional distribution calculated from Tables 13.14, 13.15, 13.16, it is straightforward to evaluate the FBAT statistic. For example, assume we have a family with two sibs and no parents. If we observed both sibs with genotype AA (or both with AB), i.e., $G = \{AA\}$ or $\{AB\}$, from Table 13.16, no information

Table 13.15 Conditional distributions or probabilities P of offspring genotypes G given that one heterozygous parent's genotype is AB

G	Conditional distribution
$\{AA\}$ or $\{AB\}$	$P = 1$.
$\{AA, AB\}$	Randomly assign AA and AB in a manner that keeps invariant the number of each.
$\{AA, BB\}$ or $\{AA, AB, BB\}$	Randomly assign $P = (1/4, 1/2, 1/4)$ to (AA, AB, BB) to each sib, discarding outcomes without at least one AA and one BB sib.
$\{AC\}$ or $\{AC, BC\}$	Randomly assign equal $P = 1/2$ to AC and BC to each sib.
$\{AB, AC\}$ or $\{AB, AC, BC\}$	Randomly assign equal $P = 1/3$ to AA, AC and BC to each sib, discarding outcomes without at least one AB and at least one AC or BC sib.
$\{AA, AC\}, \{AA, BC\},$ $\{AA, AB, AC\},$ $\{AA, AB, BC\}$ or $\{AA, AC, BC\}$	Randomly assign equal $P = 1/4$ to AA, AC, AB and BC to each sib, discarding outcomes without at least one AA and at least one AC or BC sib.
$\{AC, BD\}, \{AC, AD\},$ $\{AC, BC, BD\}$ or $\{AC, BC, BD, AD\}$	Randomly assign equal $P = 1/4$ to AC, AD, BC and BD to each sib, discarding outcomes in which either C or B is not present.

can be inferred about the parents' genotypes and such sibpairs are not informative because $P = 1$. On the other hand, if we observe one AA sib and one BB sib, i.e., $G = \{AA, BB\}$, then we know both parents' genotypes are AB. From Table 13.16, conditional on the sufficient statistic for both parents' genotypes to be missing, we requires the two sibs' genotypes to be either (AA, BB) or (BB, AA) with equal probability, which would be $1/2$ after deleting outcomes without at least one AA and one BB. Thus, $(X_{i1}, X_{i2}) = (2, 0)$ if $(G_{i1}, G_{i2}) = (AA, BB)$ for the two sibs, $(0, 2)$ if $(G_{i1}, G_{i2}) = (BB, AA)$ for the two sibs. We can then calculate $\mathrm{E}(X_{i1}|S_i) = \mathrm{E}(X_{i2}|S_i) = 2 \times (1/2) + 0 \times (1/2) = 1$ and $\mathrm{E}(X_{i1}^2|S_i) = \mathrm{E}(X_{i2}^2|S_i) = 2^2 \times (1/2) + 0^2 \times (1/2) = 2$. Thus, $\mathrm{Var}(X_{i1}|S_i) = \mathrm{Var}(X_{i2}|S_i) = 1$ and $\mathrm{Cov}(X_{i2}, X_{i2}|S_i) = -1$ because $\mathrm{E}(X_{i1}X_{i2}|S_i) = 0$. The contribution to U in Eq. (13.20) is $(Y_{i1} - Y_{i2})$ and the contribution to $\mathrm{Var}(U)$ is $(Y_{i1} - Y_{i2})^2$, assuming the first sib is AA and the second is BB. Thus, such families with both sibs affected, $Y_{i1} = Y_{i2} = 1$, will not be informative and have no contribution, but a discordant sibpair, $(Y_{i1}, Y_{i2}) = (1, 0)$ or $(Y_{i1}, Y_{i2}) = (0, 1)$, will be informative.

By conditioning on the traits and parental genotypes, the FBAT statistic does not use all the information about linkage and association that is available in the data. To use more information, one can separate the family data into two independent partitions, corresponding to the population information and the within-family information. Specifically, the full distribution of the data, which consists of the offspring phenotype, Y, the offspring genotype coding X, and the parental genotype (or the sufficient statistics for parents, S), can be partitioned into two independent parts:

$$\Pr(Y, X, S) = \Pr(X|Y, S)\Pr(Y, S).$$

Table 13.16 Conditional distributions or probabilities P of offspring genotypes G given that no parent's genotype is known

G	Conditional distribution
$\{AA\}$ or $\{AB\}$	$P = 1$.
$\{AA, AB\}$	Randomly assign AA and AB in a manner that keeps invariant the number of each.
$\{AA, BB\}$ or $\{AA, AB, BB\}$	Randomly assign equal $P = 1/3$ to AA, AB and BB to each sib, discarding outcomes without at least one AA and one BB sib.
$\{AB, AC, BC\}$	Randomly assign equal $P = 1/3$ to AB, AC and BC to each sib, discarding outcome without at least one of AB, AC and BC.
$\{AB, AC\}$	Randomly assign equal $P = 1/2$ to AB and AC to each sib, discarding outcomes without at least one AB or AC sib.
$\{AA, BC\}$, $\{AA, AB, AC\}$, $\{AA, AC, BC\}$ or $\{AA, AB, AC, BC\}$	Randomly assign equal $P = 1/4$ to AA, AB, AC and BC to each sib, discarding outcomes without at least one AA sib and without both B and C present.
$\{AC, BD\}$	Randomly assign equal $P = 1/2$ to AC and BD to each sib, discarding outcomes without at least one AC and one BD sib.
$\{AC, BC, BD\}$ or $\{AC, BC, AD, BD\}$	Randomly assign equal $P = 1/4$ to AC, BC, AD and BD to each sib, discarding outcomes that do not contain at least three of the four alleles A, B, C and D.

Under the null hypothesis, we can replace $\Pr(X|Y, S)$ by $\Pr(X|S)$. If Y is a quantitative trait, we can model $\Pr(Y, S)$ using a conditional mean model that is given by the linear regression model

$$E(Y) = \mu + \beta E(X|S). \tag{13.22}$$

This conditional mean model has been suggested for screening the genetic markers in GWAS. Markers are then selected for the next step based on the conditional power of the FBAT analysis.

13.5.4 FBAT Website and Software

FBAT has a website (http://www.biostat.harvard.edu/~fbat/default.html), which contains a brief introduction to what analyses FBAT does. The software for using FBAT can also be downloaded from http://www.biostat.harvard.edu/~fbat/fbat.htm for different computing platforms. The documentation for using FBAT, key references and applications of FBAT can be found at the FBAT website.

We have introduced some basic features and uses of FBAT. Based on the website of FBAT, FBAT can do many statistical analyses for family-based designs, including (i) analyzing family data with different traits, e.g., a binary trait, a quantitative trait, a time to event trait, and multiple traits; (ii) analyzing both autosomal and X chromosomes; (iii) testing diallelic and multiallelic markers with different genetic models; (iv) providing large sample and simulation-based exact tests for testing H_0: no linkage and no association, and H_0: no association; and (v) testing haplotypes and multiple markers, and providing estimates of haplotype frequencies and pairwise LD between markers.

13.6 Bibliographical Comments

Model-based methods to test for linkage were studied by Morton [185] more than half a century ago. These methods were mainly developed to identify genetic susceptibilities for Mendelian diseases. For more complex diseases with incomplete penetrances, methods have been developed to analyze large family data or pedigrees (Sect. 13.1). The Elston-Stewart algorithm (Elston and Stewart [75]) is an efficient recursive approach to calculate a likelihood function for large pedigrees with a small number of markers. Monte-Carlo Markov Chain methods for pedigree analysis are summarized in Thompson [272].

Alternatively, model-free methods based on IBD sharing are simple (Sect. 13.2). Estimating IBD sharing probabilities is important to model-free methods (Sect. 13.2.1). The Lander-Green algorithm can be used to estimate IBD sharing probabilities for various family structure in a multipoint fashion (Lander and Green [158] and Kruglyak et al. [153]). Haseman and Elston [118] developed the HE regression model to detect linkage using the quantitative traits of two sibs (Sect. 13.2.3). The original HE model is based on the squared trait difference of two sibs. Wright [304] found a full likelihood of sibpair data as a function of both a sum and a difference of the trait values. Using both the sibpair trait sum and difference as dependent variables was proposed by Drigalenko [63] (Sect. 13.2.4). In the revisited HE regression, Elston et al. [72] adopted this idea and used the overall mean-centered cross-product of sibpair traits as a measure of trait similarity. As the variances of the squared trait sum and squared trait difference may not be the same, Forrest [88]; Shete et al. [241]; Visscher and Hopper [281]; and Xu et al. [308] considered using different weighting methods for the squared sum and squared difference of the trait values, so that two different estimates of he same slope for the regression would be used. In addition to the linkage analysis using sibpairs, regression-based linkage analysis has been extended to other pairs using the GEE method (Chen et al. [33]; Olson and Wijsman [199]). Chen et al. [33] linked the different types of the working covariance matrix in GEEs to the different HE regression analyses and variance component methods. A two-level HE method for quantitative trait linkage was developed by Wang and Elston [291].

Hopper and Mathews [124] and Lange et al. [159]) are good references for the variance component model (Sect. 13.2.5). For the extension to a general pedigree, refer to Almasy and Blangero [8]. The idea of expressing the correlation of two traits in terms of the additive variance and kinship coefficient is due to Blangero et al. [17], which was used for estimating the missing heritability using GWAS data by Yang et al. [310]. In the variance component model, for the LRT to have a mixture of chi-squared distributions with different degrees of freedom under non-standard situations, refer to Self and Liang [238] and Self et al. [239] and, for using the Score and Wald tests, refer to Blangero et al. [17].

In Sect. 13.2.6, linkage analysis based on IBD sharing by sibpairs was studied. Blackwelder and Elston [16] and Knapp et al. [147] compared the mean and proportion tests and their properties. Schaid and Nick [232] proposed to use the maximum of the mean and proportion tests as a robust test. The triangle constraints for IBD sharing probabilities in Fig. 13.3 were obtained and studied by Faraway [83], Holmans [123] and Whittemore and Tu [303]. In particular, Whittemore and Tu [303] proposed the simple "minmax" test, which has the minimum of the worst (maximum) power loss due to using a wrong model, indexed by the parameter w in the family of statistics $T(w)$. Extension of the IBD sharing by sibpairs to sib-triples was considered by Whittemore and Tu [303], who also obtained constraints on the IBD sharing probabilities by sib-triples. The simple test statistic based on the midpoint $w = 0.5$ was proposed by Feingold and Siegmund [84]. The two-degree-of-freedom statistic or the MLS was proposed by Risch [213, 214], while Morton [186] and Risch [215] discussed how to convert the MLS to a one-degree-of-freedom test. Collins et al. [41] and Whittemore and Tu [303] also compared the power performance of these two tests. Extending to multi-locus models was studied by Cordell et al. [45, 46]; and Dupuis et al. [65].

The TDT was first proposed by Spielman et al. [255] (Sect. 13.3) to test linkage in the presence of association. Both the MGRR and HHRR tests were studied in Terwilliger and Ott [267], and the GHRR test was named by Falk and Rubinstein [81]. The matched design for analyzing transmitted/nontransmitted alleles was discussed in Schaid and Sommer [235] and Zhao [326]. Some comparisons between the TDT and HHRR and the impact of population stratification on the HHRR test can be found in Schaid and Sommer [235] and Terwilliger and Ott [267]. Spielman and Ewens [253] examined the TDT and population structure and showed that the TDT is a valid test of linkage regardless of population structure, and that it is not a valid test of association with multiple sibs. The joint probabilities of the transmitted and nontransmitted alleles in Table 13.9 were obtained in Ott [200]. Schaid [228] developed methods to test association using general conditional probabilities of offspring genotypes given mating type and given that the offspring is affected, using which some two-degree-of-freedom LRT and Score tests can be derived. This conditional likelihood method is also used to derive the conditional probabilities in Table 13.10.

A robust linkage test using the MERT was considered by Gastwirth and Friedlin [97]. They showed that the MERT of the family of normally distributed statistics $\{T(w) : w \in [0, 1/2]\}$ is the MERT of the extreme pair $T(0)$ and $T(1/2)$, and that the MERT is equivalent to the "minmax" test proposed by Whittemore and Tu [303]. See also reviews of this subject in Shih and Whittemore [242]. The conditional probabilities of affected offspring genotypes given parental genotypes of

Schaid [228] were used to derive one-degree-of-freedom Score tests assuming a genetic model (Schaid and Sommer [234]). Zheng et al. [333] extended this to a family of genetic models indexed by $x \in [0, 1]$ and obtained the family of robust tests $\{Z(x) : x \in [0, 1]\}$ given in (13.19). They also considered MERT and maximum tests, including MAX2, which takes the maximum of the extreme pair and MAX3, given in Sect. 13.4.2. The proof that the existence of the extreme pair for $\{Z(x) : x \in [0, 1]\}$ was given in Zheng et al. [332], which is also outlined in Problem 13.4. The CLRTs using trios were studied by Zheng et al. [331] and Troendle et al. [275] with different alternative spaces. Due to constrained alternative spaces, the CLRTs follow mixtures of chi-squared distributions. A recent adaptive approach to use deviation from HWE in trios to select an underlying genetic model followed by testing association using $Z(x^*)$ with a selected model x^* was considered by Yuan et al. [314]. A review of robust procedures with applications to linkage analysis using affected sibpairs and association tests using trios is provided by Joo et al. [136].

Most of the material on FBAT presented in Sect. 13.5 is based on Laird and Lange [155] and Rabinowitz and Laird [210]. The latter contains detailed discussion of using a sufficient statistic in FBAT. Using the empirical variance to estimate $\mathrm{Var}(U)$ in Sect. 13.5.1 was suggested by Lake et al. [157]. Applying FBAT to multiallelic markers and multiple traits was covered by Laird and Lange [155]. Rabinowitz and Laird [210] listed all the conditional distributions when testing for linkage and for association in the presence of linkage. For testing association in the presence of linkage, we need to condition on the distribution of IBD observed among the offspring. Here we listed some conditional distributions for testing linkage from nuclear families of arbitrary size, in Tables 13.14, 13.15, 13.16. The five-member family figure, Fig. 13.5, is similar to the one considered by Horvath et al. [125] under the null hypothesis of no linkage. Herbert et al. [120] and Van Steen et al. [280] used (13.22) to screen genetic markers in the first stage analysis of GWAS for a quantitative trait, and then tested a small number of selected markers in the second stage. We have focused on the application of FBAT to parent-offspring trios (Sect. 13.5.2). FBAT has also been extended to analyze haplotype data and perform a multivariate test to handle multivariate traits, using what is called the FBAT-GEE statistic (Laird and Lange [155]).

Beside the original TDT and FBAT, there have been many other approaches developed to analyze family data, including a conditional analysis incorporating a polygenic component in family data for quantitative traits (Zhu and Elston [347, 348]), the pedigree disequilibrium test (Martin et al. [180]), and the QTDT, a TDT for a quantitative trait (Abecasis et al. [1]). It is generally considered that the TDT-type methods are less powerful than unrelated population-based case-control approaches, although the latter may suffer confounding due to population structure (Zhu et al. [349]).

13.7 Problems

13.1 Using the results in Table 13.2, verify

(1) $E(g_{ij}) = 0$ for $i = 1, 2$;
(2) $Var(g_{ij}) = 2p(1 - p)$ for $i = 1, 2$; and
(3) Derive $Cov(g_{1j}, g_{2j}|i = 1)$.

13.2 In testing linkage based on IBD sharing by affected sibpairs,

(1) For a given a, show that the Score test $Z_{ST}(a)$ can be written as in (13.17).
(2) Show that $Z_{ST}(a)$ and $T(w)$ are equivalent with a one-to-one function between a and w.
(3) Show that the asymptotic null correlation of $Z_{ST}(a_1)$ and $Z_{ST}(a_2)$, for $a_1 \neq a_2$, is as given in (13.18).

13.3 In association analysis using parent-offspring trios, show that the Score test can be written as in (13.19).

13.4 TDT-type robust tests and the extreme pair (Zheng et al. [332]).

(1) The parameterization of the GRRs (λ_1, λ_2) used in Sect. 13.4.2 is not unique. Consider $\lambda_1 = 1 + r \sin\theta$ and $\lambda_2 = 1 + r \cos\theta$, where $r \geq 0$ and $\theta \in [0, \pi/4]$ is a nuisance parameter ($\pi = 180°$). Show that the Score test for $H_0 : r = 0$ for a given θ can be written as

$$Z(\theta) = \frac{d\cos\theta + e\sin\theta}{\sqrt{I(\theta)}} = \frac{d\cos\theta + e\sin\theta}{\sqrt{a\cos^2\theta + c\sin^2\theta - b\sin(2\theta)}},$$

where $a = n_2/4 + 2n_4/16$, $b = n_2/4 + n_4/8$, $c = (n_2 + n_4 + n_5)/4$, $d = (n_{22} - n_2/2) + (n_{42} - n_4/4)$ and $e = (n_{21} - n_2/2) + (n_{41} - n_4/2) + (n_{51} - n_5/2)$. Indicate which values of $\theta \in [0, \pi/4]$ corresponds to the REC and DOM models.
(2) Find the asymptotic null correlation of $Z(\theta_1)$ and $Z(\theta_2)$ for $\theta_1, \theta_2 \in [0, \pi/4]$. Show it can be expressed as

$$\mathrm{Corr}(\theta_1, \theta_2) = \frac{\cos\theta_1 Q_1(\theta_2) + \sin\theta_1 Q_2(\theta_2)}{\sqrt{I(\theta_1)I(\theta_2)}},$$

where $Q_1(\theta) = a\cos\theta - b\sin\theta$ and $Q_2(\theta) = a\sin\theta - b\cos\theta$.
(3) Show that, for $\theta_i \in [0, \pi/4]$ ($i = 1, 2$), $\cos(\theta_1 - \theta_2) \geq \sin(\theta_1 + \theta_2)$.
(4) Using $c > a > b$ and (3), show that, for $\theta_i \in [0, \pi/4]$ ($i = 1, 2$), $\mathrm{Corr}(\theta_1, \theta_2) > 0$.
(5) For $\theta \in [0, \pi/4]$, show that $\partial\,\mathrm{Corr}(0, \theta)/\partial\theta < 0$ and $\partial\,\mathrm{Corr}(\theta, \pi/4)/\partial\theta > 0$.
(6) Let $f(\theta) = \mathrm{Corr}(0, \theta) + \mathrm{Corr}(\theta, \pi/4)$. Show that $f(\theta)$ has exactly one root $\theta^* \in [0, \pi/4]$, i.e., $f'(\theta^*) = df(\theta)/d\theta|_{\theta=\theta^*} = 0$.
(7) Show that $f'(\theta) > 0$ if $\theta < \theta^*$ and $f'(\theta) < 0$ if $\theta > \theta^*$, i.e., $f(\theta)$ has a minimum value on $[0, \pi/4]$ at either $\theta = 0$ or $\theta = \pi/4$.
(8) Use (7) to verify $\mathrm{Corr}(0, \theta) + \mathrm{Corr}(\theta, \pi/4) \geq 1 + \mathrm{Corr}(0, \pi/4)$ for any $\theta \in [0, \pi/4]$. Thus, $(Z(0), Z(\pi/4))$ is the extreme pair to construct the MERT.

References

1. Abecasis, G.R., Cardon, L.R., Cookson, W.O.: A general test of association for quantitative traits in nuclear families. Am. J. Hum. Genet. **66**, 279–292 (2000)
2. Abecasis, G.R., Cookson, W.O.: GOLD—-graphical overview of linkage disequilibrium. Bioinformatics **16**, 182–183 (2000)
3. ACCESS Research Group: Design of a case control etiologic study of sarcoidosis (ACCESS). J. Clinic. Epidemiol. **52**, 1173–1186 (1999)
4. Agresti, A.: Categorical Data Analysis. Wiley, London (1990)
5. Agresti, A.: A survey of exact inference for contingency tables. Stat. Sci. **7**, 131–177 (1992)
6. Ahn, K., Haynes, C., Kim, W., St. Fleur, R., Gordon, D., Finch, S.J.: The effects of SNP genotyping errors on power of the Cochran-Armitage linear trend test for case/control association studies. Ann. Hum. Genet. **71**, 249–261 (2007)
7. Albert, P.S., Ratnasinghe, D., Tangrea, J., Wacholder, S.: Limitations of the case-only design for identifying gene-environment interaction. Am. J. Epidemiol. **154**, 687–693 (2001)
8. Almasy, L., Blangero, J.: Multipoint quantitative-trait linkage analysis in general pedigrees. Am. J. Hum. Genet. **62**, 1198–1211 (1998)
9. Armitage, P.: Tests for linear trends in proportions and frequencies. Biometrics **11**, 375–386 (1955)
10. Astle, W., Balding, D.J.: Population structure and cryptic relatedness in genetic association studies. Stat. Sci. **24**, 451–471 (2009)
11. Bacanu, S.A., Devlin, B., Roeder, K.: The power of genomic control. Am. J. Hum. Genet. **66**, 1933–1944 (2000)
12. Balding, D.J.: A tutorial on statistical methods for population association studies. Nat. Rev. Genet. **7**, 781–791 (2006)
13. Balding, D.J., Nichols, R.A.: A method for quantifying differentiation between populations at multi-allelic loci and its implications for investigating identity and paternity. Genetica **96**, 3–12 (1995)
14. Benjamini, Y., Hochberg, Y.: Controlling the false discovery rate: a practical and powerful approach to multiple testing. J. Roy. Stat. Soc. Ser. B **57**, 289–300 (1995)
15. Benjamini, Y., Yekutieli, D.: The control of the false discovery rate in multiple testing under dependency. Ann. Stat. **29**, 1165–1188 (2001)
16. Blackwelder, W.C., Elston, R.C.: A comparison of sib-pair linkage tests for disease susceptibility loci. Genet. Epidemiol. **2**, 85–97 (1985)
17. Blangero, J., Williams, J.T., Almasy, L.: Variance component methods for detecting complex trait loci. Adv. Genet. **42**, 151–181 (2001)
18. Birnbaum, A., Laska, E.: Optimal robustness: a general method, with applications to linear estimators of location. J. Am. Stat. Assoc. **62**, 1230–1240 (1967)
19. Bose, S., Slud, E.: Maximin efficiency robust tests and some extensions. J. Stat. Plann. Infer. **46**, 105–121 (1995)

G. Zheng et al., *Analysis of Genetic Association Studies*,
Statistics for Biology and Health,
DOI 10.1007/978-1-4614-2245-7, © Springer Science+Business Media, LLC 2012

20. Bourgain, C., Abney, M., Schneider, D., Ober, C., McPeek, M.S.: Testing for Hardy-Weinberg equilibrium in samples with related individuals. Am. J. Hum. Genet. **168**, 2349–2361 (2004)
21. Breslow, N.E., Day, N.E.: Statistical Methods in Cancer Research, vol. 1: The Analysis of Case-Control Studies. IARC Scientific Publications, vol. 32 (1980)
22. Brown, D.G., Harrower, I.M.: A new integer programming formulation for the pure parsimony problem in haplotype analysis. In: Jonassen, I., Kim, J. (eds.) Workshop on Algorithms in Bioinformatics. Springer, Berlin (2004)
23. Brown, D.G., Harrower, I.M.: Integer programming approaches to haplotype inference by pure parsimony. IEEE/ACM Trans. Comput. Biol. Bioinform. **3**, 141–154 (2006)
24. Campbell, C.D., Ogburn, E.L., Lunetta, K.L., Lyon, H.N., Freedman, M.L., Groop, L.C., Altshuler, D., Ardlie, K.G., Hirschhorn, J.N.: Demonstrating stratification in a European American population. Nat. Genet. **37**, 868–872 (2005)
25. Carlin, B.P., Louis, T.A.: Bayes and Empirical Bayes Methods for Data Analysis. Chapman & Hall, England (1996)
26. Casci, T.: EPISTASIS: A network of interactors. Nat. Rev. Genet. **11**, 531 (2010)
27. Casella, G., Berger, R.L.: Statistical Inference. Duxbury Press, Belmont (1990)
28. Cavalli-Sforza, L.L., Menozzi, P., Piazza, A.: The History and Geography of Human Genes. Princeton University Press, Princeton (1994)
29. Ceppellini, R., Siniscalco, M., Smith, C.A.B.: The estimation of gene frequencies in a random mating population. Ann. Hum. Genet. **20**, 97–115 (1955)
30. Chatterjee, N., Carroll, R.J.: Semiparametric maximum likelihood estimation exploiting gene-environment independence in case-control studies. Biometrika **92**, 399–418 (2005)
31. Chen, H.S., Zhu, X., Zhao, H., Zhang, S.: Qualitative semi-parametric test for genetic associations in case-control designs under structured populations. Ann. Hum. Genet. **67**, 250–264 (2003)
32. Chen, J., Chatterjee, N.: Exploiting Hardy-Weinberg equilibrium for efficient screening of single SNP associations from case-control studies. Hum. Hered. **63**, 196–204 (2007)
33. Chen, W.M., Broman, K.W., Liang, K.Y.: Quantitative trait linkage analysis by generalized estimating equations: unification of variance components and Haseman-Elston regression. Genet. Epidemiol. **26**, 265–272 (2004)
34. Chen, X., Liu, C.T., Zhang, M., Zhang, H.: A forest-based approach to identifying gene and gene-gene interactions. Proc. Natl. Acad. Sci. USA **104**, 19199–19203 (2007)
35. Chernoff, H.: On the distribution of the likelihood ratio. Ann. Math. Stat. **25**, 573–578 (1954)
36. Chernoff, H., Lander, E.: Asymptotic distribution of the likelihood ratio test that a mixture of two binomials is a single binomial. J. Stat. Plann. Infer. **43**, 19–40 (1987)
37. Clark, A.G.: Inference of haplotypes from PCR-amplified samples of diploid populations. Mol. Biol. Evol. **7**, 111–122 (1990)
38. Clarke, G.M., Morris, A.P.: A comparison of sample size and power in case-only association studies of gene-environment interaction. Am. J. Epidemiol. **171**, 498–505 (2010)
39. Clayton, D., Hills, M.: Statistical Methods in Epidemiology. Oxford Science Publications Inc., New York (1993)
40. Cochran, W.G.: Some methods for strengthening the common chi-square tests. Biometrics **10**, 417–451 (1954)
41. Collins, A., MacLean, C.J., Morton, N.E.: Trials of the beta model for complex inheritance. Proc. Natl. Acad. Sci. USA **93**, 9177–9181 (1996)
42. Congdon, P.: Bayesian Models for Categorical Data. Wiley, England (2005)
43. Conneely, K.N., Boehnke, M.: So many correlated tests, so little time! Rapid adjustment of P values for multiple correlated tests. Am. J. Hum. Genet. **81**, 1158–1168 (2007)
44. Cordell, H.J.: Detecting gene-gene interactions that underlie human diseases. Nat. Rev. Genet. **10**, 392–404 (2009)
45. Cordell, H.J., Todd, J.A., Bennett, S.T., Kawaguchi, Y., Farrall, M.: Two-locus maximum lod score analysis of a multifactorial trait: joint consideration of IDDM2 and IDDM4 with IDDM1 in type 1 diabetes. Am. J. Hum. Genet. **57**, 920–934 (1995)

46. Cordell, H.J., Wedig, G.C., Jacobs, K.B., Elston, R.C.: Multilocus linkage tests based on affected relative pairs. Am. J. Hum. Genet. **66**, 1273–1286 (2000)
47. Cox, D.R.: Interaction. Int. Stat. Rev. **52**, 1–31 (1984)
48. Cox, D.R., Hinkley, D.V.: Theoretical Statistics. Chapman & Hall/CRC, Boca Raton (1974)
49. Crow, J.F., Kimura, H.: An Introduction to Population Genetics Theory. Burgess Publication Co, Minneapolis (1970)
50. Culverhouse, R., Klein, T., Shannon, T.: Detecting epistatic interactions contributing to quantitative traits. Genet. Epidemiol. **27**, 141–152 (2004)
51. Curnow, R.N., Morris, A.P., Whittaker, J.C.: Locating genes involved in human diseases. Appl. Stat. **47**, 63–76 (1998)
52. Czika, W., Weir, B.S.: Properties of the multiallelic trend test. Biometrics **60**, 69–74 (2004)
53. Dadd, T., Lewis, C.M., Weale, M.E.: Delta-centralization fails to control for population stratification in genetic association studies. Hum. Hered. **69**, 285–294 (2009)
54. Daly, M.J., Rioux, J.D., Schaffner, S.F., Hudson, T.J., Lander, E.S.: High-resolution haplotype structure in the human genome. Nat. Genet. **29**, 229–232 (2001)
55. Davies, R.B.: Hypothesis testing when a nuisance parameter is present only under the alternative. Biometrika **64**, 247–254 (1977)
56. Davies, R.B.: Hypothesis-testing when a nuisance parameter is present only under the alternative. Biometrika **74**, 33–43 (1987)
57. David, H.A., Nagaraja, H.N.: Order Statistics. 3rd edn. Wiley, Hoboken (2003)
58. Dempster, A., Laird, N.M., Rubin, D.: Maximum likelihood from incomplete data via the EM algorithm (with discussion). J. Roy. Stat. Soc. Ser. B **39**, 1–38 (1977)
59. Devlin, B., Risch, N.: A comparison of linkage disequilibrium measures for fine-scale mapping. Genomics **29**, 311–322 (1995)
60. Devlin, B., Roeder, K.: Genomic control for association studies. Biometrics **55**, 997–1004 (1999)
61. Donegani, M.: An adaptive and powerful randomization test. Biometrika **78**, 930–933 (1991)
62. Douglas, J.A., Boehnke, M., Lange, K.: A multipoint method for detecting genotyping errors and mutation in sibling-pair linkage data. Am. J. Hum. Genet. **66**, 1287–1297 (2000)
63. Drigalenko, E.: How sib pairs reveal linkage. Am. J. Hum. Genet. **63**, 1242–1245 (1998)
64. Dudoit, S., van der Laan, M.J.: Multiple Testing Procedures with Applications to Genomics. Springer, New York (2008)
65. Dupuis, J., Brown, P.O., Siegmund, D.O.: Statistical methods for linkage analysis of complex traits from high-resolution maps of identity by descent. Genetics **140**, 843–856 (1995)
66. Editorial in Nature Genetics: Freely associating. Nat. Genet. **22**, 1–2 (1999)
67. Edwards, A.W.F.: Foundations of Mathematical Genetics, 2nd edn. Cambridge University Press, Cambridge (2000)
68. Edwards, B.J., Haynes, C., Levenstien, M.A., Finch, S.J., Gordon, D.: Power and sample size calculations in the presence of phenotype errors for case/control genetic association studies. BMC Genet. **8**, 1–18 (2005)
69. Eitan, Y., Kashi, Y.: Direct micro-haplotyping by multiple double PCR amplifications of specific alleles (MD-PASA). Nucleic Acids Res. **30**, e62 (2002)
70. Ejigou, A., McHugh, R.: Relative risk estimation under multiple matching. Biometrika **68**, 85–91 (1981)
71. Elandt-Johnson, R.C.: Probability Models and Statistical Methods in Genetics. Wiley, New York (1971)
72. Elston, R.C., Buxbaum, S., Jacobs, K.B., Olson, J.M.: Haseman and Elston revisited. Genet. Epidemiol. **19**, 1–17 (2000)
73. Elston, R.C., Johnson, W.D.: Basic Biostatistics for Genetists and Epidemiologists. Wiley, West Sussex (2008)
74. Elston, R.C., Lin, D.Y., Zheng, G.: Multistage sampling for genetic studies. Ann. Rev. Gen. Hum. Genet. **8**, 327–342 (2007)
75. Elston, R.C., Stewart, J.: A general model for the genetic analysis of pedigree data. Hum. Hered. **21**, 523–542 (1971)

76. Emigh, T.H.: A comparison of tests for Hardy-Weinberg equilibrium. Biometrics **36**, 627–642 (1980)
77. Epstein, M.P., Allen, A.S., Satten, G.A.: A simple and improved correction for population stratification in case-control studies. Am. J. Hum. Genet. **80**, 921–930 (2007)
78. Epstein, M.P., Satten, G.A.: Inference on haplotype effects in case-control studies using unphased genotype data. Am. J. Hum. Genet. **73**, 1316–1329 (2003)
79. Evans, M., Hastings, N., Peacock, B.: Statistical Distributions. 3rd edn. Wiley, New York (2000)
80. Excoffier, L., Slatkin, M.: Maximum likelihood estimation of molecular haplotype frequencies in a diploid population. Mol. Biol. Evol. **12**, 921–927 (1995)
81. Falk, C.T., Rubinstein, P.: Haplotype relative risks: an easy reliable way to construct a proper control sample for risk calculations. Ann. Hum. Genet. **51**, 227–233 (1987)
82. Falush, D., Stephens, M., Pritchard, J.K.: Inference of population structure using multilocus genotype data: linked loci and correlated allele frequencies. Genetics **164**, 1567–1587 (2003)
83. Faraway, J.J.: Improved sib-pair linkage test for disease susceptibility loci. Genet. Epidemiol. **10**, 225–233 (1993)
84. Feingold, E., Siegmund, D.O.: Strategies for mapping heterogeneous recessive traits by allele-sharing methods. Am. J. Hum. Genet. **60**, 965–978 (1997)
85. Ferreira, T., Marchini, J.: Modeling interactions with known risk loci – a Bayesian model averaging approach. Ann. Hum. Genet. **75**, 1–9 (2011)
86. Fleiss, J.L., Levin, B., Paik, M.C.: Statistical Methods for Rates and Proportions. 3rd edn. Wiley, New York (2003)
87. Foppa, I., Spiegeiman, D.: Power and sample size calculations for case-control studies of gene-environment interactions with a polytomous exposure variable. Am. J. Epidemiol. **146**, 596–604 (1997)
88. Forrest, W.F.: Weighting improves the "new Haseman-Elston" method. Hum. Hered. **52**, 47–54 (2001)
89. Foulkes, A.S.: Applied Statistical Genetics: For Population-Based Association Studies with R. Springer, Berlin (2009)
90. Freidlin, B., Podgor, M.J., Gastwirth, J.L.: Efficiency robust tests for survival or ordered categorical data. Biometrics **55**, 883–886 (1999)
91. Freidlin, B., Zheng, G., Li, Z., Gastwirth, J.L.: Trend tests for case-control studies of genetic markers: power, sample size and robustness. Hum. Hered. **53**, 146–152 (2002) (Erratum **68**, 220 (2009))
92. Fridley, B.L., Serie, D., Jenkins, G., White, K., Bamlet, W., Potter, J.D., Goode, E.L.: Bayesian mixture models for the incorporation of prior knowledge to inform genetic association studies. Genet. Epidemiol. **34**, 418–426 (2010)
93. Gabriel, S.B., Schaffner, S.F., Nguyen, H., Moore, J.M., Roy, J., Blumenstiel, B., Higgins, J., DeFelice, M., Lochner, A., Faggart, M., Liu-Cordero, S.N., Rotimi, M., Adeyemo, A., Cooper, R., Ward, R., Lander, E.S., Daly, M.J., Atshuler, D.: The structure of haplotype blocks in the human genome. Science **296**, 2225–2229 (2002)
94. Garcia-Closas, M., Lubin, J.H.: Power and sample size calculations in case-control studies of gene-environment interactions: Comments on different approaches. Am. J. Epidemiol. **149**, 689–692 (1999)
95. Gastwirth, J.L.: On robust procedures. J. Am. Stat. Assoc. **61**, 929–948 (1966)
96. Gastwirth, J.L.: The use of maximin efficiency robust tests in combining contingency tables and survival analysis. J. Am. Stat. Assoc. **80**, 380–384 (1985)
97. Gastwirth, J.L., Freidlin, B.: On power and efficiency robust linkage tests for affected sibs. Ann. Hum. Genet. **64**, 443–453 (2000)
98. Gauderman, W.J.: Sample size requirements for matched case-control studies of gene-environment interaction. Stat. Med. **21**, 35–50 (2002)
99. Gelman, A., Carlin, J.B., Stern, H.S., Rubin, D.B.: Bayesian Data Analysis. Chapman & Hall, England (1995)

100. Genovese, G., Friedman, D.J., Ross, M.D., Lecordier, L., Uzureau, P., Freedman, B.I., Bowden, D.W., Langefeld, C.D., Oleksyk, T.K., Uscinski Knob, A.L., Bernhardy, A.J., Hicks, P.J., Nelson, G.W., Vanhollebeke, B., Winkler, C.A., Kopp, J.B., Pays, E., Pollak, M.R.: Association of Trypanolytic ApoL1 variants with kidney disease in African-Americans. Science **7**, 1–7 (2010)
101. Ghosh, A., Zou, F., Wright, F.A.: Estimating odds ratios in genome scans: An approximate conditional likelihood approach. Am. J. Hum. Genet. **82**, 1064–1074 (2008)
102. Gonzalez, J.R., Carrasco, J.L., Dudbridge, F., Armengol, L., Estivill, X., Moreno, V.: Maximizing association statistics over genetic models. Genet. Epidemiol. **32**, 246–254 (2008)
103. Gordon, D., Finch, S.J., Nothnagel, M., Ott, J.: Power and sample size calculations for case-control genetic association tests when errors are present: application to single nucleotide polymorphisms. Hum. Hered. **54**, 22–33 (2002)
104. Gorroochurn, P., Heiman, G.A., Hodge, S.E., Greenberg, D.A.: Centralizing the non-central chi-square: A new method to correct for population stratification in genetic case-control association studies. Genet. Epidemiol. **30**, 277–289 (2006)
105. Gorroochurn, P., Hodge, S.E., Heiman, G.A., Greenberg, D.A.: A unified approach for quantifying, testing and correcting population stratification in case-control association studies. Hum. Hered. **64**, 149–159 (2007)
106. Graubard, B.I., Korn, E.L.: Choice of column scores for testing independence in ordered $2 \times K$ contingency tables. Biometrics **43**, 471–476 (1987)
107. Guedj, M., Wojcik, J., Della-Chiesa, E., Nuel, G., Forner, K.: A fast, unbiased and exact allelic test for case-control association studies. Hum. Hered. **61**, 210–221 (2006)
108. Guedj, M., Nuel, G., Prum, B.: A note on allelic tests in case-control association studies. Ann. Hum. Genet. **72**, 407–409 (2008)
109. Guo, S.W., Thompson, E.A.: Performing the exact test of Hardy-Weinberg proportion for multiple alleles. Biometrics **48**, 361–372 (1992)
110. Gusfield, D.: Inference of haplotypes from samples of diploid populations: complexity and algorithms. J. Comput. Biol. **8**, 305–323 (2001)
111. Gusfield, D.: Haplotype inference by pure parsimony. In: Baesa-Yates, R., Chavez, E., Crochemore, M. (eds.) The 14th Annual Symposium on Combinatorial Pattern Matching (CPM03), pp. 144–155. Springer, Berlin/Heidelberg (2003)
112. Haldane, J.B.S.: An exact test for randomness of mating. J. Genet. **52**, 631–635 (1954)
113. Hamilton, D.C., Cole, D.E.C.: Standardizing a composite measure of linkage disequilibrium. Ann. Hum. Genet. **68**, 234–239 (2004)
114. Hanson, R.L., Looker, H.C., Ma, L., Muller, Y.L., Baier, L.J., Knowler, W.C.: Design and analysis of genetic association studies to finely map a locus identified by linkage analysis: Sample size and power calculations. Ann. Hum. Genet. **70**, 332–349 (2006)
115. Hardy, G.H.: Mendelian proportions in a mixed population. Science **28**, 49–50 (1908)
116. Harrington, D., Fleming, T.: A class of rank test procedures for censored survival data. Biometrika **69**, 553–566 (1982)
117. Hartl, D., Clark, A.G.: Principles of Population Genetics, 3rd edn. Sinauer Associates Inc., Sunderland (1997)
118. Haseman, J.K., Elston, R.C.: The investigation of linkage between a quantitative trait and a marker locus. Behav. Genet. **2**, 3–19 (1972)
119. Hawley, M., Kidd, K.: HAPLO: a program using the EM algorithm to estimate the frequencies of multi-site haplotypes. J. Hered. **86**, 409–411 (1995)
120. Herbert, A., Gerry, N.P., McQueen, M.B., Heid, I.M., Pfeufer, A., Illig, T., Wichmann, H.E., Meitinger, T., Hunter, D., Hu, F.B., et al.: A common genetic variant is associated with adult and childhood obesity. Science **312**, 279–283 (2006)
121. Hoeting, J.A., Madigan, D., Raftery, A.E., Volinsky, C.T.: Bayesian model averaging: a tutorial. Stat. Sci. **14**, 382–417
122. Hoh, J., Ott, J.: Mathematical multi-locus approaches to localizing complex human trait genes. Nat. Rev. Genet. **4**, 701–709 (2003)
123. Holmans, P.: Asymptotic properties of affected-sib-pair linkage analysis. Am. J. Hum. Genet. **52**, 362–374 (1993)

124. Hopper, J.L., Mathews, J.D.: Extensions to multivariate normal models for pedigree analysis. Ann. Hum. Genet. **46**, 373–383 (1982)
125. Horvath, S., Xu, X., Lake, S.L., Silverman, E.K., Weiss, S.T., Laird, N.M.: Family-based tests for associating haplotypes with general phenotype data: application to asthma genetics. Genet. Epidemiol. **26**, 61–69 (2004)
126. Hunter, D.J.: Gene-environment interactions in human diseases. Nat. Rev. Genet. **6**, 287–298 (2005)
127. Hunter, D.J., Kraft, P., Jacobs, K.B., Cox, D.G., Yeager, N., Hankinson, S.E., Wacholder, S., Wang, Z., Welch, R., Hutchinson, A., et al.: A genome-wide association study identifies alleles in FGFR2 associated with risk of sporadic postmenopausal breast cancer. Nat. Genet. **39**, 870–874 (2007)
128. Hurley, J.D., Engle, L.J., Davis, J.T., Welsh, A.M., Landers, J.E.: A simple, bead-based approach for multi-SNP molecular haplotyping. Nucleic Acids Res. **32**, e186 (2005)
129. Hwang, S.-J., Beaty, T.H., Liang, K.-Y., Coresh, J., Khoury, M.J.: Minimum sample size estimation to detect gene-environment interaction in case-control designs. Am. J. Epidemiol. **140**, 1029–1037 (1994)
130. Ito, T., Chiku, S., Inoue, E., Tomita, M., Morisaki, T., Morisaki, H., Kamatani, N.: Estimation of haplotype frequencies, linkage disequilibrium measures, and combination of haplotype copies in each pool by use of pooled DNA data. Am. J. Hum. Genet. **72**, 384–398 (2003)
131. Jeffries, N.O.: Ranking bias in association studies. Hum. Hered. **67**, 267–275 (2009)
132. Johnson, G.C.L., Esposito, L., Barratt, B.J., Smith, A.N., Heward, J., DiGenova, G., Veda, H., Cordell, H.J., Eaves, I.A., Dudbridge, F., Twells, R.C.J., Payne, F., Hughes, W., Nutland, S., Stevens, H., Carr, P., Tuomilehto-Wolf, E., Tunmilehto, J., Gough, S.C.L., Clayton, D.G., Todd, J.A.: Haplotype tagging for the identification of common disease genes. Nat. Genet. **29**, 233–237 (2001)
133. Johnson, V.E.: Bayes factor based on test statistics. J. R. Statist. Soc. B **67**, 689–701 (2005)
134. Johnson, V.E.: Properties of Bayes factors based on test statistics. Scand. J. Statist. **35**, 354–368 (2008)
135. Joo, J., Kwak, M., Ahn, K., Zheng, G.: A robust genome-wide scan statistic of the Wellcome Trust Case-Control Consortium. Biometrics **65**, 1115–1122 (2009)
136. Joo, J., Kwak, M., Chen, Z., Zheng, G.: Efficiency robust statistics for genetic linkage and association studies under genetic model uncertainty. Stat. Med. **29**, 158–180 (2010)
137. Joo, J., Kwak, M., Zheng, G.: Improving power for testing genetic association in case-control studies by reducing alternative space. Biometrics **66**, 266–276 (2010)
138. Jorde, L.B.: Linkage disequilibrium and the search for complex disease genes. Genome Res. **10**, 1435–1444 (2000)
139. Kang, H.M., Sul, J.H., Service, S.K., Zaitlen, N.A., Kong, S.Y., Freimer, N.B., Sabatti, C., Eskin, E.: Variance component model to account for sample structure in genome-wide association studies. Nat. Genet. **42**, 348–354 (2010)
140. Kass, R.E., Raftery, A.E.: Bayes factors. J. Am. Stat. Assoc. **90**, 773–795 (1995)
141. Ke, X., Cardon, L.R.: Efficient selective screening of haplotype tag SNPs. Bioinformatics **19**, 287–288 (2003)
142. Khouri, M.J., Beaty, T.H., Cohen, B.H.: Fundamentals of Genetic Epidemiology. Oxford University Press, London (1993)
143. Kim, S., Morris, N.J., Won, S., Elston, R.C.: Single-marker and two-marker association tests for unphased case-control genotype data, with a power comparison. Genet. Epidemiol. **34**, 67–77 (2010)
144. Klein, R.J., Zeiss, C., Chew, E.Y., Tsai, J.-Y., Sackler, R.S., Haynes, C., Henning, A.K., SanGiovanni, J.P., Mane, S.M., Mayne, S.T., Bracken, M.B., Ferris, F.L., et al.: Complement factor H polymorphism in aged-related macular degeneration. Science **308**, 385–389 (2005)
145. Knapp, M.: Re: Biased tests of association: comparisons of allele frequencies when departing from Hardy-Weinberg proportions. Am. J. Epidemiol. **154**, 287 (2001)
146. Knapp, M.: On the asymptotic equivalence of allelic and trend statistic under Hardy-Weinberg equilibrium. Ann. Hum. Genet. **72**, 589 (2008)

147. Knapp, M., Seuchter, S.A., Baur, M.P.: Linkage analysis in nuclear families. 1: Optimality criteria for affected sib-pair tests. Hum. Hered. **44**, 37–43 (1994)
148. Knowler, W.C., Williams, R.C., Pettitt, D.J., Steinberg, A.G.: Gm3;5,13,14 and type 2 diabetes mellitus: an association in American Indians with genetic admixture. Am. J. Hum. Genet. **43**, 520–526 (1988)
149. Konfortov, B.A., Bankier, A.T., Dear, P.H.: An efficient method for multi-locus molecular haplotyping. Nucleic Acids Res. **35**, e6 (2007)
150. Kooperberg, C., LeBlanc, M.: Increasing the power of identifying gene × gene interactions in genome-wide association studies. Genet. Epidemiol. **32**, 255–263 (2008)
151. Kooperberg, C., LeBlanc, M., Dai, J.Y., Rajapakse, I.: Structures and assumptions: Strategies to harness gene × gene and gene × environment interactions in GWAS. Stat. Sci. **24**, 472–488 (2009)
152. Kooperberg, C., Ruczinski, I.: Identifying interacting SNPs using Monte Carlo logic regression. Genet. Epidemiol. **28**, 157–170 (2005)
153. Kruglyak, L., Daly, M.J., Reeve-Daly, M.P., Lander, E.S.: Parametric and nonparametric linkage analysis: a unified multipoint approach. Am. J. Hum. Genet. **58**, 1347–1363 (1996)
154. Kuk, A.Y.C., Zhang, H., Yang, Y.: Computationally feasible estimation of haplotype frequencies from pooled genotype data with and without assuming Hardy-Weinberg Equilibrium. Bioinformatics **25**, 379–386 (2009)
155. Laird, N.M., Lange, C.: Family-based methods for linkage and association analysis. Adv. Genet. **60**, 219–252 (2008)
156. Lachin, J.M.: Biostatistical Methods: The Assessment of Relative Risks. Wiley, New York (2000)
157. Lake, S.L., Blacker, D., Laird, N.M.: Family-based tests of association in the presence of linkage. Am. J. Hum. Genet. **67**, 1515–1525 (2000)
158. Lander, E.S., Green, P.: Construction of multilocus genetic linkage maps in humans. Proc. Natl. Acad. Sci. USA **84**, 2363–2367 (1987)
159. Lange, K., Westlake, J., Spence, M.A.: Extensions to pedigree analysis. III. Variance components by the scoring method. Ann. Hum. Genet. **39**, 485–491 (1976)
160. Lee, S.Y. Chung, Y., Elston, R.C., Kim, Y., Park, T.: Log-linear model based multifactor dimensionality reduction method to detect gene-gene interactions. Bioinformatics **23**, 2589–2595 (2007)
161. Lee, W.C.: Case-control association studies with matching and genomic controlling. Genet. Epidemiol. **27**, 1–13 (2004)
162. Lewontin, R.C.: The interaction of selection and linkage. I. general considerations; heterotic models. Genetics **49**, 49–67 (1964)
163. Li, C.C.: Notes on relative fitness of genotypes that forms a geometric progression. Evolution **13**, 564–567 (1959)
164. Li, C.C.: Genetic equilibrium under selection. Biometrics **23**, 397–484 (1967)
165. Li, C.C.: The First Course in Population Genetics. The Boxwood Press, Pacific Grove (1976)
166. Li, J.Z., Absher, D.M., Tang, H., Southwick, A.M., Casto, A.M., Ramachandran, S., Cann, H.M., Barsh, G.S., Feldman, M., Cavalli-Sforza, L.L., Myers, R.M.: Worldwide human relationships inferred from genome-wide patterns of variation. Science **319**, 1100–1104 (2008)
167. Li, Y., Graubard, B.I.: Testing Hardy-Weinberg equilibrium and homogeneity of Hardy-Weinberg disequilibrium using complex survey data. Biometrics **65**, 1096–1104 (2009)
168. Li, Q., Zheng, G., Li, Z., Yu, K.: Efficient approximation of p-value of maximum of correlated tests with applications to genome-wide association studies. Ann. Hum. Genet. **72**, 397–406 (2008)
169. Li, Q., Zheng, G., Liang, X., Yu, K.: Robust tests for single-marker analysis in case-control genetic association studies. Ann. Hum. Genet. **73**, 245–252 (2009)
170. Li, Q., Yu, K., Li, Z., Zheng, G.: MAX-rank: a simple and robust genome-wide scan for case-control association studies. Hum. Genet. **123**, 617–623 (2008)
171. Li, W.: Three lectures on case-control genetic association analysis. Brief. Bioinform. **9**, 1–13 (2008)

172. Li, Y., Willer, C., Sanna, S., Abecasis, G.: Genotype imputation. Ann. Rev. Genomics Hum. Genet. **10**, 387–406 (2009)
173. Lin, D.Y., Zeng, D.: Likelihood-based inference on haplotype effects in genetic association studies. J. Am. Stat. Assoc. **101**, 89–104 (2006)
174. Liu, N., Zhang, K., Zhao, H.: Haplotype-association analysis. Adv. Genet. **60**, 335–405 (2008)
175. Long, J.C., Williams, R.C., Urbanek, M.: An E-M algorithm and testing strategy for multiple-locus haplotypes. Am. J. Hum. Genet. **56**, 799–810 (1995)
176. Lou, X.Y., Chen, G.B., Yan, L., Ma, J.Z., Zhu, J., Elston, R.C., Li, M.D.: A generalized combinatorial approach for detecting gene-by-gene and gene-by-environment interactions with application to nicotine dependence. Am. J. Hum. Genet. **80**, 1125–1137 (2007)
177. Lubin, J.H., Gail, M.H.: On power and sample size for studying features of the relative odds of disease. Am. J. Epidemiol. **131**, 552–566 (1990)
178. Marchini, J., Cardon, L.R., Phillips, M.S., Donnelly, P.: The effects of human population structure on large genetic association studies. Nat. Genet. **36**, 512–517 (2004)
179. Marchini, J., Donnelly, P., Cardon, L.R.: Genome-wide strategies for detecting multiple loci that influence complex diseases. Nat. Genet. **37**, 413–417 (2005)
180. Martin, E.R., Kaplan, N.L., Weir, B.S.: Tests for linkage and association in nuclear families. Am. J. Hum. Genet. **61**, 439–448 (1997)
181. Mehta, C.R., Patel, N.R.: Algorithm 643: Fexact: A FORTRAN subroutine for Fisher's exact test on unordered $r \times c$ contingency tables. ACM Trans. Math. Software **12**, 154–161 (1986)
182. McVean, G.: Linkage disequilibrium, recombination and selection. In: Balding, D.J., Bishop, M., Cannings, C. (eds.) Handbook of Statistical Genetics, 3rd edn., pp. 909–944. Wiley, New York (2007)
183. Michalatos-Beloin, S., Tishkoff, S.A., Bentley, K.L., Kidd, K.K., Ruano, G.: Molecular haplotyping of genetic markers 10 kb apart by allele-specific long-range PCR. Nucleic Acids Res. **24**, 4841–4843 (1996)
184. Moore, J.H., Gilbert, J.C., Tsai, C.T., Chiang, F.T., Holden, T., Barney, N., White, B.C.: A flexible computational framework for detecting, characterizing, and interpreting statistical patterns of epistasis in genetic studies of human disease susceptibility. J. Theor. Biol. **241**, 252–261 (2006)
185. Morton, N.E.: Sequential tests for the detection of linkage. Am. J. Hum. Genet. **7**, 277–318 (1955)
186. Morton, N.E.: Logarithm of odds (lods) for linkage in complex inheritance. Proc. Natl. Acad. Sci. USA **93**, 3471–3476 (1996)
187. Murcray, C.E., Lewinger, J.P., Gauderman, W.J.: Gene-environment interaction in genome-wide association studies. Am. J. Epidemiol. **169**, 219–226 (2009)
188. Nakachi, K., Imai, K., Hayashi, S., Watanabe, J., Kawajiri, K.: Genetic susceptibility to squamous cell carcinoma of the lung in relation to cigarette smoking dose. Cancer Res. **51**, 5177–5180 (1991)
189. Namkung, J., Kim, K., Yi, S., Chung, W., Kwon, M.S., Park, T.: New evaluation measures for multifactor dimensionality reduction classifiers in gene-gene interaction analysis. Bioinformatics **25**, 338–345 (2009)
190. Nature Genetics: Editorial: freely associating. Nat. Genet. **22**, 1–2 (1999)
191. NCI-NHGRI: Replicating genotype-phenotype associations. Nature **447**, 655–660 (2007)
192. Neuhauser, M.: Exact tests for the analysis of case-control studies of genetic markers. Hum. Hered. **54**, 151–156 (2002)
193. Nielsen, D.M., Ehm, M.G., Weir, B.S.: Detecting marker-disease association by testing for Hardy-Weinberg disequilibrium at a marker locus. Am. J. Hum. Genet. **63**, 1531–1540 (1998)
194. Nielsen, D.M., Ehm, M.G., Zaykin, D.V., Weir, B.S.: Effect of two- and three-locus linkage disequilibrium on the power to detect marker/phenotype associations. Genetics **168**, 1029–1040 (2004)
195. Nielsen, D.M., Weir, B.S.: A classical setting for associations between markers and loci affecting quantitative traits. Genet. Res. **74**, 271–277 (1999)

196. Niu, T., Qin, Z.S., Xu, X., Liu, J.S.: Bayesian haplotype inference for multiple linked single-nucleotide polymorphisms. Am. J. Hum. Genet. **70**, 157–169 (2002)
197. Niu, T.: Algorithms for inferring haplotypes. Genet. Epidemiol. **27**, 334–347 (2004)
198. Noether, G.E.: On a theorem of Pitman. Ann. Math. Stat. **26**, 64–68 (1955)
199. Olson, J.M., Wijsman, E.M.: Linkage between quantitative trait and marker loci: methods using all relative pairs. Genet. Epidemiol. **10**, 87–102 (1993)
200. Ott, J.: Statistical properties of the haplotype relative risk. Genet. Epidemiol. **6**, 127–130 (1989)
201. Pattin, K.A., White, B.C., Barney, N., Gui, J., Nelson, H.H., Kelsey, K.T., Andrew, A.S., Karagas, M.R., Moore, J.H.: A computationally efficient hypothesis testing method for epistasis analysis using multifactor dimensionality reduction. Genet. Epidemiol. **33**, 87–94 (2009)
202. Pfeiffer, R.M., Gail, M.H.: Sample size calculations for population- and family-based case-control association studies on marker genotypes. Genet. Epidemiol. **25**, 136–148 (2003)
203. Piegorsch, W.W., Weinberg, C.R., Taylor, J.A.: Non-hierarchical logistic models and case-only designs for assessing susceptibility in population-based case-control studies. Stat. Med. **13**, 153–162 (1994)
204. Prentice, R.L., Pyke, R.: Logistic disease incidence models and case-control studies. Biometrika **66**, 403–411 (1979)
205. Price, A.L., Patterson, N.J., Plenge, R.M., Weinblatt, M.E., Shadick, N.A., Reich, D.: Principal components analysis corrects for stratification in genome-wide association studies. Nat. Genet. **38**, 904–909 (2006)
206. Price, A.L., Zaitlen, N.A., Reich, D., Patterson, N.: New approaches to population stratification in genome-wide association studies. Nat. Rev. Genet. **11**, 459–463 (2010)
207. Pritchard, J.K., Stephens, M., Rosenberg, N.A., Donnelly, P.: Association mapping in structured populations. Am. J. Hum. Genet. **67**, 170–181 (2000)
208. Qin, H., Morris, N., Kang, S.J., Li, M., Tayo, B., Lyon, H., Hirschhorn, J.N., Cooper, R.S., Zhu, X.: Interrogating local population structure for fine mapping in genome wide association studies. Bioinformatics **26**, 2961–2968 (2010)
209. Qin, Z.S., Niu, T., Liu, J.S.: Partition-ligation-expectation-maximization algorithm for haplotype inference with single nucleotide polymorphisms. Am. J. Hum. Genet. **71**, 1242–1247 (2002)
210. Rabinowitz, D., Laird, N.M.: A unified approach to adjusting association tests for population admixture with arbitrary pedigree structure and arbitrary missing marker information. Hum. Hered. **50**, 211–223 (2000)
211. Reich, D.E., Goldstein, D.B.: Detecting association in a case-control study while correcting for population stratification. Genet. Epidemiol. **20**, 4–16 (2001)
212. Requena, F., Ciudad, N.M.: A major improvement to the network algorithm for Fisher's exact test in $2 \times c$ contingency tables. Comput. Stat. Data Anal. **51**, 490–498 (2006)
213. Risch, N.: Genetics of IDDM: evidence for complex inheritance with HLA. Genet. Epidemiol. **6**, 143–148 (1989)
214. Risch, N.: Linkage strategies for genetically complex traits. III. The effect of marker polymorphism on analysis of affected relative pairs. Am. J. Hum. Genet. **46**, 242–253 (1990)
215. Risch, N.: Corrections to: Linkage strategies for genetically complex traits. III. The effect of marker polymorphism on analysis of affected relative pairs. Am. J. Hum. Genet. **51**, 673–675 (1992)
216. Ritchie, M.D., Hahn, L.W., Roodi, N., Bailey, L.R., Dupont, W.D., Parl, F.F., Moore, J.H.: Multifactor-dimensionality reduction reveals high-order interactions among estrogen-metabolism genes in sporadic breast cancer. Am. J. Hum. Genet. **69**, 138–147 (2001)
217. Ritchie, M.D., Hahn, L.W., Moore, J.H.: Power of multifactor dimensionality reduction for detecting gene-gene interactions in the presence of genotyping error, missing data, phenocopy, and genetic heterogeneity. Genet. Epidemiol. **24**, 150–157 (2003)
218. Robert, C.P., Casella, G.: Monte Carlo Statistical Methods. Springer, New York (2004)

219. Rosenberg, N.A., Nordborg, M.: A general population-genetic model for the production by population structure of spurious genotype-phenotype associations in discrete, admixed or spatially distributed populations. Genetics **173**, 1665–1678 (2006)
220. Rosenberg, N.A., Pritchard, J.K., Weber, J.L., Cann, H.M., Kidd, K.K., Zhivotovsky, L.A., Feldman, M.W.: Genetic structure of human populations. Science **298**, 2381–2385 (2002)
221. Ruczinski, I., Kooperberg, C., LeBlanc, M.: Exploring interactions in highdimensional genomic data: An overview of logic regression, with applications. J. Mult. Anal. **90**, 178–195 (2004)
222. Sahai, H., Khurshid, A.: Statistics in Epidemiology: Methods, Technology, and Applications. CRC Press, Boca Raton (1996)
223. Sasieni, P.D.: From genotypes to genes: doubling the sample size. Biometrics **53**, 1253–1261 (1997)
224. Satten, G.A., Epstein, M.P.: Comparison of prospective and retrospective methods for haplotype inference in case-control studies. Genet. Epidemiol. **27**, 192–201 (2004)
225. Satten, G.A., Flanders, W.D., Yang, Q.: Accounting for unmeasured population substructure in case-control studies of genetic association using a novel latent-class model. Am. J. Hum. Genet. **68**, 466–477 (2001)
226. Sawcer, S.: Bayes factors in complex genetics. Euro. J. Hum. Genet. **18**, 746–750 (2010)
227. Scheffé, H.: The Analysis of Variance. Wiley, New York (1959)
228. Schaid, D.J.: General score tests for associations of genetic markers with disease using cases and their parents. Genet. Epidemiol. **13**, 423–449 (1996)
229. Schaid, D.J.: Relative efficiency of ambiguous vs. directly measured haplotype frequencies. Genet. Epidemiol. **23**, 426–443 (2002)
230. Schaid, D.J.: Evaluating associations of haplotypes with traits. Genet. Epidemiol. **27**, 348–364 (2004)
231. Schaid, D.J.: Power and sample size for testing association of haplotypes with complex traits. Ann. Hum. Genet. **70**, 116–130 (2005)
232. Schaid, D.J., Nick, T.G.: Sib-pair linkage tests for disease susceptibility loci: common tests vs. the asymptotically most powerful test. Genet. Epidemiol. **7**, 359–370 (1990)
233. Schaid, D.J., Jacobsen, S.J.: Biased tests of association: comparison of allele frequencies when departing from Hardy-Weinberg proportions. Am. J. Epidemiol. **149**, 706–711 (1999)
234. Schaid, D.J., Sommer, S.S.: Genotype relative risks: methods for design and analysis of candidate-gene association studies. Am. J. Hum. Genet. **53**, 1114–1126 (1993)
235. Schaid, D.J., Sommer, S.S.: Comparison of statistics for candidate-gene association studies using cases and parents. Am. J. Hum. Genet. **55**, 402–409 (1994)
236. Schwender, H., Ickstadt, K.: Identification of SNP interactions using logic regression. Biostatistics **9**, 187–198 (2008)
237. Sebastiani, P., Lazarus, R., Weiss, S.T., Kunkel, L.M., Kohane, I.S., Ramoni, M.F.: Minimal haplotype tagging. Proc. Natl. Acad. Sci. USA **100**, 9900–9905 (2003)
238. Self, S.G., Liang, K.Y.: Asymptotic properties of maximum likelihood estimators and likelihood ratio tests under nonstandard conditions. J. Am. Stat. Assoc. **82**, 605–610 (1987)
239. Self, S.G., Longton, G., Kopecky, K.J., Liang, K.Y.: On estimating HLA/disease association with application to a study of aplastic anemia. Biometrics **47**, 53–61 (1991)
240. Sham, P.: Statistics in Human Genetics. Arnold Applications of Statistics, London (1998)
241. Shete, S., Jacobs, K.B., Elston, R.C.: Adding further power to the Haseman and Elston method for detecting linkage in larger sibships: weighting sums and differences. Hum. Hered. **55**, 79–85 (2003)
242. Shih, M.C., Whittemore, A.S.: Allele-sharing among affected relatives: non-parametric methods for identifying genes. Stat. Meth. Med. Res. **10**, 27–55 (2001)
243. Shih, M.C., Whittemore, A.S.: Tests for genetic association using family data. Genet. Epidemiol. **22**, 128–145 (2002)
244. Shoukri, M.M., Lathrop, G.M.: Statistical testing of genetic linkage under heterogeneity. Biometrics **49**, 151–161 (1993)
245. Siegmund, D.O., Yakir, B.: The Statistics of Gene Mapping. Springer, New York (2007)

246. Skol, A.D., Scott, L.J., Abecasis, G.R., Boehnke, M.: Joint analysis is more efficient than replication-based analysis for two-stage genome-wide association studies. Nat. Genet. **38**, 209–213 (2006)
247. Sladek, R., Rocheleau, G., Rung, J., Dina, C., Shen, L., Serre, D., Boutin, P., Vinvent, D., Belisle, A., Hadjadj, S., Balkau, B., Heude, B., et al.: A genome-wide association study identifies novel risk loci for type 2 diabetes. Nature **445**, 881–885 (2007)
248. Slager, S.L., Schaid, D.J.: Case-control studies of genetic markers: power and sample size approximations for Armitage's test for trend. Hum. Hered. **52**, 149–153 (2001)
249. Smith, P.G., Day, N.E.: The design of case-control studies: the influence of confounding and interaction effects. Int. J. Epidemiol. **13**, 356–365 (1984)
250. Song, K., Elston, R.C.: The Hardy-Weinberg disequilibrium (HWD) measure and test statistics for a disease-susceptibility locus with multiple alleles allowing for an inbreeding coefficient (F). Genetica **119**, 269–293 (2003)
251. Song, K., Elston, R.C.: A powerful method of combining measures of association and Hardy-Weinberg disequilibrium for fine-mapping in case-control studies. Stat. Med. **25**, 105–126 (2006)
252. Song, M.S., Nicolae, D.L.: Restricted parameter space models for testing gene-gene interaction. Genet. Epidemiol. **33**, 386–393 (2009)
253. Spielman, R.S., Ewens, W.J.: The TDT and other family-based tests for linkage disequilibrium and association. Am. J. Hum. Genet. **59**, 983–989 (1996)
254. Sun, L., Bull, S.B.: Reduction of selection bias in genomewide studies by resampling. Genet. Epidemiol. **28**, 352–367 (2005)
255. Spielman, R.S., McGinnis, R.E., Ewens, W.J.: Transmission test for linkage disequilibrium: The insulin gene region and insulin-dependent diabetes mellitus (IDDM). Am. J. Hum. Genet. **52**, 506–516 (1993)
256. Spinka, C., Carroll, R.J., Chatterjee, N.: Analysis of case-control studies of genetic and environmental factors with missing genetic information and haplotype-phase ambiguity. Genet. Epidemiol. **29**, 108–127 (2005)
257. Stephens, M., Smith, N.J., Donnelly, P.: A new statistical method for haplotype reconstruction from population data. Am. J. Hum. Genet. **68**, 978–989 (2001)
258. Stephens, M., Donnelly, P.: A comparison of Bayesian methods for haplotype reconstruction from population genotype data. Am. J. Hum. Genet. **73**, 1162–1169 (2003)
259. Stephens, M., Balding, D.J.: Bayesian statistical methods for genetic association studies. Nat. Rev. Genet. **10**, 681–690
260. Storey, J.D.: A direct approach to false discovery rates. J. Roy. Stat. Soc. Ser. B **64**, 479–498 (2002)
261. Storey, J.D.: The positive false discovery rate: A Bayesian interpretation and the q-value. Ann. Stat. **31**, 2013–2035 (2003)
262. Stram, D.O., Leigh, P.C., Bretsky, P., Freedman, M., Hirschhorn, J.N., Altshuler, D., Kolonel, L.N., Henderson, B.E., Thomas, D.C.: Modeling and E-M estimation of haplotype-specific relative risks from genotype data for a case-control study of unrelated individuals. Hum. Hered. **55**, 179–190 (2003)
263. Stram, D.O., Haiman, C.A., Hirschhorn, J.N., Altshuler, D., Kolonel, L.N., Henderson, B.E., Pike, M.C.: Choosing haplotype-tagging SNPS based on unphased genotype data using a preliminary sample of unrelated subjects with an example from the Multiethnic Cohort Study. Hum. Hered. **55**, 27–36 (2003)
264. Tang, H., Choudhry, S., Mei, R., Morgan, M., Rodriguez-Cintron, W., Burchard, E.G., Risch, N.J.: Recent genetic selection in the ancestral admixture of Puerto Ricans. Am. J. Hum. Genet. **81**, 626–633 (2007)
265. Tang, H., Peng, J., Wang, P., Risch, N.J.: Estimation of individual admixture: analytical and study design considerations. Genet. Epidemiol. **28**, 289–301 (2005)
266. Tang, H., Quertermous, T., Rodriguez, B., Kardia, S.L., Zhu, X., Brown, A., Pankow, J.S., Province, M.A., Hunt, S.C., Boerwinkle, E., Schork, N.J., Risch, N.J.: Genetic structure, self-identified race/ethnicity, and confounding in case-control association studies. Am. J. Hum. Genet. **76**, 268–275 (2005)

267. Terwilliger, J.D., Ott, J.: A haplotype-based 'haplotype relative risk' approach to detecting allelic associations. Hum. Hered. **42**, 337–346 (1992)

268. The International HapMap Consortium: The international HapMap project. Nature **426**, 789–796 (2003)

269. The International HapMap Consortium: A haplotype map of the human genome. Nature **437**, 1299–1320 (2005)

270. Thomas, D.C.: Statistical Methods in Genetic Epidemiology. Oxford University Press, London (2004)

271. Thomas, D.C.: Gene-environment-wide association studies: emerging approaches. Nat. Rev. Genet. **11**, 259–272 (2010)

272. Thompson, E.A.: Pedigree Analysis in Human Genetics. Johns Hopkins University Press, Baltimore (1986)

273. Tierney, L., Kadane, J.B.: Accurate approximations for posterior moments and marginal densities. J. Am. Stat. Assoc. **81**, 82–86 (1986)

274. Tregouët, D.A., Escolano, S., Tiret, L., Mallet, A., Golmard, J.L.: A new algorithm for haplotype-based association analysis: the stochastic-EM algorithm. Ann. Hum. Genet. **68**, 165–177 (2004)

275. Troendle, J.F., Yu, K.F., Mills, J.L.: Testing for genetic association with constrained models using triads. Ann. Hum. Genet. **73**, 225–230 (2009)

276. Tzeng, J.Y., Devlin, B., Wasserman, L., Roeder, K.: On the identification of disease mutations by the analysis of haplotype similarity and goodness of fit. Am. J. Hum. Genet. **72**, 891–902 (2003)

277. Tzeng, J.Y., Wang, C.H., Kao, J.T., Hsiao, C.K.: Regression-based association analysis with clustered haplotypes through use of genotypes. Am. J. Hum. Genet. **78**, 231–242 (2006)

278. Umbach, D.M., Weinberg, C.R.: Designing and analysing case-control studies to exploit independence of genotype and exposure. Stat. Med. **16**, 1731–1743 (1997)

279. van der Vaart, A.W.: Asymptotic Statistics. Cambridge University Press, Cambridge (1998)

280. Van Steen, K., McQueen, M.B., Herbert, A., Raby, B., Lyon, H., Demeo, D.L., Murphy, A., Su, J., Datta, S., Rosenow, C., et al.: Genomic screening and replication using the same data set in family-based association testing. Nat. Genet. **37**, 683–691 (2005)

281. Visscher, P.M., Hopper, J.L.: Power of regression and maximum likelihood methods to map QTL from sib-pair and DZ twin data. Ann. Hum. Genet. **65**, 583–601 (2001)

282. Voight, B.F., Pritchard, J.K.: Confounding from cryptic relatedness in case-control association studies. PLOS Genet. **1**(3), e32 (2005)

283. Wacholder, S., Rothman, N., Caporaso, N.: Population stratification in epidemiologic studies of common genetic variants and cancer: Quantification of bias. J. Natl. Cancer Inst. **92**, 1151–1158 (2000)

284. Wakefield, J.: A Bayesian measure of the probability of false discovery in genetic epidemiology studies. Am. J. Hum. Genet. **81**, 208–227 (2007)

285. Wakefield, J.: Bayes factors for genome-wide association studies: Comparison with p-values. Genet. Epidemiol. **33**, 79–86 (2009)

286. Wakefield, J., De Vocht, F., Hung, R.L.: Bayesian mixture modeling of gene-environment and gene-gene interactions. Genet. Epidemiol. **34**, 16–25 (2010)

287. Wall, J.D., Pritchard, J.K.: Assessing the performance of the haplotype block model of linkage disequilibrium. Am. J. Hum. Genet. **73**, 502–515 (2003)

288. Wang, K., Sheffield, V.C.: A constrained-likelihood approach to marker-trait association studies. Am. J. Hum. Genet. **77**, 768–780 (2005)

289. Wang, K., Li, M., Hadley, D., Liu, R., Glessner, J., Grant, S.F.A., Hakonarson, H., Bucan, M.: PennCNV: An integrated hidden Markov model designed for high-resolution copy number variation detection in whole-genome SNP genotyping data. Genome Res. **17**, 1665–1674 (2007)

290. Wang, S., Kidd, K.K., Zhao, H.: On the use of DNA pooling to estimate haplotype frequencies. Genet. Epidemiol. **24**, 74–82 (2003)

291. Wang, T., Elston, R.C.: Two-level Haseman-Elston regression for general pedigree data analysis. Genet. Epidemiol. **29**, 12–22 (2005)

292. Wang, T., Zhu, X., Elston, R.C.: Improving power in contrasting linkage-disequilibrium patterns between cases and controls. Am. J. Hum. Genet. **80**, 911–920 (2007)
293. Wang, X., Elston, R.C., Zhu, X.: The meaning of interaction. Hum. Hered. **70**, 269–277 (2010)
294. Wang, X., Elston, R.C., Zhu, X.: Statistical interaction in human genetics: how should we model it if we are looking for biological interaction? Nat. Rev. Genet. **12**, 74 (2011)
295. Wang, W.Y.S., Barratt, B.J., Clayton, D.G., Todd, J.A.: Genome-wide association studies: Theoretical and practical concerns. Nat. Rev. Genet. **6**, 109–118 (2005)
296. Walter, S.D.: Matched case-control studies with a variable number of controls per case. Appl. Stat. **29**, 172–179 (1980)
297. Weinberg, W.: Über den Nachweis der Vererbung beim Menschen. Jahreshefte des Vereins fur vaterländische Naturkunde in Württemberg **64**, 368–382 (1908)
298. Weir, B.S.: Inferences about linkage disequilibrium. Biometrics **35**, 235–254 (1979)
299. Weir, B.S.: Genetic Data Analysis II. Sinauer Associates Inc., Sunderland (1996)
300. Weir, B.S., Cockerham, C.C.: Complete characterization of disequilibrium at two loci. In: Feldman, M.W. (ed.) Mathematical Evolutionary Theory, pp. 86–110. Princeton University Press, Princeton (1989)
301. The Wellcome Trust Case Control Consortium (WTCCC): Genome-wide association study of 14,000 cases of seven common diseases and 3,000 shared controls. Nature **447**, 661–683 (2007)
302. Whittemore, A.S.: Population structure in genetic association studies. In: 2006 Proceedings of the American Statistical Association, ASA Section on Statistics in Epidemiology [CD-ROM], ASA, Alexandria, VA, pp. 2657–2667 (2006)
303. Whittemore, A.S., Tu, I.P.: Simple, robust linkage tests for affected sibs. Am. J. Hum. Genet. **62**, 1228–1242 (1998)
304. Wright, F.A.: The phenotypic difference discards sib-pair QTL linkage information. Am. J. Hum. Genet. **60**, 740–742 (1997)
305. Wu, C., Zhang, H., Liu, X., DeWan, A., Dubrow, R., Ying, Z., Yang, Y., Ying, Z.: Detecting essential and removable interactions in genome-wide association studies. Stat. Its Interface **2**, 161–170 (2010)
306. Xiao, R., Boehnke, M.: Quantifying and correcting for the winner's curse in genetic association studies. Genet. Epidemiol. **33**, 453–462 (2009)
307. Xing, E.P., Jordan, M.I., Sharan, R.: Bayesian haplotype inference via the Dirichlet process. J. Comput. Biol. **14**, 267–284 (2007)
308. Xu, X., Weiss, S., Xu, X., Wei, L.J.: A unified Haseman-Elston method for testing linkage with quantitative traits. Am. J. Hum. Genet. **67**, 1025–1028 (2000)
309. Yamada, R., Okada, Y.: An optimal dose-effect mode trend test for SNP genotype tables. Genet. Epidemiol. **33**, 114–127 (2009)
310. Yang, J., Benyamin, B., McEvoy, B.P., Gordon, S., Henders, A.K., Nyholt, D.R., Madden, P.A., Heath, A.C., Martin, N.G., Montgomery, G.W., et al.: Common SNPs explain a large proportion of the heritability for human height. Nat. Genet. **42**, 565–569 (2010)
311. Yang, Q., Khoury, M.J., Flanders, W.D.: Sample size requirements in case-only designs to detect gene-environment interaction. Am. J. Epidemiol. **146**, 713–720 (1997)
312. Yang, Y., Zhang, J., Hoh, J., Matsuda, F., Xu, P., Lathrop, M., Ott, J.: Efficiency of single-nucleotide polymorphism haplotype estimation from pooled DNA. Proc. Natl. Acad. Sci. USA **100**, 7225–7230 (2003)
313. Yeager, M., Orr, N., Hayes, R.B., Jacobs, K.B., Kraft, P., Wacholder, S., Minichiello, M.J., Fearnhead, P., Yu, K., Chatterjee, N., et al.: Genome-wide association study of prostate cancer identifies a second risk locus at 8q24. Nat. Genet. **39**, 645–649 (2007)
314. Yuan, M., Tian, X., Zheng, G., Yang, Y.: Adaptive transmission disequilibrium test for family trio design. Stat. Appl. Genet. Molec. Biol. **8**(1), (2009). doi:10.2202/1544–6115.1451. Article 30
315. Zang, Y., Fung, F.W.K., Zheng, G.: The asymptotic powers for matched trend tests and robust matched trend tests in case-control genetic association studies. Comput. Stat. Data Anal. **54**, 65–77 (2010)

316. Zang, Y., Fung, F.W.K., Zheng, G.: Simple algorithms to calculate asymptotic null distributions for robust tests in case-control genetic association studies in R. J. Stat. Software **33**(8), (2010)
317. Zaykin, D.V., Zhivotovsky, L.A.: Ranks of genuine association in while-genome scans. Genetics **171**, 813–823 (2005)
318. Zaykin, D.V., Westfall, P.H., Young, S.S., Karnoub, M.A., Wagner, M.J., Ehm, M.G.: Testing association of statistically inferred haplotypes with discrete and continuous traits in samples of unrelated individuals. Hum. Hered. **53**, 79–91 (2002)
319. Zaykin, D.V., Meng, Z., Ehm, M.G.: Contrasting linkage-disequilibrium patterns between cases and controls as a novel association-mapping method. Am. J. Hum. Genet. **78**, 737–746 (2006)
320. Zhang, K., Deng, M., Chen, T., Waterman, M.S., Sun, F.: A dynamic programming algorithm for haplotype block partitioning. Proc. Natl. Acad. Sci. USA **99**, 7335–7339 (2002)
321. Zhang, H., Zhang, H., Zheng, G., Li, Z.: Statistical methods for haplotype-based matched case-control association studies. Genet. Epidemiol. **31**, 316–326 (2007)
322. Zhang, H., Yang, H.S., Yang, Y.: PoooL: An efficient algorithm for estimating haplotypes from large DNA pools. Bioinformatics **24**, 1942–1948 (2008)
323. Zhang, S., Zhu, X., Zhao, H.: On a semiparametric test to detect associations between quantitative traits and candidate genes using unrelated individuals. Genet. Epidemiol. **24**, 44–56 (2003)
324. Zhang, Y., Liu, J.S.: Bayesian inference of epistatic interactions in case-control studies. Nat. Genet. **39**, 1167–1173 (2007)
325. Zhang, Z., Ersoz, E., Lai, C.Q., Todhunter, R.J., Tiwari, H.K., Gore, M.A., Bradbury, P.J., Yu, J., Arnett, D.K., Ordovas, J.M., Buckler, E.S.: Mixed linear model approach adapted for genome-wide association studies. Nat. Genet. **42**, 355–360 (2010)
326. Zhao, H.: Family-based association studies. Stat. Meth. Med. Res. **9**, 563–587 (2000)
327. Zhao, J., Jin, L., Xiong, M.: Test for interaction between two unlinked loci. Am. J. Hum. Genet. **79**, 831–845 (2006)
328. Zhao, L.P., Li, S.S., Khalid, N.: A method for the assessment of disease associations with single-nucleotide polymorphism haplotypes and environmental variables in case-control studies. Am. J. Hum. Genet. **72**, 1231–1250 (2003)
329. Zheng, G.: Can the allelic test be retired from analysis of case-control association studies? Ann. Hum. Genet. **72**, 848–851 (2008)
330. Zheng, G., Chen, Z.: Comparison of maximum statistics for hypothesis testing when a nuisance parameter is present only under the alternative. Biometrics **61**, 254–258 (2005)
331. Zheng, G., Chen, Z., Li, Z.: Tests for candidate-gene association using case-parents design. Ann. Hum. Genet. **67**, 589–597 (2003)
332. Zheng, G., Freidlin, B., Gastwirth, J.L.: Obtaining robust TDT-type candidate-gene association tests for a family of genetic models. In: Proceedings of the American Statistical Association, ASA Section on Statistics in Epidemiology [CDROM], ASA, Alexandria, VA (2001)
333. Zheng, G., Freidlin, B., Gastwirth, J.L.: Robust TDT-type candidate-gene association tests. Ann. Hum. Hered. **66**, 145–155 (2002)
334. Zheng, G., Freidlin, B., Gastwirth, J.L.: Comparison of robust tests for genetic association using case-control studies. In: Rojo, J. (ed.) Optimality: The Second Erich L. Lehmann Symposium. Lecture Notes–Monograph Series, vol. 49, pp. 320–336. Institute of Mathematical Statistics, Beachwood (2006)
335. Zheng, G., Freidlin, B., Gastwirth, J.L.: Robust genomic control for association studies. Am. J. Hum. Genet. **78**, 350–356 (2006)
336. Zheng, G., Freidlin, B., Li, Z., Gastwirth, J.L.: Choice of scores in trend tests for case-control studies of candidate-gene associations. Biomet. J. **45**, 335–348 (2003)
337. Zheng, G., Gastwirth, J.L.: On estimation of the variance in Cochran-Armitage trend tests for genetic association using case-control studies. Stat. Med. **25**, 3150–3159 (2006)
338. Zheng, G., Joo, J., Yang, Y.: Pearson's test, trend test, and MAX are all trend tests with different types of scores. Ann. Hum. Genet. **73**, 133–140 (2009)

339. Zheng, G., Joo, J., Zhang, C., Geller, N.L.: Testing association for markers on the X chromosome. Genet. Epidemiol. **31**, 834–843 (2007)
340. Zheng, G., Joo, J., Zaykin, D.V., Wu, C.O., Geller, N.L.: Robust tests in genome-wide scans under incomplete linkage disequilibrium. Stat. Sci. **24**, 503–516 (2009)
341. Zheng, G. Li, Z., Gail, M.H., Gastwirth, J.L.: Impact of population substructure on trend tests for genetic case-control association studies. Biometrics **66**, 196–204 (2010)
342. Zheng, G., Marchini, J., Geller, N.L.: Introduction of the special issue: Genome-wide association studies. Stat. Sci. **24**, 387 (2009)
343. Zheng, G., Meyer, M., Li, W., Yang, Y.: Comparison of two-phase analyses for case-control genetic association studies. Stat. Med. **27**, 5054–5075 (2008)
344. Zheng, G., Ng, H.K.T.: Genetic model selection in two-phase analysis for case-control association studies. Biostatistics **9**, 391–399
345. Zheng, G., Song, K., Elston, R.C.: Adaptive two-stage analysis of genetic association in case-control designs. Hum. Hered. **63**, 175–186 (2007)
346. Zheng, G., Tian, X.: Robust trend tests for genetic association using matched case-control design. Stat. Med. **25**, 3160–3171 (2006)
347. Zhu, X., Elston, R.C.: Power comparison of regression methods to test quantitative traits for association and linkage. Genet. Epidemiol. **18**, 322–330 (2000)
348. Zhu, X., Elston, R.C.: Transmission/disequilibrium tests for quantitative traits. Genet. Epidemiol. **20**, 57–74 (2001)
349. Zhu, X., Li, S., Cooper, R.S., Elston, R.C.: A unified association analysis approach for family and unrelated samples correcting for stratification. Am. J. Hum. Genet. **82**, 352–365 (2008)
350. Zhu, X., Zhang, S., Zhao, H., Cooper, R.S.: Association mapping, using a mixture model for complex traits. Genet. Epidemiol. **23**, 181–196 (2002)
351. Ziegler, A., König, I.: A Statistical Approach to Genetic Epidemiology: Concepts and Applications. Wiley-VCH Verlag, Weinheim (2006)
352. Ziegler, A., König, I., Thompson, J.R.: Biostatistics aspects of genome-wide association studies. Biom. J. **50**, 8–28 (2008)
353. Zöllner, S., Pritchard, J.K.: Overcoming the winner's curse: Estimating penetrance parameters from case-control data. Am. J. Hum. Genet. **80**, 605–615 (2007)
354. Zöllner, S., Teslovich, T.M.: Using GWAS data to identify copy number variants contributing to common complex diseases. Stat. Sci. **24**, 530–546 (2009)
355. Zou, G.Y., Donner, A.: The merits of testing Hardy-Weinberg equilibrium in the analysis of unmatched case-control data: a cautionary note. Ann. Hum. Genet. **70**, 923–933 (2006)
356. Zucker, D.M., Lakatos, E.: Weighted log rank type statistics for comparing survival curves when there is a time lag in the effectiveness of treatment. Biometrika **77**, 853–864 (1990)

Index

G. Zheng et al., *Analysis of Genetic Association Studies*,
Statistics for Biology and Health,
DOI 10.1007/978-1-4614-2245-7, © Springer Science+Business Media, LLC 2012

Printed in the USA
CPSIA information can be obtained
at www.ICGtesting.com
CBHW052112061224
18616CB00003BA/44